Psychological Aspects of Obesity:
A Handbook

Psychological Aspects of Obesity:
A Handbook

Benjamin B. Wolman, Ph.D.
Editor

Stephen DeBerry, Ph.D.
Editorial Associate

VNR VAN NOSTRAND REINHOLD COMPANY
NEW YORK CINCINNATI TORONTO LONDON MELBOURNE

Van Nostrand Reinhold Company Regional Offices:
New York   Cincinnati

Van Nostrand Reinhold Company International Offices:
London   Toronto   Melbourne

Copyright © 1982 by Van Nostrand Reinhold Company

Library of Congress Catalog Card Number: 81-1917
ISBN: 0-442-22609-8

Manufactured in the United States of America

Published by Van Nostrand Reinhold Company
135 West 50th Street, New York, N.Y. 10020

Published simultaneously in Canada by Van Nostrand Reinhold Ltd.

15 14 13 12 11 10 9 8 7 6 5 4 3 2 1

Library of Congress Cataloging in Publication Data

Main entry under title:
Psychological Aspects of Obesity: A Handbook
    Includes index.
    1. Obesity – Psychological aspects. I. Wolman,
Benjamin B.
RC552.025023   616.3'98'0019   81-1917
ISBN O-442-22609-8   AACR2

Contributors

Edward Abramson, Ph.D.
Professor of Psychology
California State University
Chico, California

Natalie Allon, Ph.D.
Assistant Professor of Sociology
Department of Human and Social Services
Philadelphia College of Textiles
Philadelphia, Pennsylvania

F. Carrera III, M.D.
Director
Children's Mental Health Clinic
Chief, Division of Child and Adolescent Psychiatry
University of Florida

W.A. Daniel, Jr., M.D.
Professor of Pediatrics
Director, Division of Adolescent Medicine
University of Alabama
Birmingham, Alabama

Stephen DeBerry, Ph.D.
Clinical Instructor
Department of Psychiatry
Albert Einstein College of Medicine
Director, Sound-view — Throgs Neck Community Mental Health Center
New York

Allan Geliebter, Ph.D.
Assistant Professor and Chairman
Department of Psychology
Touro College and
Research Associate
Obesity Research Center
St. Lukes – Roosevelt Hospital
New York, New York

Milton Kline, Ed.D.
Director
Institute for Research in Hypnosis
Morton Prince Center for Hypnotherapy
New York, New York

David Laskowitz, Ph.D.
Chief Psychologist
Director of In-service Training
Lincoln Community Mental Health Center
Dobbs Ferry, New York

Gloria Leon, Ph.D.
Associate Professor of Psychology
University of Minnesota
Minneapolis, Minnesota

Barbara Lukert, M.D., F.A.C.P.
Professor of Medicine
Division of Endocrinology
University of Kansas
Kansas City, Kansas

Colleen S.W. Rand, Ph.D.
Assistant Professor of Psychology in Psychiatry
Shands Teaching Hospital
University of Florida
Gainesville, Florida

Judith Rodin, Ph.D.
Professor of Psychology
Yale University
New Haven, Connecticut

Janet Wollershein, Ph.D.
Professor of Psychology and Director of Clinical Psychology
University of Montana

Benjamin B. Wolman, Ph.D.
Editor-in-Chief
International Encyclopedia of Psychiatry, Psychology, Psychoanalysis, and Neurology

Preface

Fight for survival is the basic, universal drive, common to all living organisms. All organisms, from the protozoa to the most brilliant human beings, endeavor to stay alive. *To eat or not to eat* is a matter of life and death. To eat means to stay alive; to starve means to die.

Practically all living organisms — including most human beings — have self-regulatory devices that control their intake of food. Hunger and satiation are these regulatory mechanisms.

Some human beings have lost or have never developed these control mechanisms. The inability to control the intake of food and body weight is sometimes related to an inadequate functioning of the neurochemical system, but it is most often a product of inadequate functioning of the mental apparatus. The inability to control body weight is fraught with serious dangers to one's health and, in addition, exposes the obese individual to a good deal of discomfort and difficulty in relating to other people.

The discomforts and dangers of being obese are well known to everyone, and especially to the over forty million obese people in the United States. Why, then, don't they do something about it?

In fact, most of them do. They go on all sorts of "crash" diets, lose some weight, and regain it in no time. Weight control is far from being a simple and easy task. It is a challenge that many people are unable to cope with. Apparently gaining weight and the difficulty in controlling it hinge on deeper psychological issues.

The present volume, written by a team of experts, zeroes in on the psychological issues that make people gain weight and prevent them from exercising adequate control of their weight and eating habits. The book is divided in two parts: (1) Etiology and Symptomatology of Obesity and (2) Treatment of Obesity. Its aim is to be of help.

BENJAMIN B. WOLMAN

Contents

Preface   vii

1. ETIOLOGY AND SYMPTOMATOLOGY OF OBESITY

1. Biology of Obesity, Barbara Lukert   1
2. Personality and Behavioral Correlates of Obesity, Gloria R. Leon   15
3. Obesity: Why the Losing Battle? Judith Rodin   30
4. Depression and Obesity, Benjamin B. Wolman   88
5. Obesity in Adolescence, William A. Daniel, Jr.   104
6. Obesity as a Barricade Against Social Stress: An Adlerian View,
      David Laskowitz   118
7. The Stigma of Overweight in Everyday Life, Natalie Allon   130

2. TREATMENT OF OBESITY

8. Psychoanalytic Treatment of Obesity, Colleen S. W. Rand   177
9. Interactional Psychotherapy of Obesity, Benjamin B. Wolman   192
10. Behavioral Approaches to the Treatment of Obesity,
      Edward E. Abramson   207
11. Multimodal Behavioral Treatment of Obesity, Stephen DeBerry   225
12. Group Therapy in the Treatment of Obesity, Janet P. Wollersheim   241
13. Hypnotherapy in the Treatment of Obesity, Milton V. Kline   268
14. Exercise and Obesity, Allan Geliebter   291

Index   311

1
ETIOLOGY AND SYMPTOMATOLOGY OF OBESITY

1

Biology of Obesity

Barbara Lukert

Obesity is defined as an excessive accumulation of adipose tissue which contains fat stored in the form of triglyceride. The derivation of the word obese implies a single etiology of overeating. It is derived from the Latin prefix *ob-* or "over" with *edere* "to eat." This, however, is an unfair definition since many obese people may eat less than their peers but expend relatively less energy. It is difficult to determine what really constitutes excess adipose tissue, but a generally accepted definition is that an individual is obese when he exceeds his ideal body weight by more than 20 percent.

Clearly, fat must be stored in the adipose tissue as either *more* adipocytes or *larger* adipocytes, or in tissue with a mixture of cellular hyperplasia and hypertrophy. It is generally accepted that the hypercellular, hypertrophic type of obesity is usually associated with early onset, whereas hypertrophic obesity is associated with a later onset (1).

Unlike the newborn of other species, the newborn infant is endowed with an abundance of adipose tissue. Adipose tissue accounts for 10–15 percent of the body weight. Premature infants are in general leaner, which suggests that fat accumulation normally occurs during the last trimester of prenancy. The stored fat in the newborn weighs roughly 400 grams as compared to 10,000 grams to be found in the average adult adipose depot. Thus the newborn has about 1/25 the stored fat it will develop during growth and maturation. This fat is stored in about one-fifth the number of adult cells and the cells contain about one-fifth as much lipid as adult adipocytes. During the first year of life, there is a definite increase in cell size but only a slight increase in cell number. Then, there is a gradual increase in cell number and cell size, with a sharp increase in both occurring at puberty. By the stage of late adolescence, adult values are reached. There does not seem to be a critical period during which there is a sharp peak in the increased appearance of cells. If this does occur, it may be in the prenatal period of perhaps in early adolescence when the rate of appearance of cells is most rapid. All obese individuals have hypertrophic cells and the severely obese have an increase in adipose cell number as well as hypertrophy (2, 3, 4, 5, 6).

Adipocytes formed at any stage of life remain in the tissue for exceedingly long periods of time. There is no evidence that the adipocyte number can ever be decreased. Formerly obese patients who have maintained near normal body weight for many years have just as many fat cells as they had when they were at their heaviest. Adipocyte number can increase in adult animals and it is thought that during the first few weeks of life the adipocytes form a pool of incompletely differentiated cells. Overeating later in life may stimulate the completion of differentiation of those cells. In animal studies, when cells achieve a lipid content of about 1.2–1.9 micrograms, new fat cells appear. This suggests that cellular hypertrophy is the first response to demands for increased storage capacity and that it, in turn, is followed by hyperplasia.

STABILITY OF BODY WEIGHT

Several recent studies have shown a pattern of slow changes in body weight over many years, supporting the hypothesis that body weight is regulated. This is particularly well documented in cross-sectional studies in the 10-state nutrition survey of 1968–1970. This study showed that weight increases between the ages of 21 and 30 years in both men and women, with only small changes thereafter (7).

There is good experimental evidence favoring the concept of an endogenous regulatory mechanism which controls body weight. The first piece of evidence is that when mature animals are fed to reduce weight or overfed to gain weight, they spontaneously readjust their food intake when allowed to eat ad lib. When the caloric restriction is stopped or the force feeding terminated, the animal modifies its food intake to return to a body weight which is at or near the expected level. The starved animal will eat an excess amount of food until the body weight returns to its original level. Conversely, animals which are force fed will decrease their food intake and will return to normal weight. A similar experiment with overfeeding has been performed on human subjects who voluntarily overate. When the experiment ended the subjects naturally, without provocation, restricted their food intake until body weight returned to its original level. The readjustment usually took only a few weeks (9).

In another study, an effort was made to alter the total body fat content. This was done either in the mouse by removing gonadal fat, which contains about 25 percent of the fat in the animal, or in OB/OB mice in which introabdominal fat was removed. After the operation, the body weight increased and total body fat was the same in operated subjects as in the unoperated controls. This suggests that the total body fat is integrated into a single functional compartment with compensatory changes occurring in each fat depot (10).

A third line of evidence supporting the regulation of total stored calories involved studies of parabiosed animals. When one animal of a pair becomes obese following destructive lesions in the ventromedian nucleus, the normal parabiotic animal becomes thin by loss of body fat. There is a reduction in food intake in the lean rat as compared to the hyperphagic animal. This suggests that the lean animal is detecting some signal from the fat animal which indicates an increased store of calories. To compensate, the lean animal reduces its food intake, and its caloric stores of fat decrease (11).

A final kind of evidence supporting the regulation of caloric stores is derived from studies of animals with hypothalamic injuries (12). After a hypothalamic injury, there is an initial rapid rate of weight gain with marked hyperphagia. This is followed by a new stability of body weight by which food intake returns to nearly normal levels. Disturbance of this higher but plateaued weight by starvation is followed by increased caloric intake until weight is restored to the plateau from which it started. Several factors which control the regulation of total stored calories can go awry in obesity. These include the factors regulating food ingestion, those involved in the distribution or storage of calories, and those which control energy expenditure.

There is an anatomical basis for the regulation of food intake. The principal neural components which integrate this system are located in the hypothalamus. Anatomically the third ventricle divides the hypothalamus into two lateral halves. Adjacent to the third ventricle are several midline nuclei which can be subdivided into anterior, medial, and posterior groups. The ventromedian nucleus occupies the prominent position in the middle hypothalamus. Bilateral destructive lesions in this area have consistently produced obesity in all species studied. The amygdala may also serve an important function. When the basal lateral part of the amygdaloid complex is stimulated, food intake is inhibited in cats. Reciprocal effects of destruction increasing, and stimulation decreasing, food intake suggest an important role for the amygdaloid complex in the control of energy balance. In addition to the hypothalamus, food intake can be modified by stimulating or destroying the septal region of the globus pallidus, the caudate nucleus, the cingulate gyrus, and the frontal lobe. In general, stimulation and destruction have reciprocal effects (12).

It is also important to consider whether calories or taste control food intake. The normal rat will eat for calories. When the caloric density of a diet for rats is decreased by adding a bland but indigestible substance, the animals will promptly increase the volume of food which they ingest in order to maintain a constant intake of calories. This adjustment is made within 24 hours. However, under certain circumstances, the regulation is not so precise and the taste of the diet becomes as important as the caloric value. This is particularly true in the hungry or deprived animal (13).

A number of hypotheses have been advanced to account for the control of body calories. These include the glucostatic hypothesis (14), the aminostatic hypothesis (15), the lipostatic hypothesis (16), and the thermostatic hypothesis (17). Mayer postulated that the ventromedian nucleus of the hypothalamus might respond to changes in the rate of glucose utilization and thus modify food intake. This hypothesis has been supported by several observations. When gold thioglucose is injected, the gold is localized in the highest concentration in the ventromedian hypothalamus. Both injected glucose and diabetes with hyperglycemia will reduce the deposition of gold thioglucose in the ventromedian hypothalamus. When gold-containing compounds which are devoid of glucose are injected, there is no accumulation of gold in the ventral median hypothalamus; this suggests that the gold is accumulated by the cells which can transport glucose. Infusions of glucose in hungry individuals reduce the feelings of hunger as well as gastric contractions. Other maneuvers which raise blood glucose, such as the injection of glucagon, decrease hunger.

The lipostatic hypothesis was proposed by Kennedy (16). He suggested that since rats which are overfed to increase their weight or starved to reduce their body weight return to their original weight when allowed to eat spontaneously, there must be some metabolite produced from fat which accomplishes the regulation. The principal metabolites released from adipose tissue are free fatty acids and glycerol. The rapid changes in the circulating concentrations of free fatty acids and their response to variations in metabolic state make them an unlikely control signal. Glycerol, on the other hand, is released during the hydrolysis of triglycerides and adipose tissue, and is a reasonable candidate to act as a regulator. Adipose tissue cannot further metabolize glycerol; therefore, glycerol is released into the circulation in proportion to the rate of hydrolysis of triglycerides. Glycerol is then transported to the liver where it can be converted to glucose. The glucose could then provide a signal to the hepatic glucose receptors and to the brain. It has also been found that the hypothalamus metabolizes glycerol and glycerol could act directly as a possible messenger to the hypothalamus.

The thermostatic hypothesis was proposed by Browbeck; this postulates that heat production, reflected in changes of body temperature, can act as a regulator of food intake (17). This hypothesis is supported by the observation that homeothermic animals eat more in cold than in hot environments. This adaptation is regulated by the preoptic region of the anterior hypothalamus. When this area of the hypothalamus is destroyed, control of body temperature is impaired. In these animals, food intake does not show the appropriate responses to temperature. Environmental temperature appears to be an important modulator of feeding behavior and is integrated into the overall control process.

There is also a relationship between amino acid levels and food intake. Experimental animals will reduce food intake if their diet is low or devoid of a single amino acid or if there is excess of one amino acid. These adjustments in intake occur very rapidly, with 75 percent change in intake occurring the first day.

The control of body weight and the regulation of body stores have also been studied in man, but the studies, of course, are not as detailed as in experimental animals. Human subjects will adjust their intake of food to changes in caloric density but the compensation might be quite slow. Speigel observed that 2-5 days were required before adaptation began and complete adaptation did not occur even after several days (18). It is concluded that humans, like animals, eat in part for calories, but that adaptive changes in caloric density of food are slow and may be inadequate in some people.

The role of taste has been investigated by Cabanac (19). He found that humans show an alteration in taste activity after weight loss. The sensitivity of taste for varying solutions of sugar was decreased after the ingestion of glucose in normal individuals. After weight loss, however, the depression in pleasant ratings for sucrose solutions was not present. Obese subjects had higher ratings for pleasantness than lean subjects and this was unchanged by ingesting glucose. Bray, on the other hand, found an aversion to very sweet solutions by obese subjects (20).

The role of the gastrointestinal tract is signaling hunger and satiation in man has received considerable attention. Hunger is usually associated with a gastric sensation, but satiation tends to have fewer physical correlates. Satiety is more frequently described in terms of relaxation and calmness.

CELL SIZE: EFFECTS ON METABOLISM

Cell size and number may be important in energy regulation. The rate of glycerol release and the response of cells to the effects of epinephrine and insulin are very much influenced by cell size. Although there is no proven link between adipose tissue, morphology, and food intake, it is tempting to think that such a link exists, since when the markedly obese individual loses weight, there are enormous forces at work to cause regaining of weight. The impetus to regain weight seems stronger than can be accounted for by habit or psychological factors alone (22).

Table 1-1 contains a list of the endocrine and metabolic changes which have been associated with obesity (21). It is interesting to note that if a group of individuals are force fed from normal weight to above 10 percent of their ideal body weight, they require more calories per square meter to maintain that weight than does the spontaneously obese patient. Subjects who are obese either

Table 1-1. Endocrine and Metabolic Changes in Spontaneous and Experimental Obesity. I. From Excess of a Mixed Diet. II. From Adding Fat to the Diet.*

	Spontaneous Obesity	Experimental Obesity I	Experimental Obesity II
Adipose tissue			
Cell size			
Cell number		Unchanged	
Caloric balance			
Calories required to maintain obese state	1300kcal/m²	2700kcal/m²	1800kcal/m²
Return to starting weight	Rapid	Rapid	Rapid
Spontaneous physical activity			
Appetite late in the day			
Fasting concentrations in blood			
Cholesterol			
Triglycerides			Normal
Free fatty acids		Unchanged or	
Amino acids			
Glucose	N or		
Insulin			
Glucose tolerance			
Oral			
Intravenous			
Insulin release			
To oral glucose			
To i.v. glucose			
To i.v. arginine			
Evidence of insulin resistance			
Insulin: glucose ratio			
Adipose tissue metabolism sensitivity to insulin in vitro			
Forearm muscle metabolism			
insulin-stimulated glucose uptake			
insulin inhibition of release of branch chain amino acids			
Hormones possibly affecting insulin resistance			
Glucocorticoids			
Plasma cortisol	N or	Unchanged	
Cortisol production rate			
Urinary 17-hydroxycorticoids	a	a	
Growth hormone			
Response to glucose			Normal
Response to arginine			Normal
Nocturnal rise			

*From Salans, L. B. and Dougherty, J. W. Effect of insulin upon glucose metabolism by adipose cells of different size, influence of cell lipid and protein content age and nutrition state. *J. Clin. Invest.*, 1971, *50*, 1399–1410.

[a]Normal/kg body weight.
= increased
= decreased

spontaneously or due to force feeding, have an elevation in their serum cholesterol, triglycerides, free fatty acids, amino acids, glucose, and insulin levels. They also have decreased glucose tolerance. The changes in insulin and the occurrence of insulin resistance in the obese individual have been extensively studied. Both patients who are spontaneously obese and those who are force fed to obesity show a rather marked degree of peripheral resistance to insulin (22, 23). When studied in vitro, the responses of adipose tissue to insulin were diminished in association with gain in weight. Weight loss by obese subjects restores insulin response and sensitivity toward normal (24).

Cell receptors for insulin have been studied extensively in obese subjects. Results are conflicting. There may be differences in mechanism of insulin resistance between those patients with early onset hyperplastic obesity and those with late onset hypertrophic obesity. Recent studies by Olefsky have shown that insulin ,binding to adipocytes and mononuclear cells is decreased in cells from insulin-resistant, obese diabetics (23). There is a significant inverse relationship between fasting plasma insulin levels and insulin binding to adipocytes. It has also been shown that caloric restriction will increase the number of receptors on mononuclear cells in obese patients, even before a significant amount of weight has been lost (24). From a clinical standpoint it has been shown that insulin resistance is an important concomitant of obesity and may be partially overcome by weight loss.

METABOLIC CHANGES ACCOMPANYING OBESITY

Obesity is accompanied by a number of metabolic and endocrinologic changes. The alteration which has received most attention is the increase in serum insulin concentration.

The consequences of hyperinsulinemia can be divided into early and late. The first early consequence is the effect on the liver (25). Livers from obese animals present many abnormalities that are consistent with overstimulation of the parenchyma by hyperinsulinemia (see Figure 1-1). Lipogenesis is enhanced because of the enhanced activity of several lipogenic enzymes (26). Esterification of fatty acids to triglycerides increases, in part as a result of augmentation of glycerokinase activity, and oxidation of fatty acids to ketone bodies decreases. All of these changes favor a marked increase in triglyceride synthesis, with the resulting intracellular accumulation of lipids and augmentation of the secretion of triglycerides as very low-density lipoprotein. All of these changes can be reversed toward normal when hyperinsulinemia decreases with weight loss (9).

Fat cells are also overstimulated by excess insulin. Adipose tissue lipogenesis is increased because of an increase in activity of several lipogenic enzymes. Under normal conditions adipose tissue glycerokinase is extremely low, but in animals

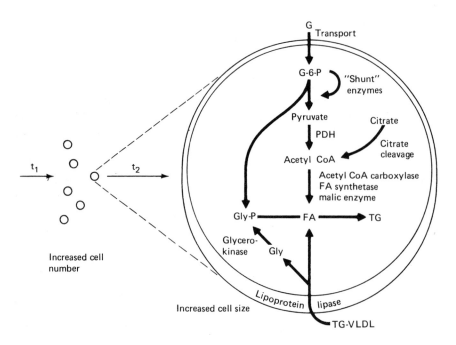

Figure 1-1. Diagram of the abnormalities prevailing in adipose tissue of obese animals. All heavy arrows indicate pathways that are increased compared to normal. All enzymes indicated have increased activity compared to normal. Abbreviations: t_1 refers to very early changes in obesity that lead to increased fat cell number; t_2 refers to early changes, due mainly to hyperinsulinaemia, that produce the anomalies indicated, with resulting increased adipocyte size. (From Assimacopoulos-Jeannet, F. and Jeanrenaud, B. Hormonal and metabolic basis of experimental obesity. *Clinics in Endocrinology and Metabolism*, 1976, 5, 347.

who are obese it may become very high with the potential of phosphorylating up to one-fifth of the available glycerol (see Figure 1-2). Lipoprotein lipase (the enzyme needed for uptake of circulating triglycerides) is also elevated. Soon after the onset of obesity, basal glucose muscle metabolism is augmented, particularly the increased incorporation of glucose into lipids. This can be further stimulated by insulin. Muscle lipoprotein lipase activity is also much greater than normal in some obese animals; this suggests that muscles from obese animals normally synthesize more lipids, but that they probably take up more of the circulating triglycerides with the resultant intracellular accumulation of fat (27, 28).

The later consequences of hyperinsulinemia in obesity may occur within a few weeks after onset of weight gain. They are characterized by the appearance of a state of insulin resistance leading to carbohydrate intolerance. There is a need for an increased insulin secretion rate to maintain a normal blood sugar.

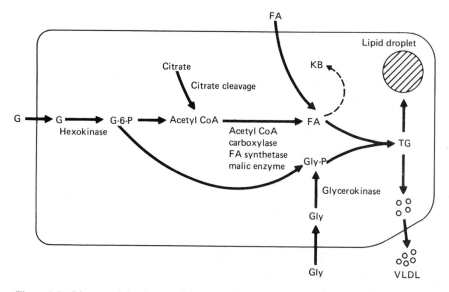

Figure 1-2. Diagram of the abnormalities prevailing in liver of obese animals. All heavy arrows indicate pathways that are increased compared to normal (dotted arrow = decreased pathway). All enzymes indicated have increased activity compared to normal. G = glucose; G-6-P = glucose-6-phosphate; FA = fatty acids; KB = ketone bodies; Gly-P = glycerophosphate; Gly = glycerol; TG = triglycerides; VLDL = very low density lipoproteins. (From Assimacopoulos-Jeannet, F. and Jeanrenaud, B. Hormonal and metabolic basis of experimental obesity. *Clinics in Endocrinology and Metabolism,* 1976, *5,* 349.

With increasing duration of obesity, the usual evolution is the appearance of fasting hyperglycemia, abnormal glucose tolerance, and poor responsiveness to exogenously administered insulin.

Two other hepatic abnormalities develop with time, further contributing to the obesity syndrome. First, the usual removal of insulin by the liver is markedly decreased in obesity and as a result more insulin can reach the periphery and reinforce hyperinsulinemia (25). Secondly, some hepatic pathways appear to become resistant to normal insulin regulation. Unlike livers from normal mice, livers of obese mice do not respond to an increased glucose load by rapidly decreasing gluconeogenesis and activating glycogen synthetase. Hepatic glucose release is thereby augmented contributing to hyperglycemia (29).

The later effects of obesity and hyperinsulinemia on adipose tissue are very complex. Basal lipogenesis remains elevated and adipose tissue becomes poorly responsive to insulin.

Later in obesity, a defect in muscle metabolism develops. Following a short-lived state of overstimulation, several types of muscle develop a state of almost complete resistance to the action of insulin (30).

Growth hormone response to a variety of stimuli is reduced in spontaneous obesity. Horton has observed that this is also true in experimental obesity in man when excess carbohydrate in a mixed diet is given but not when excess fat is added to the diet (31).

Cortisol production rates are increased in both spontaneous and experimental obesity (32). These production rates are normal in relation to body size and surface area. Serum cortisol is not found to be increased in either type of obesity, but if one looks at the urinary 17-keto- and ketogenic steroids they will be found to be elevated.

Alterations in glucagon metabolism in the obese subject have been looked for but the evidence is controversial. Some groups have found normal plasma values in obese subjects; others have found normal suppression by glucose but an increased response to intravenous arginine. Other investigators have found a diminished response to the infusion of alanine and to starvation (33, 34).

Prolactin plays an important role in lower animals; however, its role in human obesity is much more questionable. Very limited studies are available. Basal concentrations of prolactin were found to be lower than normal in four obese males, but prolactin response to insulin-induced hypoglycemia remained intact while that of growth hormone was impaired (35).

CALORIC REQUIREMENTS

There does seem to be a difference in the number of calories required by obese people to maintain body weight. Fascinating studies by Sims, in which he overfed volunteers with no family history of diabetes or obesity, found that not all of their subjects gained the amount of weight predicted from the calories ingested (9). This was especially noticeable when the calories were provided as carbohydrates. It seemed clear that individuals differed in their efficiency of weight gain. This resurrected the older theories that man can adapt to excess intake by spending calories inefficiently. In addition, it was noted that calories required to maintain the weight gain exceeded those necessary to maintain basal weight by an amount which could not readily be accounted for by the increase in body size. Several years ago, German writers referred to *Luxuskonsumption,* that is, an increase in heat production to produce a stable body weight in the face of increased caloric intake. This term was used after the turn of the century by Newman who found that he could vary his caloric intake by as much as 800 kilocalories per day while maintaining stable body weight.

A number of different mechanisms could account for the increased caloric requirements to maintain the weight gained by ingesting an excess of a mixed diet of over 1500 calories per day. Sims, in his studies, found that when basal metabolic rates and thermic effects of a standard meal were studied in two different groups of individuals, one group of overfed volunteers showed no change from a control group, whereas another group given excess carbohydrate clearly showed an increase in body temperature both overnight and in response to meals during the period of overfeeding. It would seem, then, that one adaptive mechanism to overeating is to increase the metabolic rate. This effect seems peculiar to the overeating of carbohydrate. One could postulate that obese subjects do not possess this adaptive mechanism.

Changes in thyroid function have long been invoked as a cause for obesity. Numerous investigators have measured serum thyroxine (T_4) and serum triiodothyronine (T_3) concentrations in obese subjects. Several investigators have found the serum T_3 to be proportional to body weight, with elevated levels of serum T_3 being observed in obese subjects (36). A significant decrease in serum reverse T_3 (RT_3), an isomer of T_3 with minimal physiologic activity, has also been found. Serum T_3 is believed to be generated in the pheriphery, probably in the liver by monodeiodination of T_4. Since the basal metabolic rate (BMR) remains normal in the presence of an increase in the T_3, it has been suggested that obese people may have an element of cellular resistance to T_3. Since either T_3 or RT_3 can be made in the periphery, it has been hypothesized that changes in the diet may alter the direction of this conversion, resulting in production of either active or inactive hormone. In the study by Sims, it was found that serum T_3 was reduced and RT_3 increased when carbohydrate was restricted in the diet, while the opposite was seen from feeding of excess carbohydrate. It seems likely that alterations in the metabolism of thyroid hormone are associated in some manner with carbohydrate content of the diet and are probably also related to the basic nutritional state.

The critical questions, however, are whether there is a difference in the basal metabolic rate in any of the varieties of obesity, whether the thermic response to food is impaired in obese subjects, and whether any change in the metabolism of thyroid hormone can explain the ease of weight gain. In a study by Miller of 29 obese women who were placed on 1500 kilocalories a day for three weeks, 20 lost weight and 9 maintained their weight. This group of nine who did not lose weight did have significantly lower metabolic rates. Sims studied four moderately overweight young men while they were eating approximately 1800 kilocalories of carbohydrate daily in excess of requirements for weight maintenance. The serum T_3 increased and RT_3 decreased for the group. However, the changes were not significant in two of the subjects. The two subjects who showed the expected changes also showed an increase in thermogenesis. Thyroid hormone increases the activity of mitochondrial alpha-glycerol-phosphate-dehydrogenase in adipose tissue. Bray found this enzyme activity to be reduced in the adipose tissue of obese patients (36).

These changes in thyroid hormone metabolism have important implications in the therapeutic management of obese subjects. A reduction of T_3 and an increase in conversion of T_4 to the inert RT_3 is part of a normal adaptation to restricted intake (37). This represents a survival mechanism under normal circumstances, but in the obese subject it might be detrimental.

From a practical point of view, the frequency with which meals are eaten appears to be nearly as important as the quality and quantity of food consumed. Small meals eaten at frequent intervals are associated with a significantly greater tendency to weight loss in obese subjects. The effect of this type of feeding on metabolic parameters has not been studied.

In summary, obesity is a serious metabolic problem which is accompanied by hyperinsulinemia, insulin resistance, blunted growth hormone response, and an increased rate of secretion or cortisol. The obese person appears to lack the ability to "waste" calories. The reasons for this are not clear, and the future must bring a better understanding of subtle hormonal or metabolic aberrations which may be present in obese subjects.

REFERENCES

1. Hirsch, J., Knittle, L. J., and Salans, L. B. Cell lipid content and cell number in obese and non-obese human adipose tissue. *J. Clin. Invest.,* 1966, *45,* 1023.
2. Hirsch, J. and Knittle, L. J. Cellularity of obese and non-obese adipose tissue. *Fed. Proceedings* (Federation of American Society for Experimental Biology), 1970, *29,* 1516–1521.
3. Brooke, C. G. D., Lloyd, J. K., and Wolf, O. H. Relation between age of onset of obesity and size and number of adipose cells. *Brit. Med. J.,* 1972, *2,* 25–27.
4. Boulton, T. J. C., Dunlop, M., and Court, J. M. Adipocyte growth in the first two years of life. *Austral. Ped. J.,* 1974, *10,* 301–305.
5. Dauncey, M. J. and Gairdner, D. Size of adipose cells in infancy. *Arch. Dis. Child.,* 1975, *50,* 286–290.
6. Knittle, L. J. General discussion in *Nutrient Requirements in Adolescence* (McKigney, J. I., and Munro, H. N., Eds.), p. 71–103. Cambridge, Massachusetts: M. I. T. Press, 1976.
7. Ten State Nutrition Survey 1968–1970. HEW Services on Mental Health Administration, Center for Disease Control III. Clinical, Anthropometry and Dental.
8. Bjorntorp, P. and Sjostrom, L. The composition of metabolism in vitro of adipose tissue fat cells of different sizes. *Europ. J. Clin. Invest.,* 1972, *2,* 78–84.
9. Sims, E. A. H., Danforth, E., Jr., Horton, E. S., Bray, G. A., Glennen, J. A., and Salans, L. B. Endocrine and metabolic effects of experimental obesity in man. *Recent Progress of Hormone Research,* 1973, *29,* 457.
10. Kennedy, G. C. The role of depot fat in the hypothalamic control of food intake in the rat. *Proc. Roy. Soc.,* 1953, *140,* 478.
11. Coleman, D. L. and Hummel, K. P. Effects of parabiosis of normal and genetically diabetic mice. *Am. J. Physiology,* 1969, *217,* 1298.
12. Assimacopoulos-Jeannet, F. and Jeanrenaud, B. Hormonal and metabolic basis of experimental obesity. *Clinic in Endocrinology and Metabolism,* 1976, *5*(No. 2), 337.

13. Booth, D. A., Toates, F. M., and Platt, S. U. Control system for hunger and its implications in animals and man. *Hunger: Basic Mechanisms and Clinical Implications* (Novin, D., Wyrwicka, W., and Bray, G. A., Eds.), p. 127. New York: Raven Press, 1975.
14. Mayer, J. Glucostatic mechanism of regulation of food intake. *New Engl. J. Med.,* 1953, *249*, 13.
15. Mellinkoff, S. M. and Franklandstell, Relationship between serum amino acid concentration and fluctuations in appetite. *J. Appl. Physiol.,* 1956, *8*, 335.
16. Kennedy, G. C. The role of depot fat in the hypothalamic control of food intake in the rat. *Proc. Roy. Soc.,* 1953, *140*, 570.
17. Brobeck, J. R. Food intake as a mechanism of temperature regulation. *Yale J. Biol. Med.,* 1948, *20*, 545.
18. Speigel, T. A. Caloric regulation of food intake in man. *J. Comparative Physiol. & Psychol.,* 1973, *84*, 24–37.
19. Cabanac, M. and Duclaux, R. Obesity: Absence of satiety aversion to sucrose. *Science,* 1970, *168*, 496–497.
20. Bray, G. A., Berry, R. E., and Benfield, J., Castenuovo-Tedesco, P., and Rodine, J. Food intake and taste preference for glucose and sucrose decrease after intestinal bypass surgery. *Hunger: Basic Mechanisms of Clinical Implications* (Novin, D., Wyrwicka, W., and Bray, G. A., Eds.). New York: Raven Press, 1975.
21. Salans, L. B. and Dougherty, J. W. Effect of insulin upon glucose metabolism by adipose cells of different size, influence of cell lipid and protein content age and nutrition state. *J. Clin. Invest.,* 1971, *50*, 1399–1410.
22. Salans, L. B., Bray, G. A., Cushman, S. W., Danforth, E., Jr., Glennen, J. A., Horton, E. S., and Sims, E. A. H. Glucose metabolism and the response to insulin by human adipose in spontaneous and experimental obesity, effects of dietary composition and adipose cell size. *J. Clin. Invest.,* 1974, *53*, 848–856.
23. Olefsky, J. M. Effect of fasting on insulin binding glucose transport and glucose oxidation in isolated rat adipocytes. *J. Clin. Invest.,* 1976, *57*, 1165–1172.
24. Olefsky, J. M. Effect of fasting on insulin binding glucose transport and glucose oxidation in isolated rat adipocytes. *J. Clin. Invest.,* 1976, *58*, 1450–1460.
25. Karakash, C., Assimacopoulos-Jeannet, F., and Jeanrenaud, B. An anomaly of insulin removal in perfused livers of obese, hypoglycemic (OB/OB) mice: A possible factor contributing to hyperinsulinemia. *J. Clin. Invest.,* 1976.
26. Miller, D. S. and Parsonage, S. Resistance to slimming adaptation or illusion. *Lancet,* 1975, *RMI*, 773–775.
27. Assimacopoulos-Jeannet, F., Singh, A., LeMarchand, Y., Loten, E. G., and Jeanrenaud, B. Abnormalities in lipogenesis and triglyceride secretion by perfusing livers of obese, hypoglycemic (OB/OB) mice: Relationship with hyperinsulinemia, *Diabetologia,* 1974, *10*, 155–162.
28. Rath, E. A., Hems, D. A., and Beloff-Chain, A. Lipoprotein lipase activities in tissues of normal and genetically obese (OB/OB) mice. *Diabetologia,* 1974, *10*, 261–265.
29. Koschinsky, T. H., Gries, F. A., and Herberg, L. Regulation of glycerol kinase by insulin in isolated fat cells and liver of Bar Harbour obese mice. *Diabetologia,* 1971, *7*, 316–322.
30. Kreutner, W., Springer, S. C., and Sharewood, J. E. Resistance of gluconeogenic and glycogenic pathways in obese hypoglycemic mice. *Am. J. Physiol.,* 1975, *228*, 663–671.
31. Chouverakis, C. and White, P. A. Obesity and insulin resistance in the obese hypoglycemic mouse (OB/OB). *Metabolism,* 1969, *18*, 998–1006.

32. Horton, E. S., Danforth, E., Jr., Sims, E. A. H., and Salans, L. B. Endocrine and metabolic alterations in spontaneous and experimental obesity. *Obesity in Perspective* (Bray G. A., Ed.), Folgarty International Center Series on Preventive Medicine. pp. 323–334. Washington: U. S. Government Printing Office.

33. O'Connell, M., Danforth, E., Jr., Horton, E. S., Salans, L. B., and Sims, E. A. H. Experimental obesity in man. III. Adrenocorticol function. *J. Clin. Endocrinol. Metabol.*, 1973, *36*, 323.

34. Gossain, V. V., Matute, M. L., and Kalkhoff, R. K. Relative influence of obesity in diabetes on plasma alpha cell glucagon. *J. Clin. Endocrinol. Metabol.*, 1974, *38*, 238.

35. Wise, J. K., Hendler, R., and Felig, P. Evaluation of alpha-cell function by infusion of alanine in normal diabetic and obese subjects. *N. Engl. J. Med.*, 1973, *288*, 487.

36. Copinschig, L'Hermite, M., Lecler, C. Q. R., Virasoro, E., and Robyn, C. Prolactin release after insulin induced hypoglycemia in obese subjects in the regulation of the adipose tissue mass. Proc. 4th Int. Meeting of Endocrinology, Marseille, 1973 (Vague, J., Boyer, J., and Addison, G. M., Eds.) p. 288. Amsterdam: Accepta Medica, 1978.

37. Bray, G. A. and Greenway, S. L. Pharmacologic approaches to treating the obese patient. *Clin. Endocrinol. Metabol.*, 1966, *5*, 2:455.

38. Portney, G. I., O'Brian, J. T., Bush, J., Vagenskis, A. G., Azizi, F., Arky, R., Ingbar, S. H., and Braverman, L. E. Effects of prolonged starvation on serum TSH, T_4 and T_3 concentration in man. *Clin. Res.*, 1973, *21*, 958.

2

Personality and Behavioral Correlates of Obesity

Gloria R. Leon

Obese persons have been characterized according to a number of traits or behaviors ranging from those that are fairly positive to others that are quite negative in nature. The obese have often been described as jolly, pleasure loving, weak willed, lazy, or self-indulgent. As our American culture increasingly considers thinness in women and lean muscularity in men as the ideal of physical attractiveness, obese persons seem to be responded to in an increasingly negative manner. Societal attitudes about obesity might thus exacerbate some of the problems posited as the cause of the obese state. It is therefore of interest to explore some of the psychological explanations of obesity and review the scientific evidence in support of these theories.

THEORETICAL FORMULATIONS

Psychodynamic

Psychodynamic formulations of obesity have posited the existence of problems at the oral stage of psychosexual development resulting from unresolved dependency needs (Jones, 1953). The symptom of obesity has therefore been viewed as a fixation at, or regression to, the oral stage of development, and the assumption has been that symptom removal without dealing with the underlying psychodynamic cause of the obese state will result in symptom substitution or a deterioration in the individual's emotional functioning (Alexander and Flagg, 1965;

15

Fenichel, 1945). Consonant with this viewpoint, the symptom of obesity is conceptualized as a depressive equivalent (Bruch, 1957). Therefore, removing the symptom without other treatment should result in the overt manifestation of depression.

Hilde Bruch (1958) moved from a classical psychoanalytic interpretation of eating disorders to a psychodynamic formulation based on a distinction between what she terms *developmental* and *reactive* types of obesity. She considers the former as a deep-seated disturbance resembling preschizophrenic development. Developmental obesity is conceptualized as beginning in infancy and caused by a fundamental feeling of rejection by the mother toward her child. Because of these strong feelings of rejection, the mother attempts to compensate by over-protective behaviors toward her child, including excessive feeding. Specifically, the mother is perceived as responding to all of the child's needs by the giving of food. Therefore, as the child develops, he or she is unable to distinguish between the various bodily urges and sensations. The result of the mother's food-giving behavior is that the child develops a disturbed body image and a lack of body identity, i.e., a feeling of not owning one's own body. Reactive obesity, on the other hand, is viewed as occurring primarily in adults in response to traumatic environmental circumstances. This type of obesity is not seen as so integrally involved in fundamental life relationships. However, in both types of obesity, symptom removal without dealing with the underlying causes of the disorder is posited to result in a deterioration in functioning.

Externality Theory

Schachter (1971) and colleagues (see Schachter and Rodin, 1974) carried out a series of investigations that were interpreted as demonstrating that the obese person's eating behavior is primarily determined by external cues rather than by internal cues of hunger. The eating behavior of normal weight persons was viewed as determined primarily by internal physiological states associated with hunger. Schachter and Rodin (1974) extended these feelings to propose that obese persons exhibit the trait of externality as a general personality characteristic and not as a characteristic specific to food consumption. The implications of this theory and the research cited in its support are that obese persons are not only more sensitive in their eating behavior to cues such as the smell and taste of food, the salience of the food cues, and the effort involved in obtaining the food, but that obese persons are also more responsive than normal weight persons to external cues in general. Experimental findings suggested that the obese are more distractible, show a greater influence of external cues on thinking and learning processes, show a greater responsiveness to affective stimuli, and are more responsive to a variety of highly salient external cues. However, the research supporting this theory has been equivocal, and many questions have been raised about study design, the interpretation of the findings in individual studies, generalizations made from the data, and the criteria used for defining obesity (Leon and Roth, 1977). The problems inherent in the selection of generally minimally overweight undergraduate college males as the subject population from which to generalize were also noted. Further, Rodin (Note 1) reported a lack of replication of the findings related to the externality hypothesis and obesity when clearly obese subjects were studied, i.e., those who were 50 percent or more above ideal body weight. In addition, subsequent research (Rodin, 1978) indicated that the eating behavior of normal weight persons was also highly responsive to external cues and that the characteristic of externality was not specific to obese persons. An investigation by Elman, Schroeder, and Schwartz (1977) also indicated that obese persons were not more susceptible to social influence than were normal weight persons.

Learning Theory

Learning theory explanations of obesity have centered around the concept of eating as a highly overlearned habit that has generalized to a variety of environmental cues and states of emotional arousal (Ferster, Nurnberger, and Levitt, 1962; Leon and Chamberlain, 1973b). It is posited that an association becomes established between diverse stimuli, unrelated to states of hunger, and the response of food intake. This association between environmental cues, emotional states, and food consumption was demonstrated in a study evaluating the behavioral differences between obese persons who had successfully maintained a weight loss over a one-year period and those who had regained the weight they had previously lost (Leon and Chamberlain, 1973a, 1973b). The weight regainers reported a greater frequency than the weight maintainers of eating high-calorie snacks while watching television, and they also reported a greater incidence of food consumption in response to feelings of loneliness, boredom, anger, and multiple states of emotional arousal. These findings of a relationship between emotional states and food consumption were further demonstrated in a study by Slochower (1976) in which affect reduction appeared to serve as a reinforcer in the eating behavior of obese individuals in an unlabeled high-arousal condition. The behavior modification procedures specifically developed for weight reduction are also relevant to these findings since these particular techniques are based on the strategy of bringing food consumption under the control of stimuli that are more appropriate for weight loss and the maintenance of that loss (Stuart and Davis, 1972).

Imitation learning or modeling is another influence considered important in the initial learning and later maintenance of the obese state. According to this paradigm, the repeated opportunity to observe other persons in one's family overeat and/or eat in response to cues unrelated to hunger results in the child learning a similar eating pattern. This pattern may be further maintained through parental reinforcement or social approval, i.e., the parent encouraging and praising the child for eating large quantities of food.

Genetic and Constitutional Factors

A discussion of parental influences in the development of obesity would be incomplete without mentioning genetic and constitutional factors. Mayer's (1965a) findings indicated that 40 percent of adolescents studied at age 15 who had one obese parent were obese, while 80 percent of the youngsters with two obese parents were also obese. However, only 10 percent of the adolescents whose parents were of normal weight were obese. Further, a consistency in obesity from childhood to later age periods has been demonstrated in a number of investigations (Crisp, Douglas, Ross, and Stonehill, 1970; Eid, 1970; Lloyd, Wolff, and Whalen, 1961). A review of studies of monozygotic and dyzygotic twins (Mayer, 1965b) indicated a strong influence of genetic factors in obesity, although environmental influences were also evident. These findings suggest that a predisposition toward obesity (through some as yet incompletely understood mechanism) might interact with family and other learning influences in determining patterns of food consumption. Further, evidence of the permanent development of relatively greater than average numbers of adipose cells in early childhood due to overfeeding points to another environmental influence that produces permanent constitutional changes in the obese individual (Sjostrom, 1978).

BODY IMAGE AND OBESITY

The perception and evaluation of one's body appears to be highly influenced by cultural and societal standards of appropriate body shape. The "American preoccupation with thinness" has been commented on by Bruch (1973) and others in terms of the etiology of anorexia nervosa. These standards of physical attractiveness can also be considered in relation to the negative evaluation placed on being fat in our culture. Indeed, Huenemann, Shapiro, Hampton, and Mitchell (1966) found that from ninth grade to twelfth grade, an increasing number of girls described themselves as fat and were dissatisfied with their physical appearance. This phenomenon occurred even though the proportion of girls who were objectively classified as obese remained the same over this grade range. On the other hand, boys over this same age period showed an increasingly greater concern with becoming more muscular rather than more lean. Nylander (1971) studied an adolescent population in Sweden and found that the feeling of being fat and the practice of dieting was a widespread phenomenon among girls, although uncommon among boys. Prejudice toward obese persons has been documented by Canning and Mayer (1966), Lerner and Gellert (1969), and Maddox, Back, and Liederman (1968).

The body image concept that an individual internalizes has been studied through perceptual, cognitive-evaluative, and interview procedures. The evidence concerning the permanence with which obese persons who have lost weight maintain an image of themselves as fat and unattractive has varied depending on the type of measurement instrument used (Leon and Roth, 1977). Perceptual measures of body image that require persons to estimate the size of various body parts indicate no significant difference in the accuracy of these estimations in persons of varying weights. Generally, most persons tend to overestimate their body size (Cappon and Banks, 1968; Garner, Garfinkel, Stancer, and Moldofsky, 1976; Leon, Eckert, Teed, and Buchwald, 1979; Sconbuch and Schell, 1967). Also, an age influence on the accuracy of body size estimation has been demonstrated by the increase in accuracy of visual estimations of body size when comparing youngsters of eight to nine years of age with adolescents (Halmi, Goldberg, and Cunningham, 1977; Leon, Bemis, Meland, and Nussbaum, 1978).

Cognitive-evaluative indices of body image obtained through the use of semantic-differential techniques have shown that obese persons exhibit a realistic change to a more positive evaluation of their body as weight loss progresses and their physical appearance is less deviant. Both moderately and massively obese persons were more negative in the various evaluations of their body before, as compared to after, weight loss and realistically rated the concept "Me Right Now" as heavier on a bipolar heavy-light dimension before weight loss had occurred (Leon, 1975; Leon, Eckert, Teed, and Buchwald, 1979).

Interviews with obese persons seeking psychiatric or other treatment for their weight status, however, often suggest a quite different body evaluation. Adolescents as well as adults who are obese often verbalize the feeling that their bodies are grotesque and loathsome, and concomitant with these feelings, exhibit low self-esteem and a generalized negative self-concept (Hammar, Campbell, Campbell, Moores, Sareen, Gareis, and Lucas, 1972; Schonfeld, 1964; Stunkard and Mendelson, 1967). The onset of this evaluation of one's body as extremely ugly and unattractive was found to occur during adolescence. Stunkard and Burt (1967) studied preadolescent and adolescent obese girls and did not find this marked negative body image evaluation in the preadolescent girls. The obese adolescent group, however, clearly manifested this disturbance. Further, Stunkard and Mendelson (1967) reported that a number of adults, even after weight loss, continued to think of their bodies in an extremely negative manner and became highly anxious whenever they gained just a pound or two. The investigators concluded from their research and clinical experience that body image disturbances occur in a minority of neurotic obese persons whose obesity began prior to adult life.

Body image disturbance in adult persons of normal weight with a history of juvenile onset obesity is consonant with Bruch's formulation (1957), based on her clinical experience, of the "fat-thin syndrome." This syndrome refers to formerly obese individuals who, even after having attained and maintained a normal weight level for a significant number of years, continue to think of themselves as fat and unattractive. These individuals are described as intensely preoccupied with thoughts of food, engaging in detailed planning of every eating situation, and becoming extremely anxious even if they gain a pound or two. Bruch felt that the psychodynamic reasons causing this particular syndrome were similar to the dynamics of developmental obesity, which she considered to be a serious psychopathological disorder. However, because of some type of environmental influence, these "fat-thin" individuals are able to exert control over their eating behavior. Nonetheless, Bruch feels that the psychodynamic conflicts are still those of a fat person, and the only way this control over their eating behavior can be achieved is through the constant vigilance and preoccupation with food and dieting that these persons manifest. Individuals manifesting this syndrome, however, retain the lack of body identity and the other features of the distorted body image of the developmentally obese.

In evaluating the issue of body image distortions in obese individuals, it is extremely important to bear in mind the particular subject population that has been sampled. Clearly, persons who are seeking short-term or extended psychotherapeutic help for their obesity problem and are desperately unhappy about their weight status are different on a number of dimensions from persons who are overweight and would like to lose weight, but whose weight status has not become an overriding issue in their lives. Some persons may manifest serious psychological problems that might be exacerbated by their obese state although these problems may not necessarily have caused their obesity. Further, one can question whether an extremely obese person who feels that he or she is unattractive and extremely large is indeed manifesting a body image *disturbance*, or a fairly accurate evaluation of appearance with respect to current societal standards of ideal body weight.

An important issue in discussing body image factors in obesity is the necessity of distinguishing between various types of obesity, particularly juvenile onset versus adult onset obesity. The work of the Rockefeller University group (e.g., Glucksman and Hirsch, 1969; Grinker, Hirsch, and Levin, 1973) has demonstrated striking body image and other psychological differences during weight reduction between severely obese persons with juvenile onset as compared to adult onset obesity. It would seem that the onset of obesity during the adolescent period would be an extremely crucial factor in terms of that individual's self-concept and evaluation of body image. Clearly, adolescence is a period in which there is a generalized preoccupation with one's body because the body is rapidly maturing and changing. Any deviations from the adolescent norms of appearance may be viewed with alarm and dismay by a particular youngster. It is not unusual to encounter an adolescent who is intensely preoccupied with a skin blemish or other bodily imperfection that may be only barely visible to another person. Given this preoccupation with physical appearance (Huenemann et al., 1966), juvenile onset obesity can be conceptualized as an extremely visible physical deviation not unlike any other type of physical handicap. The ramifications of this handicap may include teasing by peers and family, other aversive social interactions, and an inadequate opportunity to learn appropriate social skills. Thus, the obese youngster develops an extremely poor self-concept and body image. These negative and painful experiences, occurring as they do during a time when issues related to the body in general are highly salient, may exert a continuing psychological influence irrespective of whether the person succeeds in losing weight at a later time. These experiences and evaluations about oneself would seem to result in quite different long-term effects than those manifested in an individual whose body was not deviant during the adolescent period but who became obese after marriage, childbirth, or at some point in middle age.

PSYCHOLOGICAL CHARACTERISTICS OF OBESE PERSONS

Investigators have used a variety of psychometric tests in attempting to delineate the psychological characteristics of obese persons. However, these investigations have generally failed to find consistent psychological traits in the obese groups studied. For example, MMPI* evaluations of 116 adult males and females seen in an obesity clinic did not reveal a personality pattern that was characteristic of that group (Johnson, Swenson, and Gastineau, 1976). Instead, a diversity of profile configurations was demonstrated among the population sampled. Pomerantz, Greenberg, and Blackburn (1977) reported findings in relation to the Masculinity-Femininity (M-F) scale of the MMPI possibly suggestive of a lack of assertiveness in a randomly selected group of 40 obese persons participating in a weight reduction clinic. However, the MMPI scale showing the relatively highest elevation for the males in the Pomerantz et al. study was the Depression (D) scale. Several other investigations have also indicated relative elevations on the D scale in persons seeking treatment for obesity. (See Leon and Roth, 1977, for a more extensive review of these studies.)

Individuals who have labeled their weight status as a problem and are seeking help for weight reduction may manifest mood and general personality characteristics that are different from obese persons who are not seeking help in changing their weight status. Silverstone (1968) concluded that the prevalence of neuroticism and psychoticism was no greater in obese than nonobese persons of the same age and social class. Further, no differences were found in the frequency

---

*Minnesota Multiphasic Personality Inventory.

of psychiatric disturbance in a group of obese, hyperobese, and normal weight lower SES women in a study by Holland, Masling, and Copley (1970). Crisp and McGuiness (1976), on the other hand, found relatively lower levels of anxiety and depression in obese as compared to normal weight groups. These findings again point to the diversity of personality and mood characteristics in obese persons, whose major point of commonality may be the fact of their excess of adipose tissue. As Mendelson (1966) observed, obese individuals may vary on a continuum from those in whom emotional problems are insignificant to those in whom emotional problems are extremely severe and intricately interwoven with issues related to eating and obesity.

PSYCHOLOGICAL AND MOOD CHANGES WITH WEIGHT REDUCTION

Moderate Obesity

There has been a great deal of interest in evaluating the relationship between weight reduction and depression because of psychodynamic concepts of obesity as a depressive equivalent. Stunkard and Rush (1974) examined a number of studies in which depression was monitored during weight reduction. They concluded that if depression occurs during the weight loss period, this mood state generally results from the stress of diets that encourage rapid weight loss, as well as the stress that occurs through long-term impatient fasting regimens. Taylor, Ferguson, and Reading (1978) carefully evaluated depressive affect during a gradual weight loss program and found that weight loss did not lead to an increase in depression. They also failed to find an association between initial levels of depression or changes in depression and attrition from the weight loss program. Silverstone and Lascelles (1966) studied a group of 72 obese patients who were receiving an anorectic drug. Several persons exhibited moderate symptoms of depression during weight loss although none became severely depressed. There was no increase with weight loss in the number of persons with mild or moderate anxiety, and the amount of weight lost was not related to either the initial or the final rating of depression. Further, Graff (1965) found that weight reduction was associated with decreases in both anxiety and depression.

Massive Obesity

The development of intestinal bypass surgery for modifying massive obesity (i.e., weight levels 100 percent or more above ideal body weight) has resulted in a natural experiment for evaluating the effect of significant changes in weight over a relatively short period of time on body image and more general aspects of psychological and interpersonal functioning. The dramatic change in physical status after bypass surgery is demonstrated by Buchwald, Schwartz, and Varco's (1973) report of a 35 percent average weight loss over time following jejunoileal bypass surgery. Through this bypass procedure, persons can continue to eat substantial amounts of food and still lose weight, although Bray (1978) reported that many persons do reduce their food intake after surgery. Generally, there is a marked change in physical appearance in a relatively short period of time since the greatest amount of weight loss tends to occur during the first year after surgery.

Espmark (1975) found that a significant number of patients experienced problems of anxiety and depression subsequent to bypass surgery, including several who attempted suicide. However, the majority of follow-up studies have indicated that there is an enhancement in psychological functioning and body image attitude with weight loss. Crisp, Kalucy, Pilkington, and Gazet (1977), using both a retrospective and prospective study design, reported that many persons experienced short-term irritability, depression, tiredness, and anxiety. However, at a point two years after surgery, a significant reduction was noted in somatic complaints and in anxiety, depression, and phobias.

A group of 24 massively obese persons were evaluated six months prior to intestinal bypass surgery, and reevaluated several days before undergoing the operation (Leon, Eckert, Teed, and Buchwald, 1979). The six-month baseline testing was caried out in order to control for the confounding effects of anticipated surgery on the personality data that is obtained while the person is in the hospital awaiting surgery. A second group of 48 massively obese persons were evaluated for the first time in the hospital prior to bypass surgery, and then reevaluated at three months, six months, and one year after surgery. MMPI evaluations revealed no consistent profile configuration for the two bypass groups studied. Both group profiles were within the normal range, were not suggestive of psychological deviance, and indicated a great amount of variability in personality characteristics among the group members. Of interest was the finding that the group initially evaluated six months prior to surgery showed a decline in somatic concerns and anxiety in the hospital as they awaited surgery, which suggests that they were looking forward in a positive manner to surgery and the anticipated changes in physical appearance. The group followed for one year after surgery exhibited at the one-year follow-up a significant decline in score on the MMPI D and Si (Social Introversion) scales, and a significant increase in score on the ES (Ego Strength) scale. The mean weight loss for this group at the one-year follow-up was 93.8 pounds. Significant and consistent changes on semantic-differential ratings for the concepts "My Body Right Now" and "My Personality Right Now" occurred at each evaluation interval over the one-year period, pointing to a marked enhancement in attitudes about one's body and personality as weight loss progressed. Questionnaire data indicated a statistically significant trend over the one-year period in the direction of a generally positive change in self-attitude.

Ratings of general physical attractiveness, sexual attractiveness, sociability, satisfaction with body weight, and other measures of body image all changed in a more positive direction over time. Further, perceptual measures of body size estimation showed a realistic adjustment with weight loss.

It must be noted, however, that secondary information obtained about persons who did not respond to the follow-up inquiries in the Leon et al. (1979) investigation revealed that 16.6 percent of the follow-up group ($N = 8$) were experiencing either severe psychological or physical problems, or a combination of these problems, subsequent to bypass surgery. These findings point to the necessity in any type of follow-up investigation to make every effort to obtain as much information as possible about the nonresponders. On the whole, however, the majority of persons in this investigation showed a clear enhancement in a variety of aspects of psychological functioning. The changes in mood exhibited by these individuals suggest that the anxiety and depression often associated with obesity may possibly be a result, rather than the cause, of the obese state.

The majority of individuals in the Leon et al. investigation, as well as those in the studies reviewed by Bray (1978), were consistent in stating that they no longer felt trapped by their obesity, and they therefore felt better about themselves. However, for those persons who have not developed social skills because of their history of obesity, or for whom changes in the family system occur because they have become more assertive and independent with weight loss, a transitional period may occur as new skills are learned and new social roles both within and outside of the family are tried out. Sometimes this transitional period may be associated with marital and other interpersonal problems due to the need for other family members to reciprocally change their roles and behaviors as psychological and behavioral changes occur in the person who has undergone bypass surgery.

Cautions about undergoing intestinal bypass surgery are necessary because of the significant number of postsurgical physical side effects and complications that have been reported (see Buchwald, 1979). This surgical procedure results in a marked change in physiological functioning and should only be undertaken when it is clear that other methods of weight reduction have not been effective and significant physical risks are present due to the individual's massive obesity. Persons should also be followed very carefully subsequent to surgery so that the physical and possible psychological problems that might appear can be dealt with. Given these prescriptions, however, bypass surgery appears to be a viable alternative for many massively obese persons who have not been able to lose weight through more conservative procedures. It has been documented that extremely beneficial psychological changes can occur following surgery.

ENVIRONMENTAL FACTORS IN EATING BEHAVIOR

Investigations have been carried out evaluating whether the eating behavior of obese persons in the natural environment differs in some fundamental way from that of normal weight persons. These studies (e.g., Dodd, Birky, and Stalling, 1976; Gaul, Craighead, and Mahoney, 1975; LeBow, Goldberg, and Collins, 1977) are consistent in demonstrating that obese persons perform fewer chews per bite, spend less time consuming their meals, and thus eat at a more rapid rate than do normal weight persons. However, the eating behavior of both obese and normal weight persons has been shown to be influenced by the eating behavior of others around them. Rosenthal and Marx (1979) found that both normal weight, successful dieters and unsuccessful dieters ate more in an experimental condition in which the model ate relatively greater amounts of food. Further, both overweight and normal weight college students reflected the rate and amount of food consumed by an eating companion (Rosenthal and McSweeney, 1979). These findings by Rosenthal and her colleagues again demonstrate that both obese and normal weight persons are influenced by external cues. The data on the faster pace of eating and the larger meals that obese persons tend to order (Dodd et al., 1976) have been influential in determining some of the techniques used in behavior modification weight reduction programs. For example, one component of treatment might involve instruction in how to eat at a slower rate, take smaller bites of food, chew the food more thoroughly, etc.

The work of Herman and Polivy on restrained and unrestrained eaters (Herman and Mack, 1975; Polivy, 1976) has resulted in further knowledge about the behaviors involved in food consumption. These investigations demonstrated that both obese and normal weight persons who typically consciously restrain themselves from overeating tended to overeat after consuming or being told that they were consuming a high-calorie preload. Persons who did not typically restrain their eating behavior showed a decline in the amount of food eaten after being forced to consume a high-calorie preload. This "disinhibitory" effect on the eating behavior of the restrained eaters suggests a cognitive element that may be relevant to issues concerning the eating behavior of obese persons on a diet. Once the "taboo" is broken and the dieter eats inappropriate foods or consumes a greater number of calories than he or she had planned to eat on a particular diet, the attitude then develops that it is no longer important or one can no longer re-exert control over one's eating behavior in that particular situation. The result is that an episode of general overeating then occurs. Practitioners developing cognitive-behavioral approaches to weight reduction may find this particular attitude an important one to deal with in helping individuals to gain control over their eating behavior despite occasional setbacks.

THE ADDICTIVE PERSONALITY

The overeating pattern manifested by many obese individuals is consonant with the notion of obesity as a severe habit disturbance or an addictive behavior pattern. For some individuals, particularly the massively obese, food consumption is a continuous, strongly learned pattern similar to other types of substance abuse patterns. The addictive nature of the eating pattern of some obese individuals was demonstrated by the MMPI findings in the Leon et al. (1979) study of the massively obese. Although there was no evidence of significant psychopathology in this group, the mean score for the group on the MacAndrew scale (a specially derived MMPI scale measuring addiction proneness) was just at the threshold indicative of an addiction problem. Further, those bypass patients who one year after surgery reported that they were eating the same amount of food or more than they had eaten prior to surgery scored relatively higher on this scale than did persons who had reduced their food intake in the year following surgery. Moderately obese persons did not score in the addictive range on the MacAndrew scale, although heavy male smokers did (Leon, Kolotkin, and Korgeski, 1979). (The latter group can also be viewed as persons who abuse a particular substance, in this case tobacco.)

Behavior modification programs have had a relatively greater degree of success in terms of the long-term maintenance of weight loss than other types of weight reduction programs (Leon, 1976). These treatment outcome findings suggest that dealing through cognitive and behavioral means with the strong habit disturbance component of the obesity problem may be a viable treatment strategy. However, as with other substance abuse problems, the therapist needs to explore with the client issues such as the decision-making process, the commitment to change one's problem behaviors, and strategies for developing effective self-control techniques.

SUMMARY

Systematic investigations directed toward defining the essential elements of "the obese personality" have not been fruitful. Obese persons share with other physically deviant individuals characteristics of poor self-esteem, negative mood states, and poor self-image. For some obese individuals, the negative body image concepts appear to be amenable to modification with weight loss. The depression and poor interpersonal relationships that psychodynamically oriented theorists have suggested as the cause of obesity may often be the result, rather than the cause, of the obese state. This alternative is suggested by the general enhancement in mood and in body image attitude demonstrated by massivley obese persons who lost a significant amount of weight following intestinal bypass surgery. The formulation of obesity as a habit disturbance with specific behaviors that can be modified has implications for the further development of behavior modification programs for weight reduction.

REFERENCE NOTE

1. Rodin, J. Obesity and external responsiveness. Paper presented at the meeting of the Eastern Psychological Association, Philadelphia, April 1974.

REFERENCES

Alexander, F. and Flagg, G. W. The psychosomatic approach. *Handbook of Clinical Psychology.* (Wolman, B. B., Ed.), pp. 855-947. New York: McGraw-Hill, 1965.

Bray, G. A. Intestinal bypass surgery for obese patients: Behavioral and metabolic considerations. *The Psychiatric Clinics of North America,* 1978, *1*, 673-689.

Bruch, H. *The Importance of Overweight.* New York: Norton, 1957.

Bruch, H. Developmental obesity and schizophrenia. *Psychiatry,* 1958, *21*, 65-70.

Bruch, H. *Eating disorders: Obesity, Anorexia Nervosa, and the Person Within.* New York: Basic Books, 1973.

Buchwald, H. (Ed.). The surgical clinics of North America. *Symposium on Morbid Obesity,* 1979, *59*, 961-1180.

Buchwald, H., Schwartz, M. Z., and Varco, R. L. Surgical treatment of obesity. *Advances in Surgery,* 1973, *7*, 235-255.

Canning, H. and Mayer, J. Obesity: Its possible effect on college acceptance. *New England Journal of Medicine,* 1966, *275*, 1172-1174.

Cappon, D. and Banks, R. Distorted body perception in obesity. *Journal of Nervous and Mental Disease,* 1968, *146*, 465-467.

Crisp, A. H., Douglas, J. W. B., Ross, J. M., and Stonehill, E. Some developmental aspects of weight. *Journal of Psychosomatic Research,* 1970, *14*, 313-320.

Crisp, A. H., Kalucy, R. S., Pilkington, T. R. E., and Gazet, J-C. Some psychosocial consequences of ileojejunal bypass surgery. *American Journal of Clinical Nutrition,* 1977, *30*, 109-120.

Crisp, A. H. and McGuiness, B. Jolly fat: Relation between obesity and psychoneurosis in general population. *British Medical Journal,* 1976, *1*, 7-9.

Dodd, D. K., Birky, H. J., and Stalling, R. B. Eating behavior of obese and normal-weight females in a natural setting. *Addictive Behaviors,* 1976, *1*, 321-325.

Eid, E. E. Follow-up study of physical growth of children who had excessive weight gain in first six months of life. *British Medical Journal,* 1970, *2*, 74-76.

Elman, D., Schroeder, H. E., and Schwartz, M. F. Reciprocal social influence of obese and normal-weight persons. *Journal of Abnormal Psychology,* 1977, *86*, 408-413.

Espmark, S. Psychological adjustment before and after bypass surgery for extreme obesity – A preliminary report. *Proceedings of the First International Congress on Obesity* (Howard, A., Ed.), pp. 242-243. London: Newman Publishing, 1975.

Fenichel, O. *The Psychoanalytic Theory of Neuroses.* New York: Norton, 1945.

Ferster, C. B., Nurnberger, J. I., and Levitt, E. B. The control of eating. *The Journal of Mathetics,* 1962, *1*, 87-109.

Garner, D. M., Garfinkel, P. E., Stancer, H. C., and Moldofsky, H. Body image disturbances in anorexia nervosa and obesity. *Psychosomatic Medicine, 1976, 38*, 327-336.

Gaul, D. J., Craighead, W. E., and Mahoney, M. J. Relationship between eating rates and obesity. *Journal of Consulting and Clinical Psychology, 1975, 43*, 123-125.

Glucksman, M. L. and Hirsch, J. The response of obese patients to weight reduction: III. The perception of body size. *Psychosomatic Medicine, 1969, 131*, 1-7.

Graff, H. Overweight and emotions in the obesity clinic. *Psychosomatics, 1965, 6*, 89-94.

Grinker, J., Hirsch, J., and Levin, B. The affective responses of obese patients to weight reduction: A differentiation based on age at onset of obesity. *Psychosomatic Medicine, 1973, 35*, 57-63.

Halmi, K. A., Goldberg, S. C., and Cunningham, S. Perceptual distortion of body image in adolescent girls: Distortion of body image in adolescence. *Psychological Medicine, 1977, 7*, 253-257.

Hammar, S. L., Campbell, M. M., Campbell, V. A., Moores, N. L., Sareen, C., Gareis, F. J., and Lucas, B. An interdisciplinary study of adolescent obesity. *Journal of Pediatrics, 1972, 80*, 373-383.

Herman, C. P. and Mack, D. Restrained and unrestrained eating. *Journal of Personality, 1975, 43*, 647-660.

Holland, J., Masling, J., and Copley, D. Mental illness in lower class normal, obese and hyperobese women. *Psychosomatic Medicine, 1970, 32*, 351-357.

Huenemann, R. L., Shapiro, L. R., Hampton, M. C., and Mitchell, B. W. A longitudinal study of gross body composition and body conformation and their association with food and activity in a teen-age population. *American Journal of Clinical Nutrition, 1966, 18*, 325-338.

Johnson, S. F., Swenson, W. M., and Gastineau, C. F. Personality characteristics in obesity: Relation of MMPI profile and age of onset of obesity to success in weight reduction. *The American Journal of Clinical Nutrition, 1976, 29*, 626-632.

Jones, E. *The Life and Work of Sigmund Freud.* New York: Basic Books, 1953.

LeBow, M. D., Goldberg, P. S., and Collins, A. Eating behavior of overweight and nonoverweight persons in the natural environment. *Journal of Consulting and Clinical Psychology, 1977, 45*, 1204-1205.

Leon, G. R. Personality, body image and eating pattern changes in overweight persons after weight loss. *Journal of Clinical Psychology, 1975, 31*, 618-623.

Leon, G. R. Current directions in the treatment of obesity. *Psychological Bulletin, 1976, 83*, 557-578.

Leon, G. R., Bemis, K., Meland, M., and Nussbaum, D. Aspects of body image perception in obese and normal weight youngsters. *Journal of Abnormal Child Psychology, 1978, 6*, 361-371.

Leon, G. R. and Chamberlain, K. Emotional arousal, eating patterns and body image as differential factors associated with varying success in maintaining a weight loss. *Journal of Consulting and Clinical Psychology, 1973, 40*, 474-480. (a)

Leon, G. R. and Chamberlain, K. A comparison of daily eating habits and emotional states of overweight persons successful or unsuccessful in maintaining a weight loss. *Journal of Consulting and Clinical Psychology, 1973, 41*, 108-115. (b)

Leon, G. R., Eckert, E. D., Teed D., and Buchwald, H. Changes in body image and other psychological factors after intestinal bypass surgery for massive obesity. *Journal of Behavioral Medicine, 1979, 2*, 39-59.

Leon, G. R., Kolotkin, R., and Korgeski, G. MacAndrew addiction scale and other MMPI characteristics associated with obesity, anorexia, and smoking behavior. *Addictive Behaviors, 1979, 4*, 401-407.

Leon, G. R. and Roth. L. Obesity: Psychological causes, correlations, and speculations. *Psychological Bulletin, 1977, 84*, 117-139.

Lerner, R. M. and Gellert, E. Body build identification, preference, and aversion in children. *Developmental Psychology,* 1969, *1,* 456-462.

Lloyd, J. K., Wolff, O. H., and Whelan, W. S. Childhood obesity: A long-term study of height and weight. *British Medical Journal,* 1961, *2,* 145-148.

Maddox, G. L., Back, K. W., and Liederman, V. R. Overweight as social deviance and disability. *Journal of Health and Social Behavior,* 1968, *9,* 287-298.

Mayer, J. Obesity in adolescence. *The Medical Clinics of North America,* 1965, *49,* 421-432. (a)

Mayer, J. Genetic factors in human obesity. *Postgraduate Medicine,* 1965, *37,* A-103-A108. (b)

Mendelson, M. Psychological aspects of obesity. *International Journal of Psychiatry,* 1966, *2,* 599-616.

Nylander, I. The feeling of being fat and dieting in a school population. *Acta Socio-medica Scandinavica,* 1971, *1,* 17-26.

Polivy, J. Perception of calories and regulation of intake in restrained and unrestrained subjects. *Addictive Behaviors,* 1976, *1,* 237-243.

Pomerantz, A. S., Greenberg. I., and Blackburn, G. L. MMPI profiles of obese men and women. *Psychological Reports,* 1977, *41,* 731-734.

Rodin, J. Environmental factors in obesity. *The Psychiatric Clinics of North America,* 1978, *1,* 581-592.

Rosenthal, B. and McSweeney, F. K. Modeling influences on eating behavior. *Addictive Behaviors,* 1979, *4,* 205-214.

Rosenthal, B. and Marx, R. D. Modeling influences on the eating behavior of successful and unsuccessful dieters and untreated normal weight individuals. *Addictive Behaviors,* 1979, *4,* 215-221.

Schachter, S. Some extraordinary facts about obese humans and rats. *American Psychologist,* 1971, *26,* 129-144.

Schachter, S. and Rodin, J. *Obese Humans and Rats.* Potomac, Md.: Lawrence Erlbaum Associates, 1974.

Schonbuch, S. S. and Schell, R. E. Judgments of body appearance by fat and skinny male college students. *Perceptual and Motor Skills,* 1967, *24,* 999-1002.

Schonfeld, W. A. Body-image disturbances in adolescents with inappropriate sexual development. *American Journal of Orthopsychiatry,* 1964, *34,* 493-502.

Silverstone, J. T. Obesity. *Proceedings of the Royal Society of Medicine,* 1968, *61,* 371-375.

Silverstone, J. T. and Lascelles, B. D. Dieting and depression. *British Journal of Psychiatry,* 1966, *112,* 513-519.

Sjöström, L. The contribution of fat cells to the determination of body weight. *The Psychiatric Clinics of North America,* 1978, *1,* 493-521.

Slochower, J. Emotional labeling and overeating in obese and normal weight individuals. *Psychosomatic Medicine,* 1976, *38,* 131-139.

Stuart, R. B. and Davis, B. *Slim Chance in a Fat World: Behavioral Control of Obesity.* Champaign, Ill.: Research Press Company, 1972.

Stunkard, A. and Burt, V. Obesity and the body image: II. Age at onset of disturbances in the body image. *American Journal of Psychiatry,* 1967, *123,* 1443-1447.

Stunkard, A. and Mendelson, M. Obesity and the body image. I. Characteristics of disturbances in the body image of some obese persons. *American Journal of Psychiatry,* 1967, *123,* 1296-1300.

Stunkard, A. J. and Rush, J. Dieting and depression reexamined. A critical review of reports of untoward responses during weight reduction for obesity. *Annals of Internal Medicine,* 1974, *81,* 526-533.

Taylor, C. B., Ferguson, J. M. and Reading, J. C. Gradual weight loss and depression. *Behavior Therapy,* 1978, *9,* 622-625.

3

Obesity:
Why the Losing Battle?*

Judith Rodin

The problem of obesity has been with us for centuries. In *Henry IV* Shakespeare admonishes, "Leave gourmandising. Know the grave does gape for thee thrice wider than for other men." Of all the human frailties, obesity is perhaps the most perverse. Its penalties are so severe, the gratifications so limited, and the remedy so simple that obesity should be the most trivial of aberrations to correct, yet it is the most recalcitrant. Almost any fat person can lose weight, few can keep it off. It is this fact that makes the study of obesity so intriguing.

Although there is too much fat in obese people, fat is one of the basic chemical constituents of the body. Actually the formation of fat is an admirable evolutionary development, allowing for compact storage of energy reserves, cushioning, insulation, and even aesthetic appeal. Marvelously adapted to the energy needs of the body, fat molecules flow in and out of the adipocytes under the constant titration of hormones and enzymes, and are often tucked away in complex macromolecules which allow rapid transport in an aqueous environment. Perhaps it is surprising that abundant fat storage and consequent obesity are not more frequent if one considers the exquisite balance between food ingestion and energy output which must be maintained over many years, during which both activities tend to be somewhat casually controlled.

---

*Based on an invited address presented within the framework of Master Lectures of the American Psychological Association.

CAUSES OF OBESITY

Obesity has been called the main public health problem in the United States. Beyond the toll which it exacts in morbidity and premature death, obesity often leads to a loss of self-esteem and social stigma in an era in which Twiggy has been the highest paid model. It is clearly the case that once obesity is present, it could have strong, health-relevant pathological consequences; however, it appears likely that even extreme obesity often has no pathology as its cause. Because this is so, a medical model styled after germ theory has been shown to be inappropriate for understanding and treating obesity; it is being replaced in all sectors by a biopsychosocial model (Booth, 1976; Rodin, 1977). This model would explain not only the disregulated state of overeating but all feeding behavior, since we see eating as a multiply regulated process which is influenced by interactions among physiological, cognitive, social, and cultural variables in a control system to which they are all essential even in the disordered state of obesity. Thus obesity could arise from, or be contributed to, by a breakdown at any of these levels or a failure in feedback among two or more of these levels.

On the basis of what we currently know about the subject, only 5 percent of all obesity can be attributed to such underlying causes as brain damage, endocrine dysfunction, and hereditary diseases like the Prader-Willi syndrome (Van Itallie, 1977). The remaining 95 percent is obesity which has no apparent primary etiology. Here the biopsychosocial model is most applicable, and in recent years investigative attention has focused increasingly on this latter component. Out of this research effort, which has been multidisciplinary in scope, two different points of view about the pathogenesis of human obesity have emerged. One school of thought holds that obesity is not biologically determined but arises from certain kinds of life style and from the chronic use of food for non-nutritive purposes (Bruch, 1961; Van Itallie and Campbell, 1972). The other school proposes that obese individuals are made that way; in other words, they are biologically programmed for fat (Nisbett, 1972).

First let us consider the alternative that many human obesities are not biologically determined. In recent years, evidence has accumulated that many obese individuals become that way because of a sedentary life style and a maladaptive use of food. For example, apart from any physiological need for food, many individuals may respond to arousal states such as anxiety, boredom, or anger by eating. However, all excessive food intake is not attributable to emotional arousal. Indeed much overeating may simply result from the repeated exposure of individuals to highly palatable, readily accessible food in an environment where the requirement to expend energy in physical activity is much too low. In addition, the prevalence of obesity is strongly influenced by race and socioeconomic factors. In both adults and young children, the prevalence of obesity is higher among lower classes and among groups not well acculturated in American society (Srole, et al., 1962). These data suggest that obesity cannot be viewed merely as an individual characteristic. Instead the body weight that an individual maintains is in large part a response to social norms and pressure. Most of you who have felt even momentary weight consciousness can support this conclusion with your personal experience.

On the other hand, the best evidence that some individuals are biologically fated to be obese comes from morphologic studies of adipose tissue pioneered by Hirsch and his associates (Hirsch and Knittle, 1970). The quantity of fat stored in the body is the product of the number of fat cells that we have and their average size. Some studies suggest a genetic component to the number of fat cells (Salans et al., 1973), and others indicate that adipose cell number may also be influenced by early nutrition. Thus the notion has developed that some obesity in humans may have its origins in childhood feeding practices. For example, infants who are bottle fed may be induced to take more formula than they actually need because of the mother's preconceived notion of how much the baby should consume. Such overfeeding could stimulate adipocyte replication and favor fat cell development.

While animal models have been developed and have some utility for our understanding of obesity, their simplicity often contributes to unwarranted, simple assumptions about the etiology of human obesity. For example, there is no evidence in humans of obesity produced by a single gene, as in congenitally obese strains of rodents. Nonetheless, there is increasing evidence to indicate the influence of genetic factors in human obesity (Mayer, 1953). These affect not only total body fat but also the relative amounts of fat in abdominal and subcutaneous body tissue and its distribution on the trunk and limbs. We can just look around us to know that there is a strong familial link in obesity. The problem, of course, is that this involves both environmental and genetic factors which are often difficult to disentangle. For example, there may be a pattern of overeating in a family which has nothing to do with their inherited traits.

The causes of obesity may be multifactorial. Its onset is determined by a combination of genetic, psychological, and environmental factors, and thus far it has been difficult to disentangle the relative importance of each component. Perhaps this is the reason that for us as scientists, as well as for the overweight person, dealing with obesity sometimes feels like such a losing battle.

DEFINING OBESITY

While it might seem easy to begin by defining the condition, historically there have been a number of methodological problems associated with the definition and measurement of obesity. An important issue is the criterion used in labeling an individual obese and particularly in measuring procedures used in determining the degree of obesity in relation to some type of standard. In some instances it is simple to define obesity, particularly when the individual in question is massively obese. Such people require no sophisticated criteria to indicate this diagnosis. The heaviest reported body weight according to the *Guiness Book of World Records* was 1069 pounds in 1974. However, the rarity of individuals with extreme obesity points out the need for careful definitions of obesity and excess body weight when dealing with less obvious situations. The distinction between overweight and obesity is especially critical. Obesity is an excess of body fat, but in general body fat content increases with age, is greater in females, and decreases with physical activity. Overweight is used to denote a body weight which is higher than standard weight. Generally the standard weights are obtained from tables which provide appropriate, desirable, or satisfactory weights in relation to height. A person is overweight when his or her body weight exceeds the limits provided by these standards. At a height of 60 inches, 100 pounds is a desirable weight for a woman and 106 pounds for a man. For every extra inch above this height, 5 pounds is added to the woman's weight and 6 pounds to the man's. Another quick rule of thumb is the so-called magic 36. If your waist dimension in inches subtracted from your height in inches is less than 36, you are probably overweight. On the other hand, if your waist or circumference taken from your height is more than 36, you may be presumed to be of normal body weight. Better definitions of overweight and obesity will probably be possible in the future by also taking into account age of onset of the obesity, eating habits, diet and weight history, hereditary factors, social class, and ethnicity. These added variables are consistent with the view that obesity is a multifactorial problem.

As I stated earlier, the study of obesity has sometimes felt like a losing battle for us as scientists, but for the overweight person, there is often the constant waging of this losing battle.

Why should this be true? We might expect it to be so because of our stereotype of the obese person as someone who is lacking in will power and gluttonous. Yet we have just reviewed over 100 studies on human eating behavior which include lab and field studies that use both self-report and observational data, and there are virtually no reliable main effects differences between overweight and normal weight people for the amount eaten. The significant differences emerge in interaction with environmental factors, and we will describe some of these later. The critical point is that overweight people do not seem to be overeating all the time but rather just under different circumstances and with different styles than their leaner contemporaries. What we now know is that a large part of the problem stems from the intriguing and perverse fact that being obese increases the likelihood of staying obese. How could this be true? Let us consider a variety of contributing factors.

METABOLIC FACTORS

It now seems clear that our metabolic machinery is devised in such a way that the fatter we are, the fatter we are primed to become. How could this unfortunate state arise? First, enlarged adipocytes have greater fat making capability and are also able to store more fat. Second, overweight people tend to have elevated basal insulin levels. The hyperinsulinemia is associated almost linearly with degree of obesity, as can be seen in Figure 3-1, and it enhances fat storage. This enhanced storage occurs as follows. It is generally believed that the storage of lipid substrates in adipose tissue is regulated by insulin. In addition to having higher basal levels of insulin, the obese also show greater insulin release after a meal than normal subjects do, making it clear that they are operating with an internal environment which favors the accumulation of fat. Hyperinsulinemia has also been linked directly to increased hunger and food consumption (Woods et al., 1977).

The fat droplet of the adipocyte is composed almost entirely of triglycerides. It is triglyceride formation or lipogenesis which leads to the deposition of fat in the adipocyte. There are several factors which modify fatty acid synthesis or lipogenesis, but most relevant to our present concerns are insulin, which accelerates the rate at which glucose is metabolized by adipose cells (Kahlenberg and Kalant, 1964), and enlarged fat cells. Thus, obesity itself influences lipolysis since lipolysis is influenced by cell size. In addition, the size of the adipocyte is also a major factor which modifies its own response to insulin and glucose. Salans, Knittle, and Hirsch (1968) showed that enlarged adipocytes from obese

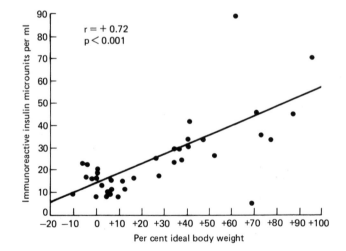

Figure 3-1.

subjects were less sensitive to the effects of insulin than small adipocytes obtained from the same subject after weight loss. They proposed that insulin resistance in obesity results in part from the enlarged fat cells.

The effect of insulin appears to reside in at least two loci: first, insulin enhances the entry of glucose into the fat cell (Bjorntorp et al., 1971; Crofford et al., 1970); then it enhances the conversion of carbon from glucose to glycogen and fatty acids. It is very clear that most overweight people are hyperinsulinemic. Shortly after the development of sensitive techniques for measuring plasma insulin by radioimmunoassay, Rabinowitz and Zierler (1962) found that obese patients had increased levels of insulin. In addition to the increase in basal secretion of insulin, obese subjects almost uniformly show an increase in secretion of insulin after administration of glucose, the metabolic end product of all ingested nutrient (Ben-David et al., 1967). Since the increased basal levels of insulin reflect enhanced secretion, the question then becomes by what mechanism the secretion is augmented. The factors which modulate insulin secretion can be divided into three groups: nutrients, hormones, and neural factors, but a prime candidate is the increased glucose concentration found in obesity since glucose level is an important factor in enhancing the secretion of insulin. The increase of glucose observed in obese individuals is most likely a reflection of their state of overnutrition, which in turn signals the pancreas to secrete more insulin.

Our pattern of food intake also influences insulin production. Food eaten rapidly or in one or two large meals makes adipose tissue more sensitive to the lipogenic effects of insulin (Leveille, 1970). Total carbohydrate and caloric intake also influence responsiveness to insulin (Bray, 1969, 1976). This has been most cogently examined by Salans and his co-workers who studied the effects of two levels of carbohydrate intake in normal weight and obese human subjects. For both groups insulin response was enhanced by a high carbohydrate diet.

Apparently there are major metabolic factors which maintain obesity by increasing the body's fat producing and fat storage capacities, but they are produced by overeating and by the style of eating and not causing it. It is now generally agreed that this point has been clearly proved by the work of Sims and his colleagues, who studied the induction of obesity in a group of volunteers in a Vermont state prison (Sims and Horton, 1968; Sims et al., 1968, 1973). These subjects ate two or three times their normal daily caloric intake and gained an average of 26 percent over their initial lean weight which they maintained for several months. The proportion of carbohydrate to fat to protein in the diet was left unchanged. The Sims study demonstrated that, with few exceptions, lean people develop endocrine and metabolic changes like those observed in spontaneous obesity when they overeat and thus increase adipose tissue mass. In addition, Horton et al. (1972) demonstrated that hyperinsulinemia and insulin resistance can be reversed in spontaneously obese subjects by caloric restriction and weight reduction. Similarly, after a restriction in caloric intake, most of the other metabolic and hormonal consequences of obesity are diminished. So we can conclude that most overweight people initially had normal responsivity, but that during active weight gain, there was enhanced lipolytic activity and metabolic and endocrine change. The studies of Sims and his colleagues clearly establish that obesity is not caused by changes in hormonal economy but rather is the cause of many of them.

INACTIVITY

A second factor which makes being obese itself contribute to the maintenance and growth of obesity is that overweight is associated with inactivity and reduced energy expenditure. This exerts its effects in two ways. First, exercise can play an important role in the response of adipocytes to insulin. Obese individuals who are exercised show evidence of improved glucose tolerance and decreased insulin levels (Bjorntorp, 1976). In fact, overall metabolism may be influenced by exercise. Second, obesity limits spontaneous physical activity and the maximal amount of work that can be performed.

Mayer and his co-workers have documented that inactivity is an important factor in obesity. In one group of studies they used time-lapse photography at summer camps to observe children swimming and playing tennis and volleyball (Bullen et al., 1964). With this technique it is possible to quantify the percentage of the picture frames involved in various degrees of activity. They found that the obese girls almost uniformly spent a smaller fraction of the time in positions of activity than did the lean girls. In swimming, for example, the obese girls tended to spend their time floating in the shallow end of the pool. The lean girls, on the other hand, spent more time in the deep end where swimming is essential to stay afloat.

Obese adults also tend to be inactive. Chirico and Stunkard (1960) used pedometers to measure the distance walked by normal and obese men and women. An obese and a lean individual of the same age and occupation were each given a pedometer to wear, and the differences in readings were used to compare the distance walked for each pair of subjects. The lean individuals on the average walked significantly further than the obese.

Obesity makes physical activity more difficult and probably less pleasurable. With less exercise, overweight people burn fewer calories and reduce metabolic activity. Again, there are some data which suggest that these factors are causal. However, without increased caloric intake, decreased physical activity alone cannot generally produce obesity. Furthermore, we have recently followed 100 outpatient obesity clinic patients for one year after weight loss and found that over

70 percent spontaneously increased activity level and energy expenditure following weight reduction. These data support the contention that inactivity may to a large extent be a consequence of, or only a small contributing factor to, causing obesity although it is clearly important in maintaining it.

EMOTIONAL AROUSAL

The third factor contributing to the maintenance of obesity once the person is fat, is the unhappiness surrounding the state itself. Studying obesity leaves me more impressed than ever with the profound psychological consequences of being overweight and its associated social stigma. Indeed, the real pathologies associated with obesity in Western society appear to be more clearly social than clinical.

Many of our norms suggest that fat people should feel mortified and ashamed for their lack of self-control. This stigmatization involves rejection and disgrace originating in a condition viewed as both a physical deformity and a behavioral aberration. Several studies have shown that people do react negatively to overweight individuals and discriminate against them (Cahnman, 1968). As Bruch (1973) suggests, overweight people are really caught in a paradox. They have attained to a large extent the fulfillment of the great American dream — a life of the same time Americans bend every effort to fight overweight, call it undesirable, and label it the "unsolved health problem of the nation." We have made excessive slimness the ideal of health and beauty.

The state of imprisonment in the role of "fatty" seems to alter one's personality, a finding also true for minority groups (Becker, 1963; Frazier, 1957; Kaplan, 1957) and for people with other physical stigmata (Kleck, Ono, and Hastorf, 1966; Linde, 1964). Even moderately overweight people behave like deviants — complying more with the requests of a nondeviant normal weight person than with one who is overweight and thus shares their deviance (Rodin and Slochower, 1974). It now seems likely that the arousal and unhappiness generated by this condition and its related consequences could lead to overeating — not in the usual psychodynamic sense but through the mechanism of arousal-induced eating.

I would like to examine the concept of a link between emotional arousal and overeating in some detail because it is such a prevalent stereotype. Indeed, there have been many who hold that emotional factors are paramount in the etiology of obesity, that persistent overeating has its basis in unresolved emotional problems, and that overeating serves as a substitute for other satisfactions. A more enlightened outlook, but one still consistent with this attitude, perceives the fat person as the victim of social and unconscious forces which compel him to persist in a repetitive self-destructive pattern. These attitudes are in keeping with psychoanalytic views that overeating probably represents an attempt to achieve substitute gratification or a defense against real or imagined anxiety resulting from emotional conflicts (Burdon and Paul, 1951; Kaplan and Kaplan, 1957; Shorvan and Richardson, 1959). These conclusions come primarily from clinical case studies which report that the obese often experience psychological and social difficulties, such as feelings of considerable social anxiety, alienation, low self-worth, mistrust, behavioral immaturity, and hypochondria (Craddock, 1969; Werkman and Greenberg, 1967). However, even the work of people who favor psychiatric explanations of obesity suggests that psychodynamic causes are far from uniform if they exist at all. It is not possible to speak of one basic personality type as characteristic for all obese people. Obesity may be associated with every conceivable psychiatric disorder, with psychosis as well as neurosis. I think that even this view is too strong since there have been many more studies (reviewed by Louderback, 1970) suggesting that the majority of overweight people are psychologically quite normal. In fact, in the lower socioeconomic groups where, as I have already indicated, the norm is some degree of overweight, there is almost no association between obesity and ill mental health. Such an association occurs more frequently in women of the upper and middle classes where the pressure to reduce is very intense.

LOSS OF WEIGHT

I believe that there has been a real failure in the clinical literature to differentiate between psychological factors related to the development of obesity and those that are created by being obese. It is indeed very distressing for people who adhere to the norms of Western urban society to be overweight. Moreover, there are certain emotional conflicts which appear to be precipitated by reducing, thus again contributing to an apparent correlation between obesity and disturbance which has been imputed with etiological significance. These studies suggest that emotional responses to dieting produce depression, anxiety, and apathy in some subjects, and responses bordering on psychotic episodes in others (Glucksman and Hirsch, 1968; Grinker et al., 1973; Swanson and Dinello, 1970). The results have been taken to suggest that for many people, overeating and obesity serve to keep a distorted psychological image intact and so, with the removal of the obese condition, the person's adjustment deteriorates. While dieting depression sometimes does occur, a psychodynamic explanation is not the only possibility. In the 1940s, Keys and his co-workers (Keys et al., 1950) studied 32 healthy young men of normal weight who lost 25 percent of their body weight in six months. These rigid dieters experienced very similar psychological symptoms to those that have been most characteristic of dieting depression (Stunkard, 1967). On most diets severe emotional disturbance seldom occurs before the patient has lost a certain amount of weight, usually 15-20 pounds or has been on the regimen more than 10 days. Thus these disturbances may at least in part be precipitated by metabolic changes. Before concluding that metabolic changes alone bring on the depression, however, we must also consider that it is simply depressing to be without food, especially for people who love to eat. They may feel deprived and crave food they can no longer have. Indeed, they are depressed by a future in which dieting will always be a way of life.

Recently we have been provided with the unique opportunity to study the psychological consequences of relatively rapid reduction of body size which allows us to better test these various hypotheses. Surgery using jejunoileal bypass that short-circuits most of the intestine produces a controlled malabsorption state and a reduction of food intake leading to a substantial and permanent weight loss in which weight stabilizes after one or two years. Surgically induced weight loss has a number of advantages for evaluating psychological impact of diminished body size. Subjects are generally extremely overweight, ranging from 250–500 pounds. Weight loss is rapid and reliable and yet it allows for continued oral gratification. It does not make prolonged demands on the patient's will power, and it usually takes place in his or her home or work environment.

In a study of the psychosocial effects of intestinal bypass surgery in severe obesity, Solow, Silverfarb, and Swift (1974) demonstrated an improvement after surgery and weight loss in mood, self-esteem, interpersonal and vocational effectiveness, body image, and activity level. There occurred a decrease in depression and also improvements in ego strength and body image that were directly proprotional to the magnitude of weight loss. The findings in this study fail to support the view (Glucksman and Hirsch, 1968) that behavioral and psychological abnormalities regularly accompany substantial reduction of adipose stores in the obese. Instead, the bypass results suggest that disturbances associated with weight loss are related to factors other than the weight loss itself. Oral deprivation or the constant stress of resisting the temptation to eat may be one such factor. Since many of the attributes described as central in the constellation associated with obesity appear surprisingly reversible in bypass patients, the obese personality, to the extent that it does exist, seems to be as much a result of obesity as a cause of it. If obesity is viewed as a symptom of psychological conflict, surgically induced weight loss seems to be a prime example of symptom removal without resolution of the antecedent conflict. The lack of any convincing evidence of the emergence of symptoms is another challenge to a simplistic psychogenic concept of obesity. At the extremes of eating disorders, in some massively obese people and in people who suffer from anorexia nervosa, there are undoubtedly real psychological disturbances. However, among the largest percentage of people who have earned the label "obese," because of a deviation of their weight from the statistical norm, psychiatric disorders appear no more prevalent than they are in a comparable number of people of normal weight.

STRESS AND ANXIETY

While I am arguing that there is no evidence linking emotional disturbance and psychopathology to overeating for a large number of overweight individuals, I would like to explore separately the contention that food consumption does increase in some people when they are aroused, anxious or fearful. Although there are some negative findings (Abramson and Wunderlich, 1972; Schachter, Goldman, and Gordon, 1968), many studies have shown that overweight people do eat more when they are aroused (Jung, 1976; McKenna, 1972; Meyer and Pudel, 1972; White, 1973). There are various reasons why we might expect that some form of stress or arousal would increase consumption for obese persons: (1) Although one explanation is that eating is ego defensive or anxiety reducing, our own review of the literature and a recent report by Leon and Roth (1977) suggest that the research evidence does not support the notion that food intake reduces anxiety. (2) A second alternative is that anxiety and arousal may be regarded as disruptors of behavior, including self-control, which then might serve to disinhibit hunger-motivated eating behavior. Increased consumption during anxiety may reflect a person's chronic hunger which is normally suppressed in an attempt to maintain weight control. Herman and Polivy (1975) have reported some tendency for normal weight chronic dieters to overeat when anxious. (3) As another explanation, I have recently suggested that increased arousal which comes from stress or anxiety may increase consumption by making an individual more responsive to salient environmental stimuli (Rodin, 1977). The study by White (1973) is especially supportive of this view.

White showed overweight and normal weight subjects four film segments at four different sessions. There were three arousal films: Lazarus' subincision film which generated distress arousal, Charlie Chaplin in *The Tramp* which provided humor arousal, and a stag film which produced sexual arousal. The fourth film, an India travelogue, was unarousing.

After viewing the film segments, participants in the study rated crackers in a different room, and the amount eaten after ten minutes was recorded. White found that the obese ate significantly more food after viewing each of the arousing films than after the nonarousing film. There were no significant differences in the amount of food eaten by normal weight persons, independent of film content. It thus appears that the obese may eat more when aroused and that the specific content of the arousal stimulus may be irrelevant to eating behavior.

There are two questions we might ask next: First, are overweight people more easily aroused and, then, what produces this link between arousal and overeating? To determine whether overweight people are hyperemotional, Rodin, Elman, and Schachter (1974) tested Columbia undergraduates — half obese, half of normal weight. In one experiment; subjects listened to one of two kinds of tapes: emotionally disturbing tapes which for ten minutes detailed either the bombing of Hiroshima or the subject's own death of leukemia, or emotionally neutral tapes which were concerned with either rain or sea shells. A few typical excerpts will allow you to judge the effectiveness of these tapes.

From Hiroshima:

Picture how the eyebrows of some were burnt off, and skin hung from their faces and hands. Others were vomiting as they walked.

Imagine trying to help someone, reaching down and grabbing him by the hands but not being able to hold him because his skin slipped off in huge, glovelike pieces into your hands.

From leukemia:

Imagine how you would feel if you could feel your body degenerating — a constant deterioration going on inside you that no one was able to stop or even slow down. You would have to be fed because you would be too weak to hold a fork. You would have to lie in bed because you would be too weak to hold up your own head.

Think about who in your family would help you, which of your friends would stand by you. . . . How would your illness affect their lives? Who would feel inconvenienced and put upon? . . . Who would be glad to see you dying in great pain and suffering?

From neutral tapes:

Think about all the varied shapes and colors of shells you've seen. Think about seeing them along the beach, about picking them up and saving an unusual one. . . . Some are rough with spiny and irregular edges that tingle when you pick them up.

Think about the rains that come in the spring and fall. Remember how sometimes it rains so hard that the sewers plug up within minutes. You may be outside and before you can reach cover you are soaked and the ground is turned to mud.

One set of tapes is concerned with deeply disturbing material; the other could be expected to leave the auditor untouched or in a lyrical, somewhat abstracted mood.

Immediately after listening to the tape, all subjects answered a series of questions about the task on which they had worked and about their perceived physiological and emotional states. On all measures, obese subjects appeared significantly more disturbed by the emotional tapes than were subjects of normal weight.

The difference does not simply reflect a tendency of the obese to exaggerate their responses because after listening to the undisturbing material the obese described themselves as significantly less emotional than normal subjects.

Next we reasoned that pain and the threat of pain are disturbing and unsettling experiences bound to make a subject edgy and tense. If the obese are more reactive and emotional than are normal weight people, the experience and anticipation of pain should be more disruptive for obese than for normal subjects. In part to consider this hypothesis, an experiment was designed to test the effects of pain on the ability of obese and normal males to learn a rather complex maze.

EXPERIMENTAL RESEARCH

To measure learning, we employed Lykken's (1957) electronic maze, which is a 20-step maze with four alternatives at each step. The maze was housed in a small metal box with four levers mounted in the front. The subject's job was to thread his way through the maze by pressing the correct sequence of levers. At each step, when the subject pressed the correct lever, a green light flashed and he automatically moved on to the next step. If the subject pressed one of the three incorrect levers, a red light flashed and an error was recorded on a counter visible to him. A light signaled when the subject had worked his way through the maze, the machine was reset, and the subject began working again until he went through the maze three times without making an error or had completed 21 trials.

Subjects experienced one of three experimental conditions — severe shock, mild shock, or no shock. Electrodes were fastened to the second and third fingers of the subject's nondominant hand to administer shock. The experiment had been explained as a study of the effects of "partial reward and punishment" on learning, and the subject was told, "You will occasionally receive a shock when you make an error. We have set up the apparatus to randomly give a shock on every few errors." In fact, the shocks were not administered randomly but were linked to one of the three incorrect levers at each step. Theoretically, a subject could learn to avoid shock by not pressing the shock lever at a given step, even if he had not learned to press the correct lever to advance. Because we wanted to minimize the possibility of upsetting the subject in the no-shock condition, electrodes were not fastened to his hand and no mention was made of shock.

The effects of electric shock on learning are presented in Table 3-1, which shows the average of the total number of errors, shocked and unshocked, made by the subjects in the course of learning (or not learning) the maze. It is evident that shock had a disruptive effect on the learning ability of obese subjects and no such effect on normal subjects. The obese made somewhat fewer errors in the no-shock condition than normal subjects and considerably more errors in the severe-shock condition. It does appear that pain interfered more with the

Table 3-1. Effects of Electric Shock on Learning.

Subjects	No Shock	Low Shock	High Shock	No vs. High Shock
	Total Number of Errors Made in:			
Normal	228.7	163.4	198.1	n.s.
Obese	189.9	228.8	286.5	<.05
p	n.s.	n.s.	<.05	
	Interaction p <.03			

ability of the obese to learn a complex task than with that of normal subjects. Altogether, three experimentally gathered facts support a view of the obese as more emotional than people of normal weight:

1. In response to a threat of painful shock, the obese describe themselves as more nervous than do normal subjects.
2. Emotionally distressing audio tapes are more upsetting to the obese than to normal subjects.
3. Painful shock interferes with the ability of the obese to learn a complex task.

Thus overweight subjects do appear more arousable than their leaner contemporaries, and it will now be demonstrated that arousal can often lead to overeating even in normal weight individuals. How might this occur? There is no evidence to date that arousal increases hunger, that it makes food taste better or that it is anxiety reducing. Instead it is most likely that arousal is a general activator which simply increases the likelihood that the most available, the most dominant, or the most reinforcing response is the one which is made. Recent behavioral (Wayner, 1974), neurobehavioral (Valenstein et al., 1976), and neuropharmacological (Antelman et al., 1976; Herberg et al., 1976) investigations lead to the suggestion that certain catecholamine-containing pathways in the brain may constitute a common neural substrate underlying a variety of different activities including eating. Arousal appears to increase catecholaminergic activity within these pathways, and external cues seem to be responsible for insuring the release of appropriate items from the behavioral repertoire. Certainly one can argue for the biological significance of a mechanism by which an aroused organism would be better off to attend and respond to salient external stimuli. A nonmonotonic relationship is expected, however, since at the extreme of arousal such attention would be, by and large, maladaptive. This line of reasoning is supported in studies with animals, showing that low doses of d-amphetamine

(Glick and Muller, 1971) and mild tail pinch (Antelman et al., 1975, 1976) reliably induce eating in sated rats. The eating behavior appears quite normal and proceeds without obvious pain. If the tail-pinch procedure continues over days, the animals gain weight, as Figure 3-2 shows.

Pharmacological studies have led to the proposal by Antelman, Fisher and their colleagues' (1976) that tail-pinch-induced eating does involve preferential facilitation of brain catecholaminergic function leading to a heightened sensitivity and responsivity to most survival-oriented and/or pre-potent environmental stimuli. They suggest that the tail pinch induces a consummatory response by heightening the valence of sensory cues from available environmental stimuli, and recently have presented data which, as I will describe later, precisely parallel our human data (Rodin, 1977; Schachter and Rodin, 1974). For example, they show that there is less tail-pinch-induced drinking for quinine-adulterated milk and greater drinking for sweetened milk than in non-tail-pinched animals. Thus the hedonic value of the external stimulus may be a key determining factor for the tail-pinch phenomenon. The dopamine-mediated disinhibitory action of the tail pinch could lower sensory motor thresholds and promote heightened sensitivity and responsivity to environmental stimuli which are salient or high in

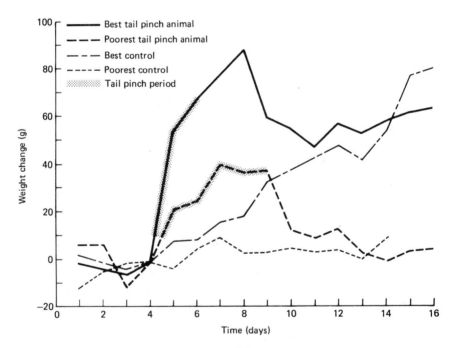

Figure 3-2.

hedonic value. I will return to these issues when discussing the phenomenon of external responsiveness, but I hope I have suggested how arousal could induce overeating without relying on a psychodynamic explanation.

I would like to explore one further mechanism by which being obese might function to maintain and increase the obesity, before going on to the primary causal factors. The final mechanism is active dieting which is prevalent among the obese. Being on a diet may itself potentiate the increased likelihood of overeating. Herman and his colleagues (Herman and Mack, 1975; Herman and Polivy, 1975) have studied self-reported restrained eaters and have come up with an intriguing finding. They report that conscious restraint is very fragile and that these consciously restrained individuals are highly vulnerable to influences which lead to increased eating. First they demonstrated that people of all weight categories could easily be classified into those who consciously restrained their eating and responsiveness to external cues, and those who did not. A simple questionnaire allowed assessment of these differences.

They then placed both restrained and unrestrained eaters in the following situation (Herman and Mack, 1975). The study was presumably a taste experiment in which subjects were required to taste either 0, 1, or 2 large milk shakes. In the next phase of the study, subjects were encouraged to "taste" as much as they wanted from a large dish of ice cream.

The results showed a fascinating turn of events. When normally restrained eaters were required, as part of the study, to finish two large milk shakes, they subsequently ate greater amounts of ice cream in the following period than if they had consumed no milk shakes or one only. Apparently having drunk so much, and perceiving themselves as already having overeaten, these normally restrained people gave up their restraint on consumption. Subjects who reported less conscious restraint of their eating behaved in exactly the opposite fashion. For them, consuming greater amounts of milk shakes *suppressed* subsequent ice cream consumption. Further data (Polivy, 1976) support the contention that this counterregulation is a cognitive effect; the experimental separation of perceived from actual calories in the preload revealed that dieters only overate after they thought they had consumed a high-calorie preload and not when they actually did.

Let us summarize the data reviewed thus far. What I have been suggesting is that overweight people are caught in a bind once they become fat. Their enlarged adipocytes and hyperinsulinemia prime their metabolic apparatus to make and store fat. Their obesity increases their physical inactivity which further affects metabolism as well as influencing energy expenditure. They also seem to need fewer calories to maintain high levels of body weight than do individuals currently overeating to achieve the same weight (Bray, 1976). They are unhappy because of social pressure and stigmatization, and appear more arousable. Increased levels of arousal may in turn promote overeating by making them more responsive to salient environmental food cues. Finally, their obese condition produces numerous diet attempts, and it seems perversely true that such conscious dietary restraint makes them more likely to overeat under conditions of distraction, alcohol consumption, and increased emotionality.

These then are factors which we now know are largely consequences of obesity, serving to maintain and promote overeating or increased fat storage. Since popular attitudes and some scientific literature have confused these factors as causes, it has been critical to discuss them first. While obviously, metabolic and endocrine dysfunction, inactivity and psychopathology may sometimes be causally implicated in certain cases of obesity, in large part they appear to have their greatest role after the obesity has developed. Clearly our next step is to consider current views of what the causal factors involved in obesity might be.

GENETIC FACTORS

The first possible factor is genetic. In family studies determining the incidence of overweight in the parents of obese individuals, the familial contribution is striking. For example, Gurney (1936) showed that when both parents were stout, 73 percent of the offspring were stout, whereas only 9 percent were stout when both parents were lean. With only one stout parent, 41 percent of the offspring were stout.

In other analyses, it seems clearer that the inherited traits — if there are any — may be for body type rather than, or in addition to, body composition. Withers (1964) showed that fathers transmitted somatotypic traits for mesomorphy to their sons and daughters, whereas mothers transmitted both endomorphy (roundness) and ectomorphy (leanness) to both sons and daughters. While these studies suggest some contribution of genetic factors, studies using identical twins have enabled us to begin to determine how much of the variance can be accounted for by genetic factors. Several such studies have examined many parameters in identical twins and found that body weight was the most variable. Newman et al. (1937) found that among 50 pairs of identical twins reared together, the mean difference in body weight averaged 4.1 pounds, with only one pair showing a difference in body weight of more than 12 pounds. Among 19 pairs of identical twins reared separately, however, the mean deviation in body weight was 9.9 pounds, more than twice that for twins reared in the same family. Five of these 19 pairs had a more than 12-pound difference in body weight, indicating that environmental factors play an important role in the appearance of obesity in genetically disposed individuals.

Rony (1940) extended these observations further by examining the deviation in body weight of 10 pairs of lean identical twins and 8 pairs of obese twins.

The body weight deviated by less than 3 percent in 8 of the 10 lean pairs, but in only one of the 8 obese pairs was the difference in body weight that small. Thus while it is clear that there is polygenic inheritance involved in the transmission of human obesity, environmental factors may play a role of overriding importance in genetically predisposed individuals. It is certainly the case that environmental factors appear to be more important in determining body weight than in determining height or even IQ.

I have, until now, been alluding to the increasing accumulation of evidence pointing to the significant role which environmental factors play in the development and maintenance of obesity. Let us now examine the data which suggest that whatever its genetic determinants and its biochemical pathways, obesity is to an unusual degree under social and environmental control. Stunkard, and his co-workers (see Stunkard, 1975) clearly documented that differences in social environment have important implications for the development and maintenance of obesity. First they indicated that there is a marked inverse relationship between socioeconomic status and the prevalence of obesity. This is demonstrated in Figure 3-3.

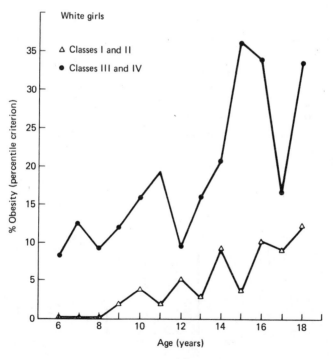

Figure 3-3.

SOCIOECONOMIC STUDIES

The analyses of this study (Stunkard, 1975) — a survey of midtown Manhattan — enabled causal inferences to be drawn about the influence of socioeconomic status. This was achieved by ascertaining not only the socioeconomic status of the respondents at the time of the study, but also that of their parents when the respondents were eight years old. Although a subject's obesity might influence his own current social class, it is unlikely that his disability in adult life could have influenced his parents' social class. Therefore, associations between the social class of the respondent's parents and his obesity can be viewed as causal. Figure 3-4 shows that such associations were almost as powerful as those between the social class of the respondents and their obesity. In addition, Stunkard demonstrated that obesity was more prevalent among downwardly mobile subjects than those who remained in the social class of their parents. It was also the case that the longer a person's family had been in this country, the less likely he was to be obese. Religious affiliation was still another social factor linked to obesity. The greatest prevalence of obesity was among Jews, followed by Roman Catholics and Protestants. Among Protestants the pattern is further exemplified. The largest amount of obesity is found among Baptists with a decreasing prevalence among Methodists, Lutherans, and Episcopalians. When hearing these data at Stunkard's testimony before the Senate Select Subcommittee on Nutrition, Senator McGovern asked, "Does that have anything to do with who's getting the most bread from heaven?"

All of these data suggest that with increasing affluence, social attitudes, fads, and fashions exert great control on eating and weight. It is for this reason that social class, level of acculturation and generation, and religion — all major aspects of one's social environment — are so strongly related to obesity.

Let us now move to the effects of the more immediate environmental influences. It is likely for humans that habits and preferences as well as immediate food cues and cognitions play a major role in eating at any particular meal, al-

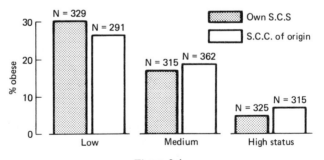

Figure 3-4.

though long-term weight regulation may be under greater biological control. All of us are responsive to the sight of well-prepared food, to fragrant aromas, and to the time of day, and sometimes these environmental stimuli which trigger eating may have nothing or very little to do with our state of physiological deprivation. While everyone occasionally overeats in the presence of tempting external food cues such as these, it appears that many overweight people are highly, sometimes uncontrollably, responsive to external food-relevant stimuli.

COGNITIVE FACTORS

In a series of studies, Schachter, Nisbett, and their colleagues reported in the late 1960s that the eating behavior of their overweight subjects was greatly influenced by the passage of time (Schachter and Gross, 1968), the taste and sight of food (Decke, 1971; Nisbett, 1968b), and the sight and number of highly palatable food cues present. For example, Nisbett (1968a) demonstrated that when one sandwich was visible but more were available nearby, overweight subjects ate almost one sandwich less than when three sandwiches were visually prominent. There was no differential effect for normal weight persons. The Nisbett study suggested that the prominence of immediate food cues would compel eating in the obese and was consistent with an earlier demonstration that overweight people reported themselves as less hungry on a religious occasion when food cues were minimal (Goldman, Jaffa, and Schachter, 1968). Ross (1974) directly tested this notion. As Figure 3-5 shows, he found that obese subjects ate twice as

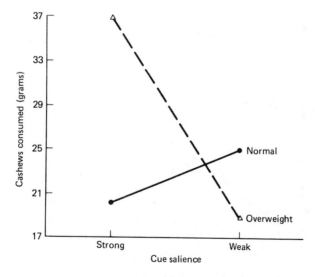

Figure 3-5.

many cashews when lights were brightly focused on the nuts as when they were dimmed, while normal weight subjects were less influenced by the visual salience manipulation. Cognitive salience — thinking about nuts or not — also had a greater effect on the eating behavior of the obese than it did on people of normal weight.

On the basis of this and related studies, Schachter and I (Schachter and Rodin, 1974) proposed that the eating behavior of the obese, under conditions of high cue or cognitive salience, appears stimulus bound. In other words, a food-relevant cue above a given level of prominence appears more likely to trigger an eating response in an overweight than in a normal weight person. This hypothetical relationship is shown in Figure 3-6. In addition, when eating behavior is elicited, it is likely to reflect heightened responsiveness. The obese do not simply eat, they overeat once they are "turned on" by potent stimuli. Overweight people eat more than normal weight people at each meal (Beaudoin and Mayer, 1953; Johnson, Burke, and Mayer, 1956), a time when food cues are undoubtedly more prominent. They also eat fewer meals (Beaudoin and Mayer, 1953; Johnson et al., 1956; Schachter and Rodin, 1974), presumably because food-relevant stimuli must be sufficiently potent before eating is elicited. Similarly, overweight people apparently do more impulse buying at the supermarket after they have just eaten, a time when thoughts of food are no doubt most prominent for them (Nisbett and Kanouse, 1969). I have also demonstrated (Rodin, 1975a) that overeating is stimulated in overweight people by thinking about food and by recent memories of very good meals.

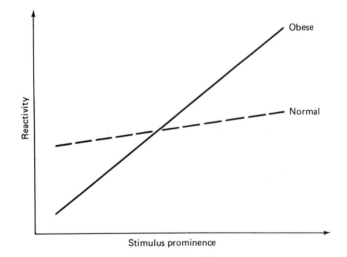

Figure 3-6.

There are two important qualifications regarding the visual salience of food cues and obesity. First, while it seems intuitively reasonable to expect that the sight of other people eating would also trigger eating in the obese, attempts to demonstrate this experimentally have been largely unsuccessful (Nisbett and Storms, 1975). I think that this is probably a result of social pressure and embarrassment. Second, there is evidence that some normal weight individuals are also responsive to cue salience (Levitz, 1975; Rodin and Slochower, 1976). I would like to stress that everyone is responsive to external cues to some extent and, as I will demonstrate below, this responsiveness can lead to overeating and obesity in some individuals.

During the last several years, my students and I have attempted to define external responsiveness and to assess its role in the development and maintenance of obesity. We began by demonstrating that many overweight subjects are highly responsive to a wide variety of external stimuli and that overeating is just one aspect of this tendency. The following is a brief outline of these results:

1. On the average, overweight subjects have quicker latency to respond to complex external stimuli, lower (i.e., more sensitive) tachistoscopic recognition thresholds, and better immediate recall for food- and non-food-relevant cues than normal weight subjects (Rodin, Herman, and Schachter, 1974; Rodin and Slochower, 1976; Rodin, Slochower, and Fleming, 1977).

2. Overweight subjects are more distracted than normal subjects by prominent irrelevant stimuli whether the primary task which provides the measure of distraction is intended or incidental (Rodin, 1973; Rodin and Slochower, 1974). Figure 3-7 demonstrates how proofreading accuracy is impaired for overweight

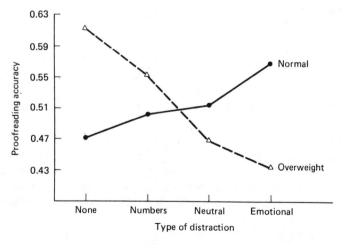

Figure 3-7.

subjects, but not for those of normal weight, with increasingly compelling distraction. This distraction appears to be due to an inability to divide attention between salient sensory inputs (Rodin and Goodman, 1976).

3. Overweight individuals require idea-generating external stimuli to produce original images, and when such cues are absent, the obese are relatively uncreative (Rodin and Rubin, 1976; Rodin and Singer, 1976).

4. Rodin and Singer (1976) examined the pattern of lateral eyeshift response to questions requiring reflection and self-generated imaginal processes to test further differences in information processing. Differential engagement of the hemispheres of the brain is presumably manifest during thought by lateral eyeshift in the direction contralateral to the hemisphere primarily involved in the cognitive task. Overweight subjects were more likely to process reflective material in the verbal mode rather than through imagery. In addition, the obese appeared to have a greater need to avoid rich environmental stimuli in order to process internal imagery material or verbal sequences stored in long-term memory.

5. The experiments reviewed thus far all suggest a heightened sensitivity to, and processing of, external stimuli on the part of the obese, but were not not directed to questioning whether their relative unresponsiveness to internal signals also extends beyond eating behavior. To consider this issue for a nonconsummatory behavior, differences in time perception were examined since the experience of time is frequently assumed to have both internal biological and cognitive components. Several studies of time have suggested a time base identified with some internal periodic biological clock (Dimond, 1964; Hammer, 1966; Hoagland, 1933; Ochberg et al., 1964), while others, notably Ornstein's experiments (1969), have led to a cognitive, information-processing model of time perception.

It was predicted that if the obese are both unresponsive to internal events and heavily dependent on external cues, the periodicity associated with internal biological rhythms such as metabolism (Francois, 1927; Hoagland, 1933) should provide relatively little time-relevant information for them, while external, cognitive variables should be quite important. If this line of reasoning is correct, there should be clear weight group differences in time perception when there are no relevant external cues at all. Without salient external information, the duration judgments of the obese should be highly variable and inaccurate relative to the estimates of normal weight subjects. The first experiment tested the prediction of increased variability and inaccuracy for the obese in the absence of time-relevant external cues; in other words, when subjects had to rely solely on internal cues (Study 1).

In the context of an experiment investigating physiological responses to complex stimuli, overweight and normal weight subjects sat in a darkened room in silence for 15 minutes while presumed physiological baseline measures were being taken. They were instructed to think about anything they wished during this period and told that they would later be asked to report their thoughts in order to evaluate the physiological data. At the end of 15 minutes, each subject was asked to complete a number of physiological and attention questions including the time-relevant measure. This item asked subjects to judge the duration of the interval on a 60-minute scale.

We found that while the mean time estimates of body overweight and normal weight treatment conditions were close to the actual 15 minutes, the groups differed greatly in variability. The means and standard deviation for each group are presented in Figure 3-8. As predicted, the responses of obese subjects were highly variable, while normal weight subjects showed much less variability.

In this study there were no explicit external cues for the passage of time. However, providing such information should affect judgments of temporal duration in the obese, if they are more influenced than normal subjects by time-relevant external cues. A second experiment specifically examined the effects of

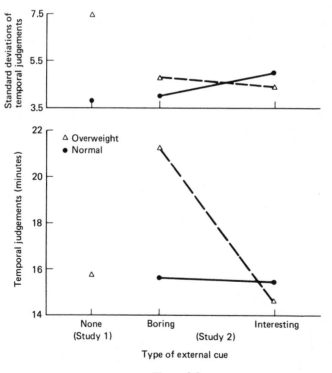

Figure 3-8.

manipulating external cues — in this case for interest and boredom — on over-weight and normal weight subjects (Study 2).

Essentially the procedure was identical to that in the first experiment with the following changes: one group of heavy and one group of normal weight sub-jects listened to an interesting tape recording for 15 minutes, and one group in each weight category heard a boring tape. The interesting sequence was taken from a recording of *Richard Nixon, Superstar,* a humorous monologue by the comedian David Frye. The passage had been rated as entertaining and interest-ing by a group of 20 judges — 10 overweight and 10 of normal weight. The same group rated as highly boring a passage read from a textbook entitled *Geography of the Pacific,* and we used this sequence for the boring stimulus. The passages were as similar as possible in number of separate ideas or codable units as well as in length. Following the 15-minute session, subjects answered several questions about their perceived physiological responses and judged the length of the inter-val on a 60-minute scale.

While the weight groups did not differ in their judgments of how interesting or boring the tapes were, their assessments of temporal duration did reveal signif-icant differences. The data presented in Figure 3-8 indicate that overweight subjects were far more affected than normal weight subjects by the manipulation of external time-relevant cues. They judged the length of the interval to be longer when the tape was boring, and somewhat shorter when the tape was interesting, than normal subjects. In addition, the data show that when salient external time-relevant cues were present, there was little of the group variability among obese subjects that was found in Study 1.

In light of these findings, we next turned to a consideration of how these differences in time perception would affect behavior since, it will be recalled, Schachter and Gross (1968) directly manipulated passage of time and found that it influenced eating behavior of overweight subjects more than that of normal subjects.

By combining the Schachter and Gross findings with the results of the present studies, the effects on eating behavior of events which slow and speed perceived time may be readily predicted. If more time seems to elapse for the obese when they are bored, and if the passage of time is a powerful cue for eating, overweight people should eat sooner when bored than when they have been doing something absorbing. This prediction should hold not only for boredom and interest but for any cognitive manipulation which affects perceived passage of time for the obese. When considering boredom, however, an additional factor may be opera-tive. Overweight individuals may simply be more likely to think about food when they are bored and, as Ross (1974) has shown, obese subjects instructed to think about food do eat considerably more than normal subjects.

To test these questions, amount eaten and latency to eat were measured after overweight and normal weight subjects had listened to either boring or interesting tapes. These were simply 50-minute excerpts from the identical sources of material used for Study 2: *Geography of the Pacific* and *Richard Nixon, Superstar*. Since thinking about food may also be a response to boredom in the obese, a control group was also tested after having been explicitly focused on food-relevant thoughts in the preceding period. These subjects heard a 50-minute tape taken from M. F. K. Fisher's *With Bold Knife and Fork* which describes the social and gastronomic activities surrounding a banquet attended by renowned French gourmets.

Testing occurred during midafternoon, after lunch and well before dinner. As in the previous two experiments, the study was explained as an investigation of physiological responses to complex auditory stimuli. Each subject was told to listen to the tape for one-half hour and then take a break during which time he could relax, drink some milk shake which was provided, leaf through magazines, or simply sit quietly. He was specifically instructed, "It is critical that you do not take a break until you think that exactly one-half hour has passed and then call the experimenter as soon as you are ready to begin the next part." Thus, a strong experimental demand was placed on being as accurate as possible in the judgment of elapsed time. The subject was further instructed to shut off the tape recorder when he began his break which, unknown to him, also simultaneously stopped a timer.

The milk shake was a frozen prepared mix to which milk was added. A full gallon in an opaque plastic container was available, and each subject could fill his glass as many times as he liked. The milk shake container was stored in a refrigerator in the room and was not visible while the tape was playing.

Although each subject believed that he was controlling the length of the break, only 10 minutes were actually allowed. If the subject signaled that he was ready before 10 minutes had elapsed, the experimenter explained that he had a few more things to do and would return shortly. If a subject had not yet terminated the break, he was stopped after 10 minutes.

The results shown in Figure 3-9 replicate, with a different dependent variable, the temporal duration judgment data obtained in the second study. Obese subjects hearing the boring tape appear to have judged time as passing slowly and, therefore, began their break sooner than those hearing the two interesting tapes. Normal weight subjects, on the other hand, took a break at about the same time, no matter which tape they heard. The time perception of overweight subjects was not significantly affected, however, by whether the interesting tapes were relevant or irrelevant to food.

In contrast, the amount of milk shake actually consumed by overweight subjects was greatly influenced by whether or not the tape was food relevant. The means for number of ounces drunk by each treatment group are presented in Figure 3-10. When the obese were listening to a description of gastronomic delights, they subsequently drank almost twice as much milk shake as they did when listen-

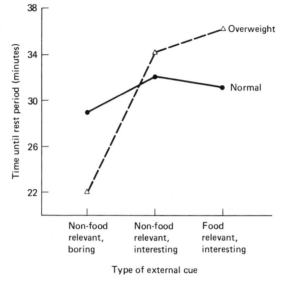

Figure 3-9.

ing to an interesting humorous monologue. Similarly, listening to the food-relevant tape also had a significantly greater effect on the amount drunk by obese subjects than did listening to a boring tape. None of these contrasts were significant for normal weight subjects, although they tended to drink least after hearing the food-relevant tape.

These data suggest that overweight subjects may eat more frequently when bored because initiation of eating is influenced by perceived passage of time, and time passes more slowly for the obese than for normal subjects when both are bored. Similarly, overweight subjects may eat less frequently than normal weight subjects when involved in something absorbing. That these results are not simply a function of the obese thinking more about food when bored is revealed in two ways. If thinking about food makes an overweight person likely to eat sooner, subjects in the food-relevant-interesting tape condition should have begun their break first, thus having the shortest latency to eat. Instead they had the longest. Second, differences in amount eaten also suggest that bored subjects did not behave like those who were specifically thinking about food. Obese subjects, hearing non-food-relevant tapes, whether boring or interesting, ate significantly less than subjects listening to the food-relevant material. This result is surprising in light of the common complaint of overweight people that they eat more when they are bored. The present data suggest that, rather than eating more food during each eating instance, they may simply eat more frequently (Rodin, 1975a).

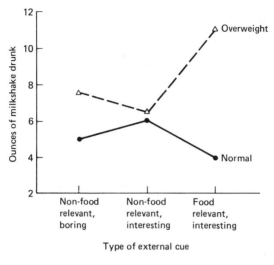

Figure 3-10.

EXTERNAL RESPONSIVENESS

We also considered questions of generalizability regarding populations from which subjects had been drawn. For the most part, all of the early work on obesity and external responsiveness tested moderately overweight (+15 to +40 percent) college-age, generally upper-middle-class white students. Thus there were several issues, outlined below, about the generality of these effects.

Degree of Overweight

Both we (Rodin, Herman, and Schachter, 1974) and Nisbett (1972) had obtained data from a few greatly obese subjects indicating that they were no more responsive to food and non-food external stimuli than normal subjects. During the course of our subsequent studies we tested the external responsiveness of several hundred individuals who varied in degree of overweight. In all our studies we found that there were people in every weight category who were extremely responsive and those who were not. Across all weight groups. degree of overweight was almost totally unrelated to degree of external responsiveness. Using externality scores standardized on the entire sample in each study, we did find, however, that when group averages were compared, moderately overweight subjects were more external than either the normal weight or the extremely obese. This finding was consistent from study to study and was true for consumption of good-tasting milk shakes (Rodin, 1975b), ratings of the palatability of increasingly sweet-tasting glucose solutions (Rodin, Moskowitz, and Bray, 1976), ratings of the palatability of milk shakes which differed in sweetness but not in caloric value (Rodin, 1975b), responsiveness to preloads of varying caloric density (Rodin, Moskowitz, and Bray, 1976), and eating and noneating responses to manipulations of external cue salience (Rodin, Slochower, and Fleming, 1977). Moderately overweight subjects also appeared most willing to work to obtain a highly preferred milk shake when permitted to sample it first. However, the actual ease or difficulty of ingesting the milk shake (manipulated by straw width) once they obtained it, had a greater impact on their preference ratings and level of consumption than it did for either normal subjects or the extremely obese (Rodin, 1975b).

Since the many experiments that have studied the relationship between obesity and externality varied greatly in how overweight the subjects were, some of the highly conflicting results which have been reported in the literature may be more understandable. Moreover, since we have demonstrated in our recent studies that there are some externally responsive individuals in every weight category, it may be insufficient to group subjects only on the basis of weight, especially current weight, without at least obtaining a weight history. This could explain the Nisbett and Temoshok (1976) finding that our measures of external responsiveness were only somewhat related to obesity in their sample. Their finding that these measures do not correlate with paper and pencil measures *descriptively* related to externality (e.g., field dependence, I-E, and automatization), however, is not surprising. We (Rodin and Goodman, 1976) have recently demonstrated that externality represents an active, processing relationship with external cues rather than a passive, compelled response to these cues.

Weight Stability

It has been suggested that obesity is determined by a genetically fixed set point for fatness (Nisbett, 1972). Whether or not this is so, we question the validity of Nisbett's operational definition. He used degree of overweight as the index of nearness to or distance from set point and found that subjects classified as below set point appeared more influenced by good and bad taste than those considered at set point. However, to us there appeared to be no a priori reason to assume that people who are 40 percent or more overweight are acutally closer to their own biological set point than those who are 20 percent overweight, that is, if degree of appropriate adipose tissue mass is continuously and normally distributed in the population. Indeed, it is possible that some 40 percent individuals are above their set point, a state whose physiological implications are unspecified. These considerations suggested that degree of overweight may not be the best way to isolate set-point differences.

In one of our experiments (Rodin, 1975b) we inferred closeness to set point from long-term weight stability. We assumed that individuals who reported no dietary restrictions and whose weight (by our actual measurement) showed little yearly fluctuation were closer to their biological set point than others whose weights were very unstable. Differences in responsiveness to taste between subjects of various weights which were either stable or unstable were then examined.

As one can see from Figure 3-11, the date replicated Nisbett's (1972) results at the empirical level. Extremely overweight subjects behaved more like normal subjects and less like the moderately obese. However, when set point was defined in terms of weight stability rather than degree of overweight, set-point differences within weight groups had very little effect. They were not related to differences in hedonic ratings or to differences in food intake, as long as consumption involved little effort. While others may disagree that stability of weight is the best measure of set point, the very disagreement points even more clearly to the problem. It is difficult a priori to specify each individual's set point and consequently to infer distance from it. Therefore, I strongly suggest that the heuristic value of this notion as a predictor for, and explanation of, eating and regulatory behavior is questionable, although its descriptive value may be great.

Age and Socioeconomic Status

We used summer camps for normal weight and overweight girls to extend the range of subjects tested to as young as nine years old. We also used outpatient clinic populations at Harbor General Hospital in Torrance, California (Bray et

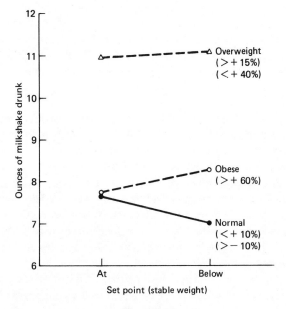

Figure 3-11.

al., 1976; Rodin et al., 1976) and a self-help obesity group in New Haven (Rodin, Slochower, and Fleming, 1977) to extend the range to as old as sixty. These latter two populations also included Blacks, people of Latin and Chinese origin, and people with as little as ninth-grade education. In all cases, the generality of the externality-overweight relationship was maintained. On the average, moderately overweight subjects were more external than those who were either extremely obese or normal weight, although there were some externally responsive people in every weight category.

Several investigators have tried to explain the relationship between overweight and responsiveness to external cues. Singh (1973) suggested that obese persons appear more externally responsive than the nonobese because they have a generalized deficiency in response inhibition. Hence, in all those situations where an ongoing response is to be terminated, the overweight continue to respond longer than the normal weight. The Singh hypothesis places the emphasis on termination, while minimizing the importance of responsiveness to environmental cues as a factor relevant to initiation of eating. These notions would not be inconsistent with one another, however.

In a theoretically more ambitious alternative, Nisbett (1972) contended that many overweight people are biologically programmed to be fat and are externally responsive because they are typically (as a result of dieting because of social pressure) in a state of physiological deprivation. Thus they are below what Nisbett calls their "biological set point." Greater attention to external cues, he argues, is a characteristic of all hungry organisms. Nisbett (1972) presents evidence suggesting that some physiological and behavioral responses of overweight people are comparable to those of normal weight people when they are food deprived. These data are most convincing with respect to taste responsiveness. This hypothesis has greater generality than earlier ones because it assumes that under certain conditions, all organisms become more responsive to external, nonvisceral cues.

In a different view, Rodin (1976a) suggested that external responsiveness may play a role in the etiology of obesity. This assumption is bolstered by more recent findings that both juvenile and adult onset obese individuals do not change in their responsiveness to food- and non-food-relevant external cues after considerable weight loss (Rodin, Slochower, and Fleming, 1977). In children attending summer weight reduction camps and adults losing weight while attending outpatient clinics or self-help groups, externality neither increases (as the Nisbett, 1972, hypothesis would predict) nor decreases systematically with weight loss. We concluded from these data that responsiveness to cognitive and environmental cues is not simply a function of degree of obesity per se, nor is it a function of physiological deprivation resulting from dieting. While it is quite possible that overweight people are physiologically hungry, this does not appear to be a sufficient explanation for their external responsiveness. Indeed, in a study measuring the effects of short-term, 24-hour deprivation, similar results were obtained (Fleming, 1975). After a 24-hour fast, hungry normal weight individuals were not significantly more responsive to external stimuli than they were prior to deprivation.

The Rodin et al. (1977) data show clearly that responsiveness to visual and cognitive cues does not change with weight loss and deprivation. Because of these results, we began to question whether taste should be considered an external cue since it does appear to be influenced by deprivation and satiety. In the early studies of Schachter (1968, 1971), Nisbett (1968b, 1972) and their associates, good taste was viewed in the same way as the sight of good food or the time of day. But as Pfaffmann (1960) has suggested, taste and other oropharyngeal stimuli have strong projections to the limbic and brainstem structures serving motivation, and visual stimuli do not. In addition, the hypothalamic receptor sites of stimulation by taste and smell are quite different from the receptor sites for visual cues. For example, Rolls (1976) has recently reported specific and different neurons firing to the sight of food and to the taste of food in deprived animals. Finally, taste can serve as an unconditioned stimulus for learning and appears to have more direct biological significance for the organism than visual or auditory stimuli (Garcia and Hankins, 1974; Rozin and Kalat, 1971).

Let us summarize the implications of separating taste from purely external cues for feeding. Since palatability is influenced by deprivation and satiety, it may be that taste responsiveness reflects long- and/or short-term changes in the energy state of the organism. Responsiveness to visual and cognitive cues in the environment, on the other hand, would be unrelated to the energy state of the organism but instead may be determined by his level of acute arousal or chronic arousability, as I suggested earlier.

To consider these hypotheses, we (Rodin, Slochower, and Fleming, Study 4, 1977) tested overweight women who were members of various local weight reduction clubs and a control group of normal weight women being treated at an outpatient clinic. It is significant to note that all subjects were both older and more varied in terms of socioeconomic status than subjects in earlier studies. On the basis of pretesting, overweight women who were highest or lowest in responsiveness to external, non-food-relevant cues were selected as subjects. The experiment then examined how, *for a particular subject*, weight loss influenced consumption in response to conditions of high versus low visual and cognitive food cue salience (holding palatability moderate) compared to the conditions of high versus low palatability (holding cue salience moderate).

Those overweight subjects who were selected on the basis of high responsiveness to non-food-relevant external stimuli were also significantly more responsive to manipulations of cognitive-visual food cues than either low external overweight or normal weight subjects. Weight loss did not reliably change degree of responsiveness to visual salience for any group. The pattern of findings for the palatability manipulation was different in several respects. First, high and low external overweight groups were more influenced by palatability differences than the normal subjects prior to weight loss, and they were not different from one another. Second, they became even more taste responsive following weight reduction. Generally, increased responsiveness was reflected in exaggerated consumption of the highly palatable food rather than increased rejection of the poor-tasting food. From these data we concluded that external cue responsiveness does not appear to result from obesity or from deprivation per se, while responsiveness to taste stimuli may indeed reflect these parameters. The findings provide a way to reconcile our hypothesis with Nisbett's (1972) by demonstrating an improtant difference between taste sensitivity and what we would call responsiveness to cognitive-visual external cues.

The thrust of these findings suggests that responsiveness to external cues does not change with weight loss. We then considered that it may precede and predispose an individual toward overeating and weight gain in a food-abundant environment. To test this hypothesis, Rodin and Slochower (1976) selected an eight-week summer camp for girls. This was not a diet camp and the food was abundant, attractively prepared, and served "family style." Candy and other treats sent by parents were plentiful in each cabin and could also be purchased at any time at the camp canteen. It was predicted that the more external a child was, the more her eating behavior would be influenced by the shift to abundant food cues which coming to camp represented. This, in turn, would affect her weight. In contrast, nonexternal children were expected to be more responsive to internal physiological signals and thus maintain a relatively constant body weight independent of alterations in the environment. The strong test of this hypothesis was provided by studying normal weight people with no history of overweight.

We found a significant positive correlation between externality and weight gain from the first to the last week, suggesting that the children who were responsive to external cues subsequently gained the most weight. Activity level and emotional adjustment were not related to weight change. The finding that there are normal weight external children who behave as do the moderately obese lends further support to the notion that externality is not purely a function of overweight but instead reflects the underlying tendency toward hyperresponsiveness.

We were pleased with these findings but puzzled over why some external children were already overweight when they arrived at camp and others were not. Perhaps externally responsive people who maintain normal weight are those who are responsive to major shifts in food cues that produce short-term weight gain but for whom long-term regulation is responsive to other factors. "Externals" who have become overweight are those individuals whose long-term regulatory mechanisms do not inhibit the continued weight gain which results from heightened responsiveness. Although we have no data which directly test this issue, there are some patterns of weight gain differences which are suggestive. Of the overweight campers who gained weight, 86 percent reached their highest weight at week 8. Of those normals who gained, 70 percent reached their highest weights before week 8 and then began to lose. While the novelty of the food environment was diminishing over time, it is also possible that long-term regulatory mechanisms were taking over. Such mechanisms could be biological, psychological, or both.

INTERNAL REGULATORY CUES

While our research has pursued the role of external stimuli in influencing feeding for overweight individuals, Schachter's early hypothesis also suggested that overweight people are, at the same time, underresponsive to internal regulatory cues. He based this assessment on the following data:

Stunkard and Koch (1964) first demonstrated that while all people commonly experienced stomach contractions, overweight people were less likely than the nonobese to correlate this gastric motility with the conscious experience of hunger. Schachter and his colleagues (1971, 1974) then questioned what implications this finding might have for eating itself. The novelty of these studies attracted wide attention since they required that hunger be manipulated and that food be available but at the same time that subjects be unaware that their eating was being measured. When crackers were offered as part of a presumed taste test, Schachter, Goldman, and Gordon (1969) found that, if full or fearful, normal weight people ate less than when they were hungry or unafraid. Both satiety and fear change internal state by reducing gastric motility and raising blood sugar level. For obese subjects, on the other hand, these manipulations had no effect on the number of crackers eaten. Subsequent attempts to replicate this phenomenon, however, found no significant difference in the number of crackers eaten by obese or normal subjects as a function of prior deprivation (Price and Grinker, 1973; Singh, 1973), and a recent study suggested that when deprivation did have an effect on the obese, it created a bad mood which lowered both food preference and consumption (Tom and Rucker, 1975).

Despite this and other lack of evidence for the internality hypothesis, the internal versus external view is cited in some form in almost every introductory psychology textbook. Yet it now appears that the injunction of extreme discontinuity between internal-physiological and external-environmental stimuli may have been premature, especially with regard to eating behavior.

There are now many indications that the internal versus external view is far too simple a description of, or explanation for, obese-normal differences. First, the development of this dichotomy was greatly influenced by the studies of Stunkard and Koch (1964) which reported high correlations between hunger and gastric contractions for normal subjects but not for many overweight individuals. On this basis, Schachter (1968) argued that the eating behavior of people of normal weight was more influenced by internal signals like gastric motility but that motility was not a hunger cue for the obese. However, in reviewing the role of the gastrointestinal tract in the regulation of food intake, Janowitz (1967, p. 220) concluded that while deficits of nutrients give rise to a complex of sensations which includes the epigastric hunger pang, gastric hunger contractions appear to be a dispensable component since eating proceeds normally in their absence. In. fact, he claims that "at present, no published data exist about any species that indicate whether or not *food intake* or other hunger-motivated behavioral parameters are actually correlated with gastric hunger contractions." Thus, relying heavily on gastric motility as an important internal signal which might predict differential feeding behavior in overweight and normal weight persons meant relying on a cue which does not appear to play a crucial role in the initiation of feeding.

The second kind of evidence taken as a lack of internal responsiveness in the obese came from studies demonstrating their failure to respond to caloric preloading as accurately as did normal subjects (Nisbett, 1968; Pliner, 1974; Schachter, Goldman, and Gordon, 1968). However, it may simply be that the level of caloric preload used in these and other comparable studies was insufficient to be detected by the overweight subjects. For example, Nisbett has suggested that many overweight individuals are physiologically deprived because of dieting or at least because of conscious restraint of their eating. If they are literally starving, they would overeat whether they had already received a 200 or 500 calorie preload since neither of these would be sufficient to satisfy their current nutritional needs. Thus, their short-term feeding could actually be seen as highly responsive to their internal physiological state at the moment.

One does not have to accept the Nisbett hypothesis to predict that overweight and normal weight individuals should not be equally responsive to preloading manipulations. As I have indicated, the corpulent person demonstrates a number of metabolic and endocrine abnormalities, generally as a result of overeating and adiposity (Sims et al., 1973). Because of these weight-related metabolic differences, overweight people may be responding to different levels or kinds of internal signals. This, in turn, could make them responsive to a different level of caloric preload than people or normal weight, but not unresponsive.

Third, as concluded by the Dahlem Workshop on Human Feeding Behavior (Wooley et al., 1976), there is now a great deal of evidence that normal subjects also show far from perfect internal regulation. Despite evidence that experimental animals are able to adapt relatively promptly and accurately to caloric dilution, studies with normal weight humans have shown that only some subjects are able to compensate over several days for changes in the caloric density of liquid diets, and in nearly all cases, consumption is sluggish and incomplete (Campbell et al., 1971; Jordan, 1969; Spiegel, 1973; O. Wooley, 1971). For most people, regardless of their body weight, internal signals do not appropriately guide eating behavior toward stable caloric intake in the short run either, unless cognitive or external cues regarding amount are also present (Spiegel, 1973; S. Wooley, 1972).

The studies which have used a preload test meal paradigm are also difficult to assess because the test meal forces the initiation of eating in a situation in which the natural response might have been to delay eating. Once a meal is begun, there is a tendency to continue eating until satiety. Thus, probability of eating cannot be equated with amount consumed in such experimental probes. The temporal features of eating therefore still have to be examined in order to understand the integrated relationship between those internal-physiological and external variables which influence both the initiation and the termination of feeding.

Thus there are clear difficulties, outlined above, with a view which dichotomizes internal and external controls and then uses this distinction to explain differences between overweight and normal weight people. External cues trigger eating against a background of certain physiological conditions. In most studies, overweight individuals have consumed more than normal subjects, but often not everything, suggesting that consumption may influence responsiveness to external stimuli either by changing the perceived palatability of the food stimulus (Cabanac, 1971) or through some other postabsorptive consequence of food. Indeed, internal factors may play an important role in modulating response to sensory or external signals. An explicit link between these factors has been drawn by Cabanac and his associates (Cabanac, 1971; Cabanac and Duclaux, 1970) who demonstrated that the pleasantness of sweet taste is determined, in part, by the nutritional needs of the organism. Sweet taste appears especially good when the individual is deprived, and it appears relatively unpleasant after satiety. There have been several studies examining the effects of body weight and/or deprivation on palatability (Grinker, 1976; Nisbett, 1968b, 1972; Rodin, 1975b; Rodin, Moskowitz, and Bray, 1976) which show that levels of acute and chronic energy supply do indeed affect palatability. These relationships are complex however and depend in part on the way the energy deficit is accomplished, the current level of body weight, and the type of food being tasted.

It now also seems likely that external stimuli directly influence internal physiological states. We pursued this question in our laboratory when we asked whether heightened external responsiveness could lead to overeating by triggering a physiological response. As one example of such a process, Teitelbaum and his co-workers (Wolgin, Cytawa and Teitelbaum, 1976) suggest that external and sensory stimuli (taste, smell, sight of food) have a general activating component which energizes the organism in addition to their directing and incentive value. They argue that this arousal plays a crucial role in the control of feeding, and that lack of activation may be a contributing factor to the lack of interest in food seen in animals with lateral hypothalamic (LH) lesions. As I described earlier, arousing the animal in other ways, such as tail pinch or amphetamine, also leads to voluntary approach to food and vigorous eating. In addition, as our research shows, heightened arousal and activation – derived from, or at least in the presence of, salient external food stimuli – could lead to overeating.

HYPOTHALAMIC LESIONS

This view takes on special significance in light of the recent data of Marshall (1975, 1976) who tested animals with unilateral ventromedial hypothalamic (VMH) lesions. Since the neural region on one side of the brain is responsive to the external environment on the contralateral side, Marshall varied the location of food-dispensing dishes for these animals. He first found that 13 of the 14 rats with unilateral damage showed an increase in responsiveness to contralateral sensory stimuli of all kinds; they showed increased orienting, exaggerated response to whisker touch, head turning, increased biting of noxious stimuli, and aggressive responses to attack. Most important, when eating, the unilateral animals began taking a significantly greater proportion of their daily food from the contralateral food dish. This suggests that the lesion itself was enhancing cue responsiveness. In other words, medial damage might produce hyperresponsiveness, which influences the animal's reactivity to external stimuli, which in turn influences feeding. Gibson and Gazzaniga (1971) noted a similar finding in split brain monkeys with unilateral hypothalamic damage. Such monkeys overate only when using the eye which projected to the hemisphere with the ventromedial lesion, suggesting that external visual cues were what influenced overeating.

These physiological data are consistent with our earlier work (Schachter and Rodin, 1974) in which we compared the behavior of overweight humans to animals with electrolytic lesions in the ventromedial region of the hypothalamus. In this monograph, we suggested that both the VMH-lesioned rat and the obese human might share a pattern of increased arousal and hyperresponsiveness to the external cues associated with food and non-food stimuli.

First, we considered finickiness. Though the lesioned animal is obese, it is also particularly sensitive to the effects of the texture or taste of its diet (Carlisle and Stellar, 1969; Corbit and Stellar, 1964; Teitelbaum, 1955). If quinine is added to its food, it eats far less than a normal animal whose food has been similarly tainted. On the other hand, if dextrose or lard is added to its normal food (they are apparently tasty to a rat) the lesioned animal eats far in excess of its regular intake or that of a control rat whose food has also been enriched. This is also true for obese humans (Decke, 1971; Nisbett, 1968b; Rodin, 1975b).

The eating habits of lesioned animals have been thoroughly studied as well. Static obese rats eat on the average slightly but not considerably more than normal rats (Teitelbaum and Campbell, 1958). They also eat fewer meals per day, eat more per meal, and eat more rapidly than do normal animals (Teitelbaum and Campbell, 1958). For each of these facts there are parallel data for overweight humans (Beaudoin and Mayer, 1953; Ross et al., 1971; Schachter and Rodin, 1974). In addition, Schachter and Rodin (1974) identified behavior unrelated to food consumption in which it was possible to draw somewhat more fanciful, though still not ridiculous, comparisons between species. For example, studies of gross activity using stabilimeter cages or activity wheels have demonstrated that the lesioned animal is markedly less active than the normal animal (Teitelbaum, 1957). This does not indicate only that the lesioned animal has trouble dragging its immense bulk around the cage. The dynamic hyperphagic rat, though not yet fat, is quite as lethargic as his obese counterpart (Teitelbaum, 1957). The same is true for overweight humans (Bullen, Reed, and Mayer, 1964; Johnson, Burke, and Mayer, 1956; Mayer, 1965).

We then identified still other types of behavior that were described in the literature for ventromedial lesioned animals and tested for these in obese humans. These were: (1) that the VMH animal is hyperemotional, easily startled, excitable, and difficult to handle (Eichelman, 1971; Wheatley, 1944), (2) that the lesioned animal is better at avoidance of painful stimuli than its normal counterpart (Grossman, 1972; Levine and Soliday, 1960; McAdam and Kaelber, 1966; Sechzer, Turner, and Liebelt, 1966), (3) that the lesioned animal appears to be more sensitive to pain (Kaada, Rasmussen, and Kveim, 1962; Turner, Sechzer, and Liebelt, 1967), and (4) that although the lesioned animal will eat large quantities of easily available food, it will not always work to get food (Miller, Bailey, and Stevenson, 1950). For each type of behavior, a parallel was found in obese humans.

Marshall suggested that medial damage might produce hyperresponsiveness by increasing the activity within catacholamine-containing systems, such as the nigrostriatal bundle, which runs through the hypothalamus. This is the system, as I described earlier, which contributes to broad, nonspecific components of arousal, and it is clear that motivated behaviors have a general component of arousal which may be characterized by increased alertness and sensitivity to relevant sensory stimuli.

These converging lines of evidence may be summarized as follows: activation and arousal by external stimuli are related to the return of normal feeding in LH-lesioned animals, and hyperarousal in response to external stimuli appears to be related to overeating in VMH-lesioned animals, in tail-pinch-induced animals, and in many overweight people. In each of these groups, heightened responsiveness to external stimuli leads to weight gain over time. The neurochemical pathways involved in these responses are involved in the general arousal of the organism and its specific responsiveness to hedonically valued external stimuli. As Striker and Zigmond (1976) have suggested, an external stimulus would thus be seen as having two effects — a specific one which activates neurons that are involved in eliciting some appropriate motivational state and a nonspecific one which removes a gate and thereby permits such responses to actually occur. Thus an individual could literally be turned on by an external stimulus. The neurochemical link between responsivity, arousal, and feeding systems has exciting implications for the study of external responsiveness in human obesity.

At present I am certainly not arguing for the underlying anatomical or neurochemical dysfunction of these responses in humans. However, others have proposed, notably Maddi (1968) and Thayer (1967), that there are large individual differences with regard to both rate of activation change and level of activation. This may be especially important with regard to eating.

This hypothesis would also explain inconsistencies in understanding the motivational state of the VMH hyperphagic animal. Rather than decreasing hunger drive as we first believed, it now appears that VMH damage enhances food motivation. This seems clear now since the food-motivated performance of the VMH animals is greatly influenced by the type of schedule used, the level of deprivation, pretraining variables, and the nature of the reward. These data suggest that not only homeostatic variables but also hedonic factors greatly influence the development and maintenance of the VMH syndrome.

In addition to general arousal, the second role of external cues on internal processes would arise from the effects of these cues on metabolic events. We reasoned that insulin release would be a likely candidate for such an intervening physiological mechanism. It is involved in increased ingestion and in increased storage of nutrients as fat.

RELEASE OF INSULIN

In rats, Nicolaidis (1968) and Steffens (1970) have both demonstrated an early release of insulin in response to gustatory stimuli, and recently Woods and his colleagues (1977) reported that rats develop the tendency to secrete insulin in the presence of stimuli that reliably predict the opportunity to eat. In some instances this was time of day, and in others, odor. Most directly relevant, however, was the report of Parra-Covarrubias and his co-workers (1971), that obese adolescents tended to secrete insulin at the sight and smell of food. In this study, however, no normal weight persons were tested and the first blood sample was taken after 5 minutes, thus eliminating the possibility of assessing an early insulin response if it were to occur.

To consider this hypothesis, we have followed the same basic procedure in several studies. All subjects are nondiabetic with normal glucose tolerance. Subjects are advised to eat least 40 percent of their diets as carbohydrate for three days prior to the study. They come to the laboratory at lunch time, having eaten nothing since dinner at 7 P.M. on the previous evening. In order to minimize stress, an indwelling catheter is placed under local xylocaine anesthesia in an antecubital vein and kept open with a slow intravenous drip of saline solution. After three control blood samples are taken, a partly cooked beefsteak is brought in and grilled, crackling in a frying pan in front of the subject, to provide rich visual and olfactory cues. Try to picture yourself sitting there, hungry — watching, hearing, and smelling a big juicy steak which the experimenters have promised that you will soon be able to eat.

Small continuous blood samples are taken for the first 10 minutes and then again at 15 and 20 minutes after the presentation of the steak. At -3, +3, and +20, subjects rate their hunger, and at +3, and +20 they rate how appetizing the steak looks — in other words, how much they would like to eat it at that moment.

Figure 3-12 shows some pilot data, based on only three overweight (+18 to +60 percent OW) and four normal weight (-6 to +8 percent OW) subjects. The mean fasting plasma immunoreactive insulin level was 18.7 μU/ml in the obese compared to 10.4 in the normal weight subjects, and the data are expressed as change scores from basal. We see a biphasic secretion of insulin: both an early phase which peaks at 2-3 minutes and a later phase rising again at 15 and 20 minutes after stimulus introduction.

If this is a real effect, the first possibility is that it is due to the cell — either because the B cell has been reset by obesity or because the obese are hyperinsulinemic. Since insulin release obeys the law of initial values, hyperinsulinemia

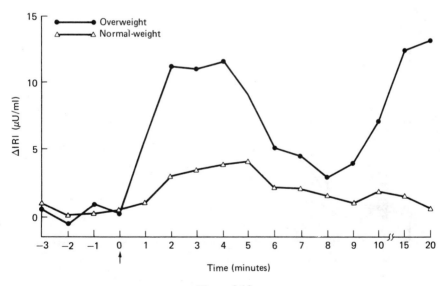

Figure 3-12.

alone could have made them more responsive. However, since a hypocaloric diet and the resultant weight loss lead to a drop in basal insulin to normal levels, we replicated the first study using several subject groups including dieted, formerly overweight people.

Eleven stabilized overweight subjects were selected. Five were highly responsive to food-relevant environmental stimuli as assessed by prior ingestion and performance measures used reliably in our laboratory, and six were not externally responsive according to these measures. Both groups had high basal insulin levels, averaging 20.4 and 23.2, respectively. There were five nonexternally responsive, normal weight subjects with an average basal insulin of 11.6, and five formerly overweight subjects who were currently within normal weight range and whose basal insulin levels averaged 12.6 — well within the normal range.

Figure 3-13 shows some contribution of hyperinsulinemia but more from external responsiveness. In other words, those individuals, regardless of current weight, whose feeding behavior is most responsive to environmental stimuli associated with food, show the greatest insulin response to the sight and smell and sound of the grilling steak.

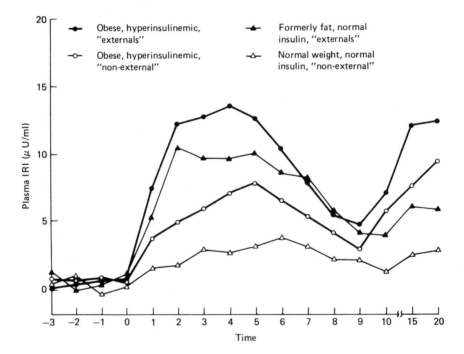

Figure 3-13.

In the next experiment, we asked whether the magnitude of the hormonal response was correlated with the palatability of the food stimulus. Palatability was determined in advance by presenting a pilot group of subjects with a list of foods and asking them to rate how much they would like to eat some of that right now. This time the foods presented were all carbohydrates. All pilot subjects had been fasted overnight and so were in a state of deprivation identical to that which would be used in the study itself.

The experimental subjects ($n = 10$) were tested on two separate days with presentations of food at palatability levels 1, 5, 9, and no food. Two were presented each day, separated by one-half hour in counterbalanced order and in a double blind procedure in which the food stimulus or an empty plate was presented.

As Table 3-2 shows, the overweight subjects had an insulin response which was significantly more affected by palatability than the normal subjects. Here we have a very crucial indication of a disregulated feedback loop. As described earlier, insulin release is related to increased hunger and feeding as well as being responsible for fat storage. If externally responsive people oversecrete insulin in the presence of compelling food cues, they might eat more calories in order to balance this hormonal and metabolic output and they might also store more of the food in fat.

HYPERRESPONSIVENESS

I have spent a great deal of time exploring the role of external factors in the development and maintenance of obesity because they have provided us with such exciting data. Indeed, our findings at the summer camp indicate that there are normal weight externals who behave as do the moderately obese; this lends further support to the notion that externality is not purely a function of overweight, but instead reflects the underlying tendency towards hyperresponsiveness.

Given that it contributes to overeating, how might this responsiveness to environmental stimuli develop? Is it innate or is it learned? In an interesting animal study, Gross (1968) tested the role of early nutritional experience upon

Table 3-2. Peak Change in Plasma Insulin within 5 Minutes after Stimulus Presentation (μU/ml).

Group	No Food	Palatability 1	5	9
Overweight externals	3	-2	7	13
Normal weight nonexternals	0	1	3	6

the development of external responsiveness. Gross directly manipulated the early environmental conditions of weanling rats by exposing them to conditions of constant and randomly varied deprivation intervals. Animals fed on a schedule of random deprivation were expected to be in a state in which energy depletion would be complicated by uncertainty regarding the future availability of food. In order to maximize the effects of scarcity and unpredictability experienced by the animals, it was decided to expose them to these conditions for a considerable length of time. Gross created three groups of experimental animals immediately after weaning. One group was allowed to eat freely, the second group was placed on a 22-hour deprivation schedule in which they were fed once every 22 hours, and the third group was placed on a random deprivation schedule in which they were fed on the average of every 22 hours with the time of deprivation ranging from 8 to 48 hours. All animals were kept on these schedules for 100 days. Gross found that rats maintained under conditions of randomly varied deprivation were highly responsive to variations in the taste and caloric density of their diets. This was interpreted as an increase in external control in the randomly deprived rats as compared to animals having regularly available food. After 100 days the animals were allowed to feed when they chose, and Gross found that even under conditions of abundance the randomly deprived animals continued to exhibit externally oriented responses to dietary variations. Most interesting, the rats that had been randomly deprived also demonstrated a pattern of external control, reflected in a measure of responsiveness to external food cues that did not involve eating. Gross tested this by measuring the amount of time they remained in contact with food in an open field although they were not allowed to eat the food. This is reminiscent of the observations of nonconsummatory food-relevant activity reported by Nisbett and Kanouse (1969) who showed that the supermarket shopping of obese humans was unrelated to deprivation state. Like these human shoppers, Gross' randomly deprived rats exhibited an interest in food independent of internal state of depletion or satiety. The animals seemed to have hungry eyes.

What then can we conclude from Gross' study about the ontology of external control in obese humans? An externally imposed schedule combining both scarcity and unpredictability might be expected to encourage dependence on external cues for the regulation of eating. Given the uncertainty of such a schedule, it would be best to eat whenever possible, regardless of internal needs. For a neonate, these conditions may well produce a lasting pattern of external control. This speculation leads us to suppose that in societies where food is normally scarce, a large proportion of the population would exhibit external control of eating. The presence of this pattern in ecologies of scarcity would not necessarily have the same association with obesity that has been found in our food-abundant society, however. Gross reports that this expectation of patterns of external control among people living in conditions of constant scarcity and unpredictability is observed in the Yanamano Indians of Brazil. When food is available, they eat continuously. Social life is centered on food and when food is plentiful the Yanamanos feast even to the point of vomiting. Yet the males of the tribe also seem to be able to spend days in the jungle without being discomforted by pangs of hunger. The conclusions drawn from Gross' study are that regardless of factors such as heredity, the imposition of irregular feeding and scarcity could facilitate external control. Although most human neonates in our society do not live in an environment of scarcity, many may live in a very unpredictable food environment. These data add to our cataloging of the important role that environmental factors play in the production and control of obesity.

OVERFEEDING

In addition to genetics and to social and external cues, nutrition appears to be another major causative factor in obesity. Most important is the type of diet. Manipulation of the diet to contribute to obesity can be accomplished in one of two ways: by changing the frequency of eating or by changing the composition of the diet. Animal studies show that eating two times a day rather than their normal six to eight times, makes rats fatter (Leveille, 1970). The same appears to be true for humans in many cases (Fabry et al., 1964). Body fat also increases as fat in the diet increases, especially in proportion to the amount of carbohydrate eaten. The greatest accumulation of fat occurs when protein intake is separated from the intake of carbohydrate and fat (Cohn et al., 1965).

In humans, studies have shown that overfeeding may be of particular importance in the onset of childhood obesity (Fomon, 1971). Experimental studies by Knittle and Hirsch (1968) have shown that the total number of adipocytes in rats can be permanently modified by infant nutrition. Thus, as Figure 3-14 demonstrates, similar nutritional experiences in humans may have prime importance in producing the hyperplasia and hypertrophy of adipose tissue found in obese humans. The treatment of obesity may therefore lie in its prevention early in life through the control of factors that influence adipose cell division and enlargement.

Knittle (1975) has demonstrated that critical adipose tissue development occurs somewhere between birth and two years of age in obese children, and that this time has important consequences for the future development of the adult fat depot. By age two, obese children have more and larger fat cells than normal children. After age two, weight loss in obese children does nothing to alter the number of adipose cells. Decreases in body fat are accomplished solely by a reduction of adipose cell size without significant changes in cell number. Thus, even in children, once a particular adipose cell number is achieved it cannot be

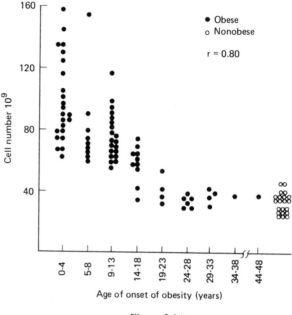

Figure 3-14.

decreased by dietary restriction, and these children usually become overweight adults. This fact is demonstrated clearly in Table 3-3. The permanent excess of fat making machinery and high lipogenic capacity that the once-obese child always carries with him may be the physical underpinning for the high rate of recidivism in weight reduction programs.

The importance of these studies is great. The total number of fat cells that we carry into adult life is at least partially dependent upon early childhood feeding and may directly influence our current eating as well. Recently, Hirsch and his co-workers (Faust, Johnson and Hirsch, 1977a, 1977b) have demonstrated in an elegant series of studies that if infant rats have some of their subcutaneous fat

Table 3-3. Prognosis of Childhood Obesity.*

Overweight Adults	Childhood Weight Status (%)	
	Average	Overweight
Males	42	86
Females	18	80

*From Abraham and Nordsieck *Public Health Reports*, 1960, *75*, 263–273.

deposits removed surgically, there is a regenerative response, especially if the rats are fed a diet high in fat. After weaning, however, the regenerative response is less likely to occur, and lipectomy, in this case leading to a reduced fat cell number, also leads to decreased overeating and obesity in animals fed a highly palatable diet. So it seems that when the capacity for fat storage is reduced because the lost tissue does not regenerate, it leads to less spontaneous overeating even in the presence of highly palatable food stimuli.

While I have focused thus far on the development of the disorders of eating which result in obesity, our understanding of these processes relies in part on our understanding of the mechanisms controlling normal eating. The final set of causative factors could arise from dysfunctions of the neural and peripheral regions involved in the regulation of eating. These various regions are shown in Figure 3-15.

NEUROLOGY OF HUNGER

The foundations for the study of the neurology of hunger were established in the 1940s and 1950s. The stereotaxic technique used by investigators during this period enabled them to make fundamental discoveries of the effects of lesions and stimulation of the hypothalamus on food intake. The interpretation of these findings and the theoretical models which evolved were strongly influenced by two great traditions in physiology — the tradition of Cannon and the tradition of Sherington. It was concluded that the lateral hypothalamus was an appetite center, and the ventromedial hypothalamus a satiety center. Mogenson (1976) has described the general approach to the study of the neural mechanisms of hunger that have been found during the last two or three decades. In Figure 3-16, the asterisks identify the aspects that have received the most attention. The more asterisks, the greater is the degree of interest by investigators. The major efforts have been studies of the integrative system, particularly the hypothalamus and the limbic structures, and studies of feeding behavior per se by behavioral scientists. Although there has been a continuing interest in signals and receptors, the number of studies is considerably fewer. The question marks designate aspects for which there is little or no definitive evidence.

The dual-center model has served well but is not untenable in light of recent research. Unfortunately, an alternative model of the central control of food intake is not currently available to take its place. This represents a major unresolved problem in research on eating behavior. The identification of the lateral hypothalamus as the feeding center was due to the discovery of the aphagia syndrome produced by LH destruction. It is now known that this syndrome is largely but not completely the result of damage to the dopaminergic (DA) nigrostriatal pathway. Much research has therefore focused on this pathway, and the lateral hy-

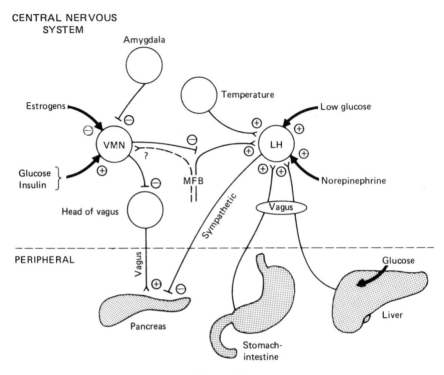

Figure 3-15.

pothalamus has in a sense fallen from grace. Stricker and Zigmond (1976) have explained the behavioral phenomena so familiar in this syndrome as a result of the fact that animals sustaining excessive damage to the nigrostriatal DA bundle coursing through the lateral hypothalamus have fundamental problems of remaining alert and sustaining arousal in response to sensory stimulation; indeed, this may underlie the intital aphagia and adipsia which is demonstrated.

Although LH neurons are not responsible for the aphagia syndrome, it is still clear that some of them are involved in the regulation of food intake. Sensory stimuli such as the taste and sight of food have been shown through electrophysiological studies by Rolls and his associates (1976) to trigger the firing of hypothalamic neurons. Thus, LH brain regions may be directly responsive to sensory food-relevant stimuli.

The ventromedial hypothalamus has also been extensively studied since early demonstrations of bilateral lesions in the ventromedial nuclei in the hypothalamus produced animals that for a time ate large quantities of food and grew extraordinarily fat. Classic descriptions of the lesioned animal present a creature that

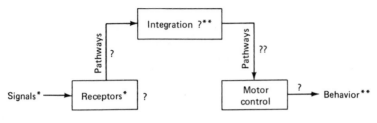

Figure 3-16.

staggers over to the food hopper almost immediately after its operation and begins shoveling in food. Recently, however, our understanding of this syndrome too has been drastically revised in light of new data. Hypothalamic hyperphagia, while it has been long associated with the ventromedial nucleus, now appears not to involve this nucleus directly in the syndrome. Rather, current evidence indicates that the hyperphagia and obesity result from damage to a longitudinally situated pathway which passes by the ventromedial nucleus. The research of Grossman, Scalfani, Gold, and others demonstrating that diencephalic or midbrain knife cuts can produce dramatic increases or decreases of feeding, with the ventromedial nucleus remaining intact, has provided new insight into the location of these pathways. However, where the pathway originates and terminates, and its relationship to recently discovered monoamine pathways, are as yet unclear and are the subject of ongoing research.

The importance of peripheral signals in the regulation of feeding, and therefore their disregulation in obesity, should also not be overlooked. Some forms of overeating and overweight may arise because of a failure of peripheral factors to regulate feeding. These peripheral factors can be grouped into gastrointestinal factors, humoral factors, and nutrient changes which are communicated directly through the blood stream. Let us look first at gastrointestinal factors. The ingestion of food could serve to inhibit food intake in one of three ways: (1) by distension of the gastrointestinal tract during the ingestion of food which may activate neural pathways to the nervous system, (2) by ingestion of food which may trigger the release of hormones from the gastrointestinal tract, and (3) by early absorption of nutrients which may signal an end to eating.

There are several possible neural signals that could inhibit food intake. Paintal (1954) has shown that stretch receptors are present in the stomach wall and they send neural impulses to the brain through the vagus nerve. Iggo (1957) has demonstrated the presence of receptors that are sensitive to the acidity of the gastric content, and Sharma and Nasset (1962) have shown that there are receptors in the wall of the small intestine that respond to the presence of glucose or amino acids in the lumen. Afferent impulses from the gastrointestinal tract have not been thoroughly investigated, and there are no studies as yet in which a complete vagal nerve section has been done on an animal in a single operation. Although there are some difficulties with the surgical procedures, it appears to be basically true that feeding behavior can remain normal if neural connections between the brain and the gut have been substantially reduced. This observation makes it unlikely that a strictly neural mechanism controls food intake at the peripheral level. However, it does not argue that nerves are not involved in the regulation of feeding behavior in the intact animal. The nerves modulate secretion, motility, and blood flow, all of which may play some role in the regulation of feeding behavior.

Humoral or hormonal mechanisms are a second way in which food in the gastrointestinal tract might provide signals to stop eating. When 50 percent of the blood from satiated rats was cross-transfused into hungry rats, food intake was depressed for up to three hours (Davis et al., 1969). This implies some circulating factor influencing food intake. Gibbs, Young, and Smith (1973) have recently suggested that the gastrointestinal hormone cholecystokinin may be one of these humoral factors. Hormones outside the gastrointestinal tract (such as insulin), glucose, and amino acids also appear to be involved in the regulation of feeding behavior.

The third possible communication route is through the blood stream. Several authors have presented theories that one or another nutrient is involved in controlling feeding behavior. The most prominent theory is that food intake is controlled by the presence or absence of an arteriovenous difference in blood sugar level (Mayer, 1955). Other theorists have proposed that absorbed amino acids or amount of body fat controls food intake (Kennedy, 1953). The latter theory is not specific about the way in which body fat is monitored, but one conceivable mechanism is that the brain senses the level of free fatty acid in the blood. However, the importance of absorbed nutrients for the short-term regulation of food intake is minimized by the results of studies with crossed intestined rats (Koopmans, 1977). In these studies food eaten by one rat enters its stomach and travels through some of its duodenum before crossing into the intestines of the other rat. About equal amounts of glucose and amino acids are absorbed into the blood stream by both rats, yet the fed rat is fully satiated and the unfed rat remains quite hungry, despite the nearly equal absorption of food into the two rats. Thus food intake does not appear to be controlled by the amount of absorbed nutrient. Some general change in energy flow, however, may still be an important controlling factor, as Booth (1976) and Friedman and Stricker (1976) have recently observed.

Apparently obesity is due to overeating — either currently and/or during childhood. But what leads to overeating? Understanding the complex relationship between physiological mechanisms and behavior has allowed us to rule out several contributing factors and focus on others. Schwartz (1977) has suggested a general model which could be applied to understand the disregulation of eating.

People might overeat because the brain itself has been programmed, either initially through genetics, or subsequently through learning, to respond inappropriately to stimuli in the internal environment or because the peripheral organs themselves may be hypo- or hyperreactive to the neural stimulation coming from the brain, again either genetically or because of maturational influences. An example of a maturational influence and the most likely candidate, of course, is overeating itself, which could reset the operation of the peripheral organs and the feedback mechanisms between peripheral and central sites.

It is also possible that the negative feedback derived from the peripheral organs may be inappropriate. In other words, it is possible for the protective negative feedback systems to become less effective, or in extreme cases inactivated. While this again could occur as a function of some genetic contribution, it is certain to occur as a function of overeating itself.

It may be that stimuli from the environment are so potent that the person is forced to ignore the feedback from his internal digestive organs or metabolic state. The potency of the stimuli could be their intrinsic hedonic and arousal value, the set or setting in which the individual finds himself, or the cultural rules regulating eating in a particular period or for a particular group. It may be, in addition, that the brain is programmed either genetically or through learning to respond inappropriately to stimuli present in the external environment. Finally, the state of the individual himself could make him more vulnerable or responsive to environmental stimuli, particularly states such as hunger or arousal.

REFERENCES

Abramson, E. D. and Wunderlich, R. A. Anxiety, fear and eating: a test of the psychosomatic concept of obesity. *Journal of Abnormal Psychology*, 1972, *79*, 317-321.

Adolph, E. F. *Am. J. Physiol.*, 1947, *151*, 110-125.

Antelman, S. M., Rowland, N. E., and Fisher, A. E. Stimulation bound ingestive behavior: A view from the tail. *Physiology and Behavior*, 1975, *17*, 743-748.

Antelman, S. M., Rowland, N. E., and Fisher, A. E. Stress related recovery from lateral hypothalmic aphagia. *Brain Research*, 1976, *102*, 346-350.

Beaudoin, R. and Mayer, J. Food intakes of obese and non-obese women. *Journal of the American Dietetic Association*, 1953, *29*, 29-33.

Becker, H. S. *Outsiders: Studies in the Sociology of Deviance.* New York: The Free Press, 1963.

Ben-David, M., Dikstein, S., Bismuth, G. and Salman, F. G. Antihypercholesterotemic effect of dehydroepiandrosterone in rats. *Proc. Soc. Exptl. Biol. Med.*, 1967, *125*, 1136-1140.

Bjorntorp, P. Effects of physical conditioning in obesity. *Obesity in Perspective* (Bray, G. A., Ed.), Fogarty International Center Series of Preventative Medicine, Vol. II, Part II. Washington, D. C.: U.S., Government Printing Office, 1976.

Bjorntorp, P., Berchtold, P., Holm, J. and Larsson, B. The glucose uptake of human adipose tissue in obesity. *Europ. J. Clin. Invest.*, 1971, *1*, 480-485.

Booth, D. A. Approaches to feeding control. *Appetite and Food Intake* (Silverstone, T., Ed.). Braunschweig: Pergamon Press, 1976.

Bray, G. A. Effect of diet and triiodothyronine on the activity of sn-glycerol-3-phosphate dehydrogenase and on the metabolism of glucose and syruvate by adipose tissue of obese patients. *Journal of Clinical Investigation*, 1969, *48*, 1413-1422.

Bray, G. A. The overweight patient. *Advances in Internal Medicine* (Stollerman, G. H., Ed.), Vol. 21. Year Book Medical Publishers, 1976.

Bray, G. A., Barry, R. E., Benfield, J., Castelnuovo-Tedesco, P. and Rodin, J. Food intake and taste preferences for glucose and sucrose decrease after intestinal bypass surgery. *Hunger: Basic Mechanisms and Clinical Implications* (Novin, D., Wyrwicka, W., and Bray, G. A., Eds.), New York: Raven Press, 1976.

Bruch, H. Conceptual confusion in eating disorders. *Journal of Nervous and Mental Disease*, 1961, *133*, 46.

Bruch, H. *Eating Disorders*. New York: Basic Books, 1973.

Bullen, B. A., Reed, R. B., and Mayer, J. Physical activity of obese and non-obese adolescent girls, appraised by motion picture sampling. *American Journal of Clinical Nutrition*, 1964, *14*, 211-223.

Burdon, A. P. and Paul, L. Obesity: A review of the literature, stressing its psychodynamic approach. *Psychiatric Quarterly*, 1951, *25*, 568-580.

Cabanac, M. Physiological role of pleasure. *Science*, 1971, *173*, 1103-1107.

Cabanac, M. and Duclaux, R. Obesity: Absence of satiety aversion to sucrose. *Science*, 1970, *168*, 469-497.

Cahnman, W. J. The stigma of obesity. *Sociological Quarterly*, 1968, *9*, 283-299.

Campbell, R. G., Hashin, S. A., and Van Itallie, T. B. Studies of food-intake regulation in man: Responses to variations in nutritive density in lean and obese subjects. *New England Journal of Medicine*, 1971, *285*, 1402-1407.

Carlisle, H. and Stellar, E. Caloric regulation and food intake preference in normal hyperphagic and aphagic rats. *Journal of Comparative and Physiological Psychology*, 1969, *69*, 107-114.

Chirico, A. M. and Stunkard, A. J. Physical activity and human obesity. *New England Journal of Medicine*, 1960, *263*, 935-940.

Cohn, C., Joseph, D., Bell, L., and Allweiss, M. D. Studies on the effects of feeding frequency and dietary composition on fat deposition. *Annals of the New York Academy of Sciences*, 1965, *131*, 507-518.

Corbit, J. and Stellar, E. Palatability, food intake, and obesity and normal and hyperphagic rats. *Journal of Comparative and Physiological Psychology*, 1964, *58*, 63-69.

Craddock, D. *Obesity and Its Management*. London: Livingston, 1969.

Crofford, O. B., Minemura, T., and Kono, T. Insulin-receptor interaction in isolated fat cells. *Adv. Enzyme Regul.*, 1970, *8*, 219-238.

Davis, J. D., Gallagher, R. L., Ladove, R. L., and Turausky, A. J. *Journal of Comparative and Physiological Psychology*, 1969, *67*, 407-414.

Decke, E. Effects of taste on the eating behavior of obese and normal persons. *Emotion, Obesity, and Cume.* (Schachter, S., Ed.). New York: Academic Press, 1971.

Dimond, S. J. The structural basis of timing. *Psychological Bulletin*, 1964, *62*, 348-350.

Eichelman, B. Effect of subcortical lesions or shock-induced aggression in the rat. *Journal of Comparative and Physiological Psychology*, 1971, *74*, 331-339.

Faust, I. M., Johnson, P. R., and Hirsch, J. Adipose tissue regeneration following lipectomy. *Science*, 1977, *197*, 391. (a)

Faust, I. M., Johnson, P. R., and Hirsch, J. Surgical removal of adipose tissue alters feeding behavior and the development of obesity in rats. *Science*, 1977, *197*, 393. (b)

Fleming, B. Effects of short-term deprivation of the external responsiveness of overweight and normal-weight subjects. Unpublished senior honor thesis, Yale University, 1975.

Fomon, S. J. A pediatrician looks at early nutrition. *Bull. N.Y. Acad. Med.*, 1971, *47* 569-578.

Francois, M. Contributions a l'étude de sense du temps: La température internal comme facteur de variations de l'appréciation subjective des durées. *Année Psychologie*, 1927, *28*, 186-204.

Frazier, F. E. *The Negro in the United States*. New York: MacMillan, 1957.

Friedman, M. I. and Stricker, E. M. *Psychological Review*, 1976, *83*, 409-431.

Garcia, J. and Hankins, W. G. The evolution of bitter and the acquisition of toxphobia. *Fifth International Symposium on Olfaction and Taste* (Denton, D., Ed.), 1974.

Gibbs, J., Young, R C., and Smith, G. P. *Journal of Comparative and Physiological Psychology*, 1973, *84*, 488.

Gibson, A. R. and Gazzaniga, M. S. Hemispheric differences in eating behavior in split-brain monkeys. *Physiologist*, 1971, *14*, 150.

Glick, S. D. and Muller, R. U. Paradoxical effects of low doses of *d*-amphetamine in rats. *Psychopharmacologia*, 1971, *22*, 396-402.

Glucksman, M. L. and Hirsch, J. The response of obese patients to weight reduction: A clinical evaluation of behavior. *Psychosomatic Medicine*, 1968, *30*, 1-11.

Goldman, R., Jaffa, M., and Schachter, S. Yom Kippur, Air France, dormitory food, and eating behavior of obese and normal persons. *Journal of Personality and Social Psychology*, 1968, *10*, 117-123.

Grinker, J. Taste factors in human and animal obesity. *Hunger: Basic Mechanisms and Clinical Implications* (Novin, D., Wyrwicka, W., and Bray, G. A., Eds.). New York: Raven Press, 1976.

Grinker, J., Hirsch, J., and Levin, B. The affective response of obese patients to weight reduction: A differentiation based on age of onset of obesity. *Psychosomatic Medicine*, 1973, *35*, 57-62.

Gross, L. The effects of early feeding experience on external responsiveness. Unpublished doctoral dissertation, Columbia University, 1968.

Grossman, S. P. Aggression, avoidance and reaction to novel environment in female rats with ventromedial hypothalamic lesions. *Journal of Comparative and Physiological Psychology*, 1972, *78*, 274-283.

Gurney, R. Hereditary factor in obesity. *Arch. Intern. Med.*, 1936, *57*, 557-561.

Hammer, K. Experimental evidence for the biological clock. *The Voices of Time* (Fraser, J. J., Ed.). Brazillier, 1966.

Herberg, L. J., Franklin, K. B. J., and Stephens, D. N. The hypothalamic 'set-point' in experimental obesity. *Recent Advances in Obesity Research* (Howard, A., Ed.). London: Newman Publications, 1975.

Herman, C. P. and Mack, D. Restrained and unrestrained eating. *Journal of Personality*, 1975, *43*, 647-660.

Herman, C. P. and Polivy, J. Anxiety, restraint and eating behavior. *Journal of Abnormal Psychology*, 1975, *84*, 666-672.

Hirsch, J. and Knittle, J. L. Cellularity of obese and nonobese human adipose tissue. *Fed. Proc.*, 1970, *29*, 1516-1521.

Hoagland, H. The physiological control of judgments of duration: Evidence for a chemical clock. *Journal of Genetic Psychology*, 1933, *9*, 267-287.

Horton, E. S., Danforth, E., Jr., Sims, E. A. H., and Salans, L. B. Correlation of forearm muscle and adipose tissue metabolism in obesity before and after weight loss. *Clinical Research*, 1972, *20*, 548.

Janowitz, H. D. Role of the gastrointestinal tract in the regulation of food intake. *Handbook of Physiology: Alimentary Canal, I* (Code, C. F., Ed.). Washington, D.C.: American Physiological Society, 1967.

Johnson, M. L., Burke, B. S., and Mayer, J. Relative importance of inactivity and overeating in the energy balance of obese high school girls. *American Journal of Clinical Nutrition*, 1956, *4*, 37-44.

Jordan, H. A. Voluntary intragastric feeding: Oral and gastric contributions to food intake and hunger in man. *Journal of Comparative and Physiological Psychology*, 1969, *68*, 498-506.

Jung, F. 1976. Untersuchungen zur Nahrungsaufnahme von Kindern and Neugeborenen unter besonderer Beruckichtigung psychischer Aktivierung. *Math. -Nat. Diss. Gottingen.*

Kaada, B. R., Rasmussen, E. W., and Kveim, O. Impaired acquisition of passive avoidance behavior by subcallosal, septal, hypothalamic and insular lesions in rats. *Journal of Comparative and Physiological Psychology*, 1962, *55*, 661-670.

Kahlenberg, A. and Kalant, N. The effect of insulin on human adipose tissue. *Canadian Journal of Biochemistry*, 1964, *42*, 1623-1635.

Kaplan, B. *The Eternal Stranger: A Study of Jewish Life in the Small Community*. New York: Bookman Associates, 1957.

Kaplan, H. I. and Kaplan, H. S. The psychosomatic concept of obesity. *Journal of Nervous and Mental Disease*, 1957, *125*, 181-189.

Kennedy, G. C. The role of depot fat in the hypothalamic control of food intake in the rat. *Proc. Roy. Soc., London*, 1953, *140*, 578-592.

Keys, A., Brozek, J., Henschel, A., Mickelson, D., and Taylor, H. *The Biology of Human Starvation*. Minneapolis: University of Minnesota Press, 1950.

Kleck, R., Ono, H., and Hastorf, A. H. The effects of physical deviancy upon face-to-face interaction. *Human Relations*, 1966, *19*, 425-436.

Knittle, J. Early influences on development of adipose tissue. *Obesity in Perspective* (Bray, G. A., Ed.). Washington, D.C.: U.S. Government Printing Office, 1975.

Knittle, J. L. and Hirsch, J. Effect of early nutrition on the development of rat epididymal fat pads: Cellularity and metabolism. *Journal of Clinical Investigation*, 1968, *47*, 2091-2098.

Koopmans, H. Talk presented to the Columbia University Appetitive Behavior Seminar, May, 1977.

Leon, G. R. and Roth, L. Obesity: Psychological causes, correlations, and speculations. *Psychological Bulletin*, 1977, *84*, No. 1, 117-139.

Leveille, G. A. Adipose tissue metabolism: Influence of periodicity of eating diet composition. *Fed. Proc.*, 1970, *29*, 1294-1301.

Levine, S. and Soliday, S. The effects of hypothalamic lesions on conditioned avoidance learning. *Journal of Comparative and Physiological Psychology*, 1960, *53*, 497-501.

Levitz, L. The susceptibility of human feeding to external controls. *Obesity in Perspective* (Bray, G. A., Ed.). Washington, D.C.: U.S. Government Printing Office, 1975.

Linde, T. F. Influence of orthopedic disability on conformity behavior. *Journal of Abnormal and Social Psychology*, 1964, *68*, 115-118.

Louderback, L. *Fat Power; Whatever You Weigh Is Right.* New York: Hawthorn Books, 1970.

Lykken, D. A study of anxiety in the sociopathic personality. *Journal of Abnormal and Social Psychology*, 1957, *55*, 6-10.

Maddi, S. R. *Personality Theories: A Comparative Analysis.* Homewood, Ill.: Dorsey Press, 1968.

Marshall, J. Increased orientation to sensory stimuli following medial hypothalamic damage in rats. *Brain Research*, 1975, *86*, 373-387.

Marshall, J. Neurochemistry of central monoamine systems as related to food intake. *Appetite and Food Intake* (Silverstone, T., Ed.). Braunschweig: Pergamon Press, 1976.

Mayer, J. Genetic, traumatic and environmental factors in the etiology of obesity. *Physiol. Rev.*, 1953, *33*, 472-508.

Mayer, J. *Annals of the New York Academy of Sciences*, 1955, *63*, 15-43.

Mayer, J. Inactivity as a major factor in adolescent obesity. *Annals of the New York Academy of Sciences*, 1965, *131*, 502-506.

McAdam, D. W. and Kaelber, W. W. Differential impairment of avoidance learning in cats with ventiomedial hypothalamic lesions. *Experimental Neurology*, 1966, *15*, 293-298.

McKenna, R. J. Some effects of anxiety level and food cues on the eating behavior of obese and normal subjects. *Journal of Personality and Social Psychology*, 1972, *221*, 311-319.

Meyer, J. E. and Pudel, U. Experimental studies on food intake in obese and normal weight subjects. *Journal of Psychosomatic Research.* 1972, *16*, 305-308.

Miller, N. E., Bailey, C. J., and Stevenson, J. A. F. Decreased hunger but increased food intake resulting from hypothalamic lesions. *Science*, 1950, *112*, 256-259.

Mogenson, G. J. Neural mechanisms of hunger. *Hunger: Basic Mechanisms and Clinical Implications* (Novin, D., Wyrwicka, W., and Bray, G. A., Eds.). New York: Raven Press, 1976.

Newman, H. H., Freeman, F. N., and Holzinger, K. N. *Twins: A Study of Heredity and Environment.* Chicago, University of Chicago Press, 1937.

Nicolaidis, S. Early systematic responses to orogastric stimulation in the regulation of food and water balance: Functional and electrophysiological data. *Annals of the New York Academy of Sciences*, 1969, *157*, 1176-1203.

Nisbett, R. E. Determinants of food intake in human obesity. *Science*, 1968, *159*, 1254-1255. (a)

Nisbett, R. E. Taste, deprivation and weight determinants of eating behavior. *Journal of Personality and Social Psychology*, 1968, *10* 107-116. (b)

Nisbett, R. E. Hunger, obesity and the ventiomedial hypothalamus. *Psychological Review*, 1972, *79*, 433-453.

Nisbett, R. E. and Kanouse, D. Obesity, food deprivation and supermarket shopping behavior. *Journal of Personality and Social Psychology*, 1969, *12*, 289-294.

Nisbett, R. E. and Storms, M. D. Cognitive, social, physiological determinants of food intake. *Cognitive Modification of Emotional Behavior* (London, H. and Nisbett, R. E., Eds.). Chicago: Aldine, 1975.

Nisbett, R. E. and Temoshok, L. Is there an external cognitive style? *Journal of Personality and Social Psychology*, 1976, *33*, 36-47.

Ochberg, F. M., Pollack, I. W., and Meyer, E. Correlation of pulse and time judgment. *Perceptual Motor Skills*, 1964, *19*, 861-862.

Ornstein, R. *On the Experience of Time.* Middlesex, England: Penguin, 1969.

Paintal, A. S. *J. Physiology (London)*, 1954, *126*, 255-265.

Parra-Covarrubias, A., Rivera-Rodriguez, I., and Almaraz-Vgalde, A. Cephalic phase of insulin secretion in obese adolescents. *Diabetes*, 1971, *20*, 800-802.

Pfaffmann, C. The pleasures of sensation. *Psychological Review*, 1960, *65*, 253–268.

Pliner, P. On the generalizability of the externality hypothesis. *Obese Humans and Rats* (Schachter, S., and Rodin, J., Eds.). Washington, D.C.: Erlbaum/Halsted, 1974.

Polivy, J. Perception of calories and regulation of intake in restrained and unrestrained subjects. *Addictive Behaviors*, 1976, *1*, 237–243.

Price, J. M. and Grinker, J. Effects of degree of obesity, food deprivation and palatability on eating behavior of humans. *Journal of Comparative and Physiological Psychology*, 1973, *85*, 265–271.

Rabinowitz, D. and Zeirler, K. L. Forearm metabolism in obesity and its response to intra-arterial insulin. Characterization of insulin resistance and evidence for adaptive hyperinsulinism. *Journal of Clinical Investigation*, 1962, *41*: 2173–2181.

Rodin, J. Effects of distraction on the performance of obese and normal subjects. *Journal of Comparative and Physiological Psychology*, 1973, *83*, 68–78.

Rodin, J. Causes and consequences of time perception differences in overweight and normal-weight people. *Journal of Personality and Social Psychology*, 1975, *31*, 898–910. (a)

Rodin, J. The effects of obesity and set point on taste responsiveness and intake in humans. *Journal of Comparative and Physiological Psychology*, 1975, *89*. (b)

Rodin, J. The relationship between external responsiveness and the development and maintenance of obesity. *Hunger: Basic Mechanisms and Clinical Implications* (Novin, D., Wyrwicka, W., and Bray, G. A., Eds.). New York: Raven Press, 1976.

Rodin, J. Research on eating behavior and obesity: Where does it fit in personality and social psychology. *Personality and Social Psychology Bulletin*, 1977, *3* No. 3.

Rodin, J., Bray, G. A., Atkinson, R. L., Dahms, W. T., Greenway, F. L., Hamilton, K., and Molitch, M. Predictors of successful weight loss in an outpatient obesity clinic. *International Journal of Obesity*, 1977, *1*, 79–87.

Rodin, J., Elman, D., and Schachter, S. Emotionality and obesity. *Obese Humans and Rats* (Schachter, S., and Rodin, J., Eds.). Washington, D.C.: Erlbaum/Wiley, 1974.

Rodin, J. and Goodman, N. R. Selective attention in overweight and normal weight individuals. Unpublished manuscript, Yale University, 1976.

Rodin, J., Herman, C. P., and Schachter, S. Obesity and various tests of external sensitivity. *Obese Humans and Rats* (Schachter, S., and Rodin, J., Eds.). Washington, D.C.: Erlbaum/Halsted, 1974.

Rodin, J., Moskowitz, H. R., and Bray, G. A. Relationship between obesity, weight loss and taste responsiveness. *Physiology and Behavior*, 1976, *17*, 591–597.

Rodin, J. and Rubin, S. Creativity differences in overweight and normal-weight persons. Unpublished manuscript, Yale University, 1976.

Rodin, J. and Singer, J. Eye-shift, thought and obesity. *Journal of Personality*, 1976, *44*, 594–610.

Rodin, J. and Slochower, J. Fat chance for a favor: Obese-normal differences in compliance and incidental learning. *Journal of Personality and Social Psychology*, 1974, *29*, 557–565.

Rodin, J. and Slochower, J. Externality in the nonobese: The effects of environmental responsiveness on weight. *Journal of Personality and Social Psychology*, 1976, *29*, 557–565.

Rodin, J., Slochower, J., and Fleming, B. The effects of degree of obesity, age of onset, and energy deficit on external responsiveness. *Journal of Comparative and Physiological Psychology*, 1977, *91*, No. 3, 586–597.

Rolls, E. T., Burton, M. J., and Mora, F. Hypothalamic neuronal responses associated with the sight of food. *Brain Research*, 1976, *111*, 53–56.

Rony, H. R. *Obesity and Leanness*. Philadelphia: Lea and Febiger, 1940.

Ross, L. Effects of manipulating the salience of food upon consumption by obese and normal eaters. *Obese Humans and Rats* (Schachter, S. and Rodin, J., Eds.): Washington, D.C.: Erlbaum/Wiley, 1974.

Ross, L. D., Pliner, P., Nesbitt, P., and Schachter, S. Patterns of externality in the eating behavior of obese and normal college students. *Emotion, Obesity and Crime* (Schachter, S., Ed.). New York: Academic Press, 1971.

Rozin, P. Psychological and cultural determinants of food choice. *Appetite and Food Intake* (Silverstone, T., Ed.). Braunschweig: Pergamon Press/Vieweg, 1976.

Rozin, P. and Kalat, J. W. Specific hungers and poison avoidance as adaptive specializations of learning. *Psychological Review*, 1971, *78*, 459–486.

Salans, L. B., Cushman, S. W., and Wiseman, R. E. Studies of human adipose cell size and number in nonobese and obese patients. *Journal of Clinical Investigation*, 1973, *52*, 929.

Salans, L. B., Knittle, J. L., and Hirsch, J. The role of adipose cell size and adipose tissue insulin sensitivity in the carbohydrate intolerance of human obesity. *Journal of Clinical Investigation*, 1968, *47*, 153–165.

Schachter, S. Obesity and eating. *Science*, 1968, *161*, 751–756.

Schachter, S. *Emotion, Obesity, and Crime.* New York: Academic Press, 1971.

Schachter, S., Friedman, L., and Handler, J. Who eats with chopsticks? *Obese Humans and Rats* (Schachter, S., and Rodin, J., Eds.). Washington, D.C.: Erlbaum/Wiley, 1974.

Schachter, S., Goldman, R., and Gordon, A. Effects of fear, food deprivation and obesity on eating. *Journal of Personality and Social Psychology*, 1968, *10*, 91–97.

Schachter, S. and Gross, L. Manipulated time and eating behavior. *Journal of Personality and Social Psychology*, 1968, *10*, 98–106.

Schachter, S. and Rodin, J. *Obese Humans and Rats.* Washington, D.C.: Erlbaum/Halsted, 1974.

Schwartz, G. E. Psychosomatic disorders and biofeedback: Psychobiological model of disregulation. *Psychopathology: Experimental Models* (Maser, J. and Seligman, M., Eds.). San Francisco: W. H. Freeman and Company, 1977.

Sechzer, J. A., Turner, S. G., and Leibelt, R. A. Motivation and learning in mice after gold thioglucose-induced hypothalamic lesions. *Psychonomic Science*, 1966, *4*, 259–260.

Sharma, R. N. and Nasset, E. S. *Am. J. Physiol.*, 1962, *202*, 725–730.

Shields, J. *Monozygotic twins brought up apart and brought up together: An investigation into the genetic and environmental causes of variation in personality.* London: Oxford University Press, 1962.

Shorvan, H. J. and Richardson, J. S. Sudden obesity and psychological trauma. *British Medical Journal*, 1949, *2*.

Sims, E. A. H., Danforth, E., Jr., Horton, E. S., Bray, G. A., Glennon, J. A., and Salans, L. B. Endocrine and metabolic effects of experimental obesity in man. *Recent Progress in Hormonal Research*, 1973, *29*, 457–496.

Sims, E. A. H., Goldman, R. F., Gluck, C. M., Horton, E. S., Kelleher, P. C., and Rowe, D. W. Experimental obesity in man. *Transcripts of the Association of American Psychiatrists*, 1968, *81*, 153–170.

Sims, E. A. H. and Horton, E. S. Endocrine and metabolic adaptation to obestiy and starvation. *American Journal of Clinical Nutrition*, 1968, *21*, 1455–1470.

Singh, D. Role of response habits and cognitive factors in determination of behavior of obese humans. *Journal of Personality and Social Psychology*, 1973, *27*, 220–238.

Solow, C., Silberfarb, P. M., and Swift, K. Psychosocial effects of intestinal bypass surgery for severe obesity. *New England Journal of Medicine*, 1974, *290*, 300–304.

Spiegel, T. Calorie regulation of food intake in man. *Journal of Comparative and Physiological Psychology*, 1973, *83*, 24–37.

Srole, L., Langner, T. S., Michael, S. T., Opler, M. K., and Rennie, T. A. C. *Mental Health in the Metropolis: The Mid-town Manhattan Study*, New York: McGraw-Hill, 1962.

Steffens, A. B. Plasma insulin content in relation to blood glucose level and meal pattern in the normal and hypothalamic hyperphagic rat. *Physiology and Behavior*, 1970, *5*, 147–151.

Stricker, E. M. and Zigmond, M. J. Brain catecholamines and the lateral hypothalamic syndrome. *Hunger: Basic Mechanisms and Clinical Implications* (Novin, D., Ed.). New York: Raven Press, 1976.

Stunkard, A. J. Obesity. *Comprehensive Textbook of Psychiatry* (Freedman, A. M., Kaplan, H. I., Kaplan, H. S., Eds.) 1st ed., Baltimore: Williams and Wilkins, 1967.

Stunkard, A. J. Presidential Address – 1974: From explanation to action in psychosomatic medicine: The case of obesity. *Psychosomatic Medicine*, 1975, *37* No. 3.

Stunkard, A. J. and Koch, C. The interpretation of gastric motility: I. Apparent bias in the reports of hunger by obese persons. *Archives of General Psychiatry*, 1964, *11*, 74–82.

Swanson, D. W. and Dinello, F. A. Follow-up of patients starved for obesity. *Psychosomatic Medicine*, 1970, *32*, 209–214.

Teitelbaum, P. Sensory control of hypothalamic hyperphagia. *Journal of Comparative and Physiological Psychology*, 1955, *48*, 156–163.

Teitelbaum, P. Random and food directed activity in hyperphagic and normal rats. *Journal of Comparative and Physiological Psychology*, 1957, *50*, 486–490.

Teitelbaum, P. and Campbell, B. A. Ingestion patterns in hyperphagic and normal rats. *Journal of Comparative and Physiological Psychology*, 1957, *51*, 135–140.

Thayer, R. E. Measurement of activation through self-report. *Psychological Reports*, 1967, *20*, 663–378.

Tom, G. and Rucker, M. Fat, full and happy. *Journal of Personality and Social Psychology*, 1975, *32*, 761–766.

Turner, S. G., Sechzer, J. A., and Liebelt, R. A. Sensitivity to electric shock after ventiomedial hypothalamic lesions. *Experimental Neurology*, 1967, *19*, 236–244.

Valenstein, E. S., Cox, V. C., and Kakolewski, J. W. Reexamination of the role of the hypothalamus in motiviation. *Psychological Reviews*, 1970, *77*, 16–31.

Van Itallie, T. B. Diet Related to Killer Diseases II. Hearings before the Select Committee on Nutrition and Human Needs of the United States Senate, Ninety-fifth Congress (First Session) February 1977, Part 2, Obesity, p. 44.

Van Itallie, T. B. and Campbell, R. B. Multidisciplinary approach to the problem of obesity. *Journal of the American Dietetic Association*, 1972, *61*, 385.

Wayner, M. J. Specificity of behavioral regulation. *Physiology and Behavior*, 1974, *12*, 851–869.

Werkman, S. L. and Greenberg, E. S. Personality and interest patterns in obese adolescent girls. *Psychosomatic Medicine*, 1967, *24*, 72–75.

Wheatley, M. D. The hypothalamus and affective behavior in cats. *Archives of Neurology and Psychiatry*, 1944, *52*, 296–316.

White, C. The effects of viewing film of different arousal content on the eating behavior of obese and normal weight subjects. *Dissertation Abstracts International*, 1973, *34* (5-B), 2324.

Withers, R. F. J. Problems in the genetics of human obesity. *Eugen. Rev.*, 1964, *56*, 81–90.

Wolgin, D. L., Cytawa, J., and Teitelbaum, P. The role of activation in the regulation of food intake. *Hunger: Basic Mechanisms and Clinical Implications* (Novin, D., Wyrwicka, W., and Bray, G. A., Eds.). New York: Raven Press, 1976.

Woods, S. C., Vasselli, J. R., Kaestner, E., Szakmary, G. A., Milburn, P., and Vitiello, M. V. Conditioned insulin secretion and meal feeding in rats. *Journal of Comparative and Physiological Psychology*, 1977, *91*, No. 1, 128–133.

Wooley, O. Long-term food regulation in the obese and nonobese. *Psychosomatic Medicine*, 1971, *33*, 436.

Wooley, O. and Wooley, S. C. The experimental psychology of obesity. *Obesity: Pathogenesis and Management* (Silverstone, T. and Finckam, J., Eds.). Lancaster: Medical and Technical Publishing Co., Ltd., 1975.

Wooley, S. C.   Physiologic versus cognitive factors in short-term food regulation in the obese and nonobese. *Psychosomatic Medicine*, 1972, *34*, 62.

Wooley, S. C. et al. Physiological aspects of feeding. *Appetite and Food Intake* (Silverstone, T., Ed.). Braunschweig: Pergamon Press, 1976.

4

Depression and Obesity

Benjamin B. Wolman

DEPRESSION AS A MOST FREQUENT CAUSE OF OBESITY

It is not true that obesity is always associated with or produced by a distinct type of mental disorder. In over thirty years of clinical practice I have treated obese individuals who suffered from a variety of emotional problems that could fit practically any clinical category of the *Diagnostic and Statistical Manual of the American Psychiatric Association.* Some obese patients I saw in my office were mildly neurotic, while others were manic-depressive and schizophrenic psychotics. All of them, however, suffered from various degrees of depression and were torn by feelings of helpless anger directed toward themselves.

Bruch (1977, Vol. 8, p. 97) noticed that the "absence of uniform psychological features is often cited as evidence against the etiological importance of psychological factors." The fact is that even thyroid dysfunction and resulting obesity could be related to emotional disorder (Alexander and Flagg, 1965), and psychological factors, especially depression, are most frequent causes of obesity. Several research workers arrived at a similar conclusion (Atkinson and Ringuette, 1967; Bosin, 1953; Bruch, 1957, 1961, 1973, 1977; Bychowski, 1950; Kurland, 1967; Nisbett, 1968; Reichman, 1972; Schachter, 1967; Stunkard, 1976; and others).

Some researchers have pointed to the connection between a low socioeconomic status and obesity. Stunkard (1962, 1976) compared the socioeconomic level of one thousand people with the socioeconomic level of their parents. The evidence of the connection between obesity and the level of income was overwhelming; the lower the socioeconomic status of an individual and of his parents was, the greater was the likelihood of overweight. The hypothesis that a low socioeconomic status gives rise to feelings of frustration and depression and, consequently, to obesity has been supported by several research workers, among them Goldblatt et al. (1965) who found 30 percent obesity in women of lower socioeconomic class compared to only 5 percent obesity in upper-class women.

EXOGENOUS DEPRESSION

The term depression does not indicate a clearcut clinical category. Wolman's *Dictionary of Behavioral Science* (p. 94) defines depression as a feeling of helplessness, hopelessness, inadequacy, and sadness. These feelings may be symptomatic of several mental disorders, but they also occur in normal individuals. When depression is caused by real misfortunes, failures, defeats, or losses, it is *exogenous;* when it is not related to any real events but stems from within, it is *endogenous.*

Exogenous depression can be normal provided it is, like all other normal human emotions, appropriate, proportionate, controllable, and adjustive. Achievement and victory produce elation; frustration and defeat cause depression. When depression corresponds to what has really taken place, it is *appropriate* and does not indicate poor mental health (Jacobson, 1957), but feeling unhappy in victory and enjoying defeat are morbid emotional reactions.

Joys and sorrows usually correspond to the magnitude of fortunate and unfortunate events. They are *proportionate* emotional reactions. When someone is ecstatically happy at irrelevant and minor achievements and reacts with an abysmal feeling of despair to slight difficulties and frustrations, his reactions are disproportionate and therefore pathological.

Mature adults can *control* the expression of their emotions. Infants react instantly and impulsively; so do some disturbed adults. Mature individuals are capable of a rational self-control and refrain from giving uninhibited vent to their feelings. A total loss of self-control is typical for severe psychotic disorders.

Adjustive reactions are the fourth attribute of emotional balance. It is maladjustive and abnormal to wallow in misery and perpetuate feelings of gloom and doom. Normal adults look for remedies and seek solutions to their difficulties. They learn from their experiences and try to avoid past errors.

ENDOGENOUS DEPRESSION

Quite often a patient of mine will say, "I feel miserable. I know I have no reason to feel unhappy. Everything I can think of is just fine. I have nothing to complain about, but why do I feel so miserable?"

Decrease in self-esteem and a low estimate of one's power is the common denominator of all depressive states. The less realistic this estimate is, the more pathological is the depression. In some cases depression is unrelated to the actual loss of power. This intrapsychic or endogenous depression is not a product of a real loss or defeat. It comes from within, from a peculiar intrapsychic constellation.

People who experience endogenous depression lack self-confidence, blame themselves, feel isolated and forsaken, have a pessimistic outlook on life, and feel exhausted or agitated. They are unable to sleep, they overeat or undereat, and they dwell on past events.

Endogenous depression is a symptom of mental disorder. The outstanding features of pathological depressions are (1) their endogenous origins, unrelated and disproportionate to real events, (2) unjustified self-accusations, and (3) a tendency to perpetuate the depression instead of seeking a way out. These three characteristics are irrational and often lead to even less rational confessions of uncommitted sins and the wish to be punished.

Endogenous depression may be associated with a variety of psychosociogenic as well as organic mental disorders. One must draw a clear line between a depressed epileptic and a depressed schizophrenic, that is, between depression as a symptom and depression as a clinical entity that can manifest itself on a neurotic and character neurotic level leading to a full-blown depressive psychosis, called manic-depressive or affect psychosis. I called it dysmutual disorder (Wolman, 1973).

PSYCHOANALYTIC INTERPRETATIONS

In the paper "Mourning and Melancholia," Freud (1917) compared melancholia with normal grief. Melancholia resembles mourning for it occurs after the loss of a loved person; however, unlike mourning, melancholia occurs only in individuals who are already disturbed. Melancholia is a regression from mature object relations to the earliest way of relating to objects, namely, to narcissistic identification, in which the object is not distinguished from the ego, and to the oral phase of personality development.

Psychoanalytic thinking has been particularly concerned with object loss, stressing the mechanism of introjection and identification (Fenichel, 1945).

In the 1950 and 1951 Symposia of the American Psychoanalytic Association, emphasis was placed on object loss in depression (Greenacre, 1953). Greenacre stressed "identification of the subject with the object loss." Pathogenic depression is characterized by its "intensity, excessive duration and dominance of the organism." Physical symptoms such as decreased motor activity and visceral disorder bear witness to the overall involvement in depression.

Bibring (ibid.) maintained that the basic "mechanism of depression" is a decrease in self-esteem due to one's real or imaginary partial or total helplessness. Depression is a reaction to feelings of inferiority and guilt.

Most participants of the panels stressed the role of love deprivation in early childhood. There was, however, no agreement as to whether aggression plays a central or secondary role in depression. It has been pointed out that depressives have oral fantasies and are inclined to seek oral gratification by overeating. Obese people are frustrated in their adult life and regress to the oral level. They overeat in order to fill the void in their life. Their regression brings back the pleasures of bottle or breast feeding and allows the obese person to avoid facing the hardships of adult life.

According to Bychowski (1950), compulsive eating is a result of separation anxiety. Overeating is the most complete form of introjection, that is, "cannibalistic incorporation."

The connection between loss and oral cravings has been stressed by Abraham (1911, 1924), Freud (1917), and several other psychoanalysts. It is worthwhile to mention the custom of having a big meal after a funeral, which resembles the primitive oral-cannibalistic rites. Apparently, the intake of food may serve as a substitute for unobtained love or loss of a beloved person (Bruch, 1969).

This idea was corroborated by several authors. Rothman and Becker (1970) reported cases of obesity in children after death of a parent, hospitalization of the mother, parental divorce, desertion by the father, the child's hospitalization, and being sent away to boarding school. Abandonment makes a child feel helpless, and being powerless is the core of depressive feelings, as will be explained in the following pages.

OBESITY AND THE DRIVE FOR POWER

All factors that serve survival can be put together under the name *basic needs*. Oxygen, water, food, rest, and all other factors necessary for the survival of organisms are basic needs. Survival is the common denominator of all basic needs. Thus power can be defined as the *ability to satisfy needs*. The more power one possesses, the better are one's chances for survival (Wolman, 1974).

The simplest power is the power of muscles, jaws, and claws. Intelligence, cunning, and manipulation represent a higher level of power. Material goods, mansions and vaults, huge tracts of land, and powerful fortresses are signs and insignia of power. People driven by their craving for power may acquire properties far beyond any possibility of ever using them and build unmanageable empires and unwieldly conglomerates. Success, status, conquest, wealth – all these terms point to the never-ending and futile human effort to deny human frailty and mortality.

No human being is so powerful as to be able to fight his adversaries singlehandedly. Even at the peak of power, one depends on allies.

The weaker one is, the more help one needs. Newborn infants are totally dependent upon parental support. Freud discovered the connection between the oral intake of food and all future ways and means of gratification and pleasure. Freud's discovery was corroborated by several studies, and Spitz's (1945) observations of children deprived of mothering offered solid empirical evidence for the existence of the infants' need to feel accepted. According to Spitz, the infants received adequate food and physical care, but the lack of affection and love proved to be devastating to their personality development. Similar ideas have been expressed by Sullivan (1953) and Horney (1950).

When a child feels accepted, he reacts with acceptance. Part of his libido, initially cathected (invested) in himself, turns toward people and objects which satisfy his needs. He begins to "love" them; that is, he wishes them to perpetuate their actions and to keep on satisfying him. The more satisfaction he receives, the more secure he feels. *Security is synonymous to the feeling of power;* whoever feels strong feels secure, and people feel secure whenever they believe in their power.

Infants perceive, or empathize with, people in the environment in two dimensions: *power,* which is the ability to satisfy needs, and *acceptance,* which is the willingness to do so. The mother can help; thus she is perceived as a strong person. The little brother and the old grandfather are weak, helpless onlookers. Infants turn to the strong people, but as they grow and become stronger they learn to depend on their own power.

The drive for power influences almost all human activities. Alfred Adler (1927) has interpreted the drive for power as a reaction against what he believed to be a universal feeling of inferiority. May (1969) related neurotic behavior to the drive for power. McClelland and associates (1961, 1971) stressed the importance of power motivation.

Depression is a self-directed helpless anger. It is an angry feeling of one's own weakness and helplessness. Depressed people are angry at the whole world for not helping them. They are most angry at themselves for being weak. They hate themselves for being weak and often act in a self-destructive manner, as if trying to punish themselves. *Obesity* is one of the choice *self-punitive* devices.

Depressed people are starved for love. They are hungry and insatiable. The more they get, the more they crave, and when they do not get enough — and there is never enough for them — they are angry at those who fail to give them enough and angry at themselves for being unable to get what they want. Depressed individuals are irritable, prone to anger, and at the same time overflowing and overdoing love and affection. Their hostile or friendly overdemanding and exaggerated behavior usually discourages other people and makes depressed individuals still more depressed.

Even a success in social relations leads to self-defeating maneuvers. In their innermost thoughts they do not believe that they deserve love; they feel that those who love them must be wrong or stupid or worthless. At any rate, this is never the "great love" they dreamed of, and certainly there must be something wrong with whoever gives love or with the love he or she gives to them. I had the opportunity to see several depressed patients who destroyed whatever they attained. In my book *Victims of Success* (Wolman, 1973b), I described several cases of such self-defeating behavior of people who wrecked their chances for success and happiness in their personal life and in their business and profession. In several instances, the defeat they brought upon themselves and/or the loss of a friend, lover, or marital spouse — which they themselves engineered — led to an overeating spell.

Frequently, overeating served one or both purposes: "If I can't get love, let me fill the void with food." Or, "It's all my fault! I always mess up things! Let me make myself fat and repulsive!"

The relationship between depression and overeating can take on several forms and shapes. Several patients of mine reported that whenever they suffered a real loss or defeat, they went on an overeating spell. The 35-year-old Mrs. J. rapidly gained weight when her mother died. The same happened to Mr. R. after the death of his mother.

The gain of weight is usually more persistent when the depression is endogenous. Whenever Mr. H. felt depressed, he rapidly gained weight. He somehow felt "more powerful" on a full stomach, and dieting was aggravating his depression. Mr. L. felt the same way, and any true or imaginary frustration was a clear signal to overeat. In these two cases, overeating represented a gain of power.

AFFILIATION MOTIVE AND DEPRESSION

As I have mentioned, no human being is capable of satisfying all his or her needs, and every human life starts in a state of *total dependence* on support from without. As children grow, the degree of dependence is gradually reduced, but no human being can ever attain full independence. Adulthood is not independence but interdependence, and even the most powerful individuals need allies, that is, they need to be accepted.

The need for acceptance (some authors call it affiliation) is one of the fundamental needs of practically all organic nature. Some comparative psychologists named it the "herd instinct," since a great many species group together for co-operative hunting and protection against predators. Only a few primates seem not to affiliate, among them pygmy hippos, forest dwelling moose, the aye-aye, and some orangutangs. Affiliation, cooperation, and acceptance are the various names for a behavior of helping one another in the fight for survival, that is, in getting food and whatever else organisms need and in mutual protection against enemies (Schachter, 1959). Loneliness implies weakness; having no allies makes one vulnerable and is therefore conducive to exogenous depression.

Adults' security depends on their own power first and acceptance second; children's security depends first on acceptance by others and then on their own power.

Power has been defined as the ability to satisfy needs, and survival is certainly the arch need. Acceptance has been defined as the willingness to satisfy needs of other people — that is, to help, protect, and defend.

Children must receive an adequate amount of protection in order to function freely as children. A child has the right to be a child and, as such, deserves all the parental protection and acceptance he needs to give him the feeling of security.

Children have no say in choosing their environment and influencing their opportunities. Adults have some degree of mobility; they can change jobs, place of residence, marital relations, religion, and their business, social, and political affiliations. Children are born to, and brought up by, people they did not choose, and for several years they are a captive audience in their parents' homes.

In most instances adults can create a more or less stable environment. If we exclude major catastrophies, adults can live all their lives in a certain neighborhood, practice a certain occupation, develop friendly relations with neighbors and relatives, and establish daily routines of their choice. Children do not have these options; they must move to a new neighborhood and attend a new school; they may feel uprooted whenever their parents decide to change their place of residence, the family relationships, or any other social interaction.

Adults remain adult as long as they live, whether they are young or middle-aged or old, and their behavioral patterns are more or less circumscribed by sex, age, occupation, religion, and so on. Children's behavioral patterns are in a continuous flux for *children need not remain children.*

All children wish to please their parents. This wish, conscious or unconscious, is related to the basic drive for survival. Parental approval means food and protection and the feeling of safety.

The worst childhood fear is the fear of abandonment (Wolman, 1978). As mentioned earlier, all human beings derive the feeling of security from two sources: their own power and the loyalty and power of their allies. The child's own power is negligible; the younger he is, the less power he has. His feeling of security depends on the power of his parents and their willingness to use it to protect him. Abandonment is therefore the worst thing that can happen to a child, for his supply of food and his very survival depend on parental care.

It is not enough for a child to get food now. His security depends on his belief that the food and protection will be forthcoming in the future. The newborn child is endowed with empathy, that is, the ability to perceive nonverbal signals and feel whether or not he is loved by the feeding mother or maternal substitute. This ability imbues the infant with feelings of security and euphoria, or fear and anxiety. Infants need to be loved, and they are happy when the feeding mother hugs, kisses, and speaks affectionately. When the feeding mother resents the child and thinks how great her life could be without the baby, the child empathizes with her feelings and becomes anxiety ridden, and fears mother will abandon him.

Rejection causes depression. Lonely children are depressed children. Unloved children fear abandonment, and abandonment means starvation and death.

PARENT-CHILD RELATIONSHIPS

My clinical observations indicate that practically all cases of obesity start in childhood and that the parent-child relationship plays a highly significant role in children's eating habits and obesity. Atkinson and Ringuette (1967) studied individuals whose weight was 100 percent over the average. Eighty-one percent of them started to gain weight at the age of twelve or earlier, and they became obese in adolescence or somewhat later. The authors pointed to depression, frustrations, and boredom as the causes of obesity. Eighty-six percent of these obese individuals had at least one obese family member. Bruch (1947, 1957, 1971, 1973, 1977) in her numerous publications reported the role of parental attitudes in children's obesity. Several other authors reported similar findings (Goldblatt et al., 1965; Mayer, 1968; Reichman, 1972; Rothman and Becker, 1970; Schachter and Rodin, 1974; Stunkard, 1976; and others).

Many obese people dissociate their craving for food from the normal feeling of hunger. They are preoccupied with thoughts of food all the time and they are unaware whether they are hungry or not. Stunkard (1959) and Stunkard and Koch (1964) measured the contractions of stomachs in obese individuals. The contractions recorded on the gastric baloon used by the investigators were not at all related to the craving for food of the obese individuals who frequently reported hunger irrespective of the stomach contractions.

Some authors believe that people affected with obesity have somehow failed to learn to discriminate between contractions of the stomach related to food deprivation and those related to emotional states, and that they react with craving for food whenever they are depressed or worried (Bruch, 1961, 1973).

The reason for the dissociation between hunger and intake of food is related to childhood experiences. Parental feeding supplies children with more than food, for giving food implies giving love. Loving parents feed their children, and well-fed children feel loved and thus secure. Receiving food is reassuring, and children derive a triple satisfaction from eating, for in addition to satisfying hunger and providing gustatory pleasure it is also a sign of being cared for and loved. Thus feeding provides nutrition, pleasure, and security.

Quite often parents overplay and/or misdirect the feeding process. Some parents praise children who overeat and criticize poor eaters. Normally, the amount of food taken in by an infant corresponds, more or less, to the physiological needs of the infant's organism. Some parents give the children the impression that overeating is a sign of good health, and many a mother praises the infant for finishing the bottle. The infant is rewarded for *eating without hunger*

(Stunkard, 1959, 1962, 1976) and he or she has learned to eat for a maternal smile.

Apparently some children are made to believe that the more they eat, the more their parents will love them. Children who overeat in order to please their parents gradually become conditioned to eat large quantities of food even when they are not hungry. One of my exceedingly obese patients, Ms. K. was taught by her mother to consume large amounts of food irrespective of hunger and with little attention to taste. As she grew older, she continued to overeat.

On several occasions she tried to diet with the help of all sorts of pills, but as soon as she began to lose weight she went back to overeating. The fear of maternal disapproval and guilt feelings for disobeying her mother prevented her from losing weight. Ms. K. was an adult person, but her mind was still in the grip of maternal rules and regulations. Her own superego took over the role of the nagging mother, and *losing weight made her feel guilty* and more and more depressed.

Some insecure and guilt-ridden parents try to overcome their own emotional shortcomings by an overzealous and overprotecting attitude in feeding. It is worthwhile to mention that the rejecting-accepting parents (parents who basically reject their children but, once in a while, when they are guilt ridden, shower their child with food and affection) have most often obese offspring.

Parental overprotection is not necessarily a sign of love. When a mother says to a child, "You cannot tie your shoe laces, or comb your hair, or set the table," and so on, and "I will do it for you," she actually tells the child, "You are clumsy or stupid or inadequate." Love is helping and encouraging, but overprotective parents discourage their child, prevent his or her mental growth and maturation, and plant seeds of insecurity. In most cases, the mothers of obese children tend to be domineering and overprotective women who treat their child as if he or she were an inanimate object to be used as compensation for the mother's true or imaginary troubles and ills, with no respect for the child and his needs. Food is overvalued, as if a chubby infant were to serve as evidence of his own health and his mother's love and devotion.

When the obese child reaches adolescence and is criticized by classmates and neighbors, the insecure mother often joins the critics. The obese child is torn between his already established desire to overeat in order to please the mother of yesterday and the fear of malicious criticism and ridicule by peers and by his mother today.

Bruch (1947, 1971) noticed that the overprotecting mothers are quite ambivalent toward their children and alternate their *overprotectiveness* with outbursts of hostility which produce in the child a feeling of low self-esteem, a conviction of his helplessness, and a clinging to the overprotecting mother who is really a rejecting mother.

OBESITY RELATED TO DYSMUTUAL (MANIC-DEPRESSIVE) DISORDERS

Abraham (1911, 1924) was the first psychoanalyst to interpret the manic-depressive disorder. Abraham proposed a most interesting hypothesis that unfortunately failed to attract much attention. At that time, Freud maintained that repressed sexuality leads to anxiety; Abraham hypothesized that repressed hostility leads to depression (Abraham, 1911, pp. 151). Abraham's essay, with its emphasis on hostility, has influenced my thoughts.

My studies have led me to establish a link among the various degrees of endogenous depression, viewed as a nosological entity, on a continuum of neurotic symptoms (hysterias, etc.) through hysteroid character neurosis, latent psychosis, and full-blown psychotic depression. The moods of elation and depression are reflections of shifts in the balance of libidinal cathexes from self-love to object love, from self-hate to object hate, from love to hate, and vice versa. I have called this group of disorders *dysmutual depressive,* because mutual relationships are disturbed and the underlying dynamics is that of self-depreciation, self-accusation, and self-defeating behavior (Wolman, 1973, 1979).

There has been a good deal of evidence that lack of maternal love causes severe depression and "affect hunger" (Bowlby, 1963; Spitz, 1945; and many others).

According to Alfred Adler (1927), the rejected child may try to win love by intentional suffering and escape into illness. "The discouraged child who finds that he can tyrannize best by tears will be a cry-baby, and a direct line of development leads from the cry-baby to the adult depressed patient," wrote Kurt Adler (1967, p. 332).

Frieda Fromm-Reichman (1959) found that most manic-depressives come from large families where no one is genuinely interested in the child's welfare. As a result of the lack of a true and meaningful relationship in childhood, the manic-depressive suffers from feelings of insecurity and rejection.

My clinical observations have led me to believe that depressive-dysmutual (manic-depressive) patients were exposed in childhood to a sort of *emotional seesaw* of acceptance and rejection, care and abandonment. The mothers of my severely depressed patients did not like their child; however, when the child was in serious trouble or gravely ill, the mothers turned around and showered the child with affection. These emotional swings were conducive to a self-defeating attitude in the offspring, for misery was the only way to win love.

Mothers of manic-depressives are neither kind, considerate, nor warm persons. Some are psychopathic, concerned about no one but themselves, resenting the burdens of motherhood, and often displaying violent tempers and brutality. The child who is to become a depressive psychotic is treated by his mother with rejection and sometimes with hate; in many cases, he has to compete, unsuccessfully, against a more privileged sibling. The future manic-depressive is the "Cinderella" of a family usually composed of a hostile mother, a disinterested or hostile father, and siblings favored by the mother.

The future manic-depressive is treated with outright dislike, except when he is seriously ill or in grave danger. He is the unwanted and unloved member of the family, treated like a burden and a handicap, except on those rare occasions when his sad condition forces his parents into a position of caring. In most cases, adequate maternal care is given to the infant in his first few months of life; the rejection coming somewhat later. Thus manic-depressives have a tendency to regress to infancy and even to a passive prenatal intrauterine life. Regression does not go back to the point of frustration or rejection, but below that point, to the true or imaginary era of the "lost paradise" of safety and love. In milder, neurotic cases of the dysmutual disorder (hysterias and depressive neuroses), the regression is usually to the oral stage, the main objective of which is *to win love.* Whatever behavioral and psychosomatic symptoms develop, all are geared to this goal; the dysmutual (manic-depressive) directs all his energies to gaining love.

Making oneself ugly, clumsy, and sick serves this purpose. The goal is to win love by self-defeat, and overweight is one of the choice methods.

The outstanding feature of dysmutual disorders is the "ever-hungry libido." A steady and friendly gratification of the infant's needs gradually introduces changes in the balance of cathexes. The infant receives love from the parents who give him their nondemanding love. However, when love is withheld from a child or when it is given in an unfriendly manner the infant is unable to develop proper emotional balance. Uncertain that his emotional needs will be satisfied, the infant feels permanently hungry. Thus, *manic-depressive patients consume gross quantities of food,* indicative of their oral-cannibalistic fixations. Unable to get love, they grab food.

The dysmutual is unable to love unless loved. The less love he gets, the more he needs. His feelings of being loved are usually short lived. Sooner or later he will experience the pangs of an emotional and physical hunger.

Dysmutuals overeat constantly, as if trying to fill the emotional void. They overeat to make themselves less attractive, less capable of an active life, less successful, and less healthy. They overeat in order to deepen their self-defeat, to prove to themselves that they are weak and unable to control their overweight; in the back of their minds looms the unconscious hope of gaining love by self-destructive behavior.

LOVE AND FOOD HUNGER

Emotionally balanced individuals tend to eat more when they are hungry and also when they are calm and in a good mood, and do not feel like eating when they are worried, upset, or frightened. Depressed people act in a different way. Food deprivation has little effect on the amount of food they eat, and their craving for food is the same irrespective of the amount of their previous food intake and the time lapsed. Anxiety and depression do not reduce their appetite; to the contrary, the more they are depressed, the more frequently they eat. They seem to be unsatisfied, in a close resemblance to their emotional makeup: they are love hungry and food hungry.

Schachter (1967, 1974) experimented with normal and obese people and found that obese people eat the same amount of food whether they were deprived of food or not and whether they felt secure or frightened. Normal people ate more when deprived of food and less when frightened. Apparently food deprivation does not affect the desire for food in overweight individuals. For obese people, eating does not appear to be related to any physiological condition and it is *stimulated by emotional factors,* such as anxiety, depression, fear, frustration, and so on.

OBESITY RELATED TO HYPERVECTORIAL
(SCHIZOPHRENIC) DISORDERS

As mentioned above, a depressive mood can be associated with various clinical entities. In my books and papers on schizophrenia (Wolman, 1961, 1965, 1966a, 1970, 1973) I have related the etiology of schizophrenia to peculiar intrafamilial dynamics. When two parents, disappointed and displeased with one another, expect their child to compensate for their misery and meet their emotional needs, they create a reversal of social roles and displacement of libido cathexes. The child is forced to give more love than he or she receives from the parents. Instead of the normal instrumental child-parent attitude, the child is forced to assume a precocious vectorial attitude and become, as it were, the parent of his or her parents. Thus, I called schizophrenia *Vectoriasis Praecox* (1966), and my book on schizophrenia in childhood is entitled *Children without Childhood* (1970). The child doomed to become schizophrenic is supposed to be a model child; he or she is constantly exposed to exaggerated parental expectations and demands (I called it the "overdemanded" child). However, since no child can satisfy the morbid parental demands, the efforts of the schizophrenic-to-be are doomed to fail, and a profound feeling of frustration and helplessness ensues. Schizophrenics are usually more depressed than the manic-depressive psychotics; they hate themselves for hating their parents. Some of them – the paranoid schizophrenics – project their hatred on others; catatonics, out of fear of their own anger, paralyze themselves. When the defenses collapse, schizophrenics act in uncontrollable fury. In my book *Call No Man Normal* (1973), I referred to them as "Fallen Angels." Obesity facilitates withdrawal from social relations.

Schizophrenics have wastefully overinvested emotional energy in their parents and have received very little (if anything at all) in return. They are on the verge of emotional bankruptcy, and latent schizophrenics avoid social contacts as if in order to save emotional energy. Their obesity serves as an alibi because, being obese, they have every reason to avoid derogatory comments, ridicule, and/or outright rejection. Being obese increases their feelings of hopelessness and helplessness, and they hate themselves for being so inadequate. Their obesity is a product of depression and perpetuates depression.

In some cases of latent schizophrenia, obesity serves as a defense mechanism against spending whatever emotional energy is available. Being obese and withdrawing from social interaction, latent schizophrenics unconsciously save energy and thus protect themselves against further deterioration (Wolman, 1966).

OBESITY AS SELF-DEFEAT

Depressed individuals often developed devious and morbid methods of coping with the torturous feeling of depression. Some of them turn to alcohol which makes them forget their misery. A frequent and generous intake of alcohol gives them the illusion of power. When intoxicated they believe themselves to be attractive, sociable, ready to embrace the entire world, and able to bring about an easy solution to all ills. They become elated, hyperoptimistic, and cocksure of themselves. Some of them turn to drugs which give them feelings of profound euphoria and omnipotence. This self-destructive behavior deepens their depressive moods and forces them to look toward ever-increasing and often lethal dosages. Some depressed individuals turn to food. They become *overeating addicts.*

Staying obese is one of the choice methods in the self-defeating behavior of depressed people. Being obese invites dislike, criticism, ridicule, and even ostracism. Children call an obese child "fatso" and other disparaging names. Friends and relatives are usually eager to offer unkind remarks about overweight, sugar-coated as advice and guidance.

Many obese people tend to withdraw from social contacts in order to avoid unpleasant remarks. Soon they may lose their friends and acquaintances and lead a lonely life — and eating becomes their main source of consolation and comfort. A vicious circle evolves: being overweight, they invite criticism and rejection, which induces them to avoid unpleasant encounters and seek comfort in food, which then makes them more obese, more rejected, more isolated, and so they eat more. Obesity leads to alienation, and alienation may contribute to obesity (Kurland, 1967; Wolman, 1973).

Some of my obese patients displayed an ingenious, albeit unconscious, device aimed at an irrational justification of their alleged helplessness. "Nobody can help me," said Mr. R., a gifted editor, "and I cannot help myself either. When the evening comes, I watch idiotic TV shows instead of doing something productive. In my office I am forced to work. I have to catch up with my work and I am taking some manuscripts home. Do you believe it? I didn't even open the manilla envelopes. I sit and nibble on whatever junky food I find in my refrigerator and watch TV. Why do I do it? I just can't help myself!"

The obese show defects of adaptation on many levels of development, often apparent as an overall immaturity. They also frequently show defects characterized by such words as "withdrawn" or "seclusive." Associated with this is a sense of helplessness, a conviction of inadequacy and inner ugliness, derogatory and self-destructive attitudes that are compensated for by flight in fantasies and daydreams (Bruch, 1958).

My obese patients often tell me the following story of their dieting. They did try to lose weight and went on all kinds of diets, with or without medications. Sometimes they lost weight in a short time, but regained it as fast as they lost it or even faster, for indeed they did not want to lose weight. In most instances, they wished and feared to get slim; consciously they liked the idea of losing weight, but their unconscious fear prevailed. Their obesity served as sort of an alibi for passivity and failure, and getting slim would have deprived them of the excuse of being passive. Some of my patients feared sexual relations and used their obesity as a convenient excuse. A success in dieting would have eliminated their choice defense mechanism and would force them to face their problem head on.

The failure in diet further contributes to one's feeling of helplessness. Quite often my patients bitterly complain about their lack of will power and inability to control their eating habits. This failure represents a self-fulfilling prophesy, for they wish to fail.

REFERENCES

Abraham, K. (1911). Notes on the psychoanalytic investigation and treatment of manic-depressive insanity and allied conditions. *Selected Papers on Psychoanalysis*. London: Hogarth, 1927.

Abraham, K. (1924). A short study of the development of the libido viewed in the light of mental disorders. *Selected Papers on Psychoanalysis*. New York: Basic Books, 1953.

Adler, A. *Understanding Human Nature*. New York: Greenberg, 1927.

Adler, K. Adler's individual psychology. *Psychoanalytic Techniques*. Wolman, B. B., Ed. New York: Basic Books, 1967.

Alexander, F. and Flagg, W. N. The psychosomatic approach. *Handbook of Clinical Psychology*. Wolman, B. B., Ed., pp. 855-947. New York: McGraw Hill, 1965.

Atkinson, R. M. and Ringuette, E. A survey of biographical and psychological features in extraordinary fatness. *Psychosomatic Medicine*, 1967, *29*, 121-133.

Bosin, H. W. *The Psychology of Overeating*. New York: National Vitamin Foundation, 1953.

Bruch, H. Psychological aspects of obesity. *Psychiatry*, 1947, *10*, 373-379.

Bruch, H. *The Importance of Overweight.* New York: Norton, 1957.

Bruch, H. Transformation of oral impulses in eating disorders: A conceptual approach. *Psychiatric Quarterly*, 1961, *35*, 458-470.

Bruch, H. Obesity and orality. *Contemporary Psychoanalysis*, 1969, *5*, 129-144.

Bruch, H. Family transactions in eating disorders. *Comprehensive Psychiatry*, 1971, *12*, 238-248.

Bruch, H. *Eating Disorders: Obesity, Anorexia Nervosa and the Person Within.* New York: Basic Books, 1973.

Bruch, H. Obesity and its treatment. *International Encyclopedia of Psychiatry, Psychology, Psychoanalysis, and Neurology*, Wolman, B. B. Ed., Vol. 8, 95-100. New York: Aesculapius Publishers, 1977.

Bychowski, G. On neurotic obesity. *Psychoanalytic Review*, 1950 *37*, 301-309.

Fenichel, O. *The Psychoanalytic Theory of Neurosis.* New York: Norton, 1945.

Freud, S. (1917) *Mourning and Melancholia*, Standard Edition, Vol. 14, pp. 243-258. London: Hogarth, 1962.

Fromm-Reichman, F. *Psychoanalysis and Psychotherapy.* Chicago: University Press, 1959.

Goldblatt, P. B., Moore, M. E., and Stunkard, A. J. Social factors in obesity. *Journal of the American Medical Association*, 1965, *192*, 1039-1057.

Greenacre, P. (Ed.). *Affective Disorders.* New York: International Universities Press, 1953.

Horney, K. *Neurosis and Human Growth.* New York: Norton, 1950.

Jacobson, E. On normal and pathological moods. *The Psychoanalytic Study of the Child*, 1957, *12*, 73-113.

Kurland, H. Extreme obesity: A psychophysiological disorder. *Psychosomatics*, 1967, *8*, 107-111.

May, R. *Love and Will.* New York: Norton, 1969.

Mayer, J. *Overweight: Causes, Cost and Control.* Englewood Cliffs, N.J.: Prentice Hall, 1968.

McClelland, D. C. *The Achieving Society.* Princeton, N. J.: Van Nostrand, 1961.

McClelland, D. C., Davis, W. N., Kalin, R., and Weimar, H. *Alcohol and Human Motivations.* New York: Free Press, 1971.

Mendelson, M., Weinbert, N., and Stunkard, A. J. Obesity in men: A clinical study of 25 cases. *Annals of Internal Medicine*, 1961, *54*, 660-680.

Nisbett, R. E. Taste, deprivation, and weight determinants of eating behavior. *Journal of Personality and Social Psychology*, 1968, *10*, 107-114.

Rado, S. The problem of melancholia. *International Journal of Psycho-Analysis*, 1928, *9*, 420-428.

Reichman, F. (Ed.). *Hunger and Satiety in Health and Disease.* Basel: Karger, 1972.

Rothman, M. and Becker, D. Traumatic situation in obesity. *Psychotherapy and Psychosomatics*, 1970, *18*, 372-376.

Schachter, S. *The Psychology of Affiliation.* Stanford: Stanford University Press, 1959.

Schachter, S. Cognitive effects on bodily functioning: Studies of obesity and eating. *Neurophysiology and Emotion*, (Glass, D. C., Ed.). New York: Rockefeller University Press and Russell Sage Foundation, 1967.

Schachter, S. and Rodin, J. *Obese Humans and Rats.* New York: Halstead Press, 1974.

Spitz, R. *The First Year of Life.* New York: International Universities Press, 1965.

Stunkard, A. J. Obesity and the denial of hunger. *Psychosomatic Medicine*, 1959, *21*, 281-288.

Stunkard, A. J. Research on a disease: Strategies in the study of obesity. *Physiological Correlates of Psychologic Orders.* (Rossler, R. and Greenfield, N. S., Eds.). Madison, Wisconsin: University of Wisconsin Press, 1962.

Stunkard, A. J. *The Pain of Obesity.* New York: Bull Publishing, 1976.

Stunkard, A. J. and Koch, C. The interpretation of gastric motility: I. Apparent bias in the reports of hunger by obese persons. *Archives of General Psychiatry*, 1964, *11*, 74-85.

Stunkard, A. J. and Mendelson, M. Obesity and the body image: I. Characteristics of disturbances in the body image of some obese persons. *American Journal of Psychiatry*, 1967, *10*, 123-130.

Sullivan, H. S. *Interpersonal Theory of Psychiatry.* New York: Norton, 1953.

Veroff, J. Power motivation. *International Encyclopedia of Psychiatry, Psychology, Psychoanalysis, and Neurology* (Wolman, B. B., Ed.) New York: Aesculapius Publishers, 1977.

Wolman, B. B. The fathers of schizophrenic patients. *Acta Psychotherapeutica*, 1961, *8*, 193-210.

Wolman, B. B. (Ed.). *Handbook of Clinical Psychology.* New York: McGraw Hill, 1965.

Wolman, B. B. *Vectoriasis Praecox or the Group of Schizophrenias.* Springfield: Thomas, 1966. (a)

Wolman, B. B. Doctor Jekyll and Mister Hyde: A new theory of the manic-depressive disorder. *Proceedings, New York Academy of Science*, 1966, *28*, 1020-1032. (b)

Wolman, B. B. *Children without Childhood: A Study of Childhood Schizophrenia.* New York: Grune and Stratton, 1970.

Wolman, B. B. *Dictionary of Behavioral Science.* New York: Van Nostrand Reinhold, 1972. (a)

Wolman, B. B. (Ed.) *Manual of Child Psychopathology.* New York: McGraw Hill, 1972. (b)

Wolman, B. B. *Call No Man Normal.* New York: New York: International Universities Press, 1973. (a)

Wolman, B. B. *Victims of Success.* New York: Quadrangle-New York Times, 1973. (b)

Wolman, B. B. Power and acceptance as determinants of social relations. *International Journal of Group Tensions*, 1974, *4*, 151-183.

Wolman, B. B. *Children's Fears.* New York: Grosset and Dunlap, 1978.

Wolman, B. B. (Ed.) *Clinical Diagnosis of Mental Disorders.* New York: Plenum, 1979.

5

Obesity in Adolescence

William A. Daniel, Jr.

According to biodata tables, 30 percent of the population of the United States exceeds ideal body weight. The incidence of obesity varies considerably in various populations, age groups, and according to definitions of obesity. Several nutrition surveys suggest that obesity is increasing in adolescents, that obese adults did not consistently have excessive birth weights, and that the majority of fat infants do not become obese children. However, obesity beginning in childhood is likely to continue into adolescence and adulthood. A general figure of 16 to 20 percent is usually given as the incidence of obesity in adolescents. From this, it is evident that obesity is a significant physical condition present during the adolescent years.

Questions arise as to the causes of obesity, why there is concern about excessive weight, and what the effects of obesity are on the psychological development of adolescents. The etiology of obesity is complex, multifaceted, and poorly understood. Genetic and environmental influences have been identified but their exact relationship remains unclear. There are, for example, critical periods for adipose cell development; heat production varies according to the quantity of "brown fat" in the body; economic factors are related to fatness or leanness; and parental obesity often influences the weight of children, even if they are adopted. Associations exist for obesity and certain disease states, for example, diabetes and hypertension. It has been said that suicide is the only common cause of death that does not strike earlier in the obese than the lean population.

Obesity is more frequent in affluent societies in which there are sedentary occupations and food is plentiful. Cultural factors are important and in some

*Supported in part by Interdisciplinary Adolescent Health Training Program No. 979.

areas of the world adult obesity is a sign of wealth and power. In the United States, the tycoons and politicians of the early twentieth century were stereotyped as obese and, even today, cartoons often associate power and greed with obesity. In our country and elsewhere, adults living in relative poverty are often obese, particularly women. The cultural view of obesity in our society is related to the fact that we are still youth oriented and we have further equated youth, vitality, and leanness. Just as Greek statues idealized young bodies, so do our advertisements; they portray fatness as repulsive and cause for rejection, unhappiness, or ridicule. Life is a continuum of change and we know that many obese children become obese adolescents during a time of dramatic physical, cognitive, and psychosocial growth. Thus obesity, when present, adds an additional burden to the psychological changes of adolescence. It is important, therefore, to be aware of the changes of normal adolescent growth. There are some general theories on adolescent obesity that should be mentioned prior to a discussion of the relationships of growth and obesity.

GROWTH AT ADOLESCENCE

Childhood is characterized by a relatively small, uniform, annual increase of height and weight. This slow rate of growth is associated with a feeling of the child's being in control of himself and of the environment. The stable relationships of body parts to each other and to the environment provide a feeling of comfort. With the onset of pubescence, this relationship of the body parts to the environment changes rapidly, for puberty is the only period of life, after birth, in which the velocity of growth increases.

Growth at adolescence is tripartite: physical, cognitive, and psychosocial. Each of these areas of change can affect the others, and disturbance in one can bring about disequilibrium in the overall pattern or rate of growth and development. Alterations from childhood into adolescence may be temporary or permanent, related to physical or mental handicaps or to emotional problems. In considering adolescent growth, there are further divisions, particularly in the field of psychosocial change. These are customarily spoken of as early, middle, or late adolescence, and consideration of developmental changes must be related to these stages of growth.

Physical growth is perhaps the most obvious and dramatic change seen in adolescence. Rapid increase in height, alterations of physique, the development of adult secondary sex characteristics, and the beginning of menstruation in girls and ejaculation in boys — all produce significant effects in young adolescents. Early adolescents are primarily concerned with their bodies, with normalcy. Rapid increase in height and in size of body parts disrupts the previous relationship of the body to the environment and alters the relationship of one part of the body to another. The former state of being in control of the body and the outer world no longer exists and is replaced by lack of control and by a feeling of wonder about the body. Comparison of appearance and body parts with those of peers comes about, and there may also be competitive physical acts to prove supremacy and normalcy.

As these changes take place, adolescents normally fantasize an ideal body image which is retained about a year or so after the peak height velocity of growth. When boys have developed increased muscle size, thus making them stronger than girls, and girls have reached menarche, a real body image has slowly replaced the ideal. (This is a particularly difficult development for the obese adolescent and will be discussed later.) At this stage of physical development, boys and girls continue to grow taller and heavier although at a much reduced rate (1). They again feel more comfortable with themselves, and the relation of body parts to each other and to the environment is reestablished as being under their control. Most adolescents are satisfied that their bodies are normal, although they may be dissatisfied with their appearance or the size of certain body parts. They usually accept themselves and attempt to become more attractive to peers.

During midadolescence, the realistic body image is associated with decreased concern about physique or, infrequently, becomes at least a temporary psychologic problem because of dissatisfaction with what one has become. For example, the "short man syndrome" may appear as a real hindrance to appropriate psychologic growth in adolescence. In general, midadolescence in boys is characterized by physical activity used to gain acceptance and status. Girls in this developmental period still attempt to become more attractive to the opposite sex although more and more of them are participating in sports and competing with adolescent boys.

Physical growth continues in late adolescence although it is limited. Little change in height occurs during late adolescence and, for the majority of teen-agers, body size and proportion have been accepted and no longer constitute a major concern. Using the body, whether in sports, work, or sexual relationships, is usually of greater consideration than body size or configuration.

Cognitive Growth

It is generally agreed that adolescence is associated with, or brings about, the beginning development of formal operational thinking. Early adolescents still think concretely. They base their evaluations and expectations on experiences of the past and this is often a temporary handicap. With rapid physical change in appearance, early adolescents have no basis on which to evaluate these changes. They are often confused and erroneously expect their bodies to function in former motor patterns, to appear as they did in earlier years, or to protect or hinder them in various situations. Again they often feel out of control, and their inability to conceptualize about the future, to think logically and hypothetically, can provide a temporary disruptive effect on psychosocial relationships.

By midadolescence, thinking has begun to change and self-understanding is increasing. The majority of midadolescents have a real body image and are able to think about the future, though perhaps unrealistically. They still may expect magical solutions to problems, but their thinking changes and is directed outward more than inward. During the transitional period, most adolescents feel transparent, on-stage, and they have difficulty thinking about themselves in relation to others. Such thought processes are closely related to the psychosocial changes occurring simultaneously and each affects the other.

Late adolescents think more abstractly and can form hypotheses. Although past experience is still a considerable factor in their thinking, many of them are able to evaluate possibilities and arrive at logical conclusions, even if they do not always accept them. Handicapping conditions, such as less than average intelligence, may preclude the development of formal operational thought. Some persons never attain this stage of cognitive change and, for others, it comes only during early adult life. However, in general, late adolescents demonstrate the ability to think about the future, to think abstractly, and to relate the consequences of their actions to themselves. Cognitive development is closely related to psychological growth and appropriate rates of development enhance each other, although all aspects of growth are not necessarily synchronous.

Psychosocial Growth

Any discussion of psychosocial growth of adolescents is likely to be oversimplified for each task of adolescence has many branches that can be of great importance. Traditionally these areas of growth have been: separation from the family with assumption of responsibility, sexuality, vocational preparation, and attaining ego identity.

The world of the small child is small. He is dependent upon a few adults and geographically his surroundings are familiar. Adolescence is a period of increased mobility, geographic expansion, and greater independence. Early adolescents typically vacillate between demands for freedom and parental support; they think about themselves and desire acceptance by others of the same sex. They frequently act inappropriately for adult expectations of age. Nevertheless, they do begin the process of emotional separation from the family and make attempts to implement physical separation. By midadolescence there is increased restlessness and more exploration, which brings about new experiences that require decisions and acceptance of responsibility for one's actions. The desire for freedom increases and, although this may conflict with parental wishes, most midadolescents do have more choices of action and feel more secure when outside the home. Late adolescents in general feel comfortable in their home community and various vacation sites, but anticipation of leaving home for further education or a job still causes feelings of concern and doubt. These adolescents can usually cope successfully with departure from the family. They desire such separation but continue the emotional ties, expecting support from the family and help in time of need. If an adolescent has a handicapping condition or illness such as seizures or diabetes, for example, separation may be more difficult, or it may be the long-sought chance for independence and the opportunity to break a parental dependence on the adolescent.

Sexuality

Early adolescents are fascinated by changes in secondary sex characteristics. As the body grows and proportions are altered, boys and girls wonder about these physical changes, explore themselves, compare body parts with a best friend, and think about sexual matters. Feelings previously unexperienced come about, dreams change, even a touch seems to have an erotic component, and these new sensations and thoughts must be dealt with. Some adolescents are puzzled and hide their concerns, whereas others share them with friends and may even seek information from adults. At the same time, they notice older adolescents — how they act, what they do — and their remarks about sexual matters are attentively listened to. Masturbation is discovered or learned from a friend, and nocturnal emissions are experienced by boys. Girls begin to menstruate and have more sexual thoughts; it is likely that far more of them masturbate than is reported in the literature. Most peer association is with members of the same sex, and heterosexual associations are predominantly in groups because groups provide support for individuals. Communication between the sexes is most often indirect, by passage of notes or use of the telephone, because these methods avoid personal contact. All of this gradually changes with midadolescence.

At that time, heterosexual association increases and first attempts are short lived and exploratory. As the midadolescent becomes more confident, relationships with a member of the opposite sex become longer and more intimate. Many such associations lead to some form of sexual expression such as kissing or petting. Sexual intercourse may occur in midadolescence, although the majority of reported studies show 50 percent or more of late adolescent girls remain virgins at graduation from high school. Coitus is frequently only a test for a boy or girl "to see if I could do it." Late adolescents are usually more stable and tend to have longer relationships with another adolescent of the opposite sex, whether or not intercourse is part of the association. Although many adolescents who have experienced intercourse desire to repeat the act frequently, actual coitus for most adolescents in high school is sporadic.

Part of the developmental change in sexuality is learning to love and be loved. Adolescents must learn to empathize with peers and adults, and early adolescents vacillate between support and condemnation of their friends. Teenagers are alert to how other adolescents act, dress, and think. Each group looks to an older group for guidance in these matters and particularly in sexual mores. As they become older the majority establish their own moral codes, learn to resist the pressure of peers, and come to decide what they consider appropriate for a young man or woman.

Vocation

Early adolescents in the United States have many material wants. In order to obtain these things, adolescents seek part-time jobs. It is evident to them that eventually they will need a job to support themselves, but young teenagers are severely limited in available work for pay. At this stage of development they are rarely concerned about an eventual adult vocation, and they relate working to the means of obtaining items they desire. Midadolescents have better chances of securing part-time work or jobs which have a higher rate of pay, and most teenagers attempt to find work to provide them with money to be spent as they choose. Little thought is given to an eventual vocation and such consideration comes more during late adolescence. As the end of high school nears, adolescents begin to think about a full-time job or about seeking training or education for a vocation. Choice of vocation is often difficult, frequently not approached without careful consideration, and often not selected until the college years. Nevertheless, almost all adolescents in our country are aware that the need to work exists and that they will eventually have to find a means of livelihood.

Many factors enter into selection of a vocation: an admired adult, physical size and shape, the ease or difficulty of learning, the length of time required to attain certification, and financial resources. Boys belonging to minorities and low-income families often hope to rise above their poverty level by participating in sports. Too often they do not realize how few reach the big leagues and astronomical salaries, but sports programs of colleges and universities do offer a means of obtaining further education and training for thousands of adolescent boys. Adolescent girls from low-income families are not so fortunate, and it is often difficult for them to obtain higher education or specialized training. In addition, there are fewer vocational opportunities for girls, although this situation is changing. More and more adolescent girls expect to work when they marry and neither expect nor desire to stay home as wife and mother. This difference is evident at all financial levels, and adolescent girls are considering more seriously their choices of vocations. Teenage pregnancy alters many hopes of the future, decreases educational attainments, and often seems to lock a girl into a poverty group of society. However, in general, adolescents tend to spend little time thinking about a vocation until they are faced with the need to support themselves, and even then their wishes, decisions, and plans are often impractical.

Ego Identity

The current concept of identity holds that accomplishing the tasks of adolescence and integrating the changes in the individual's personality lead to attaining ego identity. Many times this does not occur until young adulthood, but some late adolescents seem to have come to feel that they are unique though similar to their peers and that they have within themselves the ability to cope with life, live independently, and commit themselves to achieving established goals. Whether working with a normal adolescent or one with health or emotional problems, it is necessary to know where along the path of change the individual subject is at a given time. Unrealistic expectations can prevent rapport and help by professionals, and the adolescent's disequilibrium in the major tasks and growth areas can confuse one's evaluation of an adolescent. If there is a health problem, it is necessary to know how the usual pattern of development is disrupted and how this alteration can affect not only further development but the future status of an adolescent.

PSYCHIATRIC VIEWS OF OBESITY

The classical view of obesity considered all obese adolescents as fixated in the oral stage of psychosexual development. This concept is now considered outmoded because the classical drive theories do not explain most instances of obesity. We know there are a variety of obesities and probably subgroups of adolescents who are obese for many different reasons. Research has shown obese adolescents do not have a common personality profile and their obesity does not have a common meaning.

Carrera (2) proposes that among certain obese adolescents there are psychologic factors leading to overeating which may form subgroups which are themselves distinct from those associated with psychologic factors leading to inactivity, and different from those in which psychologic factors lead to disturbances in satiety mechanisms. Bullen et al. (3) found that obese adolescent girls often had eating binges when they felt bad, were worried, depressed, left out of peer activities, bored, etc. These authors hypothesized that such eating behavior is a learned reaction rather than springing from innate drives or emotional abnormality. However, there is a broad range of emotional problems, particularly in obese adolescent girls, which often continue into adult life and affect not only self-concepts but interpersonal relationships as well (3, 4).

Bruch's classic work (5) with obese children and adolescents began with the recognition that satisfaction of inherited biological needs is closely related to emotional and mental development. Food was often used to relieve the tensions of unsolvable and often unconscious conflicts and could be equated with an insatiable desire to obtain love and as a symbol of inhibited destructive impulses. Food can also substitute for sexual gratification or represent self-indulgence. These concepts have been present in many psychiatric theories, and it is unfortunate that they may often be applied to obese persons under the assumption that all obesity is psychogenic. In the analysis of data on obese adolescents, Bruch came to consider the possibility of disturbances of perception and conception. She concluded that there is often a conceptual confusion in obese adolescents and that they have a basic conviction of being misshapen because of someone else's actions. These obese girls seemed to suffer from a real lack of identity because they felt they did not "own" their bodies. In particular, they lacked awareness of bodily urges and signals, including emotional reactions and interpersonal effectiveness. They were unable to recognize hunger and satiation. Bruch believes that body awareness must be learned and that obese adolescents have had incorrect learning experiences and, as a result, their behavior is different from nonobese adolescents (5).

Many researchers have observed and reported disturbances in families having an obese adolescent child. The child is often the scapegoat of one or both parents and occasionally of siblings. Parental overconcern with the obesity is commonly found, and it may preoccupy a parent's attention. Bullen et al. (3) found the adolescent girl in such a family to have conflict relating to separation, concern with sex on the fantasy level, and lack of heterosexual interests at the reality level, with evidence of disturbances in body image.

Carrera (2) believes that there is a need to evaluate obese teenagers to determine if psychotherapy is indicated. Risk fastors are: evidence of a pathological parent-child relationship; hypercritical family attitudes related to the patient's obesity; "compulsive" eating in response to a variety of moods and affects; withdrawal-"hate my body"-increased sensitivity triad; eating patterns including the night-eating syndrome; evidence that the adolescent is not attuned to his own feelings including bodily sensations of hunger and satiety; a lack of closeness among family members with coexistent difficulties in separation from the family; an attitude of preference for the status quo reflected in delayed involvement with the tasks of adolescence — developing a sense of individual identity, a growing independence and self-reliance, involvement in heterosexual orientation, and participation and involvement in the peer culture.

THE INTERRELATIONSHIP OF OBESITY AND ADOLESCENT GROWTH

Most clinicians consider obesity to be present if an adolescent's body weight is 20 percent or more above ideal body weight, or above the ninety-seventh percentile according to current height-weight charts. The same standards are applicable during childhood, and this is of interest because an obese child is likely to become an obese adolescent who is also likely to become an obese adult. Most children with juvenile onset of obesity not only have increased body weight but are taller than their nonobese agemates. Pubertal changes usually begin earlier among chronically obese children, and girls begin to menstruate sooner than their contemporaries. Genital size in obese males is often of great concern to the boys and to their parents, although the genitalia are almost always of normal size when suprapubic fat is pushed away.

The stability of relationships of body parts to each other and to the environment in small children has been mentioned. Normally there is a disruption of this state of being by the rapid growth of early adolescence, and there is often an associated feeling of helplessness. For obese adolescents who have been obese as children, this is doubly difficult. During late childhood most parents have made efforts to reduce the child's weight, or the child has tried to lose weight, but such efforts usually are very temporary or fail. Repeated failure to lose weight and prevent regaining weight has often produced a feeling of being unable to achieve a desired weight or desired physique; thus, a feeling of helplessness may exist before the onset of adolescence. With rapid growth and its associated feeling of helplessness about the body, many obese young adolescents feel even more helpless about their bodies, and the great changes in size and shape may bring about a feeling of hopelessness. It is not unusual for an obese adolescent to believe that he/she is powerless to do anything that might decrease weight or bring about a desired appearance.

At this same stage of development, most adolescents have an ideal body image. One may ask what constitutes an ideal body image for an adolescent who has been fat as a child. It is not unusual to find that the self-image and ego were damaged in an obese child. Hammar (6) believes that patients who become obese in very early childhood or in late adolescence often exhibit fewer distortions and have less damaged self-images than do those patients having an onset of obesity during late childhood or very early adolescence. He also found that patients who are grossly obese during early adolescence retain a mental picture of themselves during adulthood as being obese and ugly, even if they are successful in reducing and achieving a normal body weight (6). Obese adolescents have had lower scores on body image scales, and obese girls in particular cited few positive attributes about their bodies; they were dissatisfied with physical characteristics and intensely disliked their figures. Hammar also reported that these obese girls were self-deprecating, expressed more fears about themselves, and were obsessed with their obesity (7). Bruch comments that obese adolescents do not "see" themselves objectively and are more concerned with the judgment of the scale than by what they feel and observe (5).

Stunkard and Mendelson (8) examined behavioral disturbances in obese persons and found that two were specifically related to the obesity. These factors were overeating and a disturbance of body image. The latter finding occurred in obese persons who were obese as adolescents and was characterized by a feeling that the body was grotesque, often loathsome, and that others viewed it with hostility and contempt. This feeling was associated with self-consciousness and impaired social functioning, particularly in relation to members of the opposite sex. In obese adults, these disturbances were not affected by weight reductions and were improved with long-term psychotherapy. The impaired body image did not occur in obese adolescents living in families in which the parents were large and fat, and who associated overweight with strength and health. Attitudes of parents and other significant persons in which the adolescent's obesity was a cause for censure or rejection were extremely important as a probable cause of the disturbed body image.

If, indeed, overeating and a disturbance in body image are the two key factors related to obesity, we must consider them in relation to adolescence. We have previously discussed Bruch's (5) finding that many obese persons lack awareness of bodily urges and are unable to correctly recognize hunger and satiation, and that this was also associated with a disturbed body image. In general, obese adolescents were obese children, and one can speculate that this lack of recognition of hunger and satiety developed during that period of growth. Most small children are not concerned about obesity until the school years and this concern increases preceding pubescence. At that time, obesity becomes a more significant factor affecting the older child's self-concept. Almost all investigators found problems in normal weight families in which there was an obese child and the parents urged or demanded that the child lose weight. There was much criticism of obese children in such families, and often they were ridiculed or rejected, or they became the scapegoat of parents and siblings. Most older prepubertal children attempt to lose weight periodically without succeeding and enter puberty with a feeling of helplessness in achieving desired change.

If an obese adolescent has been obese as a child, has experienced frustration and failure in changing the body shape, and has been subjected to disturbing family and peer relationships, it is likely that the alteration of the relationship of body parts, the rapid changes in appearance, and the increased feeling of helplessness of adolescence will exert a greater effect than in his nonobese peers. This feeling of differentness, of not belonging, complicates resolution of the change from ideal to real body image necessary for psychosocial growth. The formation of a real body image typically occurs about a year or so after the peak of the growth spurt. Apparently, in obese adolescents it is not associated with a reappearance of the feeling of being in control, improved self-esteem, progress toward heterosexual relationships, and a lessening of self-consciousness. We propose that the disturbances of the body image so much a part of behavioral and emotional disorders of obese adults are formed or fixed during the growth spurt of early adolescence, are not resolved during midadolescence and, with the continuing lack of awareness of body urges, continue into adulthood where they persist as inhibiting factors in other areas of psychosocial development and interpersonal relationships.

There is then ample evidence that obese adolescents frequently have distorted body images, often because they have been obese as children and therefore have experienced a more intense feeling of helplessness in early adolescence. As pubertal changes begin to occur, there is usually a greater desire to conform to accepted peer standards of bodily shape, but the body changes so rapidly that the feeling of helplessness is increased and can lead to a feeling of hopelessness. This is even more tragic, for if there is no hope then often the desire to live is damaged. Hopelessness associated with the body image and low self-concept may preclude forming an ideal body image from which a real body image is derived. If the ideal body image is replaced by a feeling of always being fat and other self-deprecating feelings, that view may become a distorted body image and remain, regardless of loss of weight during the later stage of growth. Psychosocial development follows the development of a real body image and is so closely related that disturbance in appropriate image formation may delay or permanently damage the psychosocial growth of an adolescent.

Most obese adolescents, like those of average weight, seem to return to a more mature view about a year after the peak height velocity of growth. This can coincide with the awareness of a real body image even if that image is fatness. At such times of midadolescence the boy or girl attempts to come to terms with him/herself, to accept the physique, and to try to adapt to the peer group and to being a teenager in today's society. Boys have an easier time in general than do girls for they can participate in sports in which bulk is advantageous, and boys also have greater social freedom than do adolescent girls. Even so, both sexes in early adolescence explore roles less related to physical size and appearance that are accepted by peers.

Heterosexual associations begin during midadolescence, and obese girls in particular may find great difficulty in establishing such relationships or try to avoid them. Studies have shown that many obese girls tend to have an overall immaturity and are more seclusive or withdrawn. These characteristics hinder the development of heterosexual attachments and dating. We have considered that many obese adolescent girls feel unloved and unacceptable and, because one of the tasks of adolescence is to love and be loved, growth in this area can be hindered or blocked. Obese adolescents of both sexes are often excluded from peer group activities and become the butt of comments; thus, appropriate teenage social development is at least temporarily impossible. Sexuality can be affected by obesity in adolescence, and associations between the two sexes are often limited; the reverse can also occur – an obese adolescent girl, apparently searching for acceptance, may become sexually active. It should be remembered that many obese adolescent girls exhibit sexual behavior typical of nonobese teenagers and dating does not seem as important to them as might be expected. In fact, obesity in adolescence may be used as a protective mechanism to prevent having to cope with heterosexual experiences. Usually by late adolescence, obese girls do desire acceptance by boys, want to date, and begin to think about the possibility of marriage. There is often greater motivation toward weight reduction during late adolescence than in previous years as sexual fulfillment becomes a greater concern.

Family Relationships

Family characteristics and actions assume great importance during adolsecent growth. The struggle for independence and separation from the family is a normal part of growth, and families are usually supportive in bringing about change. It has been found that obese children are often used by one or the other parent as "a thing, an object whose function it is to fulfull the parent's needs, to compensate them for failures and frustrations in their own lives" (9). Bruch has also found that obese children are often of the sex opposite that wished for by the parents (10). This leads to confusion in sexual identification at a time when the adolescent is uncertain about bodily concepts, growth, and identity. Change toward a more normal weight was found in families in which the weight of the adolescent was stable and where the families showed little anxiety or punitive overconcern with the excess weight. In contrast, when families showed constant preoccupation with the obesity, there was progressive obesity and poor adjustment psychologically. Bullen et al. (3) found that disturbances in family relationships were the rule; this was often characterized by poor sociability among family members and much fighting among siblings. In these families, the obese adolescent girls were also poorly adjusted and more dependent on the family, and had separation anxiety about leaving the mother, great concern with sex on the fantasy level, and a lack of real heterosexual interests (6).

Early adolescents in particular can suffer from family disruptions and relationships which apparently delay psychological maturation and lead to continuing immaturity. Midadolescents may still feel many of these effects although the peer group begins to play a more important role. Older obese adolescents, girls more so than boys, are often more immautre than their contemporaries. However, at this stage of development, many obese adolescents wish to leave home and try their own way in the world in order to relieve tensions at home. Peers are still important to older adolescents, and those who are obese still struggle for acceptance if they have not achieved a satisfactory status. Peer relationships are often a problem for obese teenagers. Many are excluded from activities, try various roles to achieve hoped-for acceptance, and often find their greatest difficulty is in hetero-sexual relationships. Girls are more vulnerable because they usually must wait to be invited to social functions rather than choosing a male partner, and loneliness and rejection are often a part of being obese. Many fat adolescents attempt to com-pensate for being left out of peer activities and adopt a facade to hide their isolation.

Adolescents of normal weight have difficulty in setting long-range goals and preparing for the future, and the difficulty seems even greater for those young people who are and have been obese. Adolescents expect magical solutions, wish for immediate gratification, and are usually narcissistic. Unrealistic expec-tations are not fulfilled and the feeling of being helpless is often exacerbated, which causes further problems.

It should be remembered that there are degrees of obesity, that personalities differ, and that families are not the same. Although there are common charac-teristics for many obese adolescents, there is great variety and the dire predictions often do not occur. Burchinal and Eppright (11) tested the psychogenic theory of obesity for a sample of rural girls in Iowa and compared family structure variables, intelligence scores, educational achievement scores, mental health analysis scores, levels of physical activity, and sex-role identification of obese girls with their lean counterparts and found that none of the tests supported the psychogenic theory of obesity. These investigators found that heavy and obese girls tended to have overweight parents who accepted their children, loved them, and supported them.

All obese adolescents should be regarded as individuals and, according to Berblinger (12), the following questions should be considered: is the obesity a reflection of psychiatric illness; can psychological trauma or an unfilled need have caused the obesity; does a change in body image cause a shift in the self-concept and self-esteem; does the weight gain have a conscious or unconscious purpose in an interpersonal situation? To these, we would add that the stage of growth must be considered: is the adolescent past the peak height velocity of physical growth; has there been appropriate cognitive growth; where along the path from early to late psychologic development is the adolescent obese patient? All of these variables are of considerable importance in learning to know if the obese patient requires psychiatric care, only psychologic support, or medical in-tervention. It can be seen that obesity is a complex condition resulting from one or several factors and that it can lead to minor emotional problems or continue to cause psychologic or psychiatric difficulties decades later.

Although we are not concerned with treatment in this chapter, it is evident that many aspects of obesity must be considered. Because results are poor in long-term goals, one must ask the question presented at the beginning of the chapter: why is obesity considered a problem? If 30 percent of the population is obese and few fat people become and remain thin, would it be helpful emotionally to try to change the cultural criticism of obesity and promote personal acceptance of one's size? It may be that early efforts should be largely directed to help fat adolescents accept themselves, in spite of peer rejection, so they do not develop other emotional problems. Perhaps such programs could prevent unhappiness and emotional difficulties even though the obesity remains and is harmful to longevity. In essence, the question to be asked is whether the danger of emotional illness and damaged self-concept may be greater than the physiologic effects of obesity. Until methods are divised whereby weight can be lost and an ideal weight maintained permanently, the possible effects of obesity in promoting emotional problems may be of primary concern. Data show that some obese girls use principles learned in adolescence during an improved and more lasting period when they become young adults. This raises the question of whether the immaturity reported in obese adolescent girls lasts longer than in nonobese girls. And, if so, then it may be that the motivation and persistence required to lose weight and maintain the new weight cannot be expected until early adulthood. If this is true, then prevention of emotional problems may be the highest priority in management of obesity in adolescence.

REFERENCES

1. Tanner, J. M. *Growth at Adolescence,* 2nd ed. Oxford: Blackwell Scientific Publications, 1962.
2. Carrera, R., III. Obesity in adolescence. *The Psychology of Obesity – Dynamics and Treatment* (Kiell, N. Ed.), pp. 113-124. Springfield, Ill.: Thomas, 1973.
3. Bullen, B. A., Monello, L. F., Cohen, H., and Mayer, J. Attitudes towards physical activity, food and family in obese and nonobese adolescent girls. *Am. J. Clin. Nutr.,* 1964, *12*, 1.
4. Tolstrup, K. On psychogenic obesity in children, IV. *Acta Paediat.*, 1953, *42*, 289.
5. Bruch, H. Psychological aspects of overeating and obesity. *Psychosom. Med.,* 1964, *V*, 269.
6. Hammar, S. L. Juvenile obesity. *Pediatrics Digest,* Nov/Dec. 21, 1979.
7. Hammar, S. L., Campbell, M. M., Campbell, V. A., Moores, N. L., Sareen, C., Gareis, F. J., and Lucas, B. An interdisciplinary study of adolescent obesity. *J. Pediat.,* 1972, *80*, 373.
8. Stunkard, A. J. and Mendelson, M. Obesity and body image. *The Psychology of Obesity – Dynamics and Treatment,* (Kiell, N. Ed.), pp. 41-47. Springfield, Ill.: Thomas, 1973.
9. Touraine, G. Obesity in children: V. The family frame of obese children. *Psychosom. Med.,* 1940, 141.
10. Bruch, H. Psychological aspects of obesity. *Psychiat.,* 1947, *10*, 373.
11. Burchinal, L. G. and Eppright, E. S. Test of the psychogenic theory of obesity for a sample of rural girls. *Am. J. Clin. Nutr.,* 1959, *7*, 288.
12. Berblinger, L. G. Obesity and psychologic stress. *Obesity* (Wilson, N. L., Ed.), pp. 153-160. Philadelphia: Davis, 1969.

6

Obesity as a Barricade Against Social Stress: An Adlerian View

David Laskowitz

The concern with obesity in American culture derives as much from the premise that fat is ugly as it does from medical considerations. To weigh less than is comfortable has therefore become an all-American preoccupation in which people struggle to fit an idealized body type regardless of differences in individual physical endowment. In our culture, feminine attractiveness is linked with being fashionably thin, and the plump look is derogated as being matronly and dowdy. Therefore, it is ironic that obesity is more common in women than in men. This potential for generating body image conflict in women is reinforced by the caveat of the advertising media that a lasting marriage requires not only that the woman be effective as a mother, but that she maintain her sexual holding power by promoting her physical image.

Given the intense interest in this topic, a broad array of factors has been implicated in its etiology, including genetic, thermodynamic, neurogenic, and metabolic (Bruch, 1973; Hofling, 1968). This chapter will focus on psychological or psychosomatic obesity, i.e., obesity associated with personality and emotional disorders. This association may be a mix of factors including those which contribute to obesity, are in reaction to obesity, or are interactionally linked in a feedback manner which creates a vicious cycle. Efforts to typologize obesity by use of labels such as "exogenous" to refer to obesity which occurs in the presence of normal metabolism, or "reactive" in response to some precipitating external event, or "developmental" to identify the problem as one that is long lived and can be traced to the early rearing history of the patient, serve a limited descriptive and epidemiological function. Stunkard (1959) illustrates the latter purpose when he underscores the poor prognosis in juvenile (developmental) obesity, with the finding that eight out of ten remain obese as adults and less than half have disturbed body images. Likewise, a review of the literature in the search for clearly delineated psychodynamic causes of obesity has proved fruitless (Kaplan and Kaplan, 1957). The view that psychodynamic factors involved in simple obesity are nonspecific has been incorporated in the DSM-III (*Diagnostic and Statistical Manual of Mental Disorders,* Third Edition).

Stunkard (1959) sought a classification system involving a broader unit of study, namely, eating patterns, but could identify only two small subgroups, which in combination accounted for only 15 percent of the study population. These were the night-eating syndrome and the binge-eating syndrome (the latter has been referred to in the DSM-III as bulimia). Apparently 85 percent of the study population could not be clearly delineated in terms of eating pattern. In any case, the unit used in the attempted classification was based on descriptive, not explanatory, information.

The unified theory of Adler's *Individual Psychology* makes no attempt to typologize, in recognition of the vast range of personal ways in which individuals, including corpulent individuals, endeavor to master their surroundings and safeguard themselves from stress. Application of Adlerian theory and principles of treatment, however, seems particularly well suited for integrating converging clinical information on this topic.

SENSE OF INFERIORITY

Fat people often display, at least on the surface, a pervasive sense of inferiority. Since this characteristic is a key component of Adlerian theory, it is pertinent to examine its developmental roots. A child living in a world of strong adults is imprinted with a sense of relative helplessness. Under congenial rearing circumstances, this experience of marginal behavioral competence diminishes gradually as a place is found in adult society. The helplessness is characterized as relative because despite the functional immaturity of the infant, *e.g.,* his inability to move about, he can nonetheless see, hear, and smell; he is sensitive to touch and pain; and his viability is ensured by his sucking reflexes. The child is therefore an active participant in his own development.

It is in the realm of feeding behavior that the infant is faced with the first challenge involving mastery of the environment. The critical ingredient at this juncture is the extent to which the mother and infant are mutually attuned. Since the vehicle for the infant's communication is the cry, the manner in which the mother responds is of critical importance. (It is assumed that the quality of the emitted cry cue is not distorted by some perinatal handicap.) The infant provides information regarding his needs through the cries that he emits, and if these are properly interpreted, it contributes to the infant's sense of adequacy and competence. Thus the mother's appropriate response to his hunger cries, as distinguished from those that are not nutritionally linked, enables the infant to experience increasing self-awareness and self-confidence in identifying his own visceral cues. The details of this feedback learning are elaborated by Bruch (1973).

Conversely, the mother who has problems in discriminating between hunger cries and those associated with nonspecific tension states, and, who intervenes inappropriately by indiscriminately plying the infant with food, undermines the infant's self-confidence. The infant's locus of power becomes constricted as he flounders in efforts to mobilize the environment in his behalf through self-initiative. This becomes an early determinant in promoting helplessness over controlling the outcome of his biological needs. This experience can also impede other adaptational devices such as trust formation and the courage to venture forth in an exploratory manner with the mother as a secure base of operation. The child may respond with timid clinging and with excessive field-dependent behavior at a later time. The latter life-style characteristic, frequently seen with the obese, has provided the basis for formulating the external-cue hypothesis in which the fat person allegedly is more responsive to external than to visceral cues in initiating eating behavior.

Illustrative of other parental mistakes is the mother who overstuffs the baby with the intent of making him sleep a long time so that he will be less demanding. Regardless of the reason, i.e., whether it be a sense of incompetence regarding the mothering function, or resentment with having to sacrifice personal satisfactions, the mother becomes basically impervious to the baby's nonnutritional needs and his efforts at self-expression. Another genre of a mistaken mothering approach is overpowering the child with food that he has already rejected, thereby stifling his strivings for autonomy.

Various life-style alternatives may unfold from scenarios such as these. The child can either develop a sense of the importance of being "good" in conformity with the mother's ambitions, regardless of his personal needs, or he can refuse to submit and be "bad." The attempted resolution of this conflict, which may have its origins in the pre-language phase of the infant's development, shapes rudimentary attitudes and perceptions of the world. These become the raw material from which a private logic and directing goals derive. Should the infant chronically capitulate to a dominating mother, the substrate for attention-getting goals as a vehicle for survival may be laid. Behavioral maneuvers for achieving them may include acts of self-sacrifice or participation in his own victimization.

Adler underscored the strength of weakness and the variety of uses to which this strategem is put (Adler, 1951). With fat people, this mode of coping may be manifest in overeating to avoid provoking the envy of friends. They likewise repudiate competitive actions, especially in the heterosexual arena. For them, food has exaggerated value. Presumably this is linked with the early mother-child "communication" that food is a cure-all for various forms of distress. Indeed, there may be some identification with the aggressor, i.e., the overpowering mother who stuffs; this may account for the tactic of self-induced forced feeding, presumably to assuage dysphoric feelings. Food, in that sense, may serve as an antidepressant by providing reassurance that life still holds some satisfactions. It is of historic interest to note that obesity has been viewed as a depressive equivalent for some individuals, and although fat people have a higher morbidity and mortality rate, they seem to have a significantly lower suicide rate (Bruch, 1973).

Early adoption of a passive-dependent response repertoire to obtain the rewards of being "good," namely, the presence of social striving for approval and recognition from the parents, may occur in a context of submitting to a controlling mother who supervises every bite. The spill-off of a pattern of seemingly "going along with the program" is commonly observed with the overeater. The precise behavioral configuration exhibited, however, is determined by largely unconscious goals. Dreikurs (1968), in his expansion of Adlerian thinking, presented four goals which, for individuals in trouble, reflect a gradient of increasing maladjustment: the quest for attention, the display of power, the desire for revenge, and the presentation of oneself as disabled. This schema has clearcut applicability to clinical experience with the overeater. For example, strict adherence to dieting provides the occasion for socially sanctioned self-preoccupation. Paradoxically, though dieting can be used to satisfy attention-getting needs, it can also generate social distance by withdrawing the dieter's attention from others, with consequent loss of spontaneity. The very act of organizing life around the requirements of strict dieting may also serve to conveniently deflect attention and energy from other, perhaps more pressing, life tasks. The position that "nothing matters but controlling weight" can have secondary gain value.

POWER GOAL

The concept of a power goal is used in a generic sense. It is not simply *power over* with intent to dominate, but also *power to*, i.e., the desire to overcome feelings of inadequacy regarding mastery of the personal world in a self-actualizing manner. The precise manner in which power strivings are used — destructively or constructively — is in part determined by the extent to which social interest is developed. In the case of the controlling, overpowering mother who endeavors to tightly supervise her child's eating behavior with rewards and punishments, there may be a backfiring of her power manipulations. She may be setting herself up for subsequent blackmail once the child learns to exploit the politics of the dinner table. He is then able to circumvent her maneuvers and to operate from a strong bargaining position.

Recourse to the exploitation of power diplomacy has its origins in the breakdown of attention-getting mechanisms for achieving security. The seeds for power strivings, in a destructive sense, sprout in a broad range of family constellations under conditions of equally varied family climates. However, this is observed with special frequency with the individual who experiences neglect, actual or fantasied, and with the individual who has been pampered, especially when the pampering has been inconsistently provided or abruptly withdrawn.

For example, one encounters power-centered behavior with obese pampered children who, as a result of overly solicitous parental behavior, have an unrealistic sense of their worth to significant adults. They have learned that they can use their well-being as a tool for exacting specific demands. A crisis ensues when the fat child is unable to extrapolate this adaptational style to other situations and his ability to rule breaks down.

The variations in private logic which promote obesity in the service of power and strength are extensive. In the author's experience, this includes achieving dramatic weight loss (110 pounds) with a 52-year-old, cancer-phobic salesman who presented a family history of loss of significant figures from cancer. He had, therefore, become convinced that the antidote to wasting away from this dread disease was having an adipose buffer. The remarkable feature of this case was the fact that he had unsuccessfully tried to lose weight "for years" using such modalities as therapeutic starvation and behavior modification, without linking the need to hold on to weight with his fear of cancer. Once his private logic was divulged, cognitive repair had as its focus his preoccupation with the inevitability of his death.

In a related example, an obese 15-year-old boy, who came at the insistence of his mother, reported being the object of repeated bullying and ridicule four years previously when he was "thin." In contrast, because of his current size and weight, he told of being able to "pin" his opponents to the ground. This so-called solution reportedly was linked to watching TV wrestling matches with his father, who himself was not heavy. Initial therapy sessions were directed at a reality formulation involving persons like his father, who were perceived as strong without being heavy. This resulted in a decision to take karate lessons as a trade-off for losing weight. The second step involved going beyond symptom substitution and exploring the details of his seeing the world as an enemy camp, and the manner in which he contributed to this.

A kindred problem was presented by a 33-year-old, upper-class woman who had recently arrived from Italy to stay with her husband, who had been sent to the United States by his company for a period of two years. She was an only child and was pregnant for the first time. The patient was referred by her obstetrician who had become concerned with her dramatic increase in weight in the absence of an organic basis, and despite his admonishments. Interviews with her revealed the private logic that the developing fetus constituted a drain on her body resources, which was countered by stuffing herself. She had misgivings about being pregnant and had been 10 pounds overweight prior to her pregnancy. She explained that in accordance with her familial values, the plump look was considered desirable, and she secretly thought that she might have been too thin.

In the latter two instances, we have examples of excessive body weight and size associated with enhanced survival power. The failure to achieve personal security by power-oriented means, whether by passive or active tactics, together with the identification of the person responsible for frustrating these power strivings, sets the stage for behavior organized around revenge goals. Variations in the ways in which vindictive behavior is expressed are limited only by the creativity of the individual.

REVENGE MOTIVE

Illustrative of the revenge motive was a 17-year-old girl who was 40 pounds overweight. Her father was a well-groomed, meticulously dressed executive with an advertising agency, and her mother was an attractive, fashionable commercial artist. The parents were both fashion conscious and were troubled by the daughter's appearance. The father, in particular, expressed disgust with her overweight. He told of his embarrassment in bringing business acquaintances home because his daughter was "fat and sloppy and lacking in self-respect." The daughter had been put on many diets, had been sent for an endocrinologic assessment with negative results, and had attended Overeaters Anonymous meetings for six months.

In therapy the daughter, an only child, angrily told of her father "being wrapped up" in her mother and of the mother's efforts to mold her into a "carbon copy of herself." The daughter also reported that she had tried to lose weight, but that is was "too painful." She was convinced that she had a metabolic problem though test results were negative. Her rage was evident as she told of a rearing history in which she had been left with baby sitters and live-in maids while her parents were constantly socializing. She had fantasies of having been adopted and one day finding her real parents. The patient was seen individually and, in several instances, in combination with her parents. In addition to an open airing of hidden and manifest agenda items, family sessions were focused on the shared importance attached to physical image and the differences in their respective ways of using it as an adaptational device. In one session, the patient tearfully told of fantasizing that she would blow up like a balloon and burst in the midst of her parents' cocktail party. In the course of therapy, the patient became more verbally assertive and insistent that they do more things together. During this period she took a job as a volunteer with a local hospital and met a college student who worked in one of the labs. The patient lost 30 pounds in three months and was elated with her accomplishment.

A second instance involving a revenge goal pertained to a young housewife with three children who had become excessively heavy during her last pregnancy and had been unable to lose weight. The husband was chagrined and openly talked of becoming "turned off" to her sexually. In therapy she told of suspecting that her husband was having affairs (despite his denials) and indicated that the last pregnancy was totally at his insistence. She expressed anger over the fact that he was responsible for getting her pregnant and that she was tired of being pushed around. Medical assessment indicated that there was no physiological basis for her excessive weight gain.

A review of her past pattern of living presented several instances in which she would manipulate herself as an oblique way of expressing anger toward others. The husband, who was himself 35 pounds overweight, was involved in several therapy sessions. He reported being repelled by his mother, who was "obese and smelly." The husband's input was mobilized in entering a shared diet and exercise program with his wife. At the end of three months, they were both satisfied that they were losing weight, and she had begun to wear clothes that she thought he would find flattering.

Behavior organized around a revenge-seeking goal is directed at defeating an opponent, usually the person who blocked the individual's efforts at ascendancy, and at rendering that opponent powerless. A person engaged in the quest for revenge usually has pervasively negative attitudes toward life, mistrusting the motives of those around him; that is, he perceives others as operating out of power-seeking interests. Should he lose the possibility of getting back at his adversary, his sense of behavioral impotence would be complete. This provides the antecedent condition for experiencing himself as disabled. It is as though he has given up the fight. His sense of inferiority becomes an accomplished fact. He displays hopelessness, appears inept, and withdraws from activity in his own behalf. The percentage of obese people who fall into this category is hard to estimate because they are unlikely to seek psychological help. They have an extended prior history of attempted weight control, but to no avail. Their weight has gone up and down, with the net result of no significant movement in any direction. Psychodynamically, these individuals behave as if they have a vested interest in maintaining their status quo, being nonresponsive to a variety of treatment modalities.

Weight loss, for a member of this group, entails the reworking of the very fabric of his cognitive life. This involves focusing on his system of inferences which, in turn, derives from private, covert assumptions about himself, the nature of the world, and his interactions with it. Concomitant with repairing attitudes and unconscious goals which serve to further separate him from his social milieu, it is important to actively promote social interest and move him toward social stimulation. Self-help groups become important vehicles for short-circuiting social alienation and promoting social interest.

Returning to the infant-mother interactional model, there is the case in which the infant shows early evidence of resisting the mother's intrusive forced feeding in response to all cues of discomfort. The price paid by the infant for engaging in disapproved behavior, i.e., eating on his own terms, is the internalization of the stigma of being "bad" and the forfeiting of rewards associated with compliance such as love, being favored, and being considered special. There is a configuration of correlated attributes associated with a self-concept of being bad, in this instance, in the context of eating behavior. These include a propensity for shame, self-condemnation, guilt, and a defensive readiness to proclaim his innocence.

An interesting analogy is observed in studying the dynamics of the night binger. He often behaves as if he has to compartmentalize his night binging, relegating this activity to a secret life. The food is eaten as inconspicuously as possible; it is gobbled down rapidly with little chewing and with awareness that the eating pattern is abnormal. The eating binge is often followed by disparaging self-criticism and self-loathing and, subsequently, by a return to a normal eating pattern or dieting. One patient involved in night binging would routinely characterize his behavior as "good" between binges, as if food were a moral issue.

In accordance with Adlerian theory of problem development, if one is uncertain about himself in relation to the world, there may be the utilization of unrealistic, subjective impressions of people to compensate for unexpressed, and often unconscious, feelings of personal inferiority and incompleteness. Comparison with others is always invidious — with others experienced as brighter, better off, more attractive, more socially desirable, etc. This makes for separating behavior and diminishes social interest. One's personal construct is strengthened by being selectively inattentive to data that is dissonant with the basic premise that he has unacceptable flaws.

Maladjustment derives from the extent to which one erects an edifice of compensatory behavior in the service of achieving apparent superiority and overcoming feelings of personal insignificance. The process of living entails movement toward subjectively conceived objectives which, for most persons, are within reason. In the case of maladjustment, individuals set unrealistic goals to ensure their personal worth. However, the apparent advantage that they obtain is not linked with the interests of their social milieu. This becomes a source of conflict between the self and others and may be expressed in a variety of ways including withdrawal, psychosomatic reactions, and obesity.

The life-pattern reverberations originating largely, though not exclusively, from the interpersonal drama of mother-infant interaction, with special reference to the politics of feeding, set the stage for the emergence of other personal factors which determine human behavior, namely, social interest reflected in willingness to participate in mutual, cooperative endeavors. Another factor is overall activity level manifest in the degree of activity with which the individual tackles life tasks. However, mother-infant interaction, though a significant determinant of ensuing patterns of living, is nonetheless but an aspect of a more global factor, the family as a social network. This includes such variables as family structure, ordinal position, parental attitude, and family ideology.

Given the view that obesity and overeating represent a symptom pattern superimposed on a broad range of the psychiatric spectrum and that no specific configuration of psychodynamics can be identified because of the diversity of background characteristics of the obese, it is nevertheless noteworthy to examine the clustering of one of the family-linked variables, e.g., ordinal position, and its interaction with parental attitude.

THE ORDINAL POSITIONS

Five ordinal positions can be considered basic, and all others can be conceptualized as variations or combinations of these five. They are identified as an only, eldest, second, middle, and youngest child. These positions are often fluid, in that a child may have occupied one position for several years and then find himself in another. Individuals occupying any of these five basic positions, singly or in combination, are considered to have their own characteristic attitudes which color their approach to life problems. These attitudes are influenced by the period in the person's life in which a specific ordinal position was occupied, as well as the length of time and the tradition of family and culture regarding role expectations. Of the five ordinal positions indicated, there was early observation that the obese individual was more likely to be recruited from persons occupying the position of only or youngest child than from the others (Bruch and Touraine, 1950). Among the 225 obese children observed in New York from 1937 to 1940, 35 percent were only children, and 35 percent were the youngest; thus, 70 percent of the obese children were rated in a special position. In a review of some of the literature, Bruch (1973) noted that similar cross-cultural findings were reported in the Funen (a Danish island) study in which the "youngest" and "only" ordinal positions accounted for 60 percent of the 40 obese children studied. A similar investigation in Germany showed that obese men were in the position of only children with a higher incidence than men in a control group. However, the meaning of these findings is statistically obscured by the fact that these obese subjects also came from very small families, heightening the probability that ordinal positions involving "only" and "youngest" would be overly represented. Clearly, ordinal position is not in itself an etiological factor in determining food disorder. However, the prevalence of the two positions cited warrants closer examination to determine the extent to which they generate attitudes toward being-in-the-world which are congenial to the obese prone.

The only child experiences special difficulties in life. He spends his entire childhood among persons who are bigger and more proficient. He may try to gain skills in areas that will win approval, or he may solicit adult sympathy by being shy, timid, and helpless. Thus the range of characteristics include: being pampered and the center of attention; being taught to survive not through self-initiated action, but by dependency on the interventions of others; wedging between the mother and father; feeling unfairly treated when requests are not granted; becoming interested only in himself; and, if the individual is male, feeling that he will never be as strong as the father.

In contrast, the youngest child may either constantly strive to catch up because he is initially outdistanced, or he may feel inferior because he believes that the distance between his older siblings and himself cannot be bridged. An inventory of potential characteristics deriving from this experience include: behaving like an only child; not being taken seriously because he is the smallest and weakest; getting mileage from retaining the baby role and placing others in his service; either excelling in competition with siblings in a compensatory manner or evading a direct struggle for superiority; and having things done for him with a tendency to boss.

As noted from the above, the existential condition of occupying one of these two ordinal positions is conducive to developing goals and a private cognitive system organized around attention getting, power manipulations, vindictive endeavors if power-centered behavior is thwarted and, finally, the presentation of oneself as disabled if the prior two goals cannot be achieved. The success with which one attains these goals is partially contingent on the activity level from which he operates. The child with a history of resisting submission to an overly dominating mother, despite her facade of loving concern, is likely to pursue his goals at a higher energy level than the passive child who submits, accommodating his mother's needs over his own, and who behaves as if muscular activity and social contacts are associated with danger and separation. Indeed, because the obese person often operates from a passive-aggressive posture, the Adlerian therapist attempts to use action-oriented methods, once the cognitive distortions are understood, to help him develop the social dimension of his existence.

Another family network variable operating in confluence with ordinal position is parental input. Nikelly (1971) details six parental attitudes which can influence an individual's adaptational style. These are: parental overprotection, pampering, neglect, partiality, domination, and response to physical unattractiveness or handicap. The implementation of these attitudes rests on the selective emphasis of specific values and contributes to the development of an implicit family ideology. Thus, if the prevailing ideology favors the expression of tenderness, passivity and purity, but taboos aggressiveness, competitiveness and sexuality, there may be recourse to expressing these arousal needs through other means, including overeating.

The Adlerian therapist operates from the tenet that behavioral change cannot be affected until the individual understands the private assumptions and hidden goals which give meaning to his excessive consumption of food. This approach resembles the procedure of targeting in on the individual's cognitive dissonance (Zimbardo, 1969). Presumably the dissonant state exists when the individual believes that he has voluntarily committed himself to a course of action (eating) which has negative consequences (obesity) in order to satisfy some immediate motive (gratification, tension reduction, etc.). The Adlerian, however, would link the motive to a dimly envisaged (unconscious, fictional) goal which serves as the steering element of his behavior and sustains the dissonance.

The patient often behaves as if he does not want to know about what is implicit in his relationship to the interpersonal world. It is as if he has a vested interest in not facing his interpersonal poverty. The Adlerian tries to impart clarity to his cognitive operations. In addition, there is use of encouragement and action-promoting techniques to deal with social stress in incremental steps. The objective may be the defusing of his misperception of living in an enemy camp or of the mistaken notion that everyone is getting promoted while he is left back. Only when conditions of perceptual and cognitive clarity prevail can social interest be activated. Otherwise, there is little understanding of the difference between "eating to live" and "living to eat," or of the notion that "food is energy and not love." The descriptive view that the obese person has a greedy, incorporative view of the world which he perceives in terms of food and supplies, in contrast to his own self which is a void that needs desperately to be filled, has limited value. The obese person must understand that his subjective view of himself has elements of a self-fulfilling prophecy; that as long as he views himself as weak and helpless, he will feel compelled to establish dependency relations and will probably seek out people who tend to be dominating; and that he can drop his adipose shield and be a "thin" effective participant in his own destiny.

REFERENCES

Adler, A. *The Practice And Theory of Individual Psychology.* New York: Humanities Press, 1951.

American Psychiatric Association. *Diagnostic and Statistical Manual of Mental Disorders* (3rd ed.). Washington, D. C.: Division of Public Affairs, American Psychiatric Association, 1980.

Bruch, H. *Eating Disorders.* New York: Basic Books, 1973.

Bruch, H. and Touraine, G. Obesity in childhood, V: The family frame of obese children. *Psychosom. Med.*, 1940, *2*, 141-206.

Dreikurs, R. *Psychology in the Classroom.* New York: Harper and Row, 1968.

Hofling, C. K. *Textbook of Psychiatry for Medical Practice,* Ch. 5. Philadelphia: Lippincott, 1968.

Kaplan, H. I. and Kaplan, H. S. The psychosomatic concept of obesity. *J. Nerv. Ment. Dis.*, 1957, *125*, 181.

Nikelly, A. G. Fundamental concepts of maladjustment. *Techniques for Behavior Change.* (Nikelly, A. G., Ed.). Springfield, Ill,: Thomas, 1971.

Stunkard, A. J. Eating patterns and obesity. *Psychiat. Quart.*, 1959, *33*, 284-292.

Zimbardo, P. G. *The Cognitive Control of Motivation.* Glenview, Ill.: Scott, Foresman and Co., 1969.

7

The Stigma of Overweight in Everyday Life*

Natalie Allon

The dynamics of stigma in contemporary America reinforce the view of overweight as a visible and discredited handicap, somewhat distinct from the inherent properties of overweight itself. The stigmatized fat person often is regarded and treated by others as having a physical, mental, emotional, moral, or appearance impairment (Allon, 1973b). Many researchers and practitioners have noted that the stigma associated with obesity significantly contributes to generating hateful self-conceptions among those who are fat and others who strenuously try to avoid fatness (Bruch, 1973a; Buchanan, 1973; Rubin, 1979; Stunkard and Burt, 1967; Stunkard and Mendelson, 1961, 1967). The social meaning of obesity is derived in interaction with others, not from the obese attribute alone. In stigmatization, deviance becomes a label attached to a person by others, rather than being an attribute of the deviant. The stigmatizing of fat people involves the rejection and disgrace which are connected with fatness viewed as a physical deformity and as a behavioral aberration (Cahnman, 1968, p. 293). The imputing of social deviancy to the fat person and the societal response to the deviant fat person cannot be explained easily by the fat person's characteristics and behavior. The *social* assignment of an individual as a deviant fat person is frequently the crucial contingency in the emergence and maintenance of his/her deviant career (Maddox, Back, and Liederman, 1968, p. 287).

---

*I am most grateful to Vivian Mayer (Aldebaran) and Karl Niedershuh for their help in collecting some of this information.

Researchers in the psychology and physiology of overweight have stated:

Obese people, like the physically handicapped, wear their "problem" for all to see at all times, and yet unlike those groups are held responsible for their condition. They can scarcely avoid interactions with others in which weight and eating behavior are an explicit topic of discussion, concern, and criticism, or a covert determinant of others' evaluations. [Wooley, Wooley, and Dyrenforth, 1979a, 1979b, p. 18.]

PREJUDICE AND DISCRIMINATION

Using populations of high school females in two experiments, DeJong (1980) has demonstrated that derogation of the obese results from the presumption that such persons are responsible for their physical deviance. Unless the obese can provide an excuse for their weight, such as a thyroid condition, or can offer evidence of successful weight loss, their character will be impugned. Some obese persons were seen as less self-disciplined and more self-indulgent than obese persons who reported having a glandular disorder. The obese person who claimed a recent 25-pound weight loss also was viewed more positively on dimensions of self-control, although not nearly so positively as was the obese person who reported having a glandular disorder. This research concludes that many obese persons are stigmatized because they are held responsible for their fatness. The obese are assumed to be responsible for their deviant status, presumably lacking self-control and will power. They are not merely physically deviant as are physically disabled or disfigured persons, but they seem to possess a characterological stigma. Fat people are viewed as "bad" or "immoral"; supposedly, they do not want to change the errors of their ways.

The stigmatized fat person lacks full social acceptance and is deprived of his/her right to be evaluated according to his/her unique personality (Kalisch, 1975, p. 77).

The word "fatness" itself has a negative sound, somehow connoting weakness, laziness, lack of self-discipline. The word "fat" is seldom used even by health professionals, who substitute the word "obese." A prevailing attitude is that the fat person could lose weight if he really wanted to; he doesn't because he's lacking in motivation and discipline. Society's negative feelings toward obesity are more seriously reflected in its attempted denial of such an entity. Department stores catering to the larger woman display their clothes on size 10 and 12 models; television ads promoting products for weight reduction demonstrate only successes, never the failures. [Craft, 1972, p. 679.]

Straus (1966, p. 795) has commented that the obese person is made quite aware of the fact that he or she is different; in countless ways, society ignores his or her needs.

Public facilities of all kinds are designed to accentuate his discomfort. Seats in theaters, airplanes, buses and other public conveyances are too narrow. Automobile designers ignore his proportions. Even turnstiles pose problems. Whether sliding through narrow doorways, sitting in ordinary chairs which creak under his weight, moving in a crowd — in almost every aspect of living — the fat man or woman is made to feel different and is made aware of the fact that he or she doesn't really "fit."

Experts have commented upon how the media have been intentionally or unintentionally insulting to fat people. A subtle insult is contained in an advertisement by a pharmaceutical company in a journal for physicians specializing in the treatment of obesity. It shows a young doctor shaking his finger at an older overweight woman who sits with an expression of shame. Another advertisement shows a female patient protesting to the doctor that she eats like a bird, while the physician imagines the bird to be a vulture. This ad was so popular that it has been a comic opening in many professional talks. (Wooley and Wooley, 1979, p. 76.)

Commenting upon the death of Cass Elliott, or "Mama Cass," reporters stated that when the 200-pound female rock singer died, initial findings suggested that she choked to death on a ham sandwich. There were many snickers in media commentaries about her body weight and the cause of her death as part of her obituary. Such insensitivities and lack of public protest were quite poignant because Cass Elliott had publicly stated, after a much publicized weight loss, that she resented discovering that people's liking for her was so dependent upon her physical appearance, and she decided that being thin was not worth it to her. *Time* magazine chose to print a letter to the editor, commenting on the cover story on Boston Symphony conductor Sarah Caldwell, which stated that one could not regard Sarah Caldwell as anything but a big blob of blubber. In an analysis of the appearances of overweight characters in the 30 most popular American television shows, it was found that overweight females, but not males, were highly underrepresented, especially overweight white females — only 1 in 131 continuing characters and 2 in single appearances. How can the social acceptance of the obese minority be fostered by such a limited exposure? (Wooley and Wooley, 1979, pp. 76-77.)

The stigmatizing characteristic of fatness often becomes an exclusive focal point of interaction between fat and thin people. Indeed, some overweight people become so preoccupied with their obesity, often to the exclusion of other personal characteristics, that they view their experiences in the world mainly in terms of body weight (Allon, 1976; Stunkard and Mendelson, 1961). It is important to investigate samples of obese persons who do not have disturbances in their body images. Such persons have not been so concerned about how others have regarded them. Some fat persons, particularly those who became obese in adult life (rather than in childhood or adolescence), or who had secure childhoods and stable personalities, or whose family did not derogate obesity, escaped disturbed body images. In fact, when families value their childrens' overweight as a sign of strength and health, the presence of obesity may even heighten self-esteem (Bruch, 1941; Stunkard and Mendelson, 1961, p. 329). It is important to stress that other people's responses to the fat person have been and can be major contributing factors in heightening or in lowering self-esteem.

It is no wonder that with the many negative views about fat people, many fat persons are full of self-disparagement and self-hatred. They are trebly disadvantaged: (1) because they are discriminated against, (2) because they are made to feel that they deserve such discrimination, and (3) because they come to accept their treatment as just (Cahnman, 1968, p. 294). Indeed, obese adolescent girls have shown their status as minority group members by withdrawal, passivity, the expectation of rejection, and an overconcern with self-image. They are victims of prejudice, similar to various ethnic and racial minorities (Monello and Mayer, 1963). However, many members of victimized ethnic and racial minorities can frequently find people who accept and esteem them, while there is usually no group to whom the obese girl can readily turn to find such a welcome, often including rejecting family members (Mayer, 1968, pp. 122–123). Obesity has been found to be particularly difficult for adolescents to accept, because being different from peers is equal to being inferior. For the adolescent, obesity not only means unattractiveness in terms of current cultural ideals, but it also implies guilt and lack of will power. Slenderness almost to the point of emaciation seems to approximate the ideal of most adolescent girls (Dwyer, 1973; Dwyer, Feldman, and Mayer, 1970; Dwyer and Mayer, 1968).

A comment needs to be added about the uses or abuses of scientific research. In many studies, Schachter and his colleagues have found that overweight people are overresponsive to external cues in the environment and underresponsive to internal visceral cues, such as gastrointestinal contractions (Schachter, 1968, 1972; Schachter, Goldman and Gordon, 1968; Schachter and Gross, 1968; Schachter and Rodin, 1974). Not only are generalizations from Schachter and his colleagues' mainly in vitro studies to the in vivo real world almost impossible, but such generalizations can be harmful. Perhaps the danger does not reside in the hard-working and careful research efforts of Schachter and his colleagues. The difficulty arises when writers in the popular press summarize that fat people are overly sensitive to external cues in the environment. Even if an employer reading a popular account of Schachter's theories wants to give the fat woman or fat man a chance and hire him or her, the employer will think twice about hiring someone who is destined to be overly sensitive to sights, noises, smells — many distracting cues in the environment. The reader of a popular version of Schachter's theories may have a noisy office with many visual, auditory, olfactory, and interpersonal stimuli, and many sources of distraction. Such an employer probably will decide that he/she will be safer and take fewer risks in hiring the thinner potential employee who is less likely to be distracted by such everyday external cues than is the overweight person.

The health industry has depicted obesity as the prime symbol of contemporary Americans' faulty life styles. Blue Cross has run advertisements in newspapers and magazines, and spots on the radio, which partly blame overweight Americans for the high cost of health care. One full-page advertisement showed a sketch of an overweight man: his shirt buttons were straining; his abdomen hung sloppily over his belt. The caption underneath the drawing commented: "One of the reasons for the high cost of health care." Underneath the caption were graphs showing the rise in the costs of coronary care units, implying that obesity was causing more heart attacks and therefore responsible for the rise in health costs. It has been shown that obesity is not always a major cause of heart attacks. The increase in coronary care unit costs is due less to a higher incidence of heart attacks than to the proliferation of high-technology medical equipment and the profit-making activities of American health industries. This Blue Cross advertisement shows how fat people are blamed for problems and expenses created by the structure of the American medical care system and its profit orientation. Blame for the failure of the health system is shifted to individuals who really are more its victims than its perpetrators. (Millman, 1980, pp. 88–89.)

Overweight people seem to experience prejudice and discrimination in many areas of life. The life insurance industry as a whole does charge differential rates for the obese individual. The Build and Blood Pressure Studies play an important role in this area, for they define the life risk which is statistically present for the overweight. The life insurance companies literally are betting against the deaths of those who are insured. When the odds of dying of those insured are increased, the companies attempt to shorten these odds. Most companies have not written differential, high-risk policies unless the applicants are at least 20 percent overweight. (Tucker, 1980, p. 57.) Some obese people have reported that the excuse (be it true or false) that "our insurance company will not cover you" is a widely used technique for refusing an employment application. Also, some medical insurance plans will not cover obesity-related claims or pay for expenses incurred for weight reduction. (Tucker, 1980, p. 58.)

Obese individuals have had much difficulty finding clothes in appropriate size ranges, in attractive styles which are more than simple body coverings, and at reasonable prices. Clothes for the overweight are not universally available.

Department stores often do not carry a full range of sizes, and when they do, the garments are often restricted in styles and in prices. The reception of the overweight shopper is not always so pleasant. Sales clerks have been reported to ignore overweight shoppers or, even worse, make disparaging comments to them. Overweight persons have commented on being pointed at and stared at by many others. Specialty shops catering to the overweight are available mainly in the large metropolitan areas, and they are not easily accessible to all consumers. (Tucker, 1980, pp. 59-60.)

Public facilities present a major problem for some overweight persons. Seating on public transportation, especially airplanes and buses, can be quite difficult. Under CAB rules, airlines can require passengers who need two seats because of their girth to pay an extra half fare. Mass transport, such as buses and subways which use formed plastic seats, is also difficult for, and even unusable by, the very overweight. Bench seating provides little or no support for the overweight. Theater and stadium seats are narrow since they are designed to provide space for the maximum number of customers at a given performance. Restaurants, such as fast-food restaurants, especially those with booth seating, can be troublesome for the overweight. Turnstile restricted access means that very overweight individuals must request alternate entrances or face embarrassment and the potential of physical damage. (Tucker, 1980, pp. 61-62.)

In summary, Lyman (1978, p. 218) has made the following insightful remarks:

Societal opposition to gluttony manifests itself in a variety of social control devices and institutional arrangements. Although rarely organized as a group, very fat individuals at times seem to form a much beset minority, objects of calculating discrimination and bitter prejudice. Stigmatized because their addiction to food is so visible in its consequences, the obese find themselves ridiculed, rejected, and repulsed by many of those who do not overindulge. Children revile them on the streets, persons of average size refuse to date, dance or dine with them, and many businesses, government, and professional associations refuse to employ them. So great is the pressure to conform to the dictates of the slimness culture in America that occasionally an overweight person speaks out, pointing to the similarities of his condition to that of racial and national minorities. Evidence of occupational and educational discrimination against fat people includes cases wherein a civil engineer is told to lose weight or find another job, overweight schoolteachers are fired for refusing to lose weight in accordance with an administratively imposed timetable, college entrance requirements give preference to slim applicants, and the president of a major corporation states that he refuses to hire fat people because he believes that excessive weight is indicative of a general lack of discipline. For those who refuse to acquiesce to the chorus of demands, threats and medical opinions that exhort them to lose weight, a retreat into seclusion sometimes seems to mitigate the oppression. Other oppressed minorities have formed defensive group associations and structured their enforced segregated existence so as to embrace group sentiment, and in a few cases so have the overweight. However, most fat people are rarely in a position to resolve their painful situation in this manner. Lonely and isolated, the fat person, or the fat couple, perhaps finds solace alone, eating to heart's and stomach's content. Ironically, this isolation and loneliness may add considerably to the vexatious situation in which over-indulgence occurs, creating a vicious circle.

Lyman has also stated that the supposed voluntary character of food gluttony makes it seem more an act of moral defalcation rather than medical pathology. As a "victimless crime," gluttony may facilitate an early death for the glutton as well as a living death. The overindulgent eater carries on an isolated, asocial ex-istence, often deprived of the admiration, companionship, and love of his/her nongluttonous peers. (Lyman, 1978, p. 220.) The large glutton may defile his/her own body space, as he/she spreads out to take more than one person's ordi-nary allotment of territory. In terms of possibly wrecking furniture, the fat glutton's girth calls for precautions. Such a glutton makes more demands on friends and associates than others of normal size. The glutton forces others to be conscious of and careful for him/her. As a potential threat to company and convenience, the glutton may lose his/her place altogether and be relegated to isolated eating places that will contain him/her. (Lyman, 1978, p. 223.)

Tobias and Gordon (1980) have discussed how fat people are discredited and stereotyped in everyday life by family members, friends, and strangers. Fat peo-ple often are not regarded or accepted as capable human beings irrespective of their weight or weight losing patterns. Sometimes the label of "fat" so intensi-fies female adolescents' feelings of loneliness and separateness that these girls do not realize that thin people experience such feelings; therefore, the fat girls turn toward other fat people. By remaining fat, some people become somewhat com-fortable in their deviant life styles and reluctant to learn the new patterns of in-teraction which many thin people have taken for granted all their lives. In fact, years of being a fat person can result in intensely painful feelings of inadequacy and insecurity that remain long after the weight is lost.

BIAS IN COLLEGE ADMISSIONS

Canning and Mayer (1966) have done research showing a strong bias in college admissions against obese boys and even more against obese girls. The obese and nonobese youth did not differ on objective measures of intellectual ability and achievement or on the percentage who applied for college admission. An obese girl had only one-third as much chance to get into a "prestige" college, the college of her choice, or indeed any college, as a nonobese girl (Mayer, 1968, p. 91).

If obese adolescents have difficulty in attending college, a substantial proportion may experience a drop in social class, or fail to advance beyond present levels. Education, occupation, and income are social-class variables that are strongly interrelated. A vicious circle, therefore, may begin as a result of college-admission discrimination, preventing the obese from rising in the social-class system. [Canning and Mayer, 1966, p. 1174.]

In particular, Mayer (1968, p. 91) states that the obese girl who does not get into and does not go to college:

. . . is thus likely to go down in socio-economic status. Decreased likelihood of advancing socially through marriage is also an obvious penalty which the obese girl — the ugly duckling of our age — has to pay. She may thus be lower-class because she is obese, as much as or rather than, be obese because she is lower-class.

In studying obesity as an influence on high school performance, Canning and Mayer (1967) found that the obese and the nonobese youth did not differ in (1) intelligence, in terms of IQ, PSAT, and SAT scores; (2) academic grades; (3) number of days absent during the school year or number of office visits to the school nurse, therefore indicating no differences in health records; (4) plans following high school graduation, the obese being just as interested in attending college as the nonobese; and (5) enrollment in extracurricular activities. The lack of differences in obese and nonobese students, especially in the important area of grades, led to the conclusion that prejudice against obese college applicants was not so much a result of the prejudice of high school teachers as it was of admission interviewers' prejudice.

BIAS IN EMPLOYMENT PRACTICES

Beside prejudice against obese college applicants, job discrimination at various levels for different kinds of jobs clearly exists for fat people. In one population of middle-aged women (Roe and Eickwort, 1976, p. 199), the major variables accounting for the association between obesity and unemployment were secondary diseases coexisting with obesity, especially abnormal EKG, diabetes, history of gall bladder disease, and hernia. Questionnaires completed by 81 employers of women in the sample population elicited the information that 15.9 percent would not hire obese women, that 43.9 percent considered obesity as conditional medical grounds for not employing an applicant, and that a history of heart disease or high blood pressure was considered as a relative or absolute cause for nonemployment by 47.6 and 30.5 percent of employers, respectively. Also, 46.3 percent of the employers considered a history of mental disease as grounds for nonemployment, and 41.5 percent considered a history of alcoholism as grounds for nonemployment. Therefore, obesity was seen as a little worse than alcoholism and a little better than mental disease, a ranking which may partly be interpreted by the common belief that mental disease is involuntary, while obesity and alcoholism are under the control of the individual.

Two researchers (Roe and Eickwort, 1976, p. 203) have stressed that in considering why some obese women were unemployed, employer prejudice should not be underestimated. In their research, while relatively few of the employers interviewed perceived obesity as an absolute contraindication to hiring, an unwillingness to employ fat women, except under defined circumstances, was reported by almost half of those responding to the questionnaire. It was not explained whether they considered obesity to be an occupational hazard, whether they objected to the appearance of those who were grossly overweight, or whether they anticipated absenteeism as a result of illness complicating the obesity.

Employability has been found to decrease with health disability even when there has been a partial limitation in the kind or amount of work that could be performed (Haber, 1969). Probability of absenteeism and illness is a most important consideration when business owners, managers, or personnel officers were deciding whether or not to hire unskilled applicants. Such attitudes may be realistic, as they reflect those of physicians in industry. During 1968, when a Rochester-based company was seeking unskilled help, major reasons for medical rejection were obesity (defined as more than 30 percent above normal standards for height and weight), hypertension, varicose veins, and hernias. In a report on the follow-up of workers whom this company did hire, it was emphasized that absenteeism, accident, and illness records were good (Strasser, 1972, p. 269). Had the rejected applicants been hired, experience might have been otherwise (Roe and Eickwort, 1976, p. 203.)

One study (Drenick, 1973) has reported on the social benefits from weight loss after a fasting regimen. The results are given in Table 7-1. Not only was there a 21 percent increase in employment after weight loss, but there was also a pay increase for 56 percent of those who were employed prior to the study.

One experimental study (Larkin and Pines, 1979) has examined the effects of weight, isolated from other characteristics of the job applicant, and found significant stereotyping and negative treatment, both in the hiring process and in evaluation. There existed a negative stereotype of overweight persons on traits relevant to successful job performance. In a simulated work setting, this negative stereotype was associated with discriminatory hiring behavior against persons who

Table 7-1. Social Benefits from Weight Loss.*
(*n* = 105)

	Before Weight Loss		After Weight Loss	
Retired, etc.		9		9
Employed	(39%)	53	(60%) 83	(after 4 years)
Unemployed	(30%)	43 (after 2 years)	(8%) 10	
Pay greater		—	(56%) 30	(of 53 employed prior to weight loss)

*From Drenick (1973, p. 359).

were overweight. Such discriminatory hiring bias occurred despite equivalent performance on task-related selection tests — physical and mental. It was not the case that performance was misperceived or misrecalled. The overweight persons were less likely to be hired even though they were perceived to be equally competent on the tests.

In a widely reported study by the Robert Half Association (an employment agency), only 9 percent of the executives surveyed who earned between $25,000 and $50,000 each year were more than 10 pounds overweight, while 39 percent of the executives surveyed who earned between $10,000 and $20,000 each year were more than 10 pounds overweight. Therefore, an executive earning between $25,000 and $50,000 was about 75 percent less likely to be overweight than his lower-paid colleague. It was estimated that each pound of fat could cost an executive $1,000 per year. This study found not only that overweight workers made less money than their slimmer counterparts, but also that they were less likely to get top spots when promotions came around. A survey done by this employment agency four years earlier had shown more overweight executives making a top salary and fewer overweight workers in the lower group. Half said that his agency got thousands of requests from employers for executives "on the thinner side." (Fat execs get slimmer paychecks, 1974.)

Reviewing the literature, the experience of others, and his own personal experiences, Louderback (1970, p. 47) states that studies show that only 10 percent of the highest salaried executives were more than 10 pounds overweight. The corporate image that sells to the public is thinness. Employers in confidence have admitted that they do not think fat people are as efficient or can stand the hard pace of work as much as thin people. Fat employees are viewed as possibly being out sick more often than thin workers. (Louderback, 1970, p. 49.)

Louderback (1970, pp. 50-51) states that weight is also considered for jobs of typists, file clerks, receptionists, and secretaries, where the public might form an impression of the company by the employees on display. Often these aesthetic considerations of image are only admitted off the record. On the record, the health angle and a vague sense of insurance problems of the overweight are stated. The medical exam required for some employment can be a convenient subterfuge not to hire a fat person for so-called other reasons than one's overweight.

Louderback (1970, pp. 51-52) also states that fat persons are viewed as tiring easily, being more accident prone, and being more likely to become victims of chronic disease. They are frozen out of the better-paying jobs with the more prestigious firms. Weight conscious employees may raise more of a fuss about hiring a fat person than do bosses. Low-paying private employers often find overweight persons to be loyal and conscientious as a result of their trouble finding work.

In order to get or keep jobs or be promoted, people in the police and fire forces, the armed forces, and the FBI have been told to reduce (Louderback, 1970, p. 53; Mayer, 1968, pp. 86-87). Because of some hard-fought individual battles, the Civil Service is still open to the overweight (Louderback, 1970, pp. 54-55). Boards of Education have tried successfully and unsuccessfully to fire capable, devoted, overweight teachers (Louderback, 1970, pp. 55-57).

Because of complaints by Pearl M. Mittelman and others that the city is denying them jobs on the basis of obesity, Los Angeles has moved to ease the restrictions against the hiring of overweight persons (Baker, 1975). In this case there was an acknowledgement by persons involved that some overweight people might be healthy and capable, quite qualified to handle jobs. I personally testified in the state of Maryland in 1979 in support of House Joint Resolution No. 75 by Delegates Dypski, Shapiro, and Dyson concerning discrimination against fat people. This resolution urged all Maryland citizens to work toward ending unjust discrimination practices against fat people. This resolution passed through its various stages and was signed into law by the governor of Maryland; the State Commission on Human Relations has been authorized to study the problem and has issued a report stressing fat discrimination (Tucker, 1980).

Discrimination against fat people in employment as a widespread practice has perhaps not been thoroughly documented because fat people are not recognized as an oppressed minority in the economic sense. The National Association to Aid Fat Americans, Inc., with headquarters in Bellerose, New York, has records and collections of many cases of possible, probable, and actual discrimination in employment against fat people.

THE NATIONAL ASSOCIATION TO AID FAT AMERICANS, INC.

NAAFA is a nonprofit organization with a few dozen chapters in cities across the United States. It was started in 1969 by an average-sized electrical engineer from New York, a man who was attracted to fat women and who saw the suffering of his fat wife. NAAFA has provided fat people and fat admirers a comfortable social support network in a world hostile to fatness. NAAFA has a perspective which challenges many commonly held views about fatness. The organization stresses that fat can be beautiful, that fat people can feel good about themselves, and that going on a diet is not always the solution to a fat person's problems. The organization also stresses that it is all right to be fat and that what most basically needs to be changed are social attitudes and treatment of fat people. Then, indeed, the self-hatred of fat people can be lessened, if not eliminated. (Millman, 1980, p. 4.)

Commenting on their victimization, NAAFA members discuss how fat Americans have difficulties in buying nice clothes, in getting and keeping jobs, in exploitation by commercial interests, in buying health and life insurance, and in social relationships in which there often is contempt, ridicule, repugnance, and avoidance, even by medical doctors. Many NAAFA members stress that being fat does not result from a lack of will power, but that body type, heredity, early childhood habits, and metabolism contribute to obesity. Many NAAFA members believe that the so-called negative effects of overweight on health have been very exaggerated. Some say that for some people a weight loss may be desirable for health reasons. Yet many argue that the typical experience of many fat people of repeatedly losing and regaining weight may be more destructive than maintaining a stable high weight. Therefore, a central goal of the organization is to help fat people accept and respect themselves as they are so that they can live the fullest and happiest lives possible. The organization has a match-dating service and dances. Newslettters published every few months offer useful information: reviews of medical treatments for overweight, advice about how and where to buy large clothes or find wide seats in public places and in transportation, names of physicians recommended as not hostile to fat people, reviews of books about dieting and weight, items about prejudice and discrimination against fatness, and announcements of weddings between members who met through the organization. NAAFA members also engage in public demonstrations, letter-writing campaigns, and interviews with the media to call attention to activities and policies that are discriminatory or offensive to fat people. (Millman, 1980, pp. 4, 8.)

The organization does not discourage dieting. Even though the fat admirers in NAAFA are attracted to fat bodies, many women in NAAFA are not so glad to be overweight. Many have come to NAAFA because they are at the end of the conventional line. Having repeatedly failed to become and stay thin, they have decided to learn to live with, and more or less accept, who they are. Unable to pass for "normal" in the outside world, they have found a comfortable home among their own. (Millman, 1980, p. 8.) Sometimes NAAFA also tries to convince fat people not to pin their hopes on a big transformation if and when they lose weight. Also, NAAFA demands full acceptance for its members in the outside world. A major argument of NAAFA is that a person should not have to be thin to deserve the full roster of human rights and privileges; self-acceptance and acceptance by others should not be conditional on a person's weight. NAAFA argues that fat people are isolated because they are socially excluded. (Millman, 1980, pp. 43-45.)

NAAFA has adopted political terminology and slogans that proclaim its members' differences from others in a neutral or positive way and in a manner that takes issue with the majority's view of normalcy. NAAFA uses the word *fat* rather than *obese* or *overweight*, or rather than "gentle and polite euphemisms" such as fleshy, a little heavy, a little rotund, chubby, pudgy, rounded, and hefty — just as Blacks rejected the word *Negro*, and *gay* was substituted for *homosexual*. In all such cases, the motive has been to discard a label that had been applied by the oppressive majority and to use instead a name originating from the minority group itself. (Millman, 1980, p. 91.)

Radical feminists have discussed the social isolation and psychological oppression of fat women. While NAAFA asks that fat people be allowed to participate fully in society as it currently exists, these radical feminists have argued that fat oppression is part of the larger problem of sexism in contemporary America. Radical feminists have argued for a more basic transformation of society. They say that present American society stresses packaging appearances for the purposes of successful saleability, with the contents being secondary. In contrast, NAAFA members often believe in quite traditional heterosexual relationships. Both NAAFA members and radical feminists have pointed out macro-societal discrimination against fat people in social institutions and micro-discrimination in more intimate interpersonal relationships. Both groups have talked about the exploitation and derogatory views of fat people in the mass media and by the medical profession. Both groups recognize a need for consciousness raising as well as for political action. (Millman, 1980, pp. 93-94.)

LEGAL ISSUES CONCERNING FAT DISCRIMINATION*

There have been very few court cases which relate to claims of discrimination based on obesity/overweight per se. Most such cases include the notion of weight standards applying differentially to the sexes. Some examples are: *Wolf* v. *Metropolitan Dade County* (274 So. 2d 584), *Cox* v. *Delta* (CCH 14 EPD 7600), and *Smith* v. *City of East Cleveland* (363 F. Supp. 1131); see also *Gerdom* v. *Continental Airlines* (CCH 13 EPD 11 320). (Tucker, 1980, p. 67.)

Two cases have been relied on as precedent by counsel for the Pennsylvania Human Relations Commission in the case of *English* v. *Philadelphia Electric Co.*, E-12163. They are *Parolis* v. *Board of Examiners of the City of New York*

---

*I am deeply grateful to Tucker (1980) for his research and summation of these cases.

(55 Misc. 2d 545 and 285 N.Y. Supp. 2d 936) and *Blodget* v. *Board of Trustees* (20 Calif. App. 3d 183, also 97 Calif. Rpt. 406). In these cases, the refusal to hire was based only on conditions of overweight, and was found by the courts in both cases to be discriminatory (Tucker, 1980, pp. 67–68). In March, 1980, an administrative finding by the Human Relations Commission of Pennsylvania held that Philadelphia Electric Company had unlawfully discriminated against the Complainant by refusing to hire her on the basis of her non-job-related handicap or disability. In this case, it was held that severe obesity is a handicap or disability. This finding has the force of the law, unless it is appealed, whereby it may or may not be upheld. In fact, this case is now being appealed by Philadelphia Electric Company.

The only state which currently specifically includes weight and height as a protected class (Michigan) protects only in the area of employment and not under the public accommodation, education, or real estate sections of the law (Elliot-Larsen Civil Rights Act, Act. No. 453, Public Acts of 1976, Approved by Governor, January 13, 1977 as Amended by Act 162, Public Acts of 1977, and Act 153, Public Acts of 1978). It should be noted that Michigan performed no study prior to including weight and size in their law. That inclusion was the result of a highly idiosyncratic local situation involving a state legislator and the director of a state institution. (Tucker, p. 68; Appendix G.)

There have been adjudications at the administrative level in the context of agencies which operate similarly to various human relations commissions. One matter was brought under Article 15, Sections 290 through 301 of the New York Code, *State Division of Human Rights (on the complaint of Trevolia Johnson)* v. *The City of New York et al.*, (S) GCD-3656-75. There it was found by a Commissioner of the New York Division of Human Rights that a woman had been denied permanent status as an employee of the New York City Housing and Development Administration, as a result of a doctor's having rated her as "not qualified" because of obesity during the probationary period of her employment with that agency. It was found that obesity was a disability within the meaning of the law and that the New York City Civil Service Commission had unlawfully discriminated against the Complainant because of the obesity. An award of back pay and reinstatement with full benefits was made. (Fleisher, Appendix F. p. 4, as cited in Tucker, 1980.)

In *Parker* v. *CETA and Franklin County CAP*, E77-0161, the Maine Human Rights Commission found that a male excluded from employment by the respondent had been discriminated against on the basis of his weight (60 pounds "overweight") and that appropriate remedies should be granted (Fleisher, Appendix F, pp. 4–5, as cited in Tucker, 1980).

However, a similar hearing before the Montana Human Rights Commission resulted in an adjudication that obesity was not a handicap within the meaning of Montana Law (similar to Maryland's). In a case brought before it, Wisconsin Department of Industry, Labor and Human Relations was led to the same conclusion under the same theory — holding that the physical condition of the complainant was clearly and completely within his self-control, but noting that this decision should be narrowly interpreted.

As it was noted that Human Rights Commission of the state of Washington processed many complaints based on size and weight discrimination, a disability specialist from this commission said that the commission did not view overweightedness to be a disabling condition. However, there were disabling conditions which manifest themselves with overweight. Such conditions would be recognized as bona fide and would be suitable for affirmative and enforcement purposes. Overweight or obese persons would be recognized by this commission to be disabled only if the employer perceived them to be disabled or if they had a disabling condition which caused them to be so. (Fleisher, Appendix F, p. 5, as cited in Tucker, 1980.)

Many cases have been concerned with how, why, and in what ways overweight/ obesity is or is not a "handicap" or a "disability," as defined by various local and state laws and policies. Therefore, physiological, psychological, sociological, and legal possible and actual definitions of "handicap" and "disability" are being scrutinized more closely. Two cases decided under other causes of action in two separate jurisdictions are relevant. The first, decided by the Supreme Court of New York, is *Parolis* v. *Board of Examiners of the City of New York*, 55 Misc. 2d. 546, 285 N.Y.S. 2d 936 (1967). There, a school teacher was denied a license as a substitute solely because of overweight. She petitioned the Court, under Article VI of the New York State Constitution, to annul the determination of the school system's Board of Examiners that she was not qualified. In granting the petition of Ms. Parolis, the court stated that no one can reasonably deny the need to limit appointments to persons in good health when such a condition affects the ability to discharge the duties of the position. Obesity as a constitutional standard is reasonably and rationally related to fitness to perform the duties of positions such as firemen and policemen. However, standing alone, obesity is not reasonably and rationally related to the ability to teach or maintain discipline. It was considered an arbitrary and capricious determination to prevent this school teacher from having a license as a substitute solely because of her overweight. (Fleisher, Appendix F, pp. 5–6, as cited in Tucker, 1980.)

Also, a physical education teacher brought a mandamus action against the Board of Trustees of Tamalpais Union High School District in California because of a refusal to reemploy her on grounds of obesity. The First District Court of Appeals found that a lower court was incorrect in holding, as the only permissible basis for refusing to reemploy her on grounds of her obesity, that her obesity impaired her ability to function effectively as a teacher and that it would, therefore, be detrimental to the welfare of the school and/or its pupils to retain her; see *Blodgett* v. *Board of Trustees,* 20 Calif. App. 3d 183, 97 Calif. 406 (1971). (Fleisher, Appendix F, pp. 6-7, as cited in Tucker, 1980.)

Should not legal protection be extended to obese/overweight persons, to the extent that their problems may be seen as similar to or identical with those of persons with other handicaps or disabilities? Physical or mental handicaps include disabilities, infirmities, malformations or disfigurements which arise from a variety of causes. The issue is whether the following definitions of a "handicapped individual" apply to the obese/overweight person. A handicapped individual is one who has a physical, mental, or emotional handicap and whose condition is demonstrable by medically accepted techniques; the handicap substantially limits or is regarded as limiting one or more of the person's major life activities such as employment, transportation, adaptation to housing, communication, self-care, recreation, socialization, education, and vocational training; the person is *regarded* as having a handicap whether an impediment exists or not, and so is limited in life activities. (Fleicher, Appendix F, pp. 1-3, as cited in Tucker, 1980.)

Legal actions and lawsuits have begun to question the legality of weight criteria for employment or membership. Such suits revolve around the civil rights and health status of fat people. Recent federal legislation requiring employment of the physically handicapped in order to qualify for federal funding (Rehabilitation Act of 1973) might have relevance for charges of discrimination by fat people. Employers have argued that fat people are unable to do the work of thin people. Employers also have taken the position that although fat people are not physically fit for the job, they are not truly handicapped because their problem is voluntary. There indeed is debate about how voluntary fatness is; some doctors view obesity as incurable. Complex physiological, biochemical, metabolic, and psychological factors affecting fat storage may mean that overweight/obesity is not always a choice for people. Obesity/overweight as an involuntary condition has not been used as an argument much in discrimination suits, in part because few fat people want to define themselves as physically handicapped and therefore are unlikely to seek protection under the Federal Rehabilitation Act. More often, the argument for equal employment opportunity has been based on the claim that fat people are just as competent in work as are thinner people. One view has been that obesity might be defined as a physical handicap and therefore come under protective legislation. In order to decide whether obesity is a physical handicap in certain cases, employers have asked doctors to state whether a fat person might safely lose a certain amount of weight in a time period satisfactory to an employer or whether the weight problem is immutable and permanent. (Millman, 1980, pp. 91-92.)

STUDIES ON THE STIGMA OF FATNESS

There have been systematic and careful studies that have found clearcut evidence of the stigma of obesity which, at least in part, may be the basis for some of this actual discrimination. At an early age, children of both sexes develop distinct aversions to chubby bodies and preferences for athletic or lean ones. The ecto-morph refers to the long, slender body; the mesomorph, to the well-muscled, athletic build; and the endomorph, to the round, fleshy body with an emphasis on corpulence. Staffieri (1967, 1972) found that overweight and nonoverweight 6- to 10-year-old male and female children responded in very unfavorable ways to silhouettes of endomorphic children, using such words as cheats, dirty, argues, gets teased, forgets, lazy, lies, sloppy, mean, ugly, stupid, worries, fights, naughty, sad, and lonely. Of the girls, 67 percent preferred to look mesomorphic, and 33 percent to look ectomorphic; none preferred the endomorphic shape. There were also very positive responses to mesomorphy and very negative responses to endomorphy in Lerner's (1969a) study. Males, 10 to 20 years of age, believed an endomorphic adult male to "be the poorest athlete," "drink the most," "smoke three packs of cigarettes a day," "eat the most," "be the least likely to be chosen leader," and "make the worst soldier."

Lerner and Gellert (1969) in a study of 45 white, urban, kindergarten children, 5 to 6 years of age, reported that 86 percent of those children who were consis-tent in their choices showed an aversion for chubbiness when tested with headless photographs of chubby, average, and thin children in bathing suits. Lerner and Korn (1972) have reported that both chubby and average 5-, 15-, and 20-year-old males assign to endomorphic drawings descriptive phrases which they them-selves judge "bad" and to mesomorphic drawings phrases which they judge "good." In all age groups the chubby subjects viewed themselves as having more of the attributes that they associated with body types other than the endomorph, which suggests that these subjects had a rejecting attitude toward their own physique. Of the 90 chubby and 90 average males who were subjects in this study, only three, each of whom was an average 5-year-old, indicated a desire to look like the endomorphic drawing.

In these studies and others (Lerner, 1969b; Lerner and Schroeder, 1971a, 1971b), the characterization given to the endomorphic, or rounded, body type was clearly derogatory. The endomorph was described with words like lazy, mean, and dirty, while such words as strong, friendly, healthy, and brave were used to describe the mesomorph. Ectomorphs were sometimes regarded unfavor-ably, although not to the same degree or as uniformly as endomorphs. These findings are replicated across age, race, sex, socioeconomic status, and geograph-ical area of residence in the United States, and even with rural Mexican children (Lerner and Pool, 1972). They are present without regard to the perceiver's own body type; they are shared values about body shape and size that are be-lieved in general by all — fat, thin, or athletic.

Negative attitudes toward endomorphs have been shown to affect behavior toward this group. Researchers have found that male and female school children have wished to and did keep a greater personal space distance from the endomorph than from the other two body types (Lerner, 1973; Lerner, Karabenick, and Meisels, 1975). Such results are interpreted to mean that children are least comfortable with, and least likely to affiliate with, children of the endomorphic body type.

Two studies (Richardson, Hastorf, Goodman, and Dornbusch, 1961; Goodman, Richardson, Dornbusch, and Hastorf, 1963) presented child populations with six black and white line drawings which depicted a normal child, a child with a brace on the left leg and crutches, a child sitting in a wheelchair with a blanket covering both legs, a child with the left hand missing, a child with facial disfigurement on one side of the mouth, and a grossly overweight child. Subjects were asked to rank the pictures in terms of likeability of persons like those shown. Out of eight samples of mentally normal children, 10 to 11 years of age (sample size ranging from 42 to 163), seven samples ranked the obese child last; only the sample of white Jewish children of low socioeconomic status in New York City ranked the obese child anywhere but in the last third. (Goodman, Richardson, Dornbusch, and Hastorf, 1963, p. 434). The authors speculated that Jewish values associated with eating were different from those of other Americans. The well-fed, stockily built Jewish child is viewed by other Jews as one who is healthy and loved. The rankings of a ninth sample consisting of 72 adults including nurses, physical and occupational therapists, physicians, psychologists, and social workers revealed again that the obese child was ranked last, considered to be least likeable. This ranking of last showed up also when various controls were introduced for sex, age, disability of the evaluators, race, urban-rural residence, and socioeconomic status.

In another study using the same drawings (Maddox, Back, and Liederman, 1968), 200 adults deliberately chosen to sample populations presumed to value fatness or at least be tolerant of overweight people — people of low socioeconomic status, black people, and overweight people — ranked the obese child last. It was suggested that because the obese are held responsible for their condition, they are disliked. It is well to keep in mind that many studies have shown that lower income levels are associated with a higher prevalence of obesity for both white and black women. In fact, black women, regardless of income, have a higher prevalence of obesity than white women (Abraham, 1975, p. 28).

Studies involving adults as well as children, therefore have shown that overweight is viewed quite negatively by a number of people in this society. The obese were less likely to be helped out by strangers than the normal weight (Rodin and Slochower, 1974). In one study (Tipton and Browning, 1972), most helping behavior by women was offered to old and obese women rather than to old and nonobese women, with the least help offered to young obese women. In another study (Galper and Weiss, 1975), the faces of obese persons were rated significantly less likeable and less attractive than faces of normal weight persons. Female adult group dieters who felt the fat stigma expressed many tensions, fears and worries (Allon, 1975).

Some authors have speculated on what lies behind some of these negative views toward fatness and fat people. Reflecting upon and summarizing some of Keys' ideas, Maddox, Back, and Liederman (1968, p. 288) have written:

> . . . even if the reputed association between leanness and longevity were demonstrably false . . . fatness would still be assessed negatively as unaesthetic and as an indication of self-indulgence. In a society which has historically been suffused with a Protestant Ethic, one characteristic of which is a strong emphasis on impulse control, fatness suggests a kind of immorality which invites retribution. Correspondingly, the reduction of overweight and the avoidance of the contagion of gluttony implies self-denial, which ought to bring appropriate rewards, including good health. This moral orientation is, in turn, reinforced by aesthetic considerations . . . . physicians, and most middle-class individuals, consider extreme overweight unsightly.

Indeed, many group dieters whom I studied believed that fatness was the outcome of immoral self-indulgence. Group dieters used much religious language in considering themselves bad or good dieters — words such as sinner, saint, devil, angel, guilt, transgression, confession, absolution, and diet Bible — as they partook of the rituals of group dieting (Allon, 1972; 1973a; 1979b, pp. 29–81). The stigmatization of overweight often is encouraged in dieting groups, in which the atmosphere permits and even prescribes discussion of self-hatred and personal anguish resulting from one's fatness. The ugly, unhealthy, and immoral connotations of overweight are often part of the stigma stressed in the group, which is used to change behavior from deviant fat to normal thin (Allon, 1975; Laslett and Warren, 1975). Indeed, group dieters collectively reinforce each other's guilt — often the sin of not being a very attractive object on the "male market." Sometimes group dieters feel that they can alleviate such guilt by punishing themselves by paying for dieting strategies and techniques (Michaels, 1969). Group dieters confess their guilt and purge themselves of their unclean fat as they atone for their fat sin by praising thinness and attempting to lose weight in the groups. The stigma of fatness is accentuated as dieters weigh in on the group's scale and hear lecturers' sermons about the horrors of fatness and the goodness of thinness. It seems that group dieters as well as others in this society almost worship the ideal of thinness. Group dieters themselves use such religious language to describe their experiences. (Allon, 1973a; 1979b, pp. 29–81.)

The psychiatrist Szasz (1975, pp. 56–69, 96–98) has stated that with the medicalization of morals in contemporary America, dieting has replaced religious fasting as a ceremonial of purification, and the treatment of obesity has replaced the absolution for the sin of gluttony. The ceremonial function of self-purification carried on formerly by fasting and presently by dieting are concealed by technical arguments in favor of weight reduction. Szasz says that the overweight woman is merely one contemporary version of the mythology of feminine pollution who needs to be purified by dieting rites; other versions of feminine pollution included menstruation, superior sexual powers, and witchery, with their own kinds of purification.

The idea of fatness as pollution may be implied in some of the studies cited as well as in others. Matthews and Westie (1966) have reported that 144 high school students in a small midwestern city preferred to be at a greater social distance from an obese child than from handicapped children depicted by drawings. Social distance was assessed by a scale of graded statements ranging from "would exclude this type of person from my school" to "would be willing to marry this type of person."

Many of the studies cited lend support to the idea that the incidence of socially deviant overweight is a function of shared definitions of best weight and tolerable deviations from that standard (Maddox, Back, and Liederman, 1968, p. 297). Reflecting upon many of the studies cited, Wooley, Wooley, and Dyrenforth (1979, p. 83) have stated:

> These studies document the hatred of obese children by other children and by adults. The impact this hatred has on the individual child is probably irreversible. It is not only the obese child who suffers from this hatred; anti-fat attitudes learned in childhood no doubt become the basis for self-hatred among those who become overweight at later ages, and a source of anxiety and self-doubt for anyone fearful of becoming overweight.

FAT AS A WOMAN'S PROBLEM

Millman (1980, p. xi) has commented:

> . . . it is especially the case that an overweight woman is assumed to have a personal problem. She is stereotypically viewed as unfeminine, in flight from sexuality, antisocial, out of control, hostile, aggressive. One of the reasons for this assumption is that despite all the gains and insights of the women's liberation movement, women are still judged very much on the basis of physical appearance. And no matter what medical evidence we acquire to the contrary, being overweight is fundamentally viewed as an *intentional* act. In the case of women, being fat is considered such an obvious default or rebellion against being feminine that it is treated as a very significant, representative, and threatening characteristic of the individual . . . . more importantly, whether being fat is really a symptom of underlying emotional conflicts or simply the

logical outcome of bad eating habits or a particular body type, the overweight individual, especially if she is a woman, probably suffers more from the social and psychological stigma attached to obesity than she does from the actual physical condition. In a wide variety of ways she is negatively defined by her weight and excluded from full participation in the ranks of the normal.

Millman (1980, pp. 192–193) also has stated:

If in our culture, fat women come to symbolize either the mother (with whom men can be weak, demanding, dependent, infantile) or the whore (with whom men can be abusive or violently sexual without obligation or guilt), they are also the worst victims of our sex-role typing. For since they represent what is split off from the image of the ideal woman they are given none of the privileges of being a desirable woman and are also narrowly exposed to what is felt to be the worst sides of men — indeed, to what is split off from the "ideal" man.

One might well ask why fat women tolerate such abuse. For many it is because they have no choice — they feel they must take this or nothing. And for some, this sadistic treatment is felt to be deserved. Since some of the women feel guilty about their own sexuality (whether because of their precocious development and too successfully replacing their mothers or because they have learned to eroticize rejection by men because their own fathers were absent, unloving or withdrawn) the poor treatment they receive from men seems consistent with their own shame and self-hatred.

But the willingness to be a victim is not simply a product of childhood traumas and individual neurosis. These dynamics, however much they fulfill individual needs, flourish in a social context that worships the notion of an "ideal" man or woman.

Many studies have suggested that fat becomes more clearly a woman's problem from the time of adolescence onward. One study has suggested that weight may be an area of greater concern among adolescent girls than among adolescent boys, as shown by the fact that the girls studied weighed themselves more frequently than did adolescent boys. In this study (Dwyer, Feldman, Seltzer, and Mayer, 1969), most girls wanted to weigh less than they did, except the leanest, while most boys wanted to weigh more than they did, except the obese boys. Girls wanted to be smaller in general and in most particular bodily areas, except for wanting larger breasts. Perhaps the girls connected their overweight more with overfatness which they considered to be undesirable, while boys connected their overweight more with muscle and bone weight, which they considered to be desirable.

In one study, adolescent females, 11 to 19 years of age, were more dissatisfied with or more critical of their bodies than were male adolescents (Clifford,

1971). Among the body satisfaction items, the females rated weight, looks, legs, waist, and hips the lowest. The authors speculated that females may be more critical of their bodies because of the great emphasis placed upon clothing, personal adornment, and standards of appearance for women.

Some reasons why the stigma of overweight centers on female adolescents include reinforcement of sex role stereotypes (Dwyer, 1973; Dwyer, Feldman, and Mayer, 1970; Dwyer and Mayer, 1968), for example, mothers' greater anxiety about fatness in daughters rather than sons; limitations in popularity and social mobility for overweight females; weight-related aspects of appearance as more intertwined with the self-concept in females than in males; overweight as more visible in females than in males; girls attributing their overweight to fatness, with boys attributing their legitimate overweight to build components other than fat and often regarding overweight as desirable; and fashion's stress on the erotic potential of the thin body for women, with utilitarian clothes for men highlighting social status and being shapeless enough to conceal large amounts of fat.

Kalisch (1972, p. 78) has added that daughters as well as mothers may believe and find evidence for the fact that obese women in contemporary America find it more difficult to be upwardly mobile socially, relate to others, and obtain suitable marriage partners than do obese men. Reinforcing traditional sex role stereotypes, the self-concept of many American women is connected with physical desirability which is based upon thinness as the socially proper norm. Often the financial status, educational achievement, and occupation of a man affect his value more than does his appearance. Also, the shape of men's clothing conceals body form and can hide bulges, while women's clothing is designed to reveal the configuration of the body. In fact, many members of the National Association to Aid Fat Americans have told me that they have a hard time buying attractive clothing in large sizes, since stores often do not stock these sizes; some fat women have been forced to become skilled in sewing in order to be clothed.

Indeed, studies have shown female, white middle-class college students to be more aware of and concerned about their bodily appearance than were male, white middle-class college students (Kurtz, 1969). Jourard and Secord (1955) found that female college students wanted to be smaller than they were in height, weight, waist, and hips, but to be bigger than they were in the bust. None of the women rated positively all their bodily parts. They did not achieve their ideal sense of attractiveness to males.

Indeed, in one study, 59 percent of female college students who were within the desirable weight limits used by medical and behavioral investigators and therapists to define obesity rated themselves low on satisfaction with figure (Douty, Moore, and Hartford, 1974). In another study (Beck, Ward-Hull, and McLear, 1976), college women rated silhouettes of female figures with large buttocks, large breasts, and a proportionately large overall female figure as less preferred than silhouettes of figures with small buttocks, moderately small breasts, and a proportionately moderate overall or standard female figure.

The price paid by women for being obese is more than psychological and emotional. Their status and roles in the society are affected. One study (Goldblatt, Moore, and Stunkard, 1965, pp. 1042–1043) has shown that compared to nonobese women, overweight women were much less likely to achieve a higher socioeconomic status and much more likely to achieve a lower status than their parents. No such clearcut relationship was found among the men studied. The percentage of men who were thin was about the same for all three social classes, while the percentage of women who were thin was directly proportional to the social class level, that is, 9 percent, 19 percent, and 37 percent for low, middle, and high socioeconomic status, respectively. Women with low socioeconomic status were six times as likely as women with high status to develop obesity, and upwardly mobile women were almost half as likely to be obese as downwardly mobile women. The image of the slim, attractive female as portrayed throughout the popular culture leads to a selection process; in any status-conferring situation, such as marriage to a higher-status male or promotion at work, thinner women may be selected over their competitors.

Another study (Herman, 1973) has qualified some of these findings, in that lower socioeconomic status and lower educational levels are linked with a greater prevalence of obesity among women, but such a linkage is limited to those 40 years of age and over. In this study, one could hypothesize that the reason that social status differences are of little or no importance among younger women is because relatively few women put on excess weight as adults until they reach 35 or 40 years of age in contemporary America. This fact could reflect social and cultural pressures in women in all social strata to stay slim until they are married or while they are concerned with sexual attractiveness, at relatively young ages.

Beller (1977) stresses that female fleshiness and fatness from birth onward in many cross-cultural and historical settings are facts of biological life which appear to have been programmed into the species, long ago, by nature. Indeed as youth grow up, body fat increases in amount among girls as it decreases among boys (Dwyer, 1973). Because of an actual greater fat accumulation in their bodies, women in general may be more concerned about fatness than men.

VARIATIONS OF FATNESS IN DIFFERENT GROUPS OF PEOPLE

In a number of studies, there is a marked inverse relationship between socioeconomic status and the prevalence of obesity, when socioeconomic status is rated by scores based upon occupation, education, weekly income, and monthly rent. Although only 11 percent of the total United States population falls in the upper or upper-middle class, these classes contain 24 percent of all dieters (Wyden, 1965, p. 8). In some studies arising from research in midtown Manhattan, New York, the prevalence of obesity among women of lower socioeconomic status was 30 percent, falling to 16 percent among those of middle status, and to only 5 percent in the upper-status group (Goldblatt, Moore, and Stunkard, 1965; Moore, Stunkard, and Srole, 1962). The prevalence of obesity in the lower class in such studies was six times that found in the upper class. When socioeconomic status was divided into 12 classes, the differences between the lowermost and the uppermost social classes became even greater – from a low of less than 2 percent in the uppermost to a high of 37 percent in the lowermost class (Stunkard, 1975, p. 199). The differences between social classes among men were similar to those among women, but of a lesser degree. For example, men of a lower socioeconomic status showed a prevalence of obesity of 32 percent compared to that of 16 percent among upper-class men (Stunkard, 1975, p. 199).

Also, a study of white school children (Stunkard, d'Aquili, Fox, and Filion, 1972), 5 to 18 years of age, in three eastern cities, revealed that by 6 years of age, 29 percent of lower-class girls were rated obese as compared with only 3 percent of upper-class girls. The differences continued through age 18.

Also, the lower the social class of respondents' parents in such studies, the more likely were respondents to be obese. Obesity was more prevalent among subjects who were downwardly mobile socially (22 percent) than among those who remained in the social class of their parents (18 percent), and far more prevalent than among those who were upwardly mobile socially (12 percent) (Goldblatt, Moore, and Stunkard, 1965.) Indeed, the longer a woman's family had been in the United States, the less likely she was to be obese: of first-generation respondents, 24 percent were overweight in contrast to only 5 percent in the fourth generation (Goldblatt, Moore, and Stunkard, 1965).

Ethnic and religious factors also influence the prevalence of obesity. When only lower-class respondents are considered, the greater than 40 percent prevalence of obesity among Hungarian and Czech respondents means that there is a 3 to 1 differential between them and the least obese group, fourth generation Americans, who show a prevalence of only 13 percent. A larger proportion of women of Italian than British backgrounds were overweight. (Stunkard, 1975, pp. 202–203.) The greatest prevalence of obesity in some studies was among the Jews, followed by Roman Catholics and Protestants. Among Protestants, as a further illustration of the strong influence of social class, the largest amount of obesity has been found among Baptists, with a decreasing prevalence among Methodists, Lutherans, and Episcopalians. (Stunkard, 1975, p. 203.)

Black-white differences in weight levels have been measured in a few studies. In studies in which racial differences have been studied without regard to socioeconomic status, black women tend to be heavier than white women at all age levels. When economic levels are approximately the same, no marked racial differences appeared. (Division of Chronic Diseases, 1966.)

In a sample of over 10,000 persons in the United States, obesity, as measured by triceps skinfold thickness, was found to be most prevalent in women, particularly black women in the older age groups (45 to 74 years) who had a prevalence of 32.4 percent. White men had a higher prevalence of obesity than black men. The lowest prevalence of obesity, 7.7 percent, was found in black men, 45 to 74 years old. Men did have lower percentages of obesity than women. Percentages for men ranged from 7.7 percent for black men 45 to 74 years old, to 16.0 percent for white men 20 to 44 years old. For women, the ranges were from 18.9 percent for white women 20 to 44 years old, to 32.4 percent for black women 45 to 74 years old. In this study, lower income levels were associated with a higher prevalence of obesity for both white and black women. In fact, black women, regardless of income, had a higher prevalence of obesity than white women did. (Abraham, 1975, p. 28.)

In the younger age group of 20 to 44 years, higher income level was associated with a higher prevalence of obesity for white men. This association was also true for black men, although the magnitude of the difference of the percentage of obesity was small. In the older age groups, income level was less consistently associated with the prevalence of obesity. In the older age group, regardless of income level, white men had a higher prevalence of obesity than black men. Such an association was not evident in the younger age group. (Abraham, 1975, p. 28.)

Some surveys of attitudes of blacks and whites toward obesity have suggested that white women are more concerned about excess weight than black women or men of either race. It is still true that men and women of both races at several age and educational levels have given definitely negative reactions about obesity. (Maddox, Back, and Liederman, 1968, p. 287.)

One must consider, therefore, the possibility that if there are patterns of prejudice and discrimination against fat people, certain people with particular characteristics are more likely to be subjected to such attitudes and treatment. In particular, poor or lower-class black women may be more likely to be shown prejudice and discrimination than other groups of people, because, statistically speaking, such women tend to be fatter than do other groups of people.

Bruch (1957, pp. 35-59; 1973, pp. 9-23) has presented the aesthetic values of overweight as clear examples of cultural and historical relativity. The wide variety of beauty norms in different societies shows that the stigmatization of fatness as ugliness is far from a universal value (Rudofsky, 1971, pp. 99-111).

Some central conclusions can be drawn about different peoples' values of thinness and fatness. In different times and in different places, people who have struggled to achieve the rewards of food, for whom the acquisition of food has been a problem, tend to praise fatness more than thinness. When food is not a taken-for-granted part of the natural order of things, overweight is often valued as a sign of prestige and success. Success in this context is equated with beauty. One has become sufficiently rich in goods so as to acquire enough food to make one beautifully fat. [Allon, 1973b, p. 93.]

Accumulating food was a mark of great prestige in tribal preliterate societies where there was a scarcity of food (Powdermaker, 1960, p. 289). Indeed, some societies — which gauge female beauty by sheer bulk — have provided fattening houses for brides to be, aimed at creating strategically placed cushions of fat, a process which can take from several weeks to two years. An especially admired feature here is steatopygia, the overdevelopment of the subcutaneous fat that covers a woman's hind parts and upper thighs. (Rudofsky, 1971, p. 99.)
In contrast to the prestige of fatness in some societies:

. . . people who take for granted economic abundance in general, and food in particular, as a way of life tend to praise thinness more than fatness. With the opportunity for overcompensation of abundances, one literally can afford to worry about "too-muchisms," including overweight. [Allon, 1973b, p. 96.]

When there is ample and relatively inexpensive food for everybody, more leisure and a release from toil and effort through mechanization, almost nonexistent physical activity in many occupations, and passive leisure time activities, obesity is likely to exist. Such conditions are present in contemporary America (Allon, 1973b, p. 96; Powdermaker, 1960, pp. 289–291; Wagner, 1970).
In the United States today, some have viewed fatness as part of the greater problem of sexual inequality. As a social disease, fat is not about lack of self-control or lack of will power (Orbach, 1979, p. 6). Fat is an example of Ryan's (1971) blame the victim approach, whereby one blames the victims of oppression rather than its perpetrators. Orbach as a social worker and therapist has worked for some years with fat persons. She states that fat expresses a rebellion against the powerlessness of women, against women having to look and be a certain way according to ideal images of the fashion and diet industries, against it not being acceptable for women to be assertive and self-confident. Fat women try to reject the whole meat market syndrome since they want to be accepted for who they are, not for what they are supposed to look like on the outside in conforming to external standards in order to please males. (Orbach, 1979, pp. 5-9.) Questioning some of the negative connotations of fatness, Aldebaran (or Vivian Mayer) (1975, 1977) has asserted that fat people have the right to be fat and eat what they want, stating that fat people are often not fat by choice. Also, do not some people have the right to choose their bodily shapes and styles, even if such do not conform to the preferences of the majority? One cannot forget the

sociocultural and economic bases, as suggested by Stunkard (1975, p. 207) who demonstrates:

. . . a maximum prevalence of obesity occurring among the poorer members of Western urban society. This prevalence decreases with both decreasing *and* increasing affluence, but the reasons for the decreases differ dramatically. With decreasing affluence, the constraint upon the development of obesity is the lack of food. With increasing affluence, fads and fashions exert the control.

In fact, Stuart and Davis (1972, p. 15) have suggested some relationships between poverty and obesity, particularly in contemporary America:

First, it is possible that poverty may be for obesity what ragweed is for hay fever — a pathogen subtly present but not detected because of the greater prominence of other cues. By this it is suggested that poverty may lead to poor education (including education about health and nutrition), little access to the opportunity for vigorous exercise, and proscription from those aspects of the occupational hierarchy which differentially reward nonobese persons. Second, it is possible that lower socioeconomic groups may place a positive value upon obesity either as a means of survival, as an aesthetic trait, or as a counter-cultural or at least sub-cultural norm. This would imply that, denied access to the requisites of a sound diet, occupants of lower socioeconomic strata might place a positive value upon obesity either as a sign of rejection of middle-class values, a possibility which finds some support in the fact that the dominant American reference groups do seem to regard obesity as a form of social deviance.

The point is that prejudice and discrimination against fat people may mean prejudice and discrimination against some groups of people rather than others. Research has shown that certain people with various ascribed and achieved characteristics tend to be fatter than others.

THE MEDICAL PROFESSION AND THE FAT STIGMA

So far I have tried to show that there are various kinds and degrees of stigmatization of fatness in contemporary America, and that the stigma as perceived by others and as experienced by oneself is particularly intense with respect to females. It now becomes important to stress that in addition to lay people, medical doctors and other professionals serving fat people stigmatize and negatively stereotype obese and overweight persons. Medical personnel contribute to making fatness a social handicap. One study (Maddox and Liederman, 1969) has shown that doctors dislike people being fat — a dislike derived from values of middle-class society and informal experience, rather than from science and formal training. The doctors studied preferred not to manage the overweight patient and most did not. They did not expect success if they did treat the overweight. The doctors believed overweight to be unaesthetic and indicative of a lack of personal control. The doctors surveyed gave an extremely negative picture of the severely overweight person, who was described as weak willed, ugly, and awkward. The doctors evaluated the overweight more harshly than the overweight rated themselves.

In another study, Maddox, Anderson, and Bogdonoff (1966) noted a strong disinclination within their study group to record the weights of obese patients and to undertake the dietary treatment of obesity. During informal discussions, young physicians acknowledged the importance of overweight in their medical appraisal of the patient, despite their failure to record clinical findings connected with obesity. Maddox and his colleagues have suggested in their studies that doctors do not vigorously address themselves to the treatment of obesity mainly for three reasons: (1) ambivalent attitudes about obesity, (2) conflicting data about the real relevance of weight reduction to physical health, and (3) the inability to help the fat person keep off the weight lost. (Ingram, 1976b, p. 36.) In another earlier study, it was noted that physicians feel apathetic toward, and hopeless about, overweight patients losing weight; they regard the failure of their patients to lose weight as the result of uncooperativeness and gluttony (Stunkard and McLaren-Hume, 1959).

In a recent study (Breytspraak, McGee, Conger, Whatley, and Moore, 1977) based upon evaluations of interviews of female patients with vague complaints and of their family doctors, medical students rated overweight women as relatively less likeable, less seductive, more emotional, more defensive, more sincere, and warmer than women of normal weight. These students had the desire to help the overweight woman, although they believed that the overweight woman was not so likely to benefit from help. Many students viewed the overweight woman as depressed and nervous, and recommended that she see a psychiatrist or a clinical psychologist.

A study (Maiman, Wang, Becker, Finlay, and Simonson, 1979) of a group of professionals primarily specializing in nutrition and mainly involved in weight reducing programs for obese patients showed much variation in attitudes toward images of the obese, causes of obesity, and ways to lose weight. Some perceptions appeared to be responses to societal and personal evaluations of obesity rather than a result of knowledge and skills acquired through professional education. Only 13 percent of the sample reported having received any special training in treating obesity. These researchers found that successful experiences for self, family, and patients in working with weight reduction was the best predictor of more favorable attitudes toward obesity; therefore, direct and personal impressions resulted in more positive evaluations.

As a medical doctor, Rubin (1978) has commented that doctors as well as others are prejudiced in terms of fatness. Doctors can be as much the victims of cultural prejudice as the patients whom they victimize. Sometimes the doctor does not know that he/she is prejudiced. Such a lack of awareness can hurt the doctor's judgment of his/her fat patients. It can take the form of exaggerating the danger of fatness or of becoming so obsessed with the fat that doctors may neglect or even overlook other important medical problems. Fatness may be seen as the person's primary, central characteristic. Such a fat patient may lose his/her medical individuality and may be abandoned or treated sadistically or vindictively.

Millman (1980, p. xiii) has stated:

One need not deny that obesity may be unhealthy to ask why fat people are so stigmatized; people with other health problems are not condemned in the same ways. Many people who are not overweight enough to be at a health risk still suffer great diminution in the quality of their lives because of the negative interpretations attached to being overweight, and many do more harm to their health by using dangerous drugs and diets trying to reach an unrealistically thin ideal. Since physical appearance rather than health is often the motivating factor in why and how people diet, and since many suffer more from the social stigma of being overweight than from the health hazards, it should be obvious that the problem of obesity and the solutions to it involve more than medical considerations.

FAT RELATED TO ILLNESS AND DEATH

Importantly, there have been recent questions and challenges raised by physicians about the relationship between obesity and (1) high blood pressure, there being little support to regard obesity as a cause of high blood pressure so as to encourage the treatment of obesity as a useful way of managing high blood pressure (Mann, 1974a, p. 184); (2) heart diseases — with the contribution of obesity to coronary heart disease being small or nonexistent, the treatment of obesity cannot be expected to be either a logical or a promising approach to the management of coronary heart disease (Mann, 1974b, p. 227); and (3) cholesterol levels, with reports finding no correlation between cholesterol level and either obesity or high blood pressure (Mann, 1974b, p. 228). In addition to Mann's review of the literature and his conclusions, some clearcut studies have not found much of a correlation between heart problems, leading to mortality, and overweight. There is no indication of a steady gradient between mortality and degree of overweight, as one progresses from slightly overweight to markedly overweight (Borhani, Hechter, Breslow, 1963). In this study, however, smoking was clearly correlated with heart diseases. Another study concluded that there was no relationship between obesity and hypertension (Bjerkedal, 1957). Some researchers have raised questions about the relationships between obesity and disease, and have cited studies which have *not* found any clearcut relationship between obesity and diabetes mellitus, hypertension, or heart disease; in addition, no association was found between obesity and lung disease, and an inverse relationship was found between anemia and degree of obesity (Rimm, Werner, Yserloo, and Bernstein, 1975). Mayer (1968, pp. 102-104) himself cites the finding that mortality from tuberculosis and suicide has been quite low among overweight insured men and women. Mayer (1968, pp. 100-115) also stresses the fact that correlation between obesity and disease entities is not causation; for many abnormalities of bodily functions, obesity may be a coexisting, rather than a causal, feature.

The point is not that obesity is without any risk; many researchers have discovered that risk factors for health are increased in populations in excess of 30 to 40 percent overweight. Still, even if correlations are found between weight and certain diseases, such are not evidence of a causal connection, certainly in the case of one individual. Both overweight and a certain disease may result from an unknown third factor. Some factor associated with overweight, such as frequent weight loss and gain, may be the actual cause of disease, and it has been argued that weight vacillations may indeed have injurious effects on health. The status of the overweight as a stigmatized minority may generate stresses which are partly responsible for the development of diseases. (Wooley and Wooley, 1979, pp. 74-75.)

Indeed, many studies fail to consider that the psychosomatic stress and anxiety which people experience partly because of the stigma of their overweight may be the real link to physiological disorders, rather than the mere fact of overweight itself. Unfortunately, some researchers seem to dismiss such factors, partly because they are hard to measure and quantify. Likewise, genetic, biochemical, physiological, psychological, and social factors behind and before the overweight and the physical disease may lead to both entities. There is much controversy even in the physiological evidence about which comes first, the physical problem or the obesity. One must remember that the correlation of overweight with certain diseases in some individual cases does not mean that this correlation holds in *all* cases. One cannot necessarily accurately predict or prove this correlation as absolutely true in the case of one fat individual. Also, the possible correlation of overweight with certain diseases does not mean that overweight causes such diseases. Treatments which reliably produce weight loss, such as gastric and intestinal bypass, produce serious illnesses themselves, and their use may decrease longevity. (Wooley and Wooley, 1979, pp. 74-75.)

Most significantly, many studies start out with unhealthy and unhappy fat people who feel unattractive and who feel much pain because of the stigma of their overweight (Stunkard, 1976). Some studies then go on to prove the foregone conclusions that such overweight people indeed are physically and psychologically disturbed. More studies need to start out with at least some happy and healthy fat people who feel attractive and good about themselves – and who in theory and practice are fighting the stigma of fat in contemporary America. Even though such people may be hard to find in this society, with the blight of the fat stigma, I personally have met some such individuals through the National Association to Aid Fat Americans. It seems that when some fat people get together to discuss their problems, wishes, and hopes, they can begin to feel better about themselves and increase their self-esteem.

Prejudicial attitudes and practices toward obesity are so deeply ingrained in our society that they often have become an accepted, almost integral part of the type of health care which the fat person can expect to receive.* The doctor-patient relationship may become an adversary one, causing fat people to avoid or delay seeking treatment until the last possible moment. There is much evidence to support the conclusion that such procrastination may play a major role in elevating the mortality rate of the obese (Abe, 1976, p. 351).

However, the fat person is not alone in denying himself prompt medical attention. Surgeons are taught that obesity makes an operation hazardous, inelegant and time consuming; consequently, when faced with the prospect of operating on an obese patient, the surgeon will often delay treatment until the situation becomes acute. Reluctance to perform the needed Cesarian section on obese women has been directly implicated as an important cause of both maternal and infant death (Sicuranza and Tisdall, 1975). When surgery is performed, it must be accomplished with standard size equipment that is either too narrow, too weak, or too short for proper use on a fat patient (Lamberth, 1969). In addition, the surgeon is often forced to rely on trial and error in his/her procedure, since the published material on surgery in the obese is both scanty and misleading (Ahern and Goodlin, 1978). (Ideas from unpublished paper by Niedershuh, 1979.)

Indeed, one striking study of an Italian American community in Pennsylvania (Stout, Morrow, Brandt, and Wolf, 1964) shows a high incidence of overweight and an unusually low incidence of death from myocardial infarction. In this community, obesity and a generous consumption of calories, fat, and wine were actually associated with a strikingly low death rate from myocardial infarction. In this community, obesity was socially acceptable and the people seemed to enjoy life; they were happy, unpretentious, mutually supporting, and trusting. This study found the levels of heart disease and diabetes below the average for slender Americans. The Rosetans in question were for the most part fat, blue-collar Italian Americans. This study shows that fat people who do not diet and who do not endure persecution find that they are quite healthy.

---

*I am grateful to Karl Niedershuh for assistance in compiling and analyzing the following information; he is a graduate student at Goddard College who has been studying the relationship between obesity and health for years.

This study of the Rosetans highlights the possibility that the condition of overweight brings with it in our society such a very heavy social pressure to conform that persons who are overweight develop some diseases partly in response to society's condemnation of them. Between overweight as "cause" and disease as "effect" may be the important intervening variable of social stress. Such stress is in part comprised of prejudice and discrimination against fat people. Experiencing the social condemnation of fat certainly may contribute to the physiological and psychological problems of the fat person. The strain of dieting and of being "fat in a thin world" may add to and even partly cause medical conditions associated with overweight. One of the major problems in studying the health implications of obesity/overweight is that it is very difficult to find subjects who have not dieted. The study of the Rosetans is quite important for it is the only known study of the obese who are not contaminated by the stress of weight loss – indeed, the fat Rosetans are found to be quite healthy. (Tucker, 1980, pp. 26-27.)

WEIGHT LOSS AND DIETING EFFORTS

Even for those who want to lose weight, studies have shown that people have a hard time losing weight and keeping it off. A review of treatment outcome conducted in 1959 (Stunkard and McLaren-Hume) concluded that about 4 percent of patients attending outpatient clinics were successful in losing as much as 40 pounds and keeping it off for two years. A 1977 update covering many new reports has suggested little improvement, with an average weight loss of 11 pounds and generally an inadequate follow-up (Wing and Jefferey, 1978). There have been attempts to improve the success rate, for example, the controversial and sometimes fatal intestinal bypass, wiring the jaws shut for periods up to several years, brain lesioning, and fasts which have been shown to have high failure rates (Innes, Campbell, Campbell, Needle, and Munro, 1974; MacCuish, Munro, and Duncan, 1968). Early reports of behavioral treatments did suggest improved success rates, but such results have not been borne out (Wing and Jefferey, 1978). Such a discrepancy may be partly attributed to the populations treated in the early studies. When samples containing older patients with more severe obesity are studied, the great majority of patients do not achieve significant weight losses (Currey, Malcolm, Riddle, and Schachter, 1977). (Some of this literature is well summarized by Wooley and Wooley, 1979.) Wooley, Wooley, and Dyrenforth (1979b) have most thoroughly pointed out the physiological and psychological reasons for their finding that although showing superior maintenance, behavioral treatments of obesity typically produce small weight losses at a decelerating rate. They stress that the inevitability of treatment failure in many instances must be faced and efforts should be made to prevent further worsening of the obese patient's self-esteem. They rebut the view that all fat people are fat by choice.

In some research, only about 10 percent of the patients in supervised weight reduction programs maintain their original losses for as long as one year. After two years the percentage drops to 6 percent, then even lower (Beller, 1977, p. 264). There is little health benefit in the activities of most dieters who repeatedly lose and regain weight — such seesaw patterns probably put a stress on the body that itself is more unhealthy than staying overweight (Millman, 1980, p. 90).

One report found that reducing diets have a five-year failure rate of 98 to 99 percent (Feinstein, 1974, p. 86); in another, repeated dieting was acknowledged to be a cause of atherosclerosis, leading to heart attacks and strokes (Division of Chronic Diseases, 1966, p. 40). Stunkard's famous dieting depression study (1957) indicated that many people become depressed when dieting is enforced, especially those who use food to combat anxiety, loneliness, and hostility. Some of these findings may support Jordan's (1973) research, which has suggested that the problems of obesity and reducing involve equilibrium in energy balance, which is extremely resistant to measures to alter it. The persistent stability of body weight shows a stable biologic equilibrium that takes years to build up to a high level of overweight and takes a long time to return to a lower level of normal weight.

"NORMAL" EATING AND ACTIVITY

Indeed, some behavior modification and other weight reducing programs are based on the myth of teaching "normal" or "average" eating behavior. Yet many studies have in fact shown that the obese on the average do not eat any more than anybody else (Garrow, 1974; see Wooley and Wooley, 1979, pp. 69-74, for a review of some of this literature). Therefore, when fat people's overall caloric intakes are measured, they prove to be within ranges defined as normal. Furthermore, studies by Passmore and his colleagues (1955a, 1955b, 1963) found that the caloric excess needed to gain a pound of fat varies among individuals, with some fat people needing only about half as many excess calories to gain a pound compared with slim people. Studies have shown that both fat and thin people can have large or small appetites, and when food intakes of obese individuals were accurately assessed and compared with people of normal weight, the intakes were identical (Bryans, 1967).

Recent surveys of eating patterns and styles (cited in Wooley and Wooley, 1979, p. 70) have produced no evidence that, on the average, the obese differ from the lean in the timing, duration, speed and consumption, or composition of meals or snacks (Kissileff, Jordan, and Levitz, 1978; Meyer, Stunkard, and Coll, 1977). Wooley and Wooley (1979, p. 70) have stated that the point is not that all overweight people consume small amounts of food, but that intake, as well as other characteristics of eating behavior, shows the same, in fact rather large, distribution in overweight as in lean samples. For every fat person who eats a given amount, there is a person who remains lean on the same diet.

Hibscher and Herman (1976) found that dieters, regardless of weight, consume more food after a calorie-rich preload than without the preload. This eating behavior characteristically has been attributed to fat people, and has been labeled a form of compulsive eating. In this study, nondieters, both fat and thin, responded to the preload in the normal manner of eating less after it. Nondieting obese subjects showed a normal caloric compensation to forced preloading. The abandonment of attempts at weight suppression in the obese might actually produce normal behavior and physiological profiles. *Dieters* exhibited the so-called obese responses, such as absence of caloric compensation or subsequent consumption varying directly with the extent of preloading, *irrespective* of weight classification.

Some studies have shown the obese to be less physically active than the nonobese, and approximately an equal number of studies have found no differences between the obese and nonobese (Garrow, 1974). Wooley and Wooley (1979, p. 70) point out that one must be cautious in interpreting these data: because of the greater weight to be moved, the heavy person uses up more energy carrying out the same movements, and appropriate corrections must be made to determine the actual work performed. Measurement methods which do not affect normal activity levels are often inaccurate, and precise observation techniques can influence natural behavior. For example, filming adolescent girls during sports as a kind of observation is probably not representative because of the self-consciousness of the subjects.

LIFE INSURANCE COMPANY DATA

It is important to note that many doctors and others treating overweight or obese patients rely heavily on life insurance company data to determine "normal" or "ideal" weights for their patients. These data associating obesity with illness and death need to be questioned. Although there may be such an association in the statistics, the statistics do not permit the conclusion that obesity is the cause of increased illness or mortality (Cahman, 1968, p. 285; Mayer, 1968, p. 114). It is not known how representative the life insurance sample is of the general human population or of the total American population. What differences might exist in the uninsured population? Is there similarity in the mortality rates? Is there the same proportion of obese to nonobese persons? (Mayer, 1968, p. 114.) Height-weight data obtained by the National Center for Health Statistics and based on a representative sample of the adult population of the United States indicate average weights of men and women that are higher than the averages revealed by insurance data (Seltzer and Mayer, 1967).

Another defect in the insurance data concerns the initial weight of the insured subject. Often the weight is obtained by a verbal statement from the subject rather than by actual measurement, and there is no way for one to verify the accuracy of the reports or detect errors. Another possible source of error lies in the lack of standardization in the recording of deaths. Information subsequent to initial weight regarding weight gain or loss is usually not available. (Mayer, 1968, p. 114.)

A great majority of doctors, in some surveys close to 100 percent, use the "average" height-weight charts derived from the statistics compiled more recently from several million holders of life insurance policies with 256 companies in the United States and Canada (Berland and Editors of Consumer Guide, 1977, pp. 19–20). Tables of desirable weights often have been based upon the statistics of the policy holders who lived the longest. The life insurance data are based specifically on measurements of prudent people who had the money and motivation, which might have been ill health, to buy life insurance policies. Some tables have been derived from policy holders who have lived in or near cities on the Eastern seaboard, such as New York and Boston, which is a narrow sample. Many weights and heights have been recorded while people wore street clothes, including shoes. This tabulation could add up to 10 pounds of weight and one inch height per body. (Berland and Editors of Consumer Guide, 1977, pp. 19–20; Wohl and Goodhart, p. 5.)

Seltzer (1966) analyzed some life insurance data and found only a loose correlation between the desirable-weights tables and the actual mortality of policy holders. Also, the charts classified lean men as underweight and did not take into account the amount of fat on a person's body. In addition, many of the height-weight tables are blind since they take only weight according to pounds into consideration, without considering what the weight is based upon, for example, the amount of fat, muscle, and bone. Muscular football players, other athletes, and physical laborers may be overweight but underfat; many sedentary persons are quite fat but not overweight; (Berland and Editors of Consumer Guide, 1977, pp. 20–21.)

DIFFICULTY IN DEFINITIONS

By deliberating omitting definitions, I am suggesting that the words *fat, overweight,* and *obese* may be used interchangeably in a sociological sense, because the differences between the labels are blurred in interactional situations. Group dieters whom I studied who were considered to be as little as 10 or 15 pounds above their ideal weight goals felt, and in fact were, just as stigmatized by certain reference groups as those who were judged 50 or more pounds overweight.

Many data do not suggest a positive correlation between amount of supposedly excess pounds and amount of stigmatization. In fact, there is not a precise, commonly agreed upon definition of the obesity-overweight phenomenon among scientists and medical doctors. There appear to be objective as well as subjective connotations to the "fact" of obesity. My own research has suggested that some working-class Italian and Irish diet club members thought that they were quite thin if they could squeeze into a size 20, while some upper-middle-class Jewish women panicked if their size 5s started feeling tight. One study has suggested that concern about weight is the greatest among the affluent, least obese population (Dwyer and Mayer, 1970, p. 513).

Medical and life insurance charts, doctors, scientists, and self-styled experts may state numbers and percentages as criteria for overweight and obesity — a person need only be stacked against such mathematics to determine where he or she fits in the fatness to thinness continuum. Yet such a person has his or her own ideas about how fat or thin he or she is, based upon complex biographical and reference group factors. Subjective definitions of overweight often do not jibe with objective numbers.

CONCLUSIONS

Kurland, (1970, p. 20), has gone so far as to state that ". . . most physicians regard obesity as a sin and treat fat patients with disdain befitting a moral leper." He describes the result of this attitude:

Medical training emphasizing the multiple causes of obesity is generally ignored, although the list of physical disorders resulting in obesity is quite lengthy. When confronted with the obese patient, the physician often neglects to diagnose such obvious abnormalities as hypothyroidism, hyperadrenalism, and even striking hypometabolic disorders. Most patients are so scornfully regarded that they are not even afforded the benefits of a diagnostic glucose tolerance test.

Kurland (1970, p. 20) goes on to examine some of the social implications of weight loss therapy:

Physicians often request that their obese patients return to the office for a series of humiliating checks on their weight loss; during these visits they may be given no more medical attention than to be weighed on the scale and have their weight recorded by the office nurse. This demeaning procedure gives a number of clear messages. Failure to lose weight is immediately regarded as little more than concrete evidence of moral turpitude . . . . Their obesity has also seriously impaired their already limited intellect so that they are not even capable of reading a scale at home with any degree of accuracy; consequently, they must report regularly to their doctor's office in order to have the vital examination performed. Recording of weight by the office nurse and dispensing of medication in a routine rather than individual fashion again emphasizes to the patient that his physical, intellectual and moral degeneracy does not make him worthy of individual attention from his physician.

Bruch, (1973b, p. 187) a prominent psychiatrist who has studied obesity and overweight for many years, has concluded:

Depite the physical and social handicap that fatness implies, there are people who function better when they are somewhat heavy. Some of them have made strenuous efforts to lose weight, practically giving up living in order to achieve it, but having reached the prescribed lower level, they feel unfit to function in areas of living that are important to them individually, and for their social usefulness. When thin, they cannot continue their interesting and useful lives until they have regained their former weight, though it may be judged as too high by conventional standards.

There are others who stay reduced, but who cannot relax: they seem to be as preoccupied with weight and dieting after they have become slim as they were before. Their whole lives continue to be centered around their appearance and the impression they make. They represent what I have come to call the "thin fat people."

One psychoanalyst (Ingram, 1976a, p. 90) wrote a letter to the *New York Times Magazine* in which he agrees with a writer who has called obesity a social disability, but disagrees with the writer's invocation of medically harmful effects of all cases of overweight. He states that there are uncertainties and contradictions in the scientific medical literature about the relationship between obesity and physical illness. He calls for some skepticism about the medical value of weight reduction, stating that ". . . we cannot show that healthy fat people have better chances of remaining healthy if they lose weight and keep it off."

Ingram (1976c, pp. 233–234) states:

A thoroughgoing bias in Western culture impairs the psychiatric and nonpsychiatric medical care of the obese person. Inconclusive evidence concerning the causal relation between obesity and chronic disease does not deter this cultural bias from exaggerating the role that obesity is thought to play in disease process. Whatever contribution it makes to physical illness, obesity remains a substantial social disability that is frequently associated with self-hate and feelings of ineffectiveness . . . .

It is not clear that obesity is a major determinant of impaired physical or emotional health. Rather, the medical indictment of obesity seems to stem from the need to justify an intensely negative cultural bias. Casual disregard of this fact and of the complexity involving issues of etiology and treatment may signify inadequate appreciation in the psychoanalyst of the extent to which he participates in this cultural bias.

The continuing failure of medical science to devise a means to help fat persons sustain weight loss to any meaningful degree has prevented the development of studies which would show if weight reduction truly does provide uniformly enhanced physical and emotional well-being.

Indeed, Bruch, (1973a, pp. 124-128) has suggested that overeating and overweight may be less intensive and extensive disturbances than other physical and emotional problems. They may serve as useful, not too destructive defense mechanisms. Some people might need to feel big in order to lead satisfying lives. Obesity may have the positive function of being a compensatory mechanism in a frustrating and stressful life. Obesity may be a handicap, but as a defensive reaction, it is less destructive than suicide or a paralyzing deep depression. For some, overeating may be a helpful defense against anxiety, loneliness, or anger. For mildly depressed overweight patients, the immediate enjoyment of food serves as reassurance that life still holds some satisfactions.

My own research on overweight children and adolescents has led me to consider self and others' perceptions of the stigma of overweight according to the following themes: (1) overweight as an exclusive focus in social interaction; (2) overweight as a reflection of a negative body image; (3) overweight as overwhelming others with many mixed emotions; (4) overweight as clashing with other qualities of the person; (5) overweight as an equivocal and uncertain predictor of joint activity of overweight and normal weight persons; (6) overweight viewed as one's own responsibility which deserves punishment by others as well as by oneself; (7) overweight viewed as an illness and not one's own responsibility, which merits treatment and help by others, especially parents and professional experts; and (8) overweight viewed as one's own responsibility and as an illness that requires the joint efforts of oneself and others, especially parents and professional experts (Allon, 1979a). These and other views of the stigma of overweight which I have cited in this paper clearly make overweight a social handicap.

In conclusion, I would assert that one major problem is that there has been little or no systematic research on healthy, relatively happy and well-adjusted fat people, who feel attractive and good about themselves. Granted, such people may be hard to find in this society, with the blight of the stigma of overweight. However, one cannot assume that such people do not or cannot exist; perhaps more could exist if the stigma placed upon obesity were lessened or obliterated. Is it fair to use research and assertions – which assume at their very outset that fat is a negative characteristic – to discriminate against one fat individual? Quite a few researchers have built their ideas about fat being "bad" or "wrong" or "sick" into the hypotheses of their research. Is it fair to apply research which may show some correlation between obesity and ill health, based upon large samples of individuals, to one healthy and competent individual? Even if one assumes that some fat people may have physical, psychological, social, etc., problems of various kinds, is it not likely that their problems will be exacerbated by acts of discrimination? Researchers (Wooley, Wooley, and Dyrenforth, 1979a, 1979b), have shown and reviewed literature which suggests that fat is not so reversible for many fat people; many cannot readily lose weight with reasonable efforts. Does it not add insult to injury to deny employment to fat people who may quite likely not be responsible for their overweight? Stigmatization makes obesity/ overweight a social handicap.

IMPLICATIONS

There is inadequate and inconclusive evidence (such as nonrepresentative samples in life insurance data) as well as lack of hard-nosed evidence about (1) the exact relationship of obesity to illness or death, (2) the effectiveness and benefits of dieting in losing and keeping off weight, and (3) the relationship of obesity and performance abilities. In light of such questionable evidence, can one really decide not to give one fat individual a job? Even if the data were to show strong statistical correlations between obesity and negative outcomes, correlation cannot be equated with causation. For example, a third factor could be causing the obesity and the negative health problem, or an intervening variable such as per-ceptions of the stigma of obesity could exist between the obesity and the health problem; such an intervening variable might very much contribute to the health problem. (At this stage of research in obesity we do not have clearcut evidence for the existence or nonexistence of such an intervening variable.) Also, it be-comes a legal, moral, and ethical question as to whether one can apply even refined statistical regularities to a unique individual case.

We are, therefore, thrown back on the notion that decision makers are products of our society and that their values are shaped by our culture which stigmatizes the fat person. Medical practitioners, college admission officers, and employers have been shown to hold prejudiced perceptions against fat people in the context of the present American culture. Because of prejudice and discrimination, the fat person loses or does not get his/her job, without clear statistical evidence as a basis for such a loss. Because the stigma of obesity contributes to abuse on the job, the fat person is further abused in his/her own self-image. Overweight as a social stigma is tantamount to overweight being a social handicap. Therefore, initially, *any* consideration of weight in employment must be illegal, unless it is used for affirmative action purposes. In fact, if weight is negatively considered, it is illegal; in regard to affirmative action policies, overweight people as handi-capped should be given equal, if not special, consideration for jobs.

Fatness is made into a social handicap by the social stigma of fatness for which there is much evidence. Fatness is a stigma and a social handicap because in social interaction there is *de facto* prejudice and discrimination in the mind's eye. The "innocent" fat person is simply not proven "guilty" enough by any evidence which can be used to deny him or her a job. Therefore, (1) we have questionable statistical data and empirical data about the negative implications of fatness; (2) we are thrown back upon the perceptions of biased people who are products of the present American society which stigmatizes fatness; and (3) we discriminate against the stigmatized fat people who are socially handicapped by others' perceptions — such fat people are kept out of jobs and further abused in their own self-images. Is not such discrimination against the fat, socially handicapped person unethical, immoral, and illegal?

REFERENCES

Abe, R., Kumagai, M. K., Hirosaki, A., and Nakamura, T. Biological characteristics of breast cancer in obesity. *Tohoku Journal of Experimental Medicine*, 1976, *120*, 351–359.

Abraham, S. *Preliminary Findings of the First Health and Nutrition Examination Survey, United States, 1971-1972: Anthropometric and Clinical Findings.* Rockville, Md.: U.S. Dept. of Health, Education and Welfare, Public Health Service, National Center for Health Statistics, 1975.

Ahern, J. K. and Goodlin, R. C. Cesarean section in the massively obese. *Obstetrics and Gynecology*, 1978, *51*, 509–510.

Aldebaran (Mayer), Vivian. Uptight and hungry: The contradiction in psychology of fat. *RT: A Journal of Radical Therapy*, 1975, *4*, 5–6.

Aldebaran (Mayer), Vivian. Fat liberation — a luxury? An open letter to radical (and other) therapists. *State and Mind*, 1977, *5*, 34–38.

Allon, N. Group dieting interaction. Ph.D. dissertation, unpublished. Brandeis University, 1972.

Allon, N. Group dieting rituals. *Transaction/Society*, 1973, *10*, 36–42. (a)

Allon, N. The stigma of overweight in everyday life. *Obesity in Perspective.* Fogarty International Center Series on Preventive Medicine, Vol. 2, Part 2, pp. 83–102. (Bray, G. A., Ed.) Washington, D.C.: U.S. Government Printing Office, 1973. (b)

Allon, N. Latent social services in group dieting. *Soc. Problems*, 1975, *23*, 59–69.

Allon, N. Self-perceptions of the stigma of overweight in relationship to weight-losing patterns. *Amer. J. Clin. Nutrit.*, 1979, *32*, 470–480.

Allon, N. Tensions in interactions of overweight adolescent girls. *Women and Health*, 1976, *1*, 14–15, 18–23.

Allon, N. *Urban Life Styles*, pp. 29–81, Dubuque, Iowa: Brown, 1979. (b)

Baker, E. Woman challenging rules: City may ease curbs on hiring obese persons. *Los Angeles Times*, October 26, 1975, pp. 3, 26.

Beck, S. B., Ward-Hull, C. I., and McLear, P.M. Variables related to women's somatic preferences of the male and female body. *J. Person. Soc. Psychol.*, 1976, *34*, 1200–1210.

Beller, A. S. *Fat and Thin: A Natural History of Obesity.* New York: Farrar, Straus and Giroux, 1977.

Berland, T. and Editors of Consumer Guide. Rating the diets. *Consumer Guide.* Skokie, Ill.: Publications International, 1977.

Bjerkedal, T. Overweight and hypertension. *Acta. Med. Scandinav.*, 1957, *159*, 13–26.

Borhani, N. O., Hechter, H. H., and Breslow, L. Report of a ten-year follow-up study of the San Francisco longshoremen. *J. Chron. Dis.*, 1963, *16*, 1251–1266.

Breytspraak, L. M., McGee, J., Conger, J. C., Whatley, J. L., and Moore, J. T. Sensitizing medical students to impression formation processes in the patient interview. *J. Med. Educat.*, 1977, *52*, 47–54.

Bruch, H. Obesity in childhood and personality development. *Amer. J. Orthopsychiat.*, 1941, *11*, 467–474.

Bruch, H. *The Importance of Overweight.* New York: W.W. Norton, 1957.

Bruch, H. *Eating Disorders: Obesity, Anorexia Nervosa and the Person Within.* New York: Basic Books, 1973. (a)

Bruch, H. Thin fat people. *J. Amer. Med. Women's Assoc.*, 1973b, *28*, 187–188, 194–195, 208. (b)

Bryans, A. M. Childhood obesity – prelude to adult obesity. *Canad. J. Publ. Health,* 1967, *58*, 486–490.

Buchanan, J. R. Five year psychoanalytic study of obesity. *Amer. J. Psychoanalys*, 1973, *33*, 30–38.

Cahnman, W. J. The stigma of obesity. *Sociolog. Quart.*, 1968, *9*, 283–299.

Canning, H. and Mayer, J. Obesity – its possible effect on college acceptance. *New Engl. J. Med.,* 1966, *275*, 1172–1174.

Canning, H. and Mayer, J. Obesity: An influence on high school performance? *Amer. J. Clin. Nutrit.,* 1967, *20*, 352–354.

Clifford, E. Body satisfaction in adolescence. *Percept. Mot. Skills,* 1971, *33*, 119–125.

Craft, C. A. Body image and obesity. *Nurs. Clin. North Amer.*, 1972, *7*, 677–685.

Currey, H., Malcolm, R., Riddle, E., and Schacte, M. Behavioral treatment of obesity: Limitations and results with the chronically obese. *J. Amer. Med. Assoc.*, 1977, *237*, 2829–2831.

DeJong, William. The stigma of obesity: The consequences of naive assumptions concerning the causes of physical deviance. *J. Health Soc. Behav.*, 1980, *21*, 75–87.

Division of Chronic Diseases, Heart Disease Control Program. *Obesity and Health.* PHS Pub. No. 1485, 1966.

Douty, H. I., Moore, J. B., and Hartford, D. Body characteristics in relation to life adjustment, body-image and attitudes of college females. *Percept. Mot. Skills,* 1974, *39*, 499–521.

Drenick, E. J. Weight reduction by prolonged fasting. *Obesity in Perspective* (Bray, G. A., Ed.). Fogarty International Center Series on Preventive Medicine, Vol. 2, Part 2, pp. 341–360. Washington, D.C.: U.S. Government Printing Office, 1973.

Dwyer, J. T. Psychosexual aspects of weight control and dieting behavior in adolescents. *Med. Aspects Human Sexual.,* 1973, *7*, 82–108.

Dwyer, J. T., Feldman, J. J., and Mayer, J. The social psychology of dieting. *J. Health Soc. Behav.,* 1970, *11*, 269–287.

Dwyer, J. T., Feldman, J. J., Seltzer, C. C., and Mayer, J. Adolescent attitudes toward weight and appearance. *J. Nutrit. Educat.*, 1969, *1*, 14–19.

Dwyer, J. T. and Mayer, J. Potential dieters: Who are they? *J. Amer. Diet. Assoc.,* 1970, *56*, 510–514.

Fat execs get slimmer paychecks. *Industry Week,* 1974, *180*, pp. 21, 24.

Feinstein, A. How do we measure accomplishment in weight reduction? *Obesity: Causes, Consequences and Treatment* (Lasagna, Ed.), pp. 81–87. New York: L. Medcom Press, 1974.

Fleisher, R. R. Coverage of obesity under Article 49B. *Report on the Study of Weight and Size Discrimination*, Appendix F, pp. 1-7. Baltimore, Maryland: Commission on Human Relations, 1980.

Galper, R. E. and Weiss, E. Attribution of behavioral intentions to obese and normal-weight stimulus persons. *Europ. J. Soc. Psychol.*, 1975, *5*, 425-440.

Garrow, J. *Energy Balance and Obesity in Man.* New York: American Elsevier, 1974.

Goldblatt, P. B., Moore, M. E., and Stunkard, A. J. Social factors in obesity. *J. Amer. Med. Assoc.*, 1965, *192*, 1039-1044.

Goodman, N., Richardson, S. A., Dornbusch, S. M., and Hastorf, A. H. Variant reactions to physical disabilities. *Amer. Sociolog. Rev.*, 1963, *28*, 429-435.

Haber, L. D. Epidemiological factors in disability. I. Major disabling conditions. *Social Security Survey of the Disabled, 1966*, Report 6. Washington, D. C.: U. S. Dept. of Health, Education and Welfare Social Security Administration Office on Research and Statistics, 1969.

Herman, M. W. Excess weight and sociocultural characteristics. *J. Amer. Diet. Assoc.*, 1973, *63*, 161-164.

Hibscher, J. A. and Herman, C. P. Obesity, dieting and the expression of "obese" characteristics. *J. Comparat. Physiolog. Psychol.*, 1977, *91*, 374-380.

Ingram, D. H. Fat and healthy. Letter to the editor, *New York Times Magazine*, Sept. 19, 1976, p. 90. (a)

Ingram, D. H. Psychoanalytic treatment of the obese person: Part I. *Amer. J. Psychoanalys.*, 1976, *36*, 35-41. (b)

Ingram, D. H. Psychoanalytic treatment of the obese person: Part III. *Amer. J. Psychoanalys.*, 1976, *36*, 227-235. (c)

Innes, J. A., Campbell, I. W., Campbell, C. H., Needle, A. L., and Munro, J. F. Long-term follow-up of therapeutic starvation. *Brit. Med. J.*, 1974, *2*, 356-359.

Jordan, H. A. In defense of body weight. *J. Amer. Diet. Assoc.*, 1973, *62*, 17-21.

Jourard, S. M. and Secord, P. R. Body-cathexis and the ideal female figure. *J. Abnorm. Soc. Psychol.*, 1955, *50*, 243-246.

Kalisch, B. J. The stigma of obesity. *Overweight and Obesity: Causes, Fallacies, Treatment* (Hafen, B. Q., Ed.) pp. 77-80. Provo, Utah: Brigham Young University Press, 1975.

Kissileff, K., Jordan, H., and Levitz, L. Eating habits of obese and normal weight humans. *Recent Advances in Obesity Research* (Bray, G. A., Ed.) Vol. 2. London: Newman, 1978.

Kurland, H. D. Obesity: An unfashionable problem. *Psychiatr. Opinion*, 1970, *7*, 20-25.

Kurtz, R. M. Sex differences and variations in body attitudes. *J. Consult. Psychol.*, 1969, *33*, 625-629.

Lamberth, I. E. Obesity and anesthesia. *Clinic. Anesthes.*, 1968, *3*, 56-66.

Larkin, J. E. and Pines, H. A. No fat persons need apply. *Sociology of Work and Occupations*, 1979, *6*, 312-327.

Laslett, B. and Warren, C. A. B. Losing weight: The organizational promotion of behavior change. *Soc. Problems*, 1975, *23*, 69-80.

Lerner, R. M. The development of stereotyped expectancies of body build behavior relations. *Child Devel.*, 1969, *40*, 137-141. (a)

Lerner, R. M. Some female stereotypes of male body-build-behavior relations. *Percept. Mot. Skills*, 1969, *28*, 363-366. (b)

Lerner, R. M. The development of personal space schemata toward body build. *J. Psychol.*, 1973, *84*, 229-235.

Lerner, R. M. and Gellert, E. Body build indentification, preference, and aversion in children. *Devel. Psychol.*, 1969, *5*, 256-462.

Lerner, R., Karabenick, S., and Meisels, M. Effects of age and sex on the development of personal space schemata towards body build. *J. Genetic Psycholog.*, 1975, *127*, 91–101.

Lerner, R. M. and Korn, S. J. The development of body-build stereotypes in males. *Child Devel.*, 1972, *43*, 908–920.

Lerner, R. and Pool, K. Body build stereotypes: A cross-cultural comparison. *Psycholog. Reports*, 1972, *31*, 527–532.

Lerner, R. and Schroeder, C. Kindergarten children's active vocabulary about body build. *Devel. Psychol.*, 1971, *5*, 179. (a)

Lerner, R. and Schroeder, C. Physique identification, preference, and aversion in kindergarten children. *Devel. psychol.*, 1971, *5*, 538. (b)

Louderback, L. *Fat Power: Whatever You Weigh Is Right.* New York: Hawthorn Books, 1970.

Lyman, S. *The Seven Deadly Sins: Society and Evil.* New York: St. Martins Press, 1978.

MacCuish, A. C., Munro, J. F., and Duncan, L. J. P. Follow-up study of refractory obesity treated by fasting. *Brit. Med. J.*, 1968, *1*, 91–92.

Maddox, G. L., Anderson, C. F., and Bogdonoff, M. D. Overweight as a problem of medical management in a public out-patient clinic. *Amer. J. Med. Sci.*, 1966, *252*, 394–403.

Maddox, G. L., Back, K. W., and Liederman, V. R. Overweight as social deviance and disability. *J. Health Soc. Behav.*, 1968, *9*, 287–298.

Maddox, G. L. and Liederman, V. R. Overweight as a social disability with medical implications. *J. Medic. Educat.*, 1969, *44*, 214–220.

Maiman, L. A., Wang, V. L., Becker, M. H., Finlay, J., and Simonson, M. Attitudes toward obesity and the obese among professionals. *J. Amer. Diet. Assoc.*, 1979, *74*, 331–336.

Mann, G. V. The influence of obesity on health (first of two parts). *New Engl. J. Med.*, 1974, *291*, 178–185. (a)

Mann, G. V. The influence of obesity on health (second of two parts). *New Engl. J. Med.*, 1974, *291*, 226–232.

Matthews, V. and Westie, C. A preferred method for obtaining rankings: Reactions to physical handicaps. *Amer. Sociolog. Rev.*, 1966, *31*, 851–854.

Mayer, J. *Overweight: Causes, Cost and Control.* Englewood Cliffs, N. J.: Prentice-Hall, 1968.

Meyer, J., Stunkard, A., and Coll, M. Eating in public places: There is no "obese eating style," it's where you eat that matters. Paper presented at the Association for the Advancement of Behavior Therapy, Atlanta, Georgia, 1977.

Michaels, S. Rituals: Dieting. *Women: A Journal of Liberation,* 1969, *1*, 32.

Millman, M. *Such a Pretty Face: Being Fat in America.* New York: Norton, 1980.

Monello, L. F. and Mayer, J. Obese adolescent girls: An unrecognized "minority" group? *Amer. J. Clin. Nutrit.*, 1963, *13*, 35–39.

Moore, M. E., Stunkard, A. J. and Srole, L. Obesity, social class and mental illness. *J. Amer. Med. Assoc.*, 1962, *181*, 962–966.

Niedershuh, K. J. Unpublished student paper, 1979.

Obesity and Health, *Public Health Service Report*, No. 1485, p. 40. U. S. Dept. of Health, Education and Welfare, 1966.

Orbach, S. *Fat Is a Feminist Issue: The Anti-diet Guide to Permanent Weight Loss.* New York: Paddington Press, 1979.

Passmore, R., Meiklejohn, A. P., Dewar, A. D., and Thow, R. An analysis of the gain in weight of overfed thin young men. *Brit. J. Nutrit.*, 1955, *9*, 27–37. (a)

Passmore, R., Meiklejohn, A. P., Dewar, A. D., and Thow, R. K. Energy utilization in overfed thin men. *Brit. J. Nutrit.*, 1955, *9*, 20–26. (b)

Passmore, R., Strong, J. A., Swindells, Y. E., and Din, N. The effect of overfeeding on two fat young women. *Brit. J. Nutrit.*, 1963, *17*, 373-383.

Powdermaker, H. An anthropological approach to the problem of obesity. *Bull. N. Y. Acad. Medic.*, 1960, *36*, 286-295.

Richardson, S. A., Hastorf, A. H., Goodman, N., and Dornbusch, S. M. Cultural uniformity in reaction to physical disabilities. *Amer. Sociolog. Rev.*, 1961, *26*, 241-247.

Rimm, A. A., Werner, L. H., Yserloo, B. V., and Bernstein, R. A. Relationship of obesity and disease in 73,532 weight-conscious women. *Publ. Health Reports*, 1975, *90*, 44-51.

Rodin, J. and Slochower, J. Fat chance for a favor: Obese-normal differences in compliance and incidental learning. *J. Person. Soc. Psychol.*, 1974, *29*, 557-565.

Roe, D. A. and Eickwort, K. R. Relationships between obesity and associated health factors with unemployment among low income women. *J. Amer. Med. Women's Assoc.*, 1976, *31*, 193-194, 198-199, 203-204.

Rubin, T. I. *Forever Thin.* New York: Bernard Geis, 1970.

Rubin, T. I. *Alive and Fat and Thinning in America.* New York: Coward, McCann and Geoghegan, 1978.

Rudofsky, B. *The Unfashionable Human Body.* Garden City, N. Y.: Doubleday, 1971.

Ryan, W. *Blaming the Victim* (rev. ed.). New York: Vintage Books, 1976.

Schachter, S. Obesity and eating. *Science*, 1968, *161*, 751-756.

Schachter, S. Some extraordinary facts about obese humans and rats. *Amer. Psychol.*, 1971, *26*, 129-144.

Schachter, S., Goldman, R., and Gordon, A. Effect of fear, food deprivation and obesity in eating. *J. Person. Soc. Psychol.*, 1968, *10*, 91-97.

Schachter, S. and Gross, L. P. Manipulated time and eating behavior. *J. Person. Soc. Psychol.*, 1968, *10*, 98-106.

Schachter, S. and Rodin, J. *Obese Humans and Rats.* Potomac, Md.: Lawrence Erlbaum, 1974.

Seltzer, C. C. Some re-evaluations of the build and blood pressure study, 1959, as related to ponderal index, somatotype, and mortality. *New Engl. J. Med.*, 1966, *274*, 254-259.

Seltzer, C. C. and Mayer, J. How representative are the weights of insured men and women? *J. Amer. Med. Assoc.*, 1967, *201*, 221-224.

Sicuranza, B. J. and Tisdall, L. H. Cesarean section in the massively obese. *J. Reproduct. Medic.*, 1975, *14*, 10-11.

Staffieri, J. R. A study of social stereotype of body image in children. *J. Person. Soc. Psychol.*, 1967, *7*, 101-104.

Staffieri, J. R. Body build and behavioral expectancies in young females. *Devel. Psychol.*, 1972, *6*, 125-127.

Stout, C., Morrow, J., Brandt, Jr., E. N., and Wolf, S. Unusually low incidence of death from myocardial infarction: Study of an Italian American community in Pennsylvania. *J. Amer. Med. Assoc.*, 1964, *188*, 845-849, or 121-125.

Strasser, A. L. Problems in hiring disadvantaged groups. *N. Y. State J. Med.*, 1972, *72*, 268-269.

Straus, R. Public attitudes regarding problem drinking and problem eating. *Ann. N. Y. Acad. of Sci.*, 1966, *133*, 792-802.

Stuart, R. B. and Davis, B. *Slim Chance in a Fat World.* Champaign, Ill.: Research Press, 1972.

Stunkard, A. J. The "dieting depression." *Amer. J. Med.*, 1957, *23*, 77-86.

Stunkard, A. J. From explanation to action in psychosomatic medicine; the case of obesity. *Psychosomat. Med.*, 1975, *37*, 195-236.

Stunkard, A. J. *The Pain of Obesity*. Palo Alto, Calif.: Bull Publishing Co., 1976.

Stunkard, A. and Burt, V. Obesity and the body image: II. Age at onset of disturbances in the body image. *Amer. J. Psychiatr.*, 1967, *123*, 1443-1447.

Stunkard, A. J., d'Aquili, E., Fox, S., and Filion, R. D. L. Influence of social calss on obesity and thinness in children. *J. Amer. Med. Assoc.*, 1972, *221*, 579-584.

Stunkard, A. and McLaren-Hume, M. The results of treatment for obesity. *Arch. Intern. Med.*, 1959, *103*, 79-85.

Stunkard, A. and Mendelson, M. Disturbance in body image of some obese persons. *J. Amer. Diet. Assoc.*, 1961, *38*, 328-331.

Stunkard, A. and Mendelson, M. Obesity and the body image: I. Characteristics of disturbances in the body image of some obese persons. *Amer. J. Psychiatr.*, 1967, *123*, 1296-1300.

Szasz, T. *Ceremonial Chemistry: The Ritual Persecution of Drugs, Addicts and Pushers*. Garden City, New York: Anchor Press, 1975.

Tipton, R. M. and Browning, S. The influence of age and obesity on helping behavior. *Brit. J. Soc. Clin. Psychol.*, 1972, *11*, 404-406.

Tobias, A. L. and Gordon, J. B. Social consequences of obesity. *J. Amer. Dietet. Assoc.*, *76*, 338-342.

Tucker, D. H. *Report on the Study of Weight and Size Discrimination*, as directed by the legislature of the state of Maryland in House Joint Resolution 75 by the Maryland Commission on Human Relations. Baltimore, Maryland: Commission on Human Relations, 1980.

Wagner, M. G. The irony of affluence. *J. Amer. Diet. Assoc.*, 1970, *57*, 311-315.

Wing, R. R. and Jefferey, R. W. Comparison of methodology and results of out-patient treatments of obesity. *Recent Advances in Obesity Research* (Bray, G. A., Ed.) Vol. 2. London: Newman, 1978.

Wohl, M. G. and Goodhart, R. S. *Modern Nutrition in Health and Disease*. Philadelphia: Lea and Febiger, 1971.

Wooley, S. C. and Wooley, O. W. Obesity and women – I. A closer look at the facts. *Women's Studies Int. Quart.*, 1979, *2*, 69-79.

Wooley, S. C., Wooley, O. W., and Dyrenforth, S. R. Obesity and women – II. A neglected feminist topic. *Women's Studies Int. Quart.*, 1979, *2*, 81-92. (a)

Wooley, S. C., Wooley, O. W., and Dyrenforth, S. R. Theoretical, practical and social issues in behavioral treatments of obesity. *J. Applied Behavior. Analys.*, 1979, *12*, 3-25. (b)

Wyden, P. *The Overweight Society*. New York: Morrow, 1965.

2
TREATMENT OF
OBESITY

8

Psychoanalytic Treatment of Obesity

Colleen S.W. Rand

Psychoanalysts have traditionally considered obesity to be the somatic representation of an emotional conflict (Bychowski, 1950). Psychoanalysts offer to help patients deal with and potentially resolve persistent neurotic problems. Hourly sessions are held several times weekly, and treatment can continue for years. Psychoanalysts rarely, if ever, treat obesity per se: they are not "diet doctors." Obese clients are accepted as patients with the understanding that therapy will focus on psychic conflicts rather than weight. In the course of treatment, weight loss often occurs. However, weight loss is incidental to the psychoanalytic process, not the focus (Rand and Stunkard, 1977).

In 1957, Kaplan and Kaplan published an influential paper that summarized known evidence on the causes of obesity. Data supporting psychoanalytic interpretations were meager in comparison to other disciplines, and the paper effectively dismissed psychoanalysis as a useful basis for understanding and treating obesity. The following two decades saw the emergence of behavior modification as the new approach to the battle of the bulge. Concurrently, surgical intervention techniques for treatment of obesity such as the jejunoileal bypass and gastric partition were, and continue to be, developed (Halverson, 1980).

At the present time we do not know how to "cure" moderate obesity under normal living conditions (i.e., outside of hospitals, prisons, and without coercion). Both motivational and biological factors (such as enhanced metabolic efficiency after starvation) are cited as contributing to the regaining of fat after weight loss. Careful long-term follow-up studies of the last few years have effectively reduced the global enthusiasm for behavior modification oriented programs – many obese adults are unable to sustain weight lost during treatment for even a year (Stunkard and Penick, 1979). Surgical interventions are markedly more successful in producing substantial, sustained weight loss for the morbidly obese, but accompanying morbidity, mortality, and expense are so great as to justify limiting operations only to this group. Weight loss of obese patients during psychoanalytic treatment is as good as that reported in outcome studies of clients in behavior modification programs. Maintenance of this weight loss over at least an 18-month period is better (Rand and Stunkard, 1978).

Psychoanalytic treatment is not appropriate for all obese adults. It is a treatment for adults with emotional difficulties, some of whom may be obese. Psychoanalytic theory, however, may have useful ideas that can be reconsidered and incorporated into general weight loss programs. Therapists in weight reduction clinics need to be aware of the psychodynamics that can accompany obesity in order to recognize clients who might benefit from psychoanalysis or psychotherapy. Psychoanalysis or psychotherapy may be essential for some obese adults who want to lose weight; these adults should be identified and referred. If life can become less emotionally complicated, these adults may be able to deal with the issues of weight regulation on a chronic basis.

Initially, this chapter reviews briefly some basic tenets of psychoanalysis in an admittedly oversimplified way. Then data from a study of obese patients in psychoanalysis are presented. These data deal first with general characteristics of patients in psychoanalysis. Secondly, weight loss of obese patients and concurrent changes in psychopathology occurring during the course of treatment are presented; eating with emotional overtones is described in this context. Next, data dealing with psychodynamic issues of some obese patients are reported. Finally, implications for therapy are discussed.

BASIC TENETS OF PSYCHOANALYTIC THOUGHT

There are many schools of psychoanalytic thought. Each school is associated with the particular person who was influential in its establishment, e.g., Freud, Adler, Horney, Fromm, Sullivan, Klein, Jung, and Rank. Each school was established when the principal psychoanalytic author found the existing theoretical system to be unsupportable. The result is that each school presents a distinct theoretical system with an unique emphasis on some aspect of the nature of man. Some psychoanalysts today clearly identify themselves with a particular school. Other psychodynamically oriented therapists are eclectic and utilize ideas from several or all of the schools. Schools of psychoanalysis are considered psychoanalytic because they use the basic premises and orientation established by Freud: psychological determinism, the unconscious, motivation, and adaptation.*

Obesity has not been a topic of major psychoanalytic concern. Psychoanalysts within each school do treat clients who are obese. However, with the exception of Freudian psychoanalysts, there has been relatively little written about the dynamics of obesity. This section presents a very brief description of general psychoanalytic thoughts and methods. The section after this will examine materials from obese patients in psychoanalytic treatment for relevant evidence.

Psychological Determinism

The meaning of psychic determinism is that no human behavior is "accidental." In the same way that physical phenomenon can be explained, psychic events are also structured by preceding events − that is , they are "determined." In early studies of hysteria, Freud (1896) examined the particuliar behaviors of a mentally ill woman. By studying the woman's memories of past events through hypnosis, he was able to show that the patient's current symptoms were not arbitrary, but made sense in the context of her past. Freud then went on to examine common experiences of forgetting, slips of the tongue, and little mistakes. These too were found to be frequently caused by the wish or intent of the person involved, and were only accidental in the sense that the person did not consciously plan them. Both bizarre symptoms and common mistakes became understandable in terms of the psychic stresses affecting the person. Bizarre eating behaviors and obesity could thus be viewed as an indication of psychic stress.

The Unconscious

The second major premise of psychoanalysis is that a person is not aware of much of his mental life; that is, much of his or her mental life is unconscious. Unconscious processes, however, actively influence what a person does. Lives of both normal and mentally ill adults are shaped by unconscious processes. Because it is easier to distinguish unconscious processes from conscious wishes when they are in conflict, much of the early study of the unconscious processes focused on the experiences of neurotic adults.

Methods of Psychoanalysis

Adults, accustomed to being introspective, are apt to confuse unconscious processes with preconscious thoughts. "Preconscious" is the term used to describe thoughts

---

*The following presentation of the basic concepts of psychoanalytic thought is guided by the texts by Munroe (1955) and Brenner (1974).

and emotions that can be brought into awareness by reflection. There are techniques in behavior modification oriented therapies that are designed specifically to help obese clients become aware of preconscious emotional and behavioral chains that trigger eating episodes (e.g., food diary records). Information about unconscious processes, however, is held to be *not* available through simple introspection and can only be gleaned indirectly, when the normal, intentional, goal-directed qualities of mind are relaxed. Psychoanalysts routinely use the method of free association, dream materials, projective methods, and instances of resistance to gain insights into the unconscious processes of their patients. (See Appendix 1 for a brief elaboration of these methods.)

Motivation and Dynamics

Human behavior is considered to be purposive and goal directed. These goals are often profoundly influenced by unconscious processes. In Freudian psychology, infant sexuality has a preponderant role in the development of human goals. Other psychoanalytic schools recognize different organizing motivations.

The unconscious process can have mutually contradicting needs that are simultaneously pressuring a person. Our behavior reflects the dynamic interplay between primitive physical urges (the id), our realistic assessment of what is actually possible (the ego), and goals that are in accord with cultural morals (the superego). The basic idea is that the unconscious processes have a purpose and motivate an individual's conscious behaviors. For example, an adult may have a strong unconscious wish to reexperience the total maternal loving attention associated with early childhood. Symbolically, home-baked goods may represent this maternal love. The conscious eating behavior is rationalized ("I just can't resist home-baked goods"), but the adult is unaware of the more profound motivations (case report provided by a psychoanalyst participating in the survey described on page 187).

Adaptation — the Genetic Approach

Adult personality is considered to be a product of the experiences of the child. Early childhood is given special importance because the first interpersonal experiences comprise the child's entire reference world: these adaptive experiences of the child structure the dynamics of his or her mind.

Adler and Horney have emphasized the function of early experiences in establishing the *general* pattern of later experiences and social relationships. This approach is described by the adage, "As the twig is bent, so grows the tree." Freudian psychoanalytic schools emphasize stages in psychosexual development, each with unique emotional needs. The impact of experiences on adult personality depends upon the stage in which they occur. The intensity of emotional needs characteristic of a given stage usually wanes as the stage is passed and is superseded by the more mature needs of the next developmental stage. Those needs that are repressed because they are too anxiety provoking are not given a chance to be worked out; these do not mature but remain at an infantile level.

Explanations for the development of obesity are guided by a therapists theoretical orientation. A "bent twig" explanation would look for important events leading to excessive eating that occurred sometime during a patient's childhood. Stage theorists would focus on disruptive or unique psychodynamic events that occurred specifically during infancy. Those practitioners of classical psychoanalysis who rely heavily on stage concepts would search for clues to the origins of adult obesity in early oral experiences of their patients. Certain aspects of the oral stage of development have a face validity, although it has been largely discredited as an explanation of adult obesity (Kaplan and Kaplan, 1957). Because of its relevance to obesity, the oral stage of psychosexual development is briefly described in Appendix II.

SURVEY OF OBESE PATIENTS IN PSYCHOANALYSIS

The "state of the art" of treating obesity was sufficiently inadequate to prompt Dr. Albert Stunkard and myself to undertake an evaluation of obese patients in psychoanalysis. The goals were to collect patient materials that could be used to evaluate the usefulness of the basic tenets of psychoanalysis in understanding obesity and to document weight changes that might occur during treatment. Although the tens or hundreds of hours involved in psychoanalytic treatments could never be offered as a general treatment, we considered the potential knowledge of the psychodynamics of obese patients available to psychoanalysts to be truly unique.

Background

The study was initiated in 1972 under the sponsorship of the research committee of the American Academy of Psychoanalysis (Rand and Stunkard, 1977, 1978). Fifty-five percent of the members responded to an initial participation request, and one-third of these (N = 104) had one or more obese patients in individual treatment. Detailed questionnaires were mailed to these analysts for each obese patient and for a control patient of the same sex and approximate age, but of normal weight. One hundred and forty-seven questionnaires were returned: 72 analysts provided data on 84 obese and 63 nonobese adults. A year and a half later, a follow-up questionnaire was sent to participating analysts, and data on 144 patients were obtained. Slightly over half of the patients were still in treatment at this time. At the time of the first questionnaire, patients had been in treatment for a median period of 31 months (with an interquartile range of 15 to 35 months); by the time of the second survey, the median period of treatment was 42 months (interquartile range, 29 to 77 months).

General Characteristics of Patients in Psychoanalysis

The patients in this survey were similar demographically to patients in other psychoanalytic surveys (e.g., Hamberg et al., 1967; Weber et al., 1967). The large majority of patients were between 18 and 50 years old and of middle or upper-middle income status. Over 60 percent were college graduates and slightly over half were Jewish. The obese and nonobese patients were comparable on all demographic variables except marital status: significantly more obese patients were single (48 percent versus 29 percent). There were more obese women (N = 64) than men (N = 20) in psychoanalysis. Women were, on the average, 47 percent overweight and men, 42 percent.

Obese patients did not enter psychoanalytic treatment as a part of a weight loss effort: only 6 percent listed weight as their chief complaint. Depression and anxiety were reported to be the chief complaints for the majority (60 percent) of both obese and nonobese patients.

Obese patients in psychoanalysis are different from obese patients in other treatment settings. The most major difference is that obese patients in other treatment programs enter treatment specifically for their obesity, but there are also other important differences. In general, obese clients are less wealthy and less educated, more are Christian, and fewer are emotionally disturbed than patients in psychoanalysis (e.g., Goldblatt et al., 1965). By way of contrast, characteristics of a group of 80 massively obese candidates for surgery for obesity were: 40 percent were middle or upper class, 4 percent had completed college, 4 percent were Jewish, and only 20 percent had psychopathology of clinical significance (Kuldau and Rand, in press).

Overview and Statistical Note

Psychoanalytic patients in this survey entered therapy because of emotional problems with the treatment goal of ameliorating those problems. For patients whose obesity was related in some way to emotional conflicts, the expectation would be that weight loss might accompany resolution of emotional issues. In the following section we will examine analyst reports of patient progress in therapy, weight changes during therapy, and relationships between eating behaviors and weight. After that, we will present psychodynamic issues of some patients that became prominent and were dealt with in the course of therapy.

Data from the survey were analyzed using the chi-square test for significance. Chi-square values were considered to be significant if $p \leqslant .01$ unless otherwise stated. With the exception of the data on weight, men and women did not differ significantly on any of the relevant variables, and results are described as obese-nonobese differences or as obese patient characteristics.

Patient Progress, Weight Changes, and Eating Behaviors

At the time of the first survey, 80 percent of the obese patients were reported to be progressing satisfactorily. Eighteen months later, 83 percent were reported to be improved or much improved in their primary problems of anxiety, depression, etc. The mean weight loss at the time of the first survey was 4.5 ± 10.8 kilograms (53 percent of the obese patients had lost more than 4.5 kilograms, 26 percent more than 9 kilograms, and 8 percent more than 18 kilograms). The mean weight losses had increased to 9.5 ± 14.1 kilograms by the time of the 18-month follow-up survey (47 percent of the obese patients had lost more than 9 kilograms, and 19 percent more than 18 kilograms). We were not able to evaluate the relationship between weight loss and treatment directly because the large majority of obese patients both lost weight and progressed satisfactorily. However, at the time of the 18-month follow-up, dissatisfaction with therapy and failure to lose weight seemed to be associated: among patients who were no longer in treatment, significantly fewer who terminated prematurely lost weight than those whose treatment was complete.

It is legitimate to ask how psychoanalytic treatment could lead to weight loss when psychoanalysts did not prescribe diets or become involved with monitoring patients' weights. One likely possibility is the relationship analysts reported between eating behaviors of their patients and emotional stress. In this sample, many more obese patients (98 percent) than nonobese patients (43 percent) were reported to eat when they were depressed, anxious, or angry. Further, significantly more obese (79 percent) than nonobese (9 percent) had gained 10 or more pounds during periods of major life stress (e.g., marriage, divorce, occupational change, death of family member, etc.). We can hypothesize that the stress → excessive eating → weight gain sequence is modified when the level of the emotional stress experienced by a patient is reduced or when a patient learns more adaptive responses to stress than overeating.

Psychodynamics of Food, Eating, and Corpulence

Sessions of both obese and nonobese patients in psychoanalysis are characterized by a flow of countless details. Repetition of details and interpretation of details become important in understanding the psychodynamic concerns of a particular patient. Although obesity was not the primary concern of obese patients in psychoanalysis, psychodynamic themes of food, eating, and the state of obesity were far more frequently encountered in the histories and current emotional lives of obese than nonobese patients. Thematic materials reported by the surveyed analysts were divided into those concerned with childhood experiences and those that were contemporary.

Childhood Adaptations

Psychoanalytic theory attributes the origins of most basic psychic strategies to the childhood years; obesity is often considered a reflection of these childhood adaptations. This survey did not attempt to evaluate the relative importance of one period of childhood (e.g., the oral stage) to another (e.g., latency), but asked simply about parent-child relationships and childhood experiences.

One issue was if food had acquired exaggerated significance for obese patients during childhood. The differences observed uniformly suggested that food had a greater impact on the social-emotional development of more obese than nonobese patients. For example, food was used as a reward for good bahavior in the families of more obese than nonobese patients (35 percent versus 12 percent). Whereas most nonobese patients (93 percent) reported they had been given the right amount to eat, almost half of the obese patients felt they had been expected to eat too much (31 percent) or given too little (13 percent). Food was also reported to have a special dynamic role in parent-child relationships for more obese (57 percent) than nonobese (17 percent) patients. Following are two examples provided by analysts of parent-child relationships characterized by an overinvolvement with food:

> *Obese woman:* The patient's parents underwent great deprivation during the war (World War II). As a result they overfed their child and insisted on eating as a way to relieve insecurity and ill feelings.

> *Obese man:* The patient was hospitalized for tuberculosis from the time he was eighteen months old until he was four. His parents visited him weekly during this time. Among his earliest memories, he recalls that his mother fed him sweet cream on her visits. His parents became separated while he was in the hospital, although his father spent weekends with him until he was eleven or twelve. By the time the patient was seven he had considerable struggles with his mother about food. These really centered on issues of autonomy and control. His mother forced him to eat everything on his plate. As a punishment she forced him to eat meals outside the front door of their apartment.

His night eating apparently started at this time. By sneaking food, symbolically he was being his own boss.

A second issue was the importance of the obese physique during childhood. Large physical stature with assumed physical strength can be an attractive attribute to a child. When only patients with an obese parent were considered, significantly more obese (71% of 49 obese patients) than nonobese (29% of 17 nonobese patients) patients were reported to identify primarily with the obese parent ($p \leq .05$). Individual patients were also reported to have used their obesity during childhood to gain attention, to assert independence, and to avoid social interactions.

There were a few normal weight patients who were brought up in stressful, food-oriented homes. The fact that these patients did not become obese underscores the potential contribution of personal constitution: not all people who eat a lot become heavy, and some people cannot or will not eat a lot (Garrow, 1978; Sims et al., 1973).

Contemporary Dynamics

There is often an overlap in psychodynamic issues, so that, for example, themes relating to obesity are related to themes of personal acceptance and sexual attractiveness. Psychodynamics of general adult functioning in areas of weight stability and fluctuations, sexuality, and symbolic meanings of food were examined with the expectation that themes of affect, self-image, deprivation and gratification, aggression, and sexuality often would be interrelated.

Psychodynamic statements reported by psychoanalysts indicated that there were at least twelve obese patients for whom the obese state was an asset. The interplay of several themes was apparent in the descriptions of each of these patients. Following are four examples that illustrate several themes of personal advantage associated with being obese:

Obese man: The patient's obesity lets him feel "huge and powerful compared to puny-looking mortals." He also associates slenderness with being small and powerless like a child.

Obese woman: The patient has a tremendous oedipal involvement with her father. The father took showers with the patient in her adolescence. By being obese she effectively avoids being physically attractive to him. The father is a physical education teacher and places great importance on being slim and athletic.

Obese woman: Both parents are obsessed with weight, their own and their daughter's. The parents are paying for the daughter's therapy with the expressed wish that she shape up. The daughter (the patient), in turn, has been able to individuate herself by being fat (20 pounds overweight). On those occasions when she has been slender she feels (unconsciously) insecure, vulnerable, and that she has compromised her autonomy to parental pressures.

Obese man: The patient gets much narcissistic gratification over being fat. Whenever he experiences rejection he usually tries to attach the rejection to his weight problem. In fact the rejection is related frequently to his directiveness or his passivity, i.e., those qualities he has taken for identification with his mother (nagging) and his father (passivity).

For most obese patients, however, being obese was not recognized as an asset: over 90 percent wanted to lose weight. So why didn't they? Two open-ended questions on the research questionnaire dealt with the psychodynamics associated with weight gain and loss. Psychodynamic statements from 66 obese patients were used to describe general psychodynamic themes (Glucksman et al., 1978). Weight gain of obese patients was usually associated with negative emotional experiences, whereas positive psychic functioning accompanied weight loss. The most common theme reported — deprivation gratification — was associated with weight fluctuations for one-third of the patients. Feelings of deprivation (loss, separation, rejection) accompanied weight gain, whereas those of gratification (love, acceptance) accompanied weight loss. These data are consistent with the hypothesis that emotional well-being is a necessary precondition to successful weight loss for some obese patients.

Weight fluctuations either up or down were associated with specific psychodynamic themes for most obese but not most normal weight patients. Psychodynamic statements in reference to weight gain or loss were reported for only 12 normal weight patients. All but one of these statements was negative, e.g., loss of self-esteem, feeling sexually undesirable (weight loss), self-destructive with guilt about loss of control (weight gain). Both weight loss and weight gain of normal weight patients appeared to be associated with psychic distress, whereas weight loss of obese patients appeared to be associated with relief of emotional distress.

Sexual issues can also be involved in the psychodynamics of obesity. The question analysts were asked to answer was, "Is eating ever used as an avoidance of sexual relationships?" The psychodynamic connection between eating and sex was reported for significantly more obese (47 percent) than nonobese (7 percent) patients. However, it is important to note that sex was *not* related to psychodynamics of eating for more than half of the obese patients and that adequacy of sexual functioning was of primary concern to only 2 percent of the obese patients compared to 13 percent of the nonobese (Rand, 1979).

In the comments provided by analysts, it was clear that some patients ate specifically to avoid intimate involvements, others ate as a *substitute* for sex when no partner was available, and still others ate as a means to maintain their obesity and sexual unattractiveness. Following are selected examples:

Obese man: Patient eats as a substitute for sex. He eats less when he is sexually satisfied.

Obese man: Obesity turns his spouse off. Patient eats and delays going to bed until his wife is asleep.

Obese woman: On several dates the patient has avoided sexual prospects and noticed increased eating soon after. She has also found herself eating as soon as her mate talks of sex.

One-third of obese patients were reported to have specific symbolic meanings associated with eating episodes compared to only 5 percent of the normal weight patients. For many obese patients there was a continuity of themes between the psychodynamics of the obese state and symbolic associations with eating, although for some patients eating had special connotations quite apart from being obese. Symbolic meanings were very personal; many dealt with themes of security, anger, or defiance. The complexity and diversity of symbolic meanings of eating for one patient is illustrated by the analyst's description that follows:

Obese woman: The beauty of some foods would make her beautiful. She loved elaborately decorated cakes with whipped cream and swirls of food colors. Home-baked goods convey comfort and allow possessive, warm feelings inside.

When she was 13 she started to get fat. She feared that she would be punished by pregnancy for an illicit relationship. At that time, fat began to symbolize pregnancy.

By eating a lot very fast the patient symbolically tries to push down anger — swallowing and burying the anger in food. She uses food to put out the fire of anger.

Summary

Reported weight losses and maintenance of these losses of obese patients in psychoanalytic treatment were better than losses in most traditional weight reduction clinics. During treatment, both obese and nonobese patients showed marked improvement in psychopathology. Food, eating, and obesity as important themes were encountered far more frequently in the histories of obese patients and had a more important role in their adult lives than for most nonobese patients. Emotional crisis of many kinds were associated with weight gain of obese patients. Food had greater symbolic importance for obese patients. In addition, obese patients were more likely to eat than nonobese patients either when a desired sexual partner was unavailable or to avoid sexual intimacies.

DISCUSSION

Not all obese adults are appropriate candidates for either psychoanalysis or other kinds of individual psychotherapy. There are obese people who have no clinically significant psychopathology. Perhaps these are the adults who are the "success" group in traditional weight loss programs. Bruch (in Glucksman, 1972) has distinguished several groups along an obesity-psychopathology dimension. Patients with psychopathology include (1) obese people who became obese in childhood, are preoccupied with size and weight, and have difficulty with issues involving delay of gratification; (2) obese patients who learn to overeat in reaction to a loss or other psychological trauma; and (3) thin-fat adults who manage to control their obesity but are preoccupied with body size and are neurotically focused on food and eating. It is these groups of obese patients and thin-fat adults who may profit from psychotherapy.

The presence or absence of debilitating emotional problems and psychodynamic conflicts really identifies who should and should not consider psychotherapy. Therapists in conventional weight loss programs who have obese clients for whom weight appears to be just one of many personal problems might consider the appropriateness of referring these people to some kind of psychotherapy.

The basic biology of many adults is such that obesity will remain a personal problem throughout life. It is not easy to learn to live with mouth hunger or stomach hunger, and to refuse food when at some level there is a "want to eat." Eliminating or reducing emotionally motivated eating may be an important step in limiting the amount of overweight with which a person has to contend within his or her constitutional framework. Obese adults whose energies are consumed in neurotic struggles with themselves are weakened in their efforts to adopt a permanently restrained eating life style. Relief of emotional conflicts may greatly facilitate both the weight loss and the maintenance of weight loss for many of these adults.

APPENDIX I: PSYCHOANALYTIC METHODS

The method of *free association* is a therapeutic technique basic to psychoanalysis. Free association requires that a patient relax the normal monitoring of what he or she says, and share every thought or thought fragment that comes to mind. Only a small fraction of what is said has therapeutic relevance. But over tens of sessions, reoccurring fragments identify unconscious preoccupations quite clearly to the analyst. *Resistance* describes the stoppage of the associational process. Typically, a patient blocks the associational stream of thought when emotionally charged materials are approached. *Dream* materials are used as direct sources of information about unconscious preoccupations. Characteristics of dreams reflect the processes that typify "irrational" psychic life. The *life pattern* is used as an index of unconscious goals, where repeated behaviors suggest a coherence to the non-rational directives of personality. For example, repeated job difficulties, divorces, and failed diets can be an indication of the persistence of an unconscious problem. In *projective methods of psychological testing,* the tester asks the patient to describe vague, abstract test stimuli like ink blots. Interpretation is based on comparison of the patient's descriptions to common responses, and examination of the responses for patterns which may indicate unconscious pre-occupations.

APPENDIX II: FREUDIAN PSYCHOANALYTIC THEORY: THE ORAL STAGE OF PSYCHOSEXUAL DEVELOPMENT

There is a compelling association between obesity and orality. Although many psychoanalysts do not accept the stage theory of psychosexual development, a discussion of obesity would be incomplete without mention of the oral stage. Classical psychoanalytic theory has interpreted adult obesity as reflecting either unsatisfactory or uniquely satisfactory oral stage experiences.

The first area of major psychosexual importance is considered to be the mouth. It was Freud who first emphasized the dual roles of the mouth: that of being part of the physical system to provide food to the body and that of being part of the sensual system, providing pleasurable taste and tactile satisfaction.

In infancy, the recurring internal state of hunger is met when the infant accepts food offered by the mother. The sequence of hunger pains, material response, sucking, warmth, satiation, and subsequent sleeping is repeated regularly. Gradually, nursing (eating), the reduction of physical discomfort (hunger) and subsequent feelings of warmth and security (maternal love) are associated. In the course of normal development, the infant learns to distinguish internal stimuli (e.g., hunger pains) from those of the external world (e.g., maternal response). An awareness and interest in the mother as a separate person emerges during the intervals between times when physical needs are of paramount importance.

The very young infant is passive and receptive. When teeth erupt, the mouth has the potential to be used in a much more aggressive fashion (literally biting). The intensity of aggression as a competing oral motivation depends on the levels of anger and frustration of the infant. The emotional associations of eating, love and aggression are felt to derive from these oral stage experiences. The central importance of the mouth in structuring emotions and sensual satisfactions (the oral stage) wanes as anal activities and products become of intense interest (the anal stage).

The psychological achievements associated with the oral stage include learning to distinguish internal stimuli from external events, to distinguish self from other, and learning to tolerate frustration. Profound negative emotional effects can occur if an infant's early experiences are too frustrating or the distinction between internal and external events is blurred. One such effect is that eating can emerge as a strategy to satisfy emotional as well as nutritional needs.

Psychoanalysts such as Bruch (1973) and Bychoski (1950) have reported case histories of patients whose early childhood experiences were felt by them to lead to excessive eating and subsequent obesity. The kinds of experiences described included cases in which the patient as an infant was fed whenever he or she was restless (rather than put to sleep, changed, played with etc.), where the only meaningful social interactions between parent and child occurred during feeding, and where feeding was so tense, unpleasant and unpredictable that the effect was to train the infant to eat as much as he could as rapidly as possible.

REFERENCES

Brenner, C. *An Elementary Textbook of Psychoanalysis.* Revised Anchor's Book Edition. New York: Anchor Books, 1974.

Bruch, H. *Eating Disorders.* New York: Basic Books, 1973.

Bychowski, G. On neurotic obesity. *Psychoanalytic Review,* 1950, *37* (4), 301-319.

Garrow, J. S. *Energy Balance and Obesity in Man.* New York: Elsevier/North-Holland Biomedical Press, 1978.

Glucksman, M. L. Psychiatric observations on obesity. *Advances in Psychosomatic Medicine,* 1972, *7,* 194-216.

Glucksman, M. L., Rand, C. S. W., and Stunkard, A. J. Psychodynamics of obesity. *Journal of the American Academy of Psychoanalysis,* 1978, *6* (1), 103-115.

Goldblatt, P. B., Moore, M. E., and Stunkard, A. J. Social factors in obesity. *Journal of the American Medical Association,* 1965, *192* (12), 1039-1044.

Halverson, J. D. Obesity surgery in Perspective. *Surgery,* 1980, *87* (2), 119-127.

Hamburg, D. A., Bibring, G. L., Fisher, C., Stanton, A. H., Wallerstein, R. S., Weistock, H. I., and Haggard, E. Report of Ad Hoc Committee on Central Fact-gathering Data. *Journal of the American Psychoanalytic Association,* 1967, *15,* 841-861.

Kaplan, H. I. and Kaplan, H. S. The psychosomatic concept of obesity. *Journal of Nervous and Mental Diseases,* 1957, *125,* 181-201.

Kuldau, J. M. and Rand, C. S. W. Jejunoileal bypass: general and psychiatric outcome after one year. *Psychosomatics* 1980, 21(f), 534–539.

Munroe, R. L. *Schools of Psychoanalytic Thought.* New York: Holt, Rinehart and Winston, 1967.

Rand, C. S. W. Obesity and human sexuality. *Medical Aspects of Human Sexuality,* 1979, *13* (1), 140-151.

Rand, C. S. W. and Stunkard, A. J. Psychoanalysis and obesity. *The Journal of the American Academy of Psychoanalysis,* 1977, *5* (4), 459-497.

Rand, C. S. W. and Stunkard, A. J. Obesity and Psychoanalysis. *American Journal of Psychiatry,* 1978, *135* (5), 547-551.

Sims, E. A. H., Danforth, E., Jr., Horton, E. S., Bray, G. A., Glennon, J. A., and Salans, L. B., Endocrine and metabolic effects of experimental obesity in man. *Recent Progress in Hormone Research,* 1973, *29*, 457-496.

Stunkard, A. J. and Penick, S. B. Behavior modification in the treatment of obesity: The problem of maintaining weight loss. *Archives of General Psychiatry,* 1979, *36*, 801-806.

Weber, J. J., Elinson, J., and Moss, L. M. Psychoanalysis and change, a study of psychoanalytic clinic records using electronic data-processing techniques. *Archives of General Psychiatry,* 1967, *17*, 687-709.

9

Interactional Psychotherapy of Obesity

Benjamin B. Wolman

With the exception of a small minority of people with an exceedingly high metabolic rate, practically everyone in the United States *may* become obese, and unless he or she controls his or her eating habits, they *will* become obese. According to the *New York Times* of February 20, 1979, over forty million Americans are overweight.

Millions of obese people undergo a variety of self-imposed or doctor-prescribed dieting procedures. Some of these methods and techniques are described in the present volume. The dieting techniques have met with various success with various individuals (Leon, 1976; Stunkard, 1958, 1974). The initial success is usually quite spectacular, but according to Feinstein's review (1970) in a majority of cases the patients regain the weight they have lost. Apparently, treatment of obesity is not an easy task. In some cases, a radical, crash dieting may aggravate one's emotional problems. Several cases of grave mental disorders, even psychotic episodes, have been caused by crash diet (Robinson and Winnik, 1973). It seems that some mentally disturbed people consciously use obesity as a defense mechanism that prevents expenditure of an otherwise scarce emotional energy. Latent schizophrenics often develop all sorts of devices that protect them from being involved with other people. Social withdrawal in latent and manifest schizophrenia serves as an energy-saving maneuver, for schizophrenics usually have already invested too much emotional energy in their parents and other significant people. In my nosological system, schizophrenics have been described as individuals who hypercathected their emotions and have given away more than could be reasonably allowed. I compared psychotic breakdown to bankruptcy, as if it represented a case of emotional insolvency (Wolman, 1966, 1970, 1973a). I believe that many latent schizophrenics and some milder cases of minifest schizophrenia unconsciously try to prevent such a bankruptcy by social withdrawal and obesity. Loss of obesity might adversely affect their energy-saving defense mechanisms and, in some cases, produce a collapse of personality structure.

ROOTS OR BRANCHES

Over the years of my psychotherapeutic practice I have treated several obese people. The tendency to gain weight is related to a great many factors, most of them, but certainly not all, of psychological nature. Moreover, even the psychosomatic or psychophysiologic origin of obesity is not homogeneous, and one must not put all obese people into one clinical category. Scientific literature (Bruch, 1973, 1977; Mayer, 1968, 1970; Stunkard, 1958, 1974; and others) is full of contradictory empirical data and diverse theoretical explanations, and there is no reason to ascribe uniformity to obesity.

The complexity of the problem and the diversity of clinical pictures militate against simplicity and uniformity in treatment of obesity. A careful differential diagnosis of every single case and flexibility in treatment techniques are imperative. The following pages will describe one of the possible approaches with adequate room for individualization.

All patients I have treated for obesity were compulsive eaters. Overeating resembles other types of addiction such as alcoholism or drugs. In treatment of addictions I avoided a head-on confrontation with their well-entrenched compulsive drinking or, even worse, drug addiction. I do not believe that one can expect good results with a direct attack on pathological overt behavioral patterns. Usually I have assumed that the need to take drugs or alcohol is rooted in the unconscious, for consciously all of my patients agreed that it was very bad to be addicted. Their addictions were *symptoms* of deep underlying emotional problems, and eventual removal of the symptoms could not last for long if the underlying causes were left untouched.

I compared the symptoms to branches of a tree that blocks the light. Cutting the branches could not solve the problem, for sooner or later new branches would grow. In order to solve the problem one must dig out the roots, for no tree can grow without roots. As soon as the roots are out, the tree falls, and the problem is solved. And, in fact, whenever I dug out and cut away the roots of addiction, the addicts were cured. I believe that the first task of psychotherapy is to dig out and remove the roots of one's emotional problems, and the following pages will briefly describe the technique that I have been using.

THE PSYCHOTHERAPEUTIC PROCESS

One cannot help wondering why people come to us psychotherapists. Is this the old dependence on the witch doctor who was believed to perform miracles? Or is it the medical model that we are supposed to "treat" patients and give them something they do not have?

I have worked with many patients who were smarter than myself and more successful in many aspects of life. Some of them I admired for their business success (Wolman, 1973b). I have also treated intellectuals, artists, and singers whom I admired.

We, the psychotherapists, have no reason to boast; we are handymen or re-pairmen. *Our job is helping people* and our skill is limited to the ability to listen to people's troubles, understand and reinterpret them, and somehow help. Certainly the easy way out would be to hypnotize or to uncondition them. I believe, however, that both hypnosis and behavior modification belong to the medical model of treatment. The physician always does something for the patients — he treats them, gives them prescriptions, and manipulates their behavior. He tells them what to do, what diet to go on, what medications to take, or how to use their muscles. Sometimes he performs surgery or straightens their bones or their backs.

Nothing of the kind is being done in any psychotherapy based on the psycho-analytic model. In the psychoanalytic model of psychotherapy to which I am deeply indebted, the psychotherapist does not do much, for *almost the entire job is done by the patient.* We cannot work with captive audiences; we do not administer shock therapy or brain surgery; we just listen and try to understand and, somehow, something happens. What, indeed, is psychotherapy?

Psychotherapy is a process of interaction. From a sociological point of view, there are two partners, one who seeks help and the other who is supposed to offer that help. One partner feels that his life went wrong and needs some kind of adjustment, and the other believes that he can help, and the person who asks for help believes this too. Without the faith in psychotherapy, without the belief of the patient that he can be helped, he will never come to us, at least not willingly.

The process of psychotherapy is actually a split-level or two-level process. On one hand, it is an interaction of two adults; one of them has an office, calls himself M.D. or Ph.D., has passed some examinations and gotten his license or certification, and is approved by society for the job he is doing. The other can be a lawyer, a teacher, an accountant, a housewife, or a garbage collector who feels disturbed and perplexed by being disturbed. There is little chance of helping somebody unless he or she feels perplexed by being disturbed. On one level, psychotherapy is the *interaction* of two adults which resembles the type of interaction that takes place between a lawyer and his client, a dentist and his patient, an accountant and his customer. The patients believe we are competent in certain areas of life and they expect us to help them. Our patients might be great scholars or surgeons, brilliant writers, or famous singers. In the therapeutic situation, they look up to us. Outside the therapeutic situation the relationship may be reversed and we look up to them.

TRANSFERENCE

The interaction that takes place between a psychotherapist and his patient transcends the usual man-to-man relationship. We are not lawyers, dentists, or surgeons; we deal with the emotional problems of people and a particular phenomenon called transference takes place.

Transference is not just a one-way street. I believe that any kind of human relation, called by Freud "object relation," is a cathexis or an investment on one's emotions in the other person. However, while Freud stressed the point of view of the person who cathects, I have developed an additional concept which takes into consideration the person who is at the receiving end of cathexis. Thus, instead of using the term "cathexis" as described in classic psychoanalysis, I deal with the concept of "interindividual cathexis" which represents the emotional load *directed* by one person toward another and *received* by the other person. In other words, if a mother loves a child, the mother is cathecting her sublimated or neutralized libido in the child, and the child is at the receiving end. The way the child feels about it, how he perceives the mother's love, is a highly important factor in his emotional balance and personality development.

The cathectic situation in any kind of psychotherapy is also a two-way process. The patient cathects his emotions in his therapist, but the therapist cannot be totally unaware of the fact that the patient did invest some of his emotions, positive or negative, in him. A psychoanalyst or a psychoanalytically oriented psychotherapist need not assume that he has the right to deal with these cathected processes in transference always in the same way, no matter who the patient is. Alexander and French (1946) have introduced the concept of *intentional manipulation of transference* by decreasing or increasing the number of sessions. I went further than Alexander and French; I maintain that whether the therapist is aware of it or not, his behavior influences the patient's transference, thus I suggested making a more efficient use of transference (Wolman, 1967).

I believe that the nature of transference cathexis depends on the nature of the disorder. The obsessive-compulsive and schizophrenic patients (the hypervectorial type) tend toward object-hypercathexis, which means overinvolvement with others. They suffer from self-hypocathexis, inadequate cathexis in themselves (Wolman, 1973a). One may, therefore, expect a most profound and sometimes vehement positive transference phenomenon in psychotherapy with schizotype patients.

Working with a great many hypervectorial patients, I noticed how easily they become overcathected and overinvolved in the transference. Some of them worry about the therapist the way they used to worry about their parents. They notice whether he looks pale or suntanned; they worry about his future; they would like to take care of him. On the other side, the sociopaths (hyperinstrumental narcissistic patients) do not worry at all about him. They worry about themselves only. Being narcissistic, they display strong paranoid tendencies and are unable to develop a positive transference. They usually develop a negative transference attitude, blaming the analyst for their misfortunes or lack of achievement (Krauss and Krauss, 1977; Wolman, 1967).

There are no fool-proof methods for dealing with transference, but I strongly object to a uniform way of dealing with transference with no consideration of the particular clinical type of the patient. I do believe that one of the main aspects of interactional psychotherapy is *individualization* in dealing with each case.

What is happening in psychoanalytic therapy is a series of libido and destrudo cathexes in which both the patient and the psychoanalyst participate. The psychoanalyst cannot escape the fact that he likes or dislikes his patients, although he must control his countertranaference phenomena, otherwise he violates his professional ethics. However, he must be aware of the fact that he does not react the same way to all people, and *being aware of his shortcomings as an individual may make him a better therapist.*

No human being can avoid being somewhat influenced by what is going on in relationship to other people. Some patients show love for the therapist which is flattering; some patients show much hatred which may be damaging to his ego. However, one of the main duties of the psychotherapist is to be always aware of what is going on and never to be carried away by his emotions.

A responsible psychotherapist gets involved with the case of his patients for this is his moral obligation to the people who seek his help, but under no circumstances must the psychotherapist become involved with the person of the patient.

THE AIMS OF PSYCHOTHERAPY

My method is based on an assumption that every human being should be given a chance to attain full mental maturity which will enable him to live his life to its fullest extent.

The aims of psychotherapy are to help people to have the *courage to live* according to their convictions, to enable them to make the best of every possible situation, and to bring as much happiness and joy to themselves and dear ones as is humanly possible. Whenever events take an adverse course and misfortune strikes, they should not fall apart but should cope with dignity and courage with the adversities life brings them.

COURAGE AND WISDOM — THE PURPOSES OF PSYCHOTHERAPY

I believe that psychotherapeutic interaction should be divided into three phases. The first phase is psychoanalytic; this means overcoming whatever emotional obstacles and irrationalities one has developed during his lifetime and especially in early childhood. It involves the removal of infantile inhibitions and the reso-lution of infantile conflicts which cripple the personality and prevent adult individuals from acting in an adult and mature way. The resolution of past con-flicts or cutting out the roots is the first phase of interactional therapy. As soon as the psychotherapy helps to resolve the past conflicts and the patient is liberated from past handicaps and able to put his intelligence and energy toward productive use, the psychotherapy moves toward two phases which I have called "Search for Identity" and "Becoming: Self-realization," respectively.

In order to be able to find oneself, in order to be able to become a mature adult, one has to go through the analytic phase in which one acquires a good sense of reality, emotional balance, and social adjustment. The sense of reality is a necessary prerequisite for any adjustment to life and any chance of finding oneself in life. People who distort reality, who have exaggerated notions of themselves and the world, or who underestimate themselves or overestimate the obstacles can hardly if ever live a genuine life.

The emotional balance includes four factors: first, the emotional reaction must be *appropriate* to the situation. We react with sorrow to defeat and with joy to success. Disturbed people react in a paradoxical way, enjoying their de-feat and finding success unacceptable. Well-balanced emotionality is also *propor-tionate*. Disturbed individuals overreact or underreact to success and failure. The third factor in emotional balance is *self-control*. Infants and disturbed people are unable to control their emotions; mature adults are able to control their emotions and react in a way that will serve their purpose and help them in attaining their goals. The fourth factor in emotional balance is *adjustability*. No matter how deep the sorrow is or how great the joy, life goes on and one cannot live in the past. Neurotics live in the past. Well-adjusted adults never deny the past but go ahead in life with maximum wisdom and courage.

The third achievement in the analytic phase should be social adjustment. People who underwent psychotherapy should be able to develop a meaningful relationship with one or more individuals and should be able to form with others a rational give-and-take relationship which would not hurt them and would prevent him from being hurt by them. All imbalances must be corrected in the psychoanalytic phase of therapy which should result in a good sense of reality, a reasonable emotional balance, and ability to relate to people.

The analytic phase enables the individual to think clearly and to act in a realistic way, but it does not solve the problem of direction in life. What one is going to do with himself, what life should mean to him, what his goal in life is — these are the problems dealt with in the second phase of interactional psychotherapy, called the *search for identity*.

Quite often toward the end of the first phase, patients feel an abundance of energy; they feel that so much more could be done with their newly acquired energy liberated from inner conflicts. They crave self-realization and fulfillment.

The main issue to be dealt with at the second psychotherapeutic phase is the *awareness that life is a gift*. When patients ask, "Where am I going, what am I going to do with myself?" I reply with a question, "What would you like to do? Assume for a minute that you don't exist. Would it make a difference to you that today is Monday, Tuesday, or Wednesday? Whether we have today a sunny or a rainy day? Would it make any difference to you whether I am here or not? Would traffic congestion bother you?" These questions usually bring one answer, "Of course not, if I am not here, who cares?"

And this is the crucial issue: the awareness that one is the center of his own universe; that his own existence is the prerequisite of joy and sorrow, success and failure; that there is nothing more in life than life itself; that human beings are poor because they have nothing else but life and they are rich because life contains all possibilities.

Once a person accepts the fact that he or she is the center of his own universe the question is asked, "What can I do with this newly acquired self-awareness and autonomy?" One may try to do things for oneself and for others; one may try to attain goals, great and small, sublime and practical. One may decide in which direction his life will go.

Awareness of oneself is not necessarily acceptance of one's faults and errors and shortcomings. Awareness of oneself is the awareness of the fact that here are the cards that one received from heredity and experience. One must play his cards the best one can. One may use some of his defenses (Freud, 1946). For instance, compensation can be turned into a useful tool of adjusting to life. Reaction formation may not necessarily be a neurotic symptom; if one is belligerent, he may use his belligerence for conquering disease or misery and not necessarily for fighting people. One may neutralize some of his energies; one may sublimate some of his energies; one may decide that this is what he is. One does not necessarily accept all the aspects of his personality nor does he necessarily subscribe to all his possibilities. One may make a choice between various ways in life and find fulfillment for what is the most important aspect of his life.

BECOMING: SELF-REALIZATION

One can distinguish three attitudes toward other people. The first attitude is *instrumental*, that is, using people for the satisfaction of one's own needs. This narcissistic attitude is typical for an infant because he needs to be supported. As the child grows, he learns that one cannot get unless one gives, and gradually develops a *mutual* attitude based on giving and receiving. This attitude is typical for friendship, sexual relations, and marriage; each party tries to please the other and expects the same in return. The third type of attitude is giving without expecting anything in return. This *vectorial* attitude is typical for the parent-child relationship (Wolman, 1966). This attitude can be directed toward one's social, religious, and other ideals. To be a giver and a creator is the highest level of personality development.

A balanced individual should be able to function at all three levels. He is instrumental in bread-winning functions, mutual in friendship and in marriage, and vectorial in regard to his children and/or his ideals. Unfortunately, a great many individuals never outgrow the first level of instrumentalism, that is, taking care of themselves with disregard for others. Living that kind of life, the life of a cocoon, gives people the feeling of futility.

In the third phase of interactional psychotherapy one tries to help the patients to develop worthwhile goals. To be a fully developed individual, one cannot remain on an instrumental level, one should be capable of mutual relationship (marriage, sexual relations, and friendship), but one must also be able to develop the ability and the desire for giving. Getting is limited; giving is unlimited.

Consider two individuals, one who stretches out his hand to get something and the other to give, who is more happy? The one who gets is fully aware of his inadequacy, of his shortcomings, of his need to receive from others. He is weak and dependent. The one who gives has the glorious feeling of being able to give, of making other people happy. He is powerful and is aware of his power.

Not every human being can be a creative artist, but every human being can create joy and happiness for himself and for others; by giving happiness to others, he achieves the highest degree of joy and happiness for himself.

The third phase of interactional psychotherapy should enable the individual to decide in which direction he is going to utilize his energy as well as his intellectual and emotional resources. At this phase, the patients find out the meaning of their lives. They discover that they can create something and add something to life. Creating is the sign and symbol of power.

I have applied the above-described method to the treatment of obesity.

THREE CASES OF OBESITY

In the following pages I shall describe three obese patients.

The business executive, Mr. L., had a horrible childhood. He was the youngest of three children. His father worked long hours but even when he was at home he acted in an insensitive and inconsiderate manner. The mother managed to emotionally compensate her children, but when my patient was two or three years old, the mother became chronically ill. For years she was in hospitals on and off, and the child L. was at the mercy of visiting neighbors and relatives. His older brother and sister were frequently forced by the visitors and the sick mother "to take care of the baby," which they did with a good deal of overt hostility. L. resented most his mother who abandoned him; he felt sadly rejected. His rare pleasant childhood recollections were related to his grave illness. When he was ill, his bedridden mother got up from her bed, hovered over him, and showed compassion and affection: his illness and misery were rewarded.

Mr. L. started to gain weight quite early in life. When he was 11 years old his mother passed away. More or less at that time he became exceedingly obese and, inevitably, ridiculed and ostracized by his schoolmates. No one wanted to play with the fat boy.

He went through a lonely adolescence. He was a bright boy and had no difficulty in his studies in high school and in college. After graduation he accepted a menial job in a company where, to his surprise, he was rewarded for his abilities, diligence, and most probably also for his timidity and subservience to the boss.

One evening when he was 28 years old, he attended the annual Christmas party on his job. He never drank heavily, but at that party he drank enough to allow one of the office secretaries to take him to her home and seduce him. The girl got pregnant. She demanded marriage and Mr. L. succumbed to her demands and married her.

The marriage was a catastrophy. The woman literally wiped the floor with Mr. L. He felt rejected and desolate and went on a heavy eating spell. The more hostile his wife was, the more he ate, and the more he ate, the more she hated him. The heavier he got, the deeper was his depression, and the deeper his depression, the more he ate.

The unconscious purpose of Mr. L.'s obesity was to make himself so unhappy, clumsy, dejected that — in a totally unrealistic Cinderella fantasy — misery would bring redemption. He unconsciously hoped that the rejecting wife would turn into a compassionate and affectionate mother, who would shower him with love.

Mr. N.'s case was different. His inferiority feeling and depression were related to paternal and not maternal hostility. His father was in business on his own. He was an exceedingly selfish, exploitative, and dishonest individual, who had frequent extramarital sexual relations. He seduced his own daughter when she was 12 years old and kept having sex with her for years to come. Mr. N's father hated his son. As far back as Mr. N. could recall, his father ridiculed, blamed, and punished him for real or imaginary transgressions. The father never missed the opportunity to put his son down especially when N. reported any scholastic or other achievement. In short, successes invited more and more rejection.

The adolescent N. knew about his father's sexual adventures. His mother did not hide the resentment of her husband and shared it with N. who felt sorry for his mother. He could not understand her passive acceptance of her husband's escapades. N. shared his mother's resentment, and at the same time was envious of his father's conquests.

Mr. N. began to gain weight when he was 13 years old, about the time when his classmates began to date girls. Necking and petting was the main subject of conversation, and here and there a 14- or 15-year-old boy bragged about having sexual intercourse.

N. shied away from girls. "Girls would not go out with a fat pig," he rationalized. "My father was a tall, slim, good looking man, and that's why he had no difficulty with women."

Mr. N.'s obesity served a purpose. It was a sort of built-in alibi. His fear of sexual inadequacy was repressed and he had a plausible excuse for avoiding girls: they rejected him. What could he do? Once in a while he half-heartedly tried to diet, and every failure in dieting fed his depression and made him eat more and more. Being overweight was a bittersweet experience: he suffered ridicule and rejection by his peers, but he did not have to try to approach girls which would have led, so he believed, to defeat and humiliation.

The third case to be reported here is that of an attractive woman, Ms. C. Ms. C. knew she could never please her parents. They presented to her a false picture of themselves which she accepted and believed until she dared to discover the truth. This discovery came after a while, when she had made significant progress in psychotherapy. The story she told me about her parents at the first few sessions of psychotherapy could make one's heart bleed for her "poor parents." According to her initial version, her parents were saintly individuals who lived in abysmal poverty. These "poor" parents dearly loved their two daughters, but they could not help complaining about their poor health and sufferings. My patient was the older child and she took care of household chores "just to be of some help to my poor parents."

Her parents lived out of town. As Ms. C. progressed in therapy her story underwent substantial changes. Her parents owned a huge plot of land and a large house. The father had a business on his own; the parents owned two expensive cars; the mother was an active church-goer, and a frequent and generous contributor to charity. Despite their allegedly poor health, none of the parents was ever hospitalized and they rarely visited a doctor's office. On one of her visits to her parent's house my patient came across several savings books with hefty cash amounts which dispelled the myth of poverty.

My patient was badly overweight. She was a voracious eater. She was especially hungry late in the evening, three or four hours after dinner. That was the time when she was quite depressed, feeling guilty for whatever sins and errors she might or might not have committed.

As she gradually regained her childhood memory and her recollections became more vivid, her description of family meals offered some clues to her obesity. Breakfasts at home were meager; her mother was always on a diet, usually with an excuse that food is very expensive and "daddy works too hard to afford waste." Ms. C. bought lunch in school, but the parents never gave her enough money. At dinner she was criticized for eating too much.

Late in the evening, when she retired to her room hungry and depressed, she waited for her parents to retire. Then she sneaked to the refrigerator to "console" herself. At 18 years of age she left home, and the night-eating sprees became her main source of consolation for loneliness and parental rejection. She gained weight rapidly and felt guilty for being unable to diet. The more guilty and depressed she was, the more she ate, all the day, and especially at night. Overeating had become the substitute for love and companionship, and the never-failing source of more guilt, more depression — and more food.

PSYCHOTHERAPY OF OBESITY

My first task in psychotherapy with obese patients is to find out *what they are trying to attain* by being obese and unable to control their overeating. I am firmly convinced that whatever people do, they do it with a conscious or an unconscious purpose.

I rarely if ever attack directly the problem of overweight, for whatever I could say, their parents, friends, and enemies have told them many times. All obese individuals I worked with knew all the facts concerning fats, sugars, starches, and calories, and could intelligently discuss the dangers of high blood pressure and so on. They did not need to be lectured or sermonized.

My task was to find out the roots, that is, the innermost, unconscious motivation and reasons for their self-defeating behavior. This had to be done at the first phase of interactional therapy, the analytic phase.

In the above-mentioned three cases and — with appropriate modifications — in other cases, the first phase of psychotherapy was devoted not to obesity itself but to its *underlying causes*. Obesity was the symptom of deeper emotional problems, and it would have been a mistake to cut the branches, that is, attack the symptoms and leave the roots untouched. The failure of many treatment methods is related to dealing with symptoms instead of digging out their causes.

In the first, analytic phase, we dug out the underlying emotional issues in Mr. L.'s life. Mr. L. became aware of his unconscious hope to win love by making himself obese and miserable. He realized that one cannot go back to one's childhood, that his mother was dead, and that no one could love an adult man who acted like a crybaby and made himself look and behave in a most unpleasant way. It took Mr. L. a while to give up his choice defenses against being successful, and his intake of food was substantially reduced.

At the second phase Mr. L. embarked on a search for identity. Gradually he became aware of his appearance and his physical and mental potentialities. He joined a health club for swimming and exercise. He picked up jogging. He began to take pride in his appearance and physical health and then started dieting in a serious and consistent manner. His job performance also improved. He felt better about himself and displayed more assuredness and self-confidence. Soon he was promoted to a responsible executive position.

In the third phase his attitude to himself, his wife, and his daughter underwent dramatic changes. He no longer craved for a motherly love from both of them. Instead he assumed a leadership position at home and began to take care of them. He set for himself a rational rule of eating, and his persistent self-control brought adequate results.

Mr. N.'s success was less spectacular and he is still undergoing psychotherapy. His obesity was complicated by sexual anxieties and the process of therapy had, at least temporarily, circumvented obesity and concentrated on sexual issues. After all, sex represented the roots of his problems, and obesity served as a cover-up for his feeling of sexual inadequacy and his fear of failure, rejection, and humiliation.

It would be inappropriate to discuss interactional psychotherapy of sexual problems in the framework of the present volume. It will therefore suffice to say that in the first phase of psychotherapy the main emphasis was on Mr. N.'s childhood and adolescence, his relationship with the father, and his sexual fantasies and anxieties. It is worthwhile to stress that without ever discussing obesity in psychotherapeutic sessions, Mr. N. cut down his intake of food and began to lose weight.

At the second phase of psychotherapy when the patient engages in the search of his own identity, Mr. N.'s life underwent radical changes. His initial choice of occupation was influenced by his too close relationship with his mother. As soon as he began to assert himself as an individual, he decided to change his occupation. He chose a career of his own liking and much in agreement with his innate abilities. He began to pay attention to his physical appearance. He embarked on a serious and systematic diet which helped him to lose weight and enabled him to buy new and attractive suits. We are still in the middle of the second phase.

The treatment of Ms. C. went through long and complex stages. At the beginning of psychotherapy she offered gallant resistance. She simply adored her parents and felt guilty for not supporting them. Despite her rather limited income, she bought expensive gifts for Christmas, birthdays, and anniversaries. She kept on nibbling on food all day long and arranged a virtual feast for herself almost every night.

The root of her problem was overinvolvement with her parents. She carried the load of a never-ending feeling of guilt for not doing enough for her parents, and being a hypervectorial, borderline, latent schizophrenic (Wolman, 1973a), overinvolved with her parents, she became an overconscientious compulsive worker tormented by guilt feelings.

Obviously, the first task of interactional psychotherapy was not to deal with obesity but to alleviate the guilt feelings and reduce her wasteful emotional involvement with the parents. This was a long and gradual psychotherapeutic process that had to be conducted with utmost caution in order not to lay bare prematurely her defenses and provoke a nervous breakdown. Of course, this was no time to deal with her obesity!

The severing of the emotional umbilical cord took a while. As mentioned earlier, she herself began to recall instances of parental socioeconomic status, occasional extravagances, and charity to everyone except to their own children. She began to compare her own childhood experiences with those of her peers, and discovered instances of selfishness on the part of her parents. Her visits home gave additional evidence of parental financial situation and their unfair and exploitative attitude. The facts flew in face of mythology, and Ms. C. gradually developed an objective evaluation of what transpired in her childhood. The spells of excruciating guilt feelings became less frequent, of shorter duration, and gradually lost their grave impact. There was, however, little change in her night feasts; apparently, she had become conditioned to them in addition to their emotionally loaded origins.

A substantial change in her eating habits started in the second psychotherapeutic phase. Ms. C. started to look for goals and direction in her life. She refused to hold on to her job and lead the life of a robot. She found a more interesting job and developed new outlets for her energies outside working hours. She became more sociable and less afraid of entering close human relationship. She entered new situations, new avenues, and she began to cherish new ideas and outlooks on life. In her newly acquired self-assertion, her self-image changed and she started to wear attractive dresses. Needless to say, she took to serious and successful dieting.

At the third phase, she became socially conscious and active in public life, contributing her skills to a worthy cause. She married, had children, and was painfully aware of the need for fair and rational parental practices.

In some cases the psychotherapy of obesity must be postponed for a long time. The 25-year-old Ms. G. was badly overweight, but her obesity helped her to avoid social contacts she was afraid of and unable to cope with. She was schizophrenic or perhaps, as some authors call it, a borderline case. She developed paranoid ideas, blaming her relatives for hating her and thus protecting herself from having to engage in close social relationships. Like many latent schizophrenics, she was prematurely and costly hypervectorial and emotionally overinvolved with her parents (Wolman, 1970, 1973a).

After seing her a few times I arrived at the conclusion that in her case losing weight would imply laying bare her defenses. She still acted on a neurotic level, and removal of her defenses could have precipitated a nervous breakdown and overt psychosis. Thus is was necessary to postpone treatment of obesity to the time of a far-reaching strengthening of her total personality structure. In her case, obesity was a minor symptom which should wait until an overhaul of her personality would permit tackling this defense (Wolman, 1976).

REFERENCES

Alexander, F. and French, T. M. *Psychoanalytic Psychotherapy.* New York: Ronald, 1946.

Bruch, H. *Eating Disorders: Obesity, Anorexia Nervosa and the Person Within.* New York: Basic Books, 1973

Bruch, H. Obesity and its treatment. *International Encyclopedia of Psychiatry, Psychology, Psychoanalysis, and Neurology* (Wolman, B. B., Ed.), Vol. 8, pp. 95-100. New York: Aesculapius Publishers, 1977.

Feinstein, A. R. The treatment of obesity: An analysis of methods, results, and factors which influence success. *Journal of Chronic Disease,* 1970, *11,* 349-363.

Freud, A. *The Ego and the Mechanisms of Defense.* New York: International Universities Press, 1946.

Krauss, B. J. and Krauss, H. H. Sociopaths. *International Encyclopedia of Psychiatry, Psychology, Psychoanalysis, and Neurology* (Wolman, B. B., Ed), Vol. 10, pp. 362-366. New York: Aesculapius Publishers, 1977.

Leon, G. R. Current directions in the treatment of obesity. *Psychological Bulletin,* 1976, *83,* 557-578.

Mayer, J. *Overweight: Causes, Cost and Control.* Englewood Cliffs, N. J.: Prentice Hall, 1968.

Mayer, J. Some aspects of the problem of regulating food intake and obesity. *International Psychiatry Clinics,* 1970, *7,* 255-344.

Robinson, S. and Winnik, H. S. Severe psychotic disturbances following crash diet weight loss. *Archives of General Psychiatry,* 1973, *29,* 559-562.

Stunkard, A. J. The management of obesity. *New York State Journal of Medicine,* 1958, *58*, 79-87,

Stunkard, A. J. New therapies for the eating disorders. *Archives of General Psychiatry,* 1974, *26*, 391-398.

Wolman, B. B. *Vectoriasis Praecox or the Group of Schizophrenias.* Springfield, Ill.: Thomas, 1966.

Wolman, B. B. (Ed.) *Psychoanalytic Technique.* New York: Basic Books, 1967.

Wolman, B. B. *Children without Childhood: A Study of Childhood Schizophrenia.* New York: Grune and Stratton, 1970.

Wolman, B. B. *Call No Man Normal.* New York: International Universities Press, 1973. (a)

Wolman, B. B. *Victims of Success.* New York: Quadrangle-New York Times, 1973. (b)

Wolman, B. B. Principles of interactional psychotherapy. *Psychotherapy: Theory, Research and Practice.* 1975, *12*, 149-159.

Wolman, B. B. (Ed.) *The Therapist's Handbook.* New York: Van Nostrand Reinhold, 1976.

10

Behavioral Approaches to the Treatment of Obesity

Edward E. Abramson

The first application of behavioral techniques to the problem of weight reduction is generally credited to Ferster, Nurnberger, and Levitt (1962). The authors presented many of the self-control techniques that comprise current behavioral treatments. Although they mention that the program was implemented with several subjects, no outcome data were presented. Levitt (Note 1) indicated that the effects of treatment were minimal. In 1967, Richard Stuart reported the results of a similar program applied to eight overweight women. The one-year follow-up yielded weight losses ranging between 26 and 47 pounds. Although this was not a controlled experimental study, Stuart's results were a dramatic improvement over those reported in the earlier, nonbehavioral literature (Stunkard and McLaren-Hume, 1959). These results along with Stuart's clear description of treatment procedures started a massive flow of research. Despite increasing methodological sophistication, few of the researchers have been able to duplicate the clinically significant weight losses reported by Stuart.

There are now several hundred published studies of behavioral methods for weight loss. Since this literature has been extensively reviewed (Abramson, 1973, 1977a, 1977b; Bellack, 1975; Jordan and Levitz, 1975; Leon, 1976; Stuart, 1973; Stunkard, 1972, 1975; Stunkard and Mahoney, 1976), a comprehensive review of the literature will not be presented here. Instead, the behavioral techniques will be briefly described and some recent developments will be discussed.

Most treatment programs use a large number of specific techniques intended to teach the participant methods of controlling his or her pattern of eating and exercise. In addition to self-control, behavior therapists have occasionally used externally imposed reinforcement contingencies for either weight loss or behavior change and aversive methods intended to suppress some types of eating.

AVERSIVE METHODS

After some experimentation with disappointing results, aversive methods have been virtually abandoned (Abramson, 1977b). A recent study (Frohwirth and Foreyt, 1978) further substantiated the conclusion that aversive conditioning is not a viable treatment for obesity. Elsewhere (Abramson and Jones, in press) I have suggested that while aversive methods are ineffective treatments for obesity, they may be useful in modifying specific eating habits. In this study, a self-administered rubber-band snap following consumption of target food decreased the palatability and consumption of that food. If these results can be replicated and extended, aversive techniques may have a limited role as part of a comprehensive treatment.

REINFORCEMENT CONTINGENCIES

Externally imposed reinforcement contingencies (i.e., return of money for reaching weight goals) have produced significant weight losses (e.g., Mann, 1972). Nonetheless, this approach has not been widely used since most of the research has yielded unimpressive results (e.g., Abrahms and Allen, 1974) and there have been reports that participants may resort to hazardous methods of reducing (e.g., use of diuretics or laxatives). Jeffrey, Thompson, and Wing (1978) hypothesized that the monetary contingency in most of the studies was too small (typically $.50 to $3.00) to provide sufficient incentive to change long-standing habits. They required participants in three groups to deposit $200 prior to the start of treatment. All participants attended weekly self-control sessions. Participants who received $20 per week for meeting caloric intake goals or meeting weight reduction goals lost an average of 20 pounds. Participants who were reinforced for weekly attendance at the sessions were significantly less successful. Four-month follow-up data were also encouraging and there was no evidence of drastic methods of reducing. While these findings support the use of strong reinforcement contingencies, the authors note that only 15 percent of the people who originally responded to the advertisement actually agreed to participate. The $200 deposit may have served to screen out individuals who lacked the motivation or the money required for participation.

SELF-CONTROL

Self-control has emerged as the behavioral approach with the most empirical support. This type of program has been conducted in an individual consultation format (e.g., Stuart, 1967), in group counseling (e.g., Wollersheim, 1970), via written manuals (e.g., Hagen, 1974), in a university counseling center (e.g., Thorn and Boudewyns, 1976), in an inpatient clinic (e.g., Musante, 1976), in an outpatient clinic (e.g., Malcolm and Currey, 1977), and as a correspondence course (Marston, 1977). The diversity of treatment formats is matched by the variety of specific techniques that have been included in this type of treatment. The underlying theme that unites these disparate efforts is that participants are learning methods which will enable them to modify their eating and energy expenditure habits.

While most of the programs reported in the literature do not include all of these procedures, the following sections should provide a representative sample of self-control techniques.

Self-monitoring

Although they may be dedicated calorie counters, most overweight individuals are not aware of their patterns of food consumption. Self-monitoring requires that they record *all* eating and drinking along with the circumstances of consumption (e.g., location, simultaneous activities). Typically, this procedure has the effect of increasing awareness and providing the data that will be necessary to devise individual strategies for modifying specific patterns.

Stimulus Control

These procedures are based on the assumption that much of the eating of overweight people is determined by external cues such as the time of day and the sight of others eating (Schachter, 1971). The external cue hypothesis has been challenged as a cause of obesity (Leon and Roth, 1977). Although sensitivity to external cues as determinants of food intake may not differentiate obese from nonobese, there is little question that at least some of the eating of obese individuals is determined by external cues. In terms of treatment then, reduction of this type of eating would be a worthwhile goal.

Stimulus control techniques are intended to reduce the number of stimuli that can trigger eating. Typically, a review of self-monitoring forms will suggest specific stimuli to be controlled. There are, however, several suggestions that are probably useful for all participants.

1. All food must be consumed while sitting at one specified place.
2. Food must be removed from any other place in the house and kept only in the kitchen or dining room.
3. Participants must make eating a singular activity. Conversation is acceptable but reading, watching television, or engaging in other activities should not occur while eating.

Changing Eating Behaviors

These techniques are intended to interrupt the chain of eating behaviors. Two techniques used to slow the pace of eating and make it a deliberate rather than an automatic behavior are:

1. At least once during the meal, the participant should put down his or her utensils and pause for one minute.
2. After each bite, the utensils should be put down until the food has been swallowed.

These techniques are based on the assumption that there is an eating style characteristic of the obese. This assumption has been challenged (Mahoney, 1975), but research has yielded conflicting outcomes (see Stunkard and Kaplan, 1977, for a review). Since there are no risks associated with changing eating behaviors, their continued use is warranted.

Self-reinforcement

Unfortunately, the reinforcing consequences of eating (i.e., good taste and pleasant sensations of being full) are immediate, while the punishing consequence of weight gain is delayed to some ill-defined point in the future. As a result, most self-control programs attempt to include short-term reinforcers for adaptive eating. Typically, one or two specific behaviors (e.g., skipping the doughnuts at coffee break or limiting evening snacks to fewer than 100 calories) will be chosen for reinforcement instead of the larger-scale goal of weight loss. Common reinforcers include money set aside for a special purchase and enjoyable activities.

Cognitive Restructuring

Many overweight individuals begin treatment with unrealistic and self-defeating beliefs. Mahoney and Mahoney (1976) have identified three of these beliefs.

The first, inappropriate standard setting, refers to unrealistic goals which participants impose upon themselves. Many, for example, believe the numerous commercial claims for quick, effortless weight loss and are greatly disappointed when they have not lost 15 pounds at the end of the first week of treatment. The second common belief is called "cognitive claustrophobia" by the Mahoneys. This refers to the tendency to view behavior in absolute terms. Thus, the dieter will think in terms of total bans of foods (e.g., "I will never eat ice cream again"). Inevitably participants succumb to temptation, eat the forbidden food (usually to excess), and feel guilty and depressed. Finally, participants think of themselves in vague, global, negative terms. This is self-defeating since it prevents acknowledging and enjoying minor successes in treatment. Thus participants who adhere to the program still view themselves as "fat slobs" after a single incident of inappropriate eating. The task of the therapist throughout treatment is to recognize and challenge these beliefs.

In recent years the basic self-control package has been expanded to include the modification of exercise patterns and the participation of spouses in treatment. Self-control programs have also been developed for use with children. These developments will be reviewed below.

EXERCISE

While most behavioral researchers attribute obesity to a positive energy balance (i.e., calories consumed exceed calories expended), attention has been focused almost exclusively on the caloric consumption part of the equation. LeBow (1977) reviewed 103 studies appearing between 1962 and 1975, and found that less than 20 percent included an attempt to modify energy expenditure (exercise) habits. The neglect of exercise is unfortunate in light of the tendency of overweight individuals to be inactive (Bradfield and Jourdan, 1972) and the demonstrated effectiveness of exercise in reducing body fat (LeBow, 1977). Two recent studies support the inclusion of exercise in behavioral programs.

Stalonas, Johnson, and Christ (1978) found that a self-control program with either exercise or self-reinforcement produced greater weight losses at the one-year follow-up than the self-control program by itself. Dahlkoetter, Callahan, and Linton (1978) compared a control group with a behavioral group, an exercise group, and a combined treatment group. In addition to the usual measures of weight loss, the effects of treatment on physical fitness and self-concept were assessed. The three treatments resulted in more weight loss than did control procedures. The combined treatment group lost more weight than either of the single treatment groups, which did not differ from each other. On measures of physical fitness, the combination group and the exercise group showed the greatest improvement. One unusual finding of both studies: there were no dropouts. Since attrition has plagued many behavioral programs (Jeffrey, 1976), future research might be directed toward assessing the effects of exercise on participant attrition. In summary, the positive results (see also Harris and Hall-bauer, 1973) indicate that behavior therapists should devote more attention to techniques aimed at increasing energy expenditure.

SPOUSE PARTICIPATION

Another promising development is the inclusion of spouses in the treatment program. Stuart and Davis (1972) speculated that husbands have a significant role in their wives' attempts to lose weight. In 1975, McReynolds (Note 2) challenged what he termed the "one man, one fork doctrine." He reported preliminary data demonstrating the benefits of using behavioral treatments with two or more family members. Mahoney and Mahoney (1976) found a .63 correlation between therapists' ratings of social support and weight loss two years after treatment.

The first published reports of the effects of spouse participation in treatment appeared in 1978. Wilson and Brownell (1978) compared an eight-week behavioral treatment with a similar program that included a family member in the treatment process. Family members attended sessions in order to learn behaviors that would facilitate the participants' weight loss. Contrary to the authors' expectations, the inclusion of family members did not increase the effectiveness of treatment. In a more elaborate study, Brownell, Heckerman, Westlake, Hayes, and Monti (1978) compared a treatment group in which the spouse was an active participant with a group in which the spouse was willing to participate, but was not asked to, and with a group in which spouses had refused to participate. For all groups the ten weekly treatment sessions were followed by six monthly maintenance sessions. In the first group spouses were asked to model appropriate behaviors, reinforce habit change rather than weight loss, refrain from eating high-calorie foods in the presence of the overweight partner, and monitor their spouses' and their own eating. The two treatments which did not include spouses were otherwise identical to the first treatment. At the end of the ten-week period, all groups lost weight but were not significantly different from each other. At the three- and six-month follow-ups, however, participants in the group with spouse participation had lost significantly more weight than members of the other two groups. Furthermore, the magnitude of weight loss for this group was impressive. After six months, the average loss was 29.6 pounds, with two-thirds of the participants losing 20 pounds or more and 22 percent losing more than 40 pounds. These results are among the best reported in the behavioral literature.

Saccone and Israel (1978) found that participants in a self-control program in which significant others (typically spouses) reinforced desirable changes in eating behavior lost significantly more weight than participants undergoing a self-control without spouse reinforcement program. Weight loss at the end of the eight-week treatment averaged 13 pounds for participants in the significant-other reinforcement program. This reduction is not as impressive as the average loss reported by Brownell et al. (1978). There was, however considerably less spouse involvement in the Saccone and Israel study.

O'Neil, Currey, Hirsch, Riddle, Taylor, Malcolm, and Sexauer (1979) compared males and females undergoing a 12-week behavioral treatment individually or with their spouses. At the completion of treatment, both males and females showed significant weight reductions. Follow-up (9 to 14 months later) showed that females had regained almost all of their weight loss while males maintained their losses. There were no differences between participants treated individually and those treated with their spouses. The authors note, however, that spouse involvement in their study was similar to that of the Wilson and Brownell (1978) study. Although spouses attended all treatment sessions, their participation in implementing the various techniques in the home was not specifically required. In contrast, Brownell et al. (1978) and Saccone and Israel (1978) provided specific tasks to be accomplished by the spouse. It should be noted, however, that Brownell et al. found no relationship between measures of specific eating behaviors and weight loss for their spouse participation group. Thus it is possible that weight loss resulted from the continued attention of the spouse rather than from any of the techniques presented.

In a related study, Zitter and Fremouw (1978) compared an individual consequation treatment group (i.e., a portion of the monetary deposit was returned for weekly attendance and for weight loss of at least one pound) with a partner consequation group that earned additional money for the weight loss of a partner. Partners were not spouses but friends who joined the program together. The six-month follow-up showed that the individual consequation treatment was significantly more effective than the partner consequation treatment. The latter group did not differ significantly from minimal treatment controls. The authors suggest that the failure of partner consequation may be attributable to mutual reinforcement for inappropriate behaviors.

From the studies reviewed, it is clear that engineering social support for program adherence and weight loss is not straightforward. The nature of the participation as well as the relationship between the participant and his/her partner may partially determine treatment outcome. McReynolds (Note 2) reported anecdotal evidence that husband-wife pairs are beneficial but mother-daughter pairs are not. The findings of Zitter and Fremouw (1978) would suggest that treatment with a friend is also counterproductive. In view of the possible benefits of this type of treatment, further research directed toward specification of optimal treatment combinations is clearly justified.

CHILDHOOD OBESITY

Behavioral methods have previously been used with overweight children in controlled environments (Dinoff, Rickard, and Colwick, 1972; Foxx, 1972). Recently, behavioral treatments have been used with normal children in their natural environments. This type of effort appears to be especially valuable since there is some evidence that obesity can be prevented by early identification and treatment of the child at risk (Knittle and Ginsberg-Fellner, 1975). Successful treatment of childhood obesity should also prevent the poor self-concept (Sallade, 1973) and rejection (Canning and Mayer, 1966) associated with obesity.

The first study of behavioral treatment applied to normal overweight children was reported by Aragona, Cassady, and Drabman (1975). Fifteen girls between the ages of five and ten years old were assigned to either a response cost plus reinforcement, response cost only, or control groups. Parents participating in the two experimental groups deposited between $12 and $30 (depending upon family income) early in the program. For both experimental groups, treatment lasted 12 weeks. After the weekly weighing, the children were sent to a playroom while the experimenters discussed the program with the parents. Both groups received nutritional information, an exercise program consisting of daily calisthenics, and stimulus control information (e.g., eating slowly, eating in one area). The response cost component for both experimental groups entailed weekly financial penalties for missing the meeting, failure to complete charts, or failing to meet the child's weight loss goal. In addition to these procedures, the response cost plus reinforcement parents were taught to reinforce their child for daily caloric reduction, exercising, and using the stimulus control techniques. At the end of treatment the two experimental groups lost significantly more weight (response cost plus reinforcement, 11.3 pounds; response cost, 9.5 pounds) than controls who gained an average of 0.9 pound. At the 31-week follow-up the response cost plus reinforcement group's average weight loss had declined to 0.7 pound, while the response cost only group averaged a 7.3-pound gain. The failure to maintain weight losses should not be interpreted as indicating relapses after the completion of treatment. Since the children were not physically mature, it would be expected that they would increase in both height and weight during the seven-month follow-up period. Edwards (1978) has proposed an index that attempts to correct for normal increases in weight and height. Using this index, Edwards recomputed the results of the Aragona et al. study. As with the original analysis, both experimental groups were superior to the controls at the end of treatment. Unlike the original analysis, however, the use of the index yielded significant differences at the seven-month follow-up. The response cost plus reinforcement treatment was significantly more effective than no-treatment control.

The Aragona et al. (1975) study was atypical in that response cost was emphasized and there was virtually no contact between the therapists and the children. A more representative program was conducted by Rivinus, Drummond, and Combrinck-Graham (1976). In this study seven girls and three boys ranging in age from 8 to 13 were treated in a ten-week program. Children were responsible for recording food consumption, while mothers were taught modeling and reinforcement techniques. An unusual feature of this program was a weekly group supper in which low-calorie foods were presented and new eating behaviors (i.e., decreasing the rate of eating) were reinforced. The nine children completing the program averaged a 6.2-pound weight loss. The findings suggested that the children with normal weight mothers lost considerably more than children with overweight mothers. Although the study lacked a control group and two of the children had regained weight one month following treatment, the results are encouraging, especially since the children came from poor, relatively uneducated, single-parent homes.

Wheeler and Hess (1976) treated 26 children between the ages of 2 and 11 in an outpatient medical clinic. Treatment was conducted in half-hour sessions with the mother and child. The child or parent monitored eating during the two weeks prior to treatment. Treatment sessions focused on one or two problem behaviors and suggested alternative behaviors. Treatment effects were assessed in terms of changes in percentage overweight. A comparison of children treated (including those who dropped out of the program) with waiting-list controls showed significant differences. Although the findings are somewhat limited by the authors' failure to clearly specify duration of treatment and outcome in terms of weight lost, the list of common problem behaviors and suggested solutions makes this study especially valuable.

The role of parents in treatment was studied by Kingsley and Shapiro (1977). Forty 10- and 11-year-old children were assigned to either children alone, mothers alone, mother and children, or control groups. At the end of the eight-week treatment, the three experimental groups had lost significantly more than the control (an average loss of 3.5 pounds versus an average gain of 2.0 pounds) but did not differ from each other. At follow-ups six and twenty weeks after completion of treatment, the experimental groups did not differ. All evidenced weight gain appropriate for their age. Although the data did not show the superiority of any one of the experimental treatments, participants in the mother and child treatment expressed the most satisfaction with treatment.

Two studies report the results of behavioral treatments used with obese adolescents. Weiss (1977a) compared five groups: no-treatment control, conventional diet (the food exchange from Stuart and Davis, 1972), conventional diet plus self-administered reinforcers, stimulus control and stimulus control plus diet plus self-sdministered reinforcers. The 46 participants were seen individually for twelve brief (10 to 15 minute) sessions. The four treatments were superior to the no-treatment control. The stimulus control and the stimulus control plus diet plus reinforcer treatments were more effective than the other treatments at the one-year follow-up. Although the differences in weight were minimal, the one-year follow-up revealed 9.77 percent average reduction in percent overweight for the two self-control groups. Coates (cited in Brownell and Stunkard, 1978a), intensively studied two obese adolescent girls receiving behavioral treatment which included a cognitive restructuring component, and a third obese adolescent girl undergoing nonbehavioral treatment. Both treatments involved twice weekly sessions for ten weeks along with five family sessions in the home. A multiple baseline design was used to assess the effects of treatment. Unlike most behavioral studies which rely exclusively on weight change as the dependent variable, Coates had an observer monitor various eating behaviors in the participants' homes. The behavioral treatment participants lost 20.9 and 11.5 pounds, while the nonbehavioral participant gained almost 4 pounds. The observations supported the role of the behavioral techniques in promoting weight loss.

Several studies have focused on the effects of behavioral techniques on specific eating behaviors of children. Epstein, Parker, McCoy, and McGee (1976) studied three obese and three nonobese seven-year-old children. The children were observed twice a week during their school lunch period for six months. Bites, sips, concurrent activities, and putting eating utensils down were the behaviors observed. A multiple baseline design was used to demonstrate that instructions to put utensils down and praise (e.g., "You put your fork down more times than usual; that's good") had the desired effects. This manipulation resulted in decreases in bite rate and in food consumed, but because of the limited nature of the intervention it was not an effective weight reduction program. In a related study, Epstein, Masek, and Marshall (1978) manipulated prelunch activity level and nutritional training in a seven-month study of six obese black children attending a Head Start program. The children aged five and six ate both breakfast and lunch at the center. After four and one-half months of observation of eating and prelunch free play, a structured exercise program and nutrition instruction were introduced. Children were awarded stars that could be exchanged for toys for improving their food selections. Food portions were weighed to allow for calculation of total caloric intake per meal. Prelunch activity was assessed by 10-second time sampling observations. For breakfast, food choices improved with mean caloric intake per child, which decreased from 529 to 392 calories as a function of treatment. For lunch, both the exercise program and the nutritional instruction produced reductions in caloric intake. The two procedures did not differ significantly. Treatment also resulted in significant decreases in percentage overweight although the effects were not maintained at a ten-month follow-up.

The authors suggest that parental involvement may be necessary for more permanent change in behavior.

In a correlational study, Cohen, Gelfand, Dodd, Jensen, and Turner (1980) investigated some of the factors associated with long-term maintenance of weight loss. Twenty-five children who had attended a children's weight loss group one to three years earlier were classified as either regainers or maintainers. Seventeen normal weight children also participated in the study. All subjects recorded their eating and exercise behaviors for four days. Parents also monitored these behaviors for one day. The results showed that maintainers report more self-regulation of weight (e.g., "Do you compliment yourself for keeping your weight down?") and more physical exercise than either the regainers or the normal weight subjects. The regainers reported more parental control than normal weight subjects.

Although the longest follow-up reported in the literature is one year, the studies reviewed warrant cautious optimism about the behavioral treatment of childhood and adolescent obesity. While choice of dependent variable continues to be a problem for research with adults (Grimes and Franzini, 1977; Johnson and Stalonas, 1977), the evaluation of treatment of children presents additional problems. Edwards (1978) has proposed a method of taking normal growth into consideration, but there is no consensus on appropriate outcome measure. Follow-up data for children who have been treated will continue to be difficult to interpret until this problem is resolved.

The research with children has several advantages over the comparable adult literature. The samples studied were drawn from schools, clinics, or other agencies that should be representative of the population of obese children. This is in contrast to much of the adult research which has made use of a captive population of mildly overweight college students drawn from an undergraduate subject pool. Because of the relative ease of observing children in school and the availability of observers and contingency managers in the natural environment (i.e., parents), it has been possible to demonstrate that the changes in weight following treatment can be attributed to habit change as presented in the behavioral program. In this manner, the studies with children may have broader implications. Several of the studies provide some evidence that weight loss is correlated with program compliance.

CURRENT STATUS

Most of the reviews of the behavioral literature cited earlier were completed in the early or mid-1970s. At that time, the behavioral treatment of obesity was a relatively new venture and, as a result, long-term follow-up data were not available. This type of data has become more available in recent years, and unfortunately the results have tended to be disappointing. Brightwell and Sloan (1977, p. 903) reviewed more than 100 articles and found only 17 with follow-ups of 26 or more weeks. They concluded that these studies ". . . provide some evidence that a subgroup of patients so treated can maintain at least some weight loss." Several more recent studies have provided follow-up data on programs previously described in the literature. In addition, there have been several studies investigating various types of booster sessions intended to maintain losses after completion of treatment.

Jeffery, Vender, and Wing (1978) report follow-up data (12 to 18 months after completion of treatment) for the first 108 clients completing the program at the Eating Disorders Clinic of Stanford Univeristy. Weight loss at the end of treatment averaged 12.8 pounds which is consistent with the results of much of the behavioral research (Jeffery, Wing, and Stunkard, 1978). At follow-up, participants lost an additional fraction of a pound on the average. This negligible average change masked great individual variability ranging from an additional weight loss of 80 pounds to a 40-pound gain. Weight loss during treatment as well as several subject characteristics were unrelated to long-term weight loss. Self-reports indicated substantial changes in eating behaviors during treatment, but there was only a slight relationship between improved behaviors and weight loss.

Beneke, Paulsen, McReynolds, Lutz, and Kohrs (1978) report 18-month follow-up data for 33 participants who had received one of two behavioral treatments (McReynolds, Lutz, Paulsen, and Kohrs, 1976). Participants in both groups maintained about two-thirds of the 17.4-pound loss reported at the end of treatment. Consistent with the results reported in the earlier study, the group receiving a treatment based solely on stimulus control was more successful than a self-control package. No attempt was made to determine the degree to which weight loss was related to implementation of the various procedures.

What is probably the longest follow-up in the literature (three years) was reported by Gotestam (1979). Data from all eleven participants completing treatment are reported. Since participants were weighed with little prior notice they did not have an opportunity to make heroic last-minute efforts to reduce (Christensen, 1976). One participant had returned to pretreatment weight, three weighed more, and eight showed beneficial effects of treatment. As a group, however, follow-up weight was not significantly less than pretreatment weight. Self-reports indicated that only one participant continued to use the behavioral techniques regularly. A comparison between three participants who denied using the techniques and seven who used them to some extent showed significantly greater losses (18.1 pounds) for the latter group.

Several investigators have attempted to use booster sessions to promote maintenance of weight losses. Kingsley and Wilson (1978) compared a social pressure treatment with group and individually administered behavioral treatments. Half of each treatment group took part in four booster sessions after completing the eight-week treatment. All participants were weighed at three, six, nine, and twelve months following treatment. At the end of treatment, both behavioral treatments were superior to the social pressure treatment, but did not differ from each other. This relationship was not maintained throughout the follow-up. The combined behavioral treatments were no more effective than the social pressure treatment. The group behavioral treatment, however, was significantly more effective than the individual behavioral treatment. Booster sessions resulted in significantly greater weight losses at the three-month follow-up regardless of the type of treatment. This difference decreased at six months and disappeared at the nine- and twelve-month follow-ups. The findings indicate that the initial superiority of behavioral treatment was not maintained over the duration of the follow-up.

In a similar study, Hall, Bass, and Monroe (1978) compared two booster strategies with no posttreatment contact. After ten weeks of treatment (average weight loss was almost 8 pounds), participants in the minimal contact group were weighed four times. In the monitoring group, participants were instructed to continue self-monitoring and mail the monitoring forms to the therapist. Participants in the continued contact group met every two weeks to provide group support and discuss implementation of techniques learned during the original treatment. No new procedures were introduced. These sessions continued for 24 weeks beyond the completion of the formal treatment. All participants were weighed 8, 16, 24, and 42 weeks after the completion of treatment. At the first follow-up, continued contact participants lost significantly more weight than members of the minimal contact group. Similar, but less strong, relationships were found for the second and third follow-ups. Forty-two weeks after the completion of treatment there were no significant differences between groups. Although these findings contradict those of an earlier study (Hall, Hall, Borden, and Hanson, 1975), the methodological difficulties present in the earlier study cause the authors to have more confidence in the more recent study. The failure to find more enduring weight loss as a result of various types of booster sessions or continued contact has also been reported by Ashby and Wilson (1977) and by Beneke and Paulsen (1979).

In summary, the long-term effectiveness of behavioral treatments has not been demonstrated. Attempts to prolong the duration of weight loss by adding booster sessions have been successful only while the booster sessions continued. Although there is some self-report data suggesting that abandonment of techniques learned during treatment may contribute to relapse, the precise nature of the relationship between program adherence and weight loss remains unclear. While these conclusions are discouraging, it is not possible to determine whether experimental methodology or the effects of treatment are responsible for the reported outcomes. For example, treatment for all participants is concluded at the end of the predetermined program (typically 8 to 12 weeks). Most of the participants will not have met their weight reduction goals at this point. If overweight individuals set unrealistic goals for weight reduction (Mahoney and Mahoney, 1976), it is possible that the behavioral program is viewed as ineffective and not much different from the numerous partially successful diets tried previously. Under these circumstances, there would be little motivation to continue using the effortful techniques learned in treatment. While this line of reasoning is clearly speculative, it is apparent that most of the experimental literature does not assess the effects of an optimal behavioral treatment. Single subject designs focusing on specific behaviors (rather than exclusive reliance on weight change as the dependent variable) over protracted periods of time may clarify the relationships between specific behavioral interventions, consequent changes in eating and exercise behaviors and, ultimately, weight loss.

The typical study involves the comparison of two or more groups, at least one of which has received behavioral treatment. Whatever the outcome of this comparison, inevitably there is wide variability within the treatment groups. In virtually all studies, some of the participants lose meaningful amounts of weight while others do not lose or gain weight. There has been considerable research directed toward identifying variables which would predict the likelihood of successful treatment (see Weiss, 1977b, and Cooke and Meyers, 1980, for reviews). Although several variables appear to be related to treatment success, at present there have been no comprehensive attempts to individualize treatment on the basis of these variables. A second direction for future research would be the development of pretreatment screening instruments which would allow programs to be matched to the specific needs of individual participants. Thus the control of eating behaviors might be the focus of one group while increasing exercise could be the major component of another.

Behavioral treatments have yet to fulfill their earlier promise. Innovations such as emphasis on exercise and spouse participation may enhance treatment effectiveness. Truly effective treatment, however, will probably require a greater understanding of the behavioral, cognitive, and physiological factors contributing to obesity. It will then be possible to develop techniques tailored to the individual needs of participants.

REFERENCE NOTES

1. Levitt, E. B. Personal communication, September 1977.
2. McReynolds, W. T. Family behavior therapy treatment for obesity. Paper presented at the annual meeting of the Association for Advancement of Behavior Therapy, San Francisco, 1975.

REFERENCES

Abrahms, J. L. and Allen, G. J. Comparative effectiveness of situational programming, financial pay-offs and group pressure in weight reduction. *Behavior Therapy*, 1974, *5*, 391-400.

Abramson, E. E. Behavioral Approaches to Weight Control. New York: Springer, 1977. (a)

Abramson, E. E. Behavioral approaches to weight control: An updated review. *Behavior Research and Therapy*, 1977, *15*, 355-363. (b)

Abramson, E. E. and Jones, D. Reducing junk food palatability and consumption by aversive conditioning. *Addictive Behaviors*, in press.

Aragona, J., Cassady, J., and Drabman, R. S. Treating overweight children through parental training and contingency contracting. *Journal of Applied Behavior Analysis*, 1975, *8*, 269-278.

Ashby, W. A. and Wilson, G. T. Behavior therapy for obesity: Booster sessions and long-term maintenance of weight loss. *Behavior Research and Therapy*, 1975, *15*, 451-463.

Bellack, A. S. Behavior therapy for weight reduction. *Addictive Behaviors*, 1975, *1*, 73-82.

Beneke, W. N. and Paulsen, B. K. Long-term efficacy of a behavior modification weight loss program: A comparison of two follow-up maintenance weight loss strategies. *Behavior Therapy*, 1979, *10*, 8-13.

Beneke, W. M., Paulsen, B., McReynolds, W. G., and Lutz, R. N. Long-term results of two behavior modification weight loss programs using nutritionists as therapists. *Behavior Therapy*, 1978, *9*, 501-507.

Bradfield, R. B. and Jordan, M. Energy expenditure of women during weight loss. *American Journal of Clinical Nutrition*, 1972, *25*, 971-975.

Brightwell, D. R. and Sloan, C. L. Long-term results of behavior therapy for obesity. *Behavior Therapy*, 1972, *8*, 898-905.

Borwnell, K. D., Heckerman, C. L., Westlake, R. J., Hayes, S. C., and Monti, P. N. The effect of couples training and partner cooperativeness in the behavioral treatment of obesity. *Behavior Research and Therapy*, 1978, *16*, 323-333.

Brownell, K. D. and Stunkard, A. J. Behavioral treatment of obesity in children. *American Journal of Diseases of Children*, 1978, *132*, 403-412. (a)

Brownell, K. B. and Stunkard, A. J. Behavior therapy change: Uncertainties in programs for weight control. *Behavior Research and Therapy*, 1978, *16*, 301. (b)

Canning, H. and Mayer, J. Obesity — Its possible effect on college acceptance. *New England Journal of Medicine*, 1966, *275*, 1172-1174.

Christensen, A. Measuring and maintaining weight losses. *Behavior Therapy*, 1976, *7*, 709-711.

Cohen, E. A., Gelfand, D. M., Dodd, D. K., Jensen, J., and Turner, C. Self-control practices associated with weight loss maintenance in children and adolescents. *Behavior Therapy*, 1980, *11*, 26-37.

Cooke, C. J. and Meyers, A. The role of predictive variables in the behavioral treatment of obesity. *Behavioral Assessment*, 1980, *2*, 59-69.

Dahlkoetter, J., Callahan, D. J., and Linton, J. Obesity and the unbalanced energy equation: Exercise vs. eating habit change. *Journal of Consulting and Clinical Psychology*, 1979, *47*, 898-905.

Dinoff, M., Rickard, H. C., and Colwick, J. Weight reduction through successive contracts. *American Journal of Orthopsychiatry*, 1972, *42*, 110-113.

Edwards, K. A. An index for assessing weight change in children: Weight/height ratios. *Journal of Applied Behavior Analysis*, 1978, *11*, 421-429.

Epstein, L. H., Masseck, B. J., and Marshall, W. R. A nutritionally-based school program for control of eating in obese children. *Behavior Therapy*, 1978, *9*, 766-778.

Epstein, L. H., Parker, L., McCoy, J. F., and McGee, G. Descriptive analysis of eating regulation in obese and non-obese children. *Journal of Applied Behavior Analysis*, 1976, *9*, 407-415.

Ferster, C. B., Nurnberger, J. I., and Levitt, E. G. The control of eating. *Journal of Mathetics*, 1962, *1*, 87-109.

Foxx, R. Social reinforcement of weight reduction: A case report of an obese retarded adolescent. *Mental Retardation*, 1972, *10*, 21-23.

Frohwirth, R. A. and Foreyt, J. P. Aversive conditioning treatment of overweight. *Behavior Therapy*, 1978, *9*, 861-872.

Gotestam, K. G. A three year follow-up of a behavioral treatment for obesity. *Addictive Behaviors*, 1979, *4*, 179-183.

Grimes, W. B. and Franzini, L. R. Skin fold measurement techniques for estimating percentage body fat. *Journal of Behavior Therapy and Experimental Psychiatry*, 1977, *8*, 65-69.

Hall, S. M., Bass, A., and Monroe, J. Continued contact and monitoring as follow-up strategies: A long-term study of obesity. *Addictive Behaviors*, 1978, *3*, 139-147.

Hall, S. M., Hall, R. G., Borden, D. L., and Hanson, R. W. Follow-up strategies in the behavioral treatment of overweight. *Behavior Research and Therapy*, 1975, *13*, 167-172.

Jeffrey, D. E. Treatment outcome issues in obesity research. *Obesity: Behavioral Approaches To Dietary Management* (William, B. J., Martin, S., and Foreyt, J. P., Eds.). New York: Brunner/Mazel, 1976.

Jeffery, R. W., Thompson, P. D., and Wing, R. R. Effects on weight reduction of strong monetary contracts for calorie restriction for weight loss. *Behavior Research and Therapy*, 1978, *16*, 363-369.

Jeffery, R. W., Vender, M., and Wing, R. R. Weight loss and behavior change one year after behavioral treatment for obesity. *Journal of Consulting and Clinical Psychology*, 1978, *46*, 368-369.

Jeffery, R. W., Wing, R. R., and Stunkard, A. J. Behavioral treatment of obesity: The state of the art 1976. *Behavior Therapy*, 1978, *9*, 189-199.

Johnson, W. G. and Stalonas, P. Measuring skin fold thickness – A cautionary note. *Addictive Behaviors*, 1977, *2*, 105-107.

Jordan, H. A. and Levitz, L. S. A behavioral approach to the problem of obesity. *Obesity and Bariatric Medicine*, 1975, *4*, 58-69.

Kingsley, R. G. and Wilson, G. T. Behavior therapy for obesity: A comparative investigation of long-term efficacy. *Journal of Consulting and Clinical Psychology*, 1977, *45*, 288-298.

Knittle, J. L. and Ginsberg-Fellner, F. Can obesity be prevented? *Childhood Obesity* (Collipp, P. J., Ed.). Acton, Mass.: Publishing Sciences Group, 1975.

LeBow, M. D. Can lighter become thinner. *Addictive Behavior*, 1977, *2*, 87-93.

Leon, G. R. Current directions in the treatment of obesity. *Psychological Bulletin*, 1976, *83*, 557-578.

Leon, G. R. and Roth, L. Obesity: Psychological causes, correlations, and speculations. *Psychological Bulletin*, 1977, *84*, 117-139.

Mahoney, K. and Mahoney, M. J. Cognitive factors in weight reduction. *Counseling Methods* (Krumboltz, J. D. and Thorsen, C. E., Eds.). New York: Holt, Rhinehart, and Winston, 1976.

Mahoney, M. J. The obese eating style: Bites, beliefs, and behavior modification. *Addictive Behavior*, 1975, *1*, 47-53.

Mahoney, M. J. The behavioral treatment of obesity: A recognaissance. *Biofeedback and Self-regulation*, 1976, *1*, 127–133.

Mahoney, M. J. and Mahoney, K. Treatment of obesity: A clinical exploration. *Obesity: Behavior Approaches to Dietary Management* (Williams, B. J., Martin, S., and Foreyt, J. P., Eds.). New York: Brunner/Mazel, 1976.

Malcolm, R. and Currey, H. S. The dietary rehabilitation clinic for the treatment of obesity. *Behavior Therapy*, 1977, *8*, 513–514.

Marston, A. R., Marston, M. R., and Ross, J. A correspondence course behavioral program for weight reduction. *Obesity and Bariatric Medicine*, 1977, *6*, 140–147.

McReynolds, W. T., Lutz, R. N., Paulsen, B. K., and Cohrs, M. B. Weight loss resulting from two behavior modification procedures with nutritionists as therapists. *Behavior Therapy*, 1976, *7*, 283–291.

Musante, G. J. The dietary rehabilitation clinic: Evaluative report of a behavioral and dietary treatment of obesity. *Behavior Therapy*, 1976, *7*, 198–204.

O'Neil, P. M., Currey, H. S., Hirsch, A. A., Riddle, F. E., Taylor, C. I., Malcolm, R. J., and Sexauer, J. B. Effects of sex of subject and spouse involvement on weight loss in a behavioral treatment program: A retrospective investigation. *Addictive Behavior*, 1979, *4*, 167–177.

Rivinus, T. M., Drummond, T., and Combrinck-Graham, L. A group behavior treatment program for overweight children: Results of a pilot study. *Pediatric and Adolescent Endocrinology*, 1976, *1*, 55–61.

Saccone, A. J. and Israel, A. C. Effects of experimenter vs. significant other-controlled reinforcement and choice of target behavior on weight loss. *Behavior Therapy*, 1978, *9*, 271–278.

Sallade, J. A comparison of the psychological adjustment of obese and non-obese children. *Journal of Psychosomatic Research*, 1973, *17*, 89–96.

Schachter, S. Some extraordinary facts about obese humans and rats. *American Psychologist*, 1971, *26*, 129–144.

Stalonas, P. M., Johnson, W. G., and Christ, M. Behavior modification for obesity: The evaluation of exercise, contingency management, and program adherance. *Journal of Consulting and Clinical Psychology*, 1978, *46*, 463–469.

Stuart, R. B. Behavioral control of overeating. *Behavior Research and Therapy*, 1967, *5*, 357–365.

Stuart, R. B. Behavioral control of overeating: A status report. *Obesity in Perspective* (Bray, G., Ed.). Fogarty International Center Series on Preventive Medicine, Vol. 2, part 2. Bethesda, Md: DHEW Publication No. (NIH) 75:708, 1976.

Stuart, R. B. and Davis, B. *Slim Chance in A Fat World: Behavioral Control of Obesity.* Champaign, Ill: Research Press, 1972.

Stunkard, A. J. New therapy for the eating disorders: Behavior modification of obesity and anorexia nervosa. *Archives of General Psychiatry*, 1972, *26*, 391–398.

Stunkard, A. J. From explanation to action in psychosomatic medicine: The case of obesity. *Psychosomatic Medicine*, 1975, *37*, 195–236.

Stunkard, A. and Kaplan, D. Eating in public places: A review of reports of the direct observation of eating behavior. *International Journal of Obesity*, 1977, *1*, 89–101.

Stunkard, A. J. and Mahoney, M. J. Behavioral treatment of the eating disorders. *Handbook of Behavior Modification* (Litenberg, H., Ed.). Englewood Cliffs, N.J.: Prentice-Hall, 1976.

Stunkard, A. and McLaren, Hume, M. The results of treatment for obesity. *Archives of Internal Medicine*, 1959, *103*, 79–85.

Thorn, M. E. and Boudewins, P. A. A behaviorally oriented weight loss program for counseling centers. *Journal of Counseling Psychology*, 1976, *23*, 81–82.

Weiss, A. R. A behavioral approach to the treatment of adolescent obesity. *Behavior Therapy*, 1977, *8*, 720–726. (a)

Weiss, A. R. Characteristics of successful weight reducers: A brief review of predicter variables. *Addictive Behaviors*, 1977, *2*, 193–201. (b)

Wilson, G. T. Methodological considerations in treatment outcome research. *Journal of Consulting and Clinical Psychology*, 1978, *46*, 687–702.

Wilson, G. T. and Brownell, K. Behavior therapy for obesity: Including family members in the treatment process. *Behavior Therapy*, 1978, *9*, 943–945.

Zitter, R. E. and Fremouw, W. J. Individual vs. partner consequation for weight loss. *Behavior Therapy*, 1978, *9*, 808–813.

11

Multimodal Behavioral Treatment of Obesity

Stephen DeBerry

Obesity has been long recognized as a pervasive hazard of dangerous proportions, and particularly problematic is the resistance of obesity to effective and long-lasting treatment. Individuals who enter therapy probably do not remain, and for those who do weight loss is minimal and temporary. The lack of long-term effectiveness in traditional weight control therapies such as hypnosis, psycho-analysis, fad dieting or group therapy has been well noted (Jeffery, Wing, and Stunkard, 1978; Leon, 1976; Penick, Filion, Fox, and Stunkard, 1971; Stollak, 1967; Stuart, 1971). The most effective strategy to date seems to be a program of behavior modification based upon a functional analysis of behavior (Ferster, Nurnberger, and Levitt, 1962; Horan and Johnson, 1971; Jeffery et al., 1978; Mahoney, 1973, 1974; Penick et al., 1971; Stollack, 1967; Stuart, 1967, 1971, 1972; Wilson, 1978). The rationale behind such an approach is that overeating consists of learned maladaptive responses that can be modified by using classi-cal and operant methods. The goal of a behavior oriented weight control program is not so much the quantitative alteration of food intake (although this is a highly desirable by-product) but rather, the modification of eating habits in order to produce lasting change. By becoming aware of the personal contin-gencies and environmental cues under which overeating occurs, the obese person can act to change them.

Self-monitoring and self-control of eating responses have been the main focus of behavioral weight control programs (Hall, Hall, Hanson, and Borden, 1974; Romanczyk, Tracy, Wilson, and Thorpe, 1973; Stuart, 1967, 1971, 1972). These operations are often combined with an assortment of therapeutic strategies such as covert sensitization (Cautela, 1967, 1970; Diament and Wilson, 1975; Foreyt and Hagen, 1973; Janda and Rimm, 1972), self-reward (Hall et al., 1974; Horan and Johnson, 1971; Mahoney, 1974; Romanczyk et al., 1973; Stuart, 1967, 1971, 1972), therapist support and approval (Leon, 1976; Mahoney, Moura and Wade, 1973; Stuart, 1967), realistic goal setting (Mahoney, 1973, 1974; Stuart, 1967, 1971, 1972), and reeducation and bibliotherapy (Mahoney, 1974; Stuart, 1971, 1972; Stunkard and Mahoney, 1976). For a more current review of methodology, the reader is referred to the chapter on behavioral treatments (see Chapter 10).

An effective behavioral program should be empirically based and individually tailored to suit the idiosyncrasies of the patient (Jeffery et al., 1978; Kroeger, 1970; Mulligan, 1976; Stuart, 1972; Wilson, 1978). The present program utilizes the multimodal treatment approach first described by Lazarus (1973, 1976). According to Lazarus, the more areas of one's personality that are directly dealt with, the more effective therapy will be. The acronym BASIC ID (behavior, affect, sensation, imagery, cognition, interpersonal relations, drugs) was conceived in order that the therapist might have a systematic framework in which to map the most effective intervention. The ideal program would employ empirically tested techniques in each of the above areas. Lazarus (1973, p. 407) states that "durable clinical results are in direct proportion to the number of specific modalities deliberately invoked by any therapeutic system." If one considers the recalcitrant nature of obesity, it seems that a multimodal approach might represent a significant improvement in treatment strategy.

The BASIC ID is subsumed under the more general concept of multimodal behavior therapy. The multimodal approach encompasses the systematic outline of seven parameters most relevant to pathology and treatment outcome. Every therapist-patient encounter involves behaviors, affects, sensations, images, and cognitions — occurring within interpersonal relationships — and, if indicated, employing drugs. Understandably, the seven modalities are interactive and interrelated. Because obesity is so clearly a multifactorial problem involving interaction between the organism and his environment, a multimodal assessment becomes clearly indicated. The clinician, using the BASIC ID as a schematic guideline, is insured of designing an effective treatment package that focuses on all problematic areas.

Faulty assessment and inadequate problem identification constitute the major flaws in traditional obesity treatment programs. People are overweight for different reasons and from different causes. Although in the overwhelming majority of cases excessive caloric intake is the primary cause of obesity, its manifestations encompass a wide range of antecedent, behavioral, and consequent phenomena. Clearly, a sociopsychosomatic (Wolman, 1965) or systems theory approach (Kroeger, 1970) that attempts to holistically identify and treat the multiplicity of idiographic factors would be most helpful. Although ideally relevant to any diagnostic category, the holistic approach stressed in the multimodal assessment is especially suited to the treatment of obesity.

Each obese person is the unique product of a history of maladaptive learning, current deficient response repertoires, and insufficient expectations. Thus, the clinician must deal not only with present behavior but with past and future behavior as well for each person. Eating serves different functions, symbolically and physiologically. Attempts have been made to categorize the obese into homogeneous groups (Wick, 1976; Wooley, 1979). Although such efforts can be helpful they have unfortunately, in many cases, fostered general treatment strategies which are most definitely not helpful. The multimodal approach emphasizes a problem-oriented record approach, idiographic in orientation and based on individual pretreatment assessment and baseline data. Lazarus (1973, 1976) advocates the development of a multimodal profile for each patient which describes the problem and proposed treatment for each area of the BASIC ID. The remainder of this chapter will be devoted to the presentation of a case within the multimodal model.

CASE HISTORY

The patient is a 5'5½" tall, 35-year-old, single woman who at the start of the program weighed 298 pounds. Mrs. S., as I will call her, lives alone and is currently employed in a responsible high-level administrative position. As a child she was not overweight and until the age of 21 her weight fluctuated beween 120 and 140 pounds. After 21, her weight steadily increased reaching its present peak of nearly 300 pounds. The patient reported unsuccessful attempts with amphetamine therapy, psychoanalysis, dieting, and weight watchers programs. She is an active and energetic woman who does not appear to be at all handicapped by her obesity. If it were not for her weight problem, she would be an attractive woman. A recent medical examination failed to uncover any organic basis to her difficulty. Mrs. S. heard about behavior modification and decided to try it because she was tired of being fat and was afraid that she would eventually be too old to lose weight.

BASELINE ASSESSMENT

First Session

The initial interview with the patient consisted of gathering background information related to the target behavior. The procedures and orientation of behavior modification were explained and discussed with Mrs. S, and it was decided that she would be seen twice a week for a period of ten weeks. During the treatment phase a goal of losing 1–2 pounds per week was mutually agreed upon. An ultimate treatment goal would be for the patient to reach her ideal weight of 140 pounds.

Second to Fifth — Two-week Baseline

Mrs. S. was instructed in the use and rationale of the food logs (see Table 11-1). The logs recorded the time, nature, quantity, and antecedent and consequent aspects of each meal. In addition, during the baseline the patient was asked to keep a daily record of weight fluctuation. In order to decide which stimuli or behaviors could be used as reinforcers, she was asked to complete the Reinforcement Survey Schedule (Cautela and Kastenbaum, 1972). By use of the food logs, baseline data were gathered for fourteen consecutive days. During the fifth session Mrs. S. was given several articles relating to diet, obesity, and behavioral weight control programs.

After evaluating and discussing the patient's logs, it was decided that this particular weight problem was related to the following factors.

Behavior

(1) High daily caloric intake — between 2600 and 3600 calories per day; (2) excessive beer drinking — three to six 12-ounce cans daily; (3) frequent alcoholic intake — one or two mixed drinks daily; (4) continuous eating throughout the day of "junk" and high-calorie foods (this finding corresponds with Ferster's,

Table 11-1. Antecedent-Behavior-Consequence (ABC) Food Intake Analysis.

Time	Food Consumed	Calories	Length of Meal	Location and Position during Meal	Degree of Hunger (1 to 5)	Mood Prior to Meal	Activity Prior to Meal	Persons Present

1962, observation that obese women tend to eat light meals but snack frequently throughout the day); (5) lack of social reinforcers and competing alternative behaviors; (6) high percentage of fried ribs, chicken, pork, beans, sausage, bacon.

Affect

Mrs. S. maintained a relatively indifferent emotional sense concerning her obesity. That is, at the start of treatment she manifest denial in regard to her appearance. Her motivation for losing weight was, according to her, totally related to reasons of physical health. It seemed therefore that part of the problem could have been a general denial of painful affect regarding her appearance. The denial was further evident in that Mrs. S. appeared quite unaware of her level of tension and anxiety. There was, likewise, an underlying hostility which came across as an aggressive need to control the situation, i.e., the initial interview.

Sensation

As noted above, the patient was relatively tense and anxious, yet unaware of her discomfort. There seemed to be a lack of bodily awareness and a paucity of positive somatic sensations. For example, she reported little interest in pleasurable sexual feeling.

Imagery

There was a marked absence of images either in relation to what she presently looked like or how she would like to appear. When requested to imagine herself as being lighter she was unable to do so. There was likewise an inability to fantasize or evoke images of herself in various situations.

Cognitive Factors

Despite her excessive weight, Mrs. S. reported few verbal statements reflecting negative thoughts. Furthermore, she did not think about losing weight or about the consequences of overeating. Her thoughts concerning other people were indicative of repressed anger and denial, e.g., "I don't care what people think; if they don't like the way I look that's too bad."

Interpersonal Relations

Mrs. S. seemed to have no difficulty in developing relationships with men who were attracted to her despite her obesity. However, she did seem to experience difficulty in maintaining these relationships. In this area she exhibited some insight, stating that her disposition might have something to do with her inability to maintain a relationship. She reported that at times she felt lonely and alienated.

Drugs

Medication had once been tried and did not seem indicated at present.

Summary

The multimodal assessment revealed a very obese, covertly hostile 35-year-old woman with excessive anxiety and tension. Her behavior in relationship to both eating and interpersonal relations seemed deficient. Mrs. S.'s main defense mechanisms appeared to be denial and reaction formation. There was definite lack of positive images, thought, sensations, and feelings. Mrs. S. seemed to be as out of touch with her body as she was with the people she related to.

Based on information obtained from baseline assessment the multimodal profile given in Table 11-2 was developed.

TREATMENT

Self-monitoring and Self-control of Eating Behavior

Self-monitoring, self-control, and self-reward form the substantive basis of the present program. However, in keeping with the multimodal approach, particular strategies especially indicated for this patient were employed.

The basis of self-monitoring and self-control is the completion of daily food logs. The logs serve not only to increase one's awareness of eating but also as a means of identifying specific problem areas and developing appropriate control and change strategies (Stuart, 1971, 1972).

Self Reward

The self-reward aspect is designed to develop effective reinforcers that can eventually be used independent of the therapist, especially during the critical period following termination (Stuart, 1972).

Covert Sensitization

Covert sensitization (Cautela, 1970) has been proved successful in dealing with problems of obesity (Lazarus, 1971; Stuart, 1967, 1971). The technique seems

Table 11-2. Multimodal Profile.

Modality	Problem	Treatment
Behavior	High caloric intake, high percentage of alcohol and fatty foods, frequent snacking, lack of social reinforcers	Self-monitoring, self-control, self-reward, competing responses, covert sensitization, exercise, reduced caloric intake, role playing for improved social contacts
Affect	Anxiousness, muscle tension, covert hostility, denial of feelings	Deep muscle relaxation, exercise, positive imagery, discussion of feelings
Sensation	Lack of somatic awareness, anxiousness, tension	Sensate focus, deep muscle relaxation, exercise
Imagery	Lack of positive images, lack of ability to fantasize	Hypnotic, imagery, time projections
Cognition	Denial of negative thoughts, lack of awareness of dangers of obesity	Increased awareness of self and others, bibliotherapy, realistic goal setting, therapist approval and support, behavioral contracting, coverant control, time projection, positive thoughts
Interpersonal relations	Covert hostility, denial of need of others, lack of effective social behaviors	Asking a friend to cooperate in program, development and use of new social reinforcers, role playing, therapist support and approval
Drugs	Medication not indicated	

especially indicated with eating disorders related to specific food substances (e.g., ice cream, pastry) or particular situations (parties, restaurants, eating in bed, or while watching television). Stuart (1967) included covert sensitization as an adjunctive therapy in his highly successful twelve-week weight control program, claiming it to be highly specific and powerful in effect. Foreyt and Hagen (1973), report that covert sensitization can cause significant decreases in liking for certain foods.

Therapist Reassurance, Support, and Approval

Reassurance by the therapist, i.e., the therapist as a positive reinforcer, is a seldom mentioned but potent variable in therapy.

Training in Deep Muscle Relaxation

Because eating is often associated with the relief from tension (Cautela, 1966), the patient was trained in deep muscle relaxation according to the method of Lazarus (1971). Relaxation training seemed especially indicated in that the patient consumed an inordinate amount of beer which she attributed to "being wound up." (Relaxation was also an integral part of the covert sensitization procedure.)

Realistic Goal Setting

Research indicates that a weight loss goal of 1-2 pounds per week is ideal. Persons who lose weight slowly and steadily are more likely to maintain the loss than those who lose weight rapidly (Stuart, 1972).

Reeducation and Bibliotherapy

During the course of therapy, the rationale behind each technique should be explained to the patient. When the food logs are discussed, new types of foods, alternate methods of preparation, nutritional aspects, and other weight related topics should be discussed. Attempts should be made to correct or modify any of the patient's misconceptions about diet and weight (Stuart, 1972). It is sometimes helpful to give the patient relevant articles concerning the dangers of obesity and the problems of weight control. These may act as nonverbal cues when the patient is alone.

Time Projection and Positive Imagery

Time projection techniques may be used with deep muscle relaxation or mild hypnosis. Under these conditions the patient can be asked to imagine himself a month in the future being 10 pounds lighter or one clothes size smaller. It is important that statements about adhering to the program be paired with positive images. Images of being thinner, handsomer, stronger, more attractive, etc., and thoughts of the positive medical and social value of losing weight (e.g., you will live longer, have less chance of a heart attack) can be used as positive reinforcers or as part of the verbal reward system.

Cooperation of Friends and Family

This is a critical, but often overlooked, factor in any therapeutic program. Family or friends can sabotage the efforts of the best therapeutic strategy.

Competing Responses and Coverant Control

Whenever the patient feels inappropriately hungry, he should engage in a prearranged competing behavior. That is, an alternative reinforcing response should occur, so that the chain of responses leading to eating can be interrupted. Ideally, the response should be initiated as early as possible in the chain. For instance, the patient could be instructed to talk on the telephone or take a walk whenever an inappropriate eating urge occurs. When the patient mentally utilizes competing responses, the process is called coverant control (Homme, 1965). Examples of coverant control statements include: "I'm going to get a heart attack if I eat that cake," or "overeating makes it hard to breathe."

Behavioral Contracting

Harris and Bruner (1971) and Christensen (1976) have reported successfully controlling obesity by using contractual procedures. Since a program of weight control is quite specific in procedure and intent, it is of great help to decide upon a verifiable, mutual agreement.

Exercise

The patient should be encouraged to increase the amount of physical exercise in which he engages. Therapists such as Stuart (1971) stress strenuous participation in exercises, e.g., aerobics. However, often in this case it is simply sufficient to request that the patient change his physical habits, e.g., walk instead of taking elevators or escalators, stand more, get off the train or bus at an earlier stop, etc.

Caloric Modification

After the mean daily caloric intake is established the patient may be told to reduce his daily calorie intake. A general rule of thumb is that 3500 calories must be lost in order to lose one pound of body weight (Stuart, 1972). Care must be taken not to suddenly reduce the number of daily calories or to reduce them below the patient's sustenance level. In this matter the therapist should consult a physician and/or nutritionist who is aware of these issues. Caloric reduction may be achieved through dieting, increasing one's energy expenditure or, ideally, a combination of both.

Table 11-3 is a multimodal summary of the treatment sessions and strategies whose rationale has already been described. The use of self-monitoring (food

Table 11-3.

Session	Treatment Strategy	Modality Invoked
1	Intake	
2	Baseline	
3	Baseline	
4	Baseline	
5	Baseline, bibliotherapy	Cognition
6	Evaluation of baseline data	
7	1500-cal/day diet; written contractual agreement all undesirable foods removed from house, shopping only for one day at a time; telling a friend and asking him/her to cooperate	Behavior, cognition, interpersonal
8	Interrupt meal for 3-5 min	Behavior
9	Putting down utensils between bites	Behavior
10	No eating in front of TV, while reading or with friends; increase in physical exercise; taught sensate focus method	Behavior, sensation
11	Eating only at designated times	Behavior
12	Training in deep muscle relaxation, time projection, positive thoughts and images, coverant control	Behavior, affect, sensation, imagery, cognition
13	Self-reward using Chinese food and discotheque dancing	Behavior, sensation
14	Second written contract; patient asked to call or talk to a friend whenever inappropriate urge to eat occurs	Behavior, cognition, interpersonal
15	Covert sensitization – beer drinking	Behavior, affect, sensation, imagery, cognition
16	Second C.S. session for beer drinking	Behavior, affect, sensation, imagery, cognition
17	Third C.S. session for beer drinking	Behavior, affect, sensation, imagery, cognition
18	Covert sensitization for fried fatty foods, i.e., ribs, chicken, pork	Behavior, affect, sensation, imagery, cognition
19	Second C.S. session for fried foods	Behavior, affect, sensation, imagery, cognition

Table 11-3. (Continued).

Session	Treatment Strategy	Modality Invoked
20	Third C.S. session for fried foods	Behavior, affect, sensation, imagery, cognition
21	Patient leaves for 3-week vacation – a tape is made containing (1) relaxation induction, (2) time projections, positive imagery, encouragement, and support	
10½ weeks		

logs), therapist support, approval and praise, and realistic goal setting continued throughout the program.   Once a strategy was used it was maintained unless otherwise indicated.

RESULTS

Results indicate that from the time actual treatment began, i.e., at the end of the baseline period (session 6), until the end of session 21, there was a total weight loss of 26 pounds (9 percent of total body weight) over a period of eight and one-half weeks. Mean weight loss was 2.6 pounds per week for the total ten and a half weeks of the program. In addition, over the total range of ten and one-half weeks, the mean number of daily calories decreased from a baseline rate of 2814 per day to a stable level of 1500 per day. Likewise the patient's intake of three highly undesirable food categories decreased from mean daily levels of 3.2 beers per day and 2.0 cocktails per day to a level of zero per day and .3 per day, respectively. Intake of large amounts of fried foods with a high fat content decreased from a pretreatment level of 2.0 times daily to a mean program level of zero. Two other problematic behaviors also decreased: the frequency of eating dropped from 6.3 to 3.4 times per day, and the percentage of eating while watching television likewise decreased from 36 percent to 10 percent of the total meals.

DISCUSSION AND FOLLOW-UP

The essential feature of this approach was the addition of a planned multimodal strategy (BASIC ID) to already proven methods. In this respect, the author agrees with Lazarus (1973, 1976) that the more modalities deliberately invoked, the greater is the chance of lasting behavioral change.

Of particular interest was the use of covert sensitization (Cautela, 1967). Because of its highly specific nature, it was possible to examine its effect independent of the other variables. Following the first application of desensitization for beer drinking, there was a significant decrement in the number of daily beers. After the third covert sensitization session, beer drinking dropped to a zero level. (It is interesting to note that this effect generalized to drinking other alcoholic beverages as well. Without specifically exposing it to covert sensitization, the drinking of alcohol decreased from a mean of 2.0 drinks per day to a posttreatment level of .3 per day.) Similarly, the same effect was found for eating fried fatty foods. After the second covert sensitization session (session 19), the consumption of large amounts of such foods decreased significantly. The fact that remaining baseline measures showed no change further reinforces the power and specificity of covert sensitization. Covert sensitization appears to be very powerful and specific in its effect and seems indicated in treating eating responses of a highly specific nature.

Throughout the program the patient expressed enthusiasm for the methods of treatment. She did not consider it a diet because stringent restrictions were not placed on what types of foods she could eat, i.e., she was not instructed to follow dietary guidelines. Dietary control should be exerted only if there is a clear imbalance of nutrients, e.g., too great a percentage of refined carbohydrates, lack of vegetables, lack of high-protein foods. Even the covert sensitization process was not a command or an explicit restricton but, rather, an implicit suggestion and attention changer (Foreyt and Hagen, 1973). The patient felt a high degree of self-discipline and self-satisfaction over her participation in a program in which she was the principal agent of change. She perceived her own self, rather than an external authority, as being responsible. The fact that she was on a 1500-calorie diet did not seem a restriction to her but, instead, she saw it as a program change made necessary by the "scientific" evaluation of the food logs.

After the treatment phase, the patient was instructed to continue monitoring her daily caloric intake. Over the next two years the patient's food intake logs were collected and her progress monitored on a biweekly basis. During this period our meetings consisted of 15-minute sessions which concentrated on her progress and any problems she might encounter. At times our contact was by telephone. During this extensive follow-up period, the patient continued to lose weight although at a slower rate (see Table 11-4). On several occasions, plateaus were reached where she was unable to lose any more weight. This finding is consistent with the results of other studies which report that weight loss tends to decrease over time (Wilson, 1978). However, at no time did the patient gain weight or return to earlier maladaptive eating habits. Likewise, during this time she reported no adverse emotional side effects but reported instead and improvement in her social life and mental outlook. The final follow-up evaluation, 114 weeks after treatment began, proved to be highly encouraging. According to

Table 11-4. Summary of Weight Loss for Total Treatment and Follow-up Period.

	Weeks	Initial Weight	Target Weight	Weight Surplus	Post-treatment Weight	Pounds Lost	Mean Weight Reduction Quotient	Pounds Lost per Week
		WI	WT	WS	WP	WL	$\frac{WL}{WS} \times 100\%$	
Treatment	0–10	298	140	158	272	26	16.5	2.6
Follow-up	10–36	272	140	132	228	44	33	1.7
	36–62	228	140	88	205	23	26	.89
	62–88	205	140	65	195	10	15	.26
	88–114	195	140	55	185	10	18	.26

Total percentage excess weight lost:

$$100\% \ \frac{WL}{WS} = 64\%$$

Total weight reduction index:

$$\frac{WL}{WS} \times \frac{WI}{WT} \times 100\% = 152$$

Feinstein (1959, p. 442), "the best measurement of dieting success would appear to be the relationship of the patient's initial obese status to the amount of weight lost and the amount of loss that was desired." An effective index of weight reduction should relate actual weight loss to both initial weight and surplus weight. The time in which the weight loss occurred and the degree of adherence to the program are not crucial factors. Accordingly, an index was devised which takes the necessary factors into account. The weight reduction index is:

$$\frac{\text{Weight Lost}}{\text{Weight Surplus}} \times \frac{\text{Initial Weight}}{\text{Target Weight}} \times 100\%$$

Employing this criteria, Feinstein states that a final reduction index of 60 or higher indicates a successful weight loss. Table 11-4 provides treatment and follow-up data employing this index.

It is obvious that over the total period of evaluation the program can be considered a success. After 114 weeks the patient lost 63 percent of total excess weight resulting in a reduction index of 152.

The results of the present program seem to support the efficacy of a multimodal approach and the use of prolonged booster sessions in behavioral weight control programs (Stunkard and Mahoney, 1976). Since weight gains in the weeks following termination of treatment seem remarkably high, the continuous involvement of the therapist is necessary (Kline, Coleman, and Wick, 1976). In contradiction to the notion that booster sessions are not important (Ashby and Wilson, 1977), the present study lends support to the necessity and effectivness of long-term follow-up and support in the behavioral treatment of eating disorders.

REFERENCES

Ashby, W. A. and Wilson, G. T. Behavior therapy for obesity: Booster sessions and long-term maintenance of weight loss. *Behaviour Research and Therapy*, 1977, *15*, 451–464.
Baer, D. M., Wolf, M. M., and Risley, T. R. Some current dimensions of applied behavior analysis. *Journal of Applied Behavior Analysis*, 1968, *1*, 91–97.
Bandura, A. *Principles of Behavior Modification*. New York: Holt, Rhinehart, and Winston, 1969.
Bellack, A. S. Behavior therapy for weight reduction. *Addictive Behaviors*, 1975, *1*, 73–82.
Cautela, J. R. and Kastenbaum, R. P. Reinforcement survey schedule – Evaluation and current applications. *Psychological Reports*, 1967, *30*, 683–690.
Cautela, J. R. Covert reinforcement. *Behavior Therapy*, 1970, *1*, 33–50.
Christensen, A. Measuring and maintaining weight losses. *Behavior Therapy*, 1976, *7*, 709–711.
Diament, C. and Wilson, G. T. An experimental investigation of the effects of covert sensitization in an analogue eating situation. *Behavior Therapy*, 1975, *6*, 499–509.

Feinstein, A. R. The measurement of success in weight reduction: An analysis of methods and a new index. *Journal of Chronic Diseases*, 1959, *10*, 439–456.

Ferster, C. B., Nurnberger, J. I., and Levitt, E. E. The control of eating. *Journal of Mathematics*, 1962, *1*, 87–109.

Foreyt, J. P. and Hagen, R. L. Covert sensitization: Conditioning or suggestion? *Journal of Abnormal Psychology*, 1973, *82*, 17–83.

Gaul, D. J., Craighead, W. E., and Mahoney, M. J. Relationship between eating rates and obesity. *Journal of Consulting and Clinical Psychology*, 1975, *43*, 123–125.

Hall, S. M. Self-control and therapist control in the behavioral treatment of overweight women. *Behavior Research and Therapy*, 1972, *10*, 59–68.

Hall, S. M., Hall, R. G., Hanson, R. W., and Borden, B. L. Permanence of two self-managed treatments of overweight. *Journal of Consulting and Clinical Psychology*, 1974, *42*, 781–786.

Harris, M. B. Self-directed program for weight control: A pilot study. *Journal of Abnormal Psychology*, 1979, *74*, 263–270.

Harris, M. B. and Bruner, C. G. A comparison of a self-control and a contract procedure for weight control. *Behavior Research and Therapy*, 1971, *9*, 347–354.

Homme, L. E. Perspectives in Psychology – XXIV. Control of coverants, the operants of the mind. *Psychological Record*, 1965, *15*, 501–511.

Horan, J. J. and Johnson, R. G. Coverant conditioning through a self-management application of the Premack principle: Its effect on weight reduction. *Journal of Behavior Therapy and Experimental Psychiatry*, 1971, *2*, 43.

Janda, H. L. and Rimm, D. C. Covert sensitization in the treatment of obesity. *Journal of Abnormal Psychology*, 1972, *80*, 37–42.

Jeffery, R. W., Wing, R. R., and Stunkard, A. J. Behavioral treatment of obesity: The state of the art. *Behavior Therapy*, 1978, *9*, 189–199.

Kanfer, F. H. and Phillips, J. S. *Learning Foundations of Behavior Therapy*. New York: Wiley, 1970.

Kingsley, R. G. and Wilson, G. T. Behavior therapy for obesity: A comparative investigation of long-term efficacy. *Journal of Consulting and Clinical Psychology*, 1977, *45*, 288–298.

Kline, M. V., Coleman, L. L., and Wick, E. E. *Obesity, Etiology, Treatment and Management*. Springfield, Ill.: Thomas, 1976.

Kroeger, W. S. Systems approach for understanding obesity: Management by behavioral modification through hypnosis. *Psychiatric Opinion*, 1970, *1*.

Lazarus, A. A. *Behavior Therapy and Beyond*. New York: McGraw-Hill, 1971.

Lazarus, A. A. Multimodal behavior therapy: Treating the basic id. *Journal of Nervous and Mental Disease*, 1973, *156*, 404–411.

Lazarus, A. A. (Ed.), *Multimodal Behavior Therapy*. New York: Springer Press, 1976.

Leon, G. R. Current directions in the treatment of obesity. *Psychological Bulletin*, 1976, *83*, 557–578.

Lieberman, R. P. and Smith, V. A multiple baseline study of systematic desensitization in a patient with multiple phobias. *Behavior Therapy*, 1972, *2*, 597–603.

Mahoney, M. J. Self monitoring and self reward of habit change. *Behavior Therapy*, 1974, *5*, 202–216.

Mahoney, M. J., Moura, N. G. M., and Wade, T. C. Relative efficacy of self-reward, self-punishment and self-monitoring techniques for weight loss. *Journal of Consulting and Clinical Psychology*, 1973, *5*, 202–216.

Mann, R. A. The behavior-therapeutic use of contingency contracting to control an adult behavior problem: Weight control. *Journal of Applied Behavior Analysis*, 1972, *5*, 99–109.

Mulligan, R. Multimodal treatment of obesity. *Multimodal Behavior Therapy* (Lazarus, A., Ed.). New York: Springer Press, 1976.

Penick, S. B., Filion, R., Fox, S., and Stunkard, A. J. Behavior modification in the treatment of obesity. *Pyschosomatic Medicine*, 1971, *33*, 49–55.

Romanczyk, R. G., Tracey, D. A., Wilson, G. T., and Thorpe, G. L. Behavioral techniques in the treatment of obesity: A comparative analysis. *Behavior Research and Therapy*, 1973, *11*, 629–640.

Stollack, G. E. Control of obesity. *Psychotherapy: Theory, Research and Practice*, 1967, *4*, 61.

Stuart, R. B. Behavioral control over eating. *Behavior Research and Therapy*, 1967, *5*, 357–365.

Stuart, R. B. A three-dimensional program for the treatment of obesity. *Behavior Research and Therapy*, 1971, *9*, 177–186.

Stuart, R. B. and Davis, R. A. *Slim Chance in a Fat World: Behavioral Control of Obesity*. New York: Champaign Press, 1972.

Stunkard, A. J. The management of obesity. *New York State Journal of Medicine*, 1958, *58*, 79–87.

Stunkard, A. J. and Mahoney, M. J. Behavioral treatment of the eating disorders. *Handbook of Behavior Modification* (Leitenberg, H., Ed.). New York: Appleton-Century-Crofts, 1976.

Wick, E. E. Overeating patterns found in overweight and obese patients. *Obesity, Etiology, Treatment and Management* (Kline, M. V., Coleman, L. L., and Wick, E. E., Eds.). Thomas, Springfield, Ill.: 1976.

Williams, M. W. and Earlene, A. R. Teaching the obese to act and think thin. *Behavioral Medicine*, 1978, *5*, 43–48.

Wilson, G. T. Methodological considerations in the treatment outcome research on obesity. *Journal of Consulting and Clinical Psychology*, 1978, *46*, 687–702.

Wolman, B. B. *Handbook of Clinical Psychology*. New York: McGraw-Hill, 1965.

Wooley, C. S., Wooley, O. W., and Dyrenforth, S. R. Theoretical, practical and social issues in behavioral treatment of obesity. *Journal of Applied Behavior Analysis*, 1979, *12*, 3–25.

12

Group Therapy in the Treatment of Obesity*

Janet P. Wollersheim

Group treatment of obese individuals offers a number of advantages which, in many cases, result in its being the treatment of choice. Groups can be structured such that members receive considerable support from each other. Positive expectations and a degree of social pressure can be fostered and used to therapeutic advantage. Members can profit not only from the suggestions of the therapists, but also from those of other group members. Clients†are encouraged to assist others in reducing their caloric intake. In so doing, they often become aware of more effective ways to achieve their own weight reduction goals. As in other forms of group treatment, it is sometimes encouraging for clients to learn that they are not so different from others and that other members experience some of the same problems. In a group setting, the therapist has an opportunity to observe group interactions and to use them to advance treatment goals. Clients who tend to be reticent in recognizing and admitting their difficulties are often able to view their difficulties more objectively after hearing others describe their problems. Homework assignments, properly planned, are capable of being more effective when suggested by the group, rather than by the individual therapist. Weight reduction is generally recognized as a difficult and discouraging task.

---

*Portions of this chapter were adapted with minor modifications from Wollersheim, J. P. Obesity: behavioral treatment manuals, *JSAS Catalog of Selected Documents in Psychology,* 1975, *5,* 237 (Ms. No. 934).

†Since most clients in weight reducing programs are women,the female gender is used in referring to clients. The therapist is referred to by the generic "he."

Clients in group treatment can be heartened to know that others also find the task difficult, but still consider it important enough not to abandon. These and other factors contribute to indicating group therapy as the treatment of choice for many obese individuals.

The purpose of this chapter is to delineate in detail a group treatment package for obesity. The techniques described stem from a cognitive-behavioral orientation and have already been demonstrated to be effective in a number of controlled studies (Hagen, 1974; Wollersheim, 1970, 1977a, 1977b). Additionally, attention is devoted to greater emphases upon certain cognitive aspects of treatment which the author (Jeffrey and Wollersheim, Note 1) and others (Mahoney and Mahoney, 1976) have found useful in treating obese individuals.

GENERAL GUIDELINES

To effectively conduct group therapy for the obese, it is imperative that therapists be well informed and up to date on the research, issues, and facts relating to obesity, nutrition, and weight reduction. Reading volumes such as this one or similar works can accomplish this objective.

Prior to the first group therapy session, clients should be interviewed and screened. The purpose of the screening interview is to impart accurate expectations regarding the nature and goals of group treatment and to exclude those for whom such treatment is not appropriate. Individuals in the latter group would include those who are obviously psychotic or markedly unstable, persons who are convinced that their weight problem cannot be alleviated by restricting caloric intake, individuals who are not sufficiently motivated to take seriously the requirement of regular attendance at weekly meetings, and those who are currently receiving any type of psychotherapy. In this latter instance, such persons may be admitted to group treatment if their therapist sees such an experience as appropriate at that particular time.

One factor with a high potential for damaging the effectiveness of any treatment group is the problem of attrition. The best way to cope with the possibility of its becoming a problem is to concentrate upon preventing it. In the screening interview, attendance requirements should be emphasized by pointing out that each person has a responsibility to herself and to others to take this aspect of the program seriously. When a person skips therapy sessions, she is reducing her chances of effectively dealing with her weight problem since she is not only missing new material but also not availing herself of the support of the group. Additionally, an individual skipping therapy sessions makes the task of weight reduction more difficult for other group members as it is easier to become discouraged when one observes other members of the group failing to take their committment seriously. Individuals who do not feel that entry into the group requires a commitment to attend regularly, both for their own benefit and the benefit of others, are best excluded from this type of group treatment.

After group therapy sessions have commenced, the therapist must continue to work toward preventing attrition. Dispensing social reinforcement and using group pressure in a *supportive* atmosphere can be helpful. In addition, the therapist should make a supportive comment to *each* individual somewhere during the course of each meeting. If a member states to the group that she is thinking of dropping out, the individual member should be supported (i.e., reflection of feelings of discouragement, etc., along with encouragement that success is possible) and should be reminded that by coming through with meeting attendance, she will learn how to bring about weight loss and she can be an incentive to the group. In this case and in the case where the member privately tells the therapist of a desire to drop out, the therapist should arrange for a brief interview after the meeting in which he is sympathetic to the client's difficulties but confident in encouraging the client, pointing out the client's potential asset to the group and the letdown to herself and other group members that such dropping out would cause.

Starting group meetings within at least five minutes after the scheduled starting time can also help prevent attrition, since the therapist can respond to those who have come on time and thus allow the late arrivers to be noticeably late. Members arriving late should be encouraged, in a pleasant manner, to be on time next week. Absentees should be phoned by the therapist as soon as possible after the meeting they missed and before the next meeting. Phone calls should not be hostile reprimands, but rather should serve as encouragement and a prompt to attend the next meeting. If an individual refuses to attend a meeting or has missed more than two successive sessions, the therapist should endeavor to arrange a brief individual interview in which he attempts to elicit the persons's reasons for not attending meetings and tries to support and encourage attendance at the next meeting. In such instances, the therapist can briefly fill the individual in on what was missed and assure her that she will be able to fit right back in at the next session.

In both the screening interview and the first group session, the therapist should discuss the issue of confidentiality. It should be explained that the therapist himself operates under professional ethics which require confidentiality of whatever personal issues group members discuss. Group members are asked to honor confidentiality also by not discussing, outside of group meetings, what other members reveal about themselves. Individuals, however, retain the freedom to discuss their own difficulties both within and outside of group meetings. Clients should be informed that although the therapist cannot guarantee that group members will not break confidentiality, experiences with similar groups indicate that clients are usually conscientious about such matters.

In conducting group discussion, the therapist will use techniques common to many forms of group therapy, such as referring questions to the group; commenting upon difficulties in communication; drawing out implications and generalizations from one client's remarks; and pointing out similarities and differences between problems, emotions, attitudes, motives, experiences, etc. The therapist should guide discussions, but he should train clients to talk to the group and not exclusively to him.

In this program, the first 15–20 minutes of each session is devoted to the use of positive expectation and social pressure to aid with weight reduction. These procedures are modeled after those used by the national weight reducing group Take Off Pounds Sensibly (TOPS). The therapist attempts to help clients build positive expectations regarding their ability to lose weight. Additionally, the therapist fosters and uses social pressure sensitively in helping each individual reduce. The following general format is used during the initial period of each meeting to foster and utilize positive expectations and social pressure:

1. Name tags with first and last name are distributed to be worn by clients and therapist.

2. There is a weigh-in in front of group, and the weight is recorded in red on each client's graph-lined chart which is to be hung conspicuously in the room before the meeting begins.

3. As the therapist weighs each client, he announces her weight and then compares it with last week's as he records it on the chart and draws a line to connect this week and last week's weight. He dispenses positive reinforcement ("Good for you"; "Now here's a lady who's going places") and encouragement ("Keep up the good work"; "You're on your way") or negative reinforcement ("Oh, oh!" "Shame! Shame!") or encouragement ("Next week will be your week"; "You'll be down next week") as the case demands and encourages group members to do likewise. Those who have lost weight wear a star reading "Bravo" throughout the meeting, those who remain the same wear a turtle sign, and those who gained weight from the previous week wear a picture of a pig. The member who lost the most weight wears a crown.

4. After the weigh-in which should take about 10 minutes, the therapist sits down with the group members for 5–10 minutes and encourages the group by reminding them of the following: there are no magic formulas to lose weight; they have to reduce their calorie intake in a way suitable to their own living situations; they said they wanted to lose weight and they can; and they owe it to themselves and to each other to lose. The therapist and group can commend an individual who is doing especially well or pressure and playfully rib a slow member. Also the therapist can use this time to ask members factual questions about the effects of obesity, nutrition, and weight loss and/or can himself provide this information.

Two major tasks of the therapist in using these procedures are to muster motivation by stressing the effectiveness of the procedures and building and utilizing social pressure by helping members become keenly aware of the fact that they have made a commitment to each other as well as to themselves. Building a *we* feeling in the group is important. Members are to be reminded repeatedly that if they do not reduce their calorie intake and lose weight they are letting both themselves and their fellow members down. By losing weight they help themselves achieve their goal and also, by example, help their fellow members and remind them that they too should keep their commitment.

Social pressure should be used with the group as a whole and with the individual members. Individuals can and should be reminded of their commitment and obligation to the group. By building a *we*-ness spirit in the group ("You're in this together"; "You have a common goal"; "Each person's success is a success and incentive for the group"; "Each of you should be concerned and supportive to a fellow member who lags behind"), the therapist can skillfully bring social pressure to bear upon slow-moving members and use positive and negative social reinforcement (as well as the symbolic reinforcers — Bravo, Pig, Turtle, Crown) to the best advantage. Building and maintaining a competitive group spirit is desirable, but the therapist's clinical skill and sensitivity should help guide the group into developing a happy medium. Competition and social pressure must be backed up by group and therapist support, and the positive and negative reinforcements should ring a playful note. The pressures and reinforcements should be real enough to provide incentive but never so harsh as to make the group aversive and extremely threatening to the individual.

It is recommended that group size be kept within the range of eight to twenty members.

MATERIALS

In the first group meeting, all participants receive booklets giving the caloric content of foods and booklets in which to record food and caloric intake each day. They are asked to bring these booklets to each group meeting.

At each session the therapist will need the following materials:

1. his calorie book;
2. an accurate scale;
3. weight charts, masking tape, and red recording pens;
4. symbolic signs (Bravo, Pig, Turtle, Crown) and straight pins;
5. name tags and straight pins;
6. his personal notes pertaining to techniques to be implemented during that session;

7. a watch to keep track of time;
8. the group folder in which to record attendance and a summary of the session;
9. a list of the participants with names, addresses, and phone numbers.

GENERAL STRUCTURE OF GROUP SESSIONS

This treatment program is designed to be provided over a period of ten weeks with weekly meetings of 90 minutes each. Each weekly session consists of a positive expectation-social pressure phase and a discussion phase. The positive expectation-social pressure phase lasts from 15–20 minutes and follows the procedures already discussed under "General Guidelines." The discussion phase lasts from 65–70 minutes and focuses upon helping participants change their eating patterns by implementing principles derived from learning theory. The following points are to be noted with regard to the discussion phase:

1. In this phase of treatment, the therapist introduces learning theory principles to aid clients in controlling their eating behavior.

2. In the first session the therapist should present the treatment rationale as delineated in "Session-by-Session Procedures" (see pp. 8–10), and parts of this explanation ought to be repeated and emphasized from time to time.

3. Clients will be instructed in methods of recording their eating behavior in the first session. In the following sessions, the discussion phase will begin by referring to the eating records and, when possible, using the records of those who lost weight as models.

4. The first half of the discussion phase should be devoted to a review of the new techniques introduced in the previous session; the eating records should be used to exemplify how some individuals were successful in implementing the techniques and to suggest how others could successfully apply such techniques to their eating behavior. Each individual's efforts should be discussed, and misunderstandings and misapplications should be clarified and corrected. It cannot be emphasized too strongly that if the treatment is to be successful, participants must apply the techniques not merely discuss them, and it is the therapist's responsibility to see that each member's efforts are discussed in detail and that the techniques are tailored to her particular situation. Detailed discussion of each member's efforts will not be possible in each session, but each member should be given some attention in each session and periodically each person's efforts should be discussed in detail. The first half of the discussion phase should also be spent checking upon progress with the other techniques introduced up to that point, although the greater portion of time will be devoted to the more re-

cent techniques introduced in the previous session. This procedure of reviewing the new material presented in the previous session also has the advantage that a member missing a session will have an opportunity to catch up.

5. The second half of the discussion phase is to be devoted to the introduction of new techniques. Discussion here should be devoted to specific ways in which each member can apply the new techniques to her own life circumstances and eating behavior.

6. Not only the therapist, but the group members too, should help each individual decide ways in which she can specifically implement various techniques. The therapist should help group members talk to each other, rather than addressing comments mainly to him. While the therapist is to assume an active role in directing the discussion, his use of questioning and comments should be such that a good amount of purposeful discussion is carried by the members themselves.

7. The technique of shaping is introduced in the first session and is to be emphasized throughout the entire program, but especially in the first four sessions. Sessions 2 to 6 are devoted specifically to ways in which eating behavior can be changed with all techniques having been introduced by the end of the sixth session. Sessions 7 to 10 are to be devoted to detailed discussion of each individual's utilization of techniques and the correction of misunderstandings and misapplications.

8. The discussion phase may also include commenting upon facts, issues, and research relating to obesity, weight reduction, and nutrition when such comments would seem to be helpful.

9. At the end of the discussion period the therapist should give a brief summary of what has transpired, reminding members that they must *apply* the techniques and that they are expected to lose at least 2 pounds by the next session.

In conducting treatment, the therapist must take care to understand fully the learning principles and the rigor necessary in applying them advantageously. On the other hand, he must also remember that clinical skills are just as important in conducting learning theory treatment as in conducting other types of treatment. This can be accomplished by the therapist assuming and manifesting a basic attitude of inquiry. This attitude of inquiry can be expressed by commenting in the form of questions (e.g., "How might Peggy reward herself for not overeating?") and by referring remarks to the group for comments (e.g., "Nancy says she can't sleep well if she doesn't eat before going to bed: what might she do to satisfy her hunger and yet not consume too many calories?"). By shaping, eliciting appropriate responses, and making pertinent comments, the therapist should see that each problem introduced is given adequate closure in terms of appropriate suggestions and solutions having been offered.

SESSION-BY-SESSION PROCEDURES

The first 15–20 minutes of each session utilize the positive expectation-social pressure techniques. The discussion phase occupies the remaining 65–70 minutes of each 90-minute session. In each session, the first half of the discussion phase is used to review the members' utilization of techniques introduced in the previous session as well as to check progress with other techniques introduced up to that point. The second half of the session is used to introduce new techniques and help members plan how to utilize them in reducing caloric intake. What follows is specification of the format for the discussion phase of each session. The specific techniques to be used in each session are thoroughly explained in the section which begins on p. 12.

Session One

In the first session the therapist explains that the discussion in the session will be concerned with helping members to alter their eating patterns by specifically applying principles of learning which account for the way in which behavior, especially eating behavior, is developed, changed, and maintained. The participants are to be assured that the techniques and principles in which they will be instructed have been validated by considerable research and that correct application of these principles will help them develop more appropriate eating patterns and yet learn to enjoy eating more. In short, the therapist gives the members the rationale for this program based upon learning principles. He should say something along these lines.

> Any behavior or action which is learned through various experiences can also be changed through experience. Your eating patterns are habits which have been learned through the years. The program we have designed for you will teach you to unlearn inappropriate eating habits which are responsible for your weight problem. At the same time you will be learning how to apply principles which help you learn appropriate eating habits which will produce weight loss, make it possible for you to maintain that weight loss and still reap a good deal of pleasure from eating and other areas of your life.
>
> While this program will focus directly on your eating patterns, this by no means implies that we will ignore other important areas of your life which

probably influence your eating habits. For example, many people develop inappropriate eating behavior because they are not getting enough satisfaction from other important areas such as recreation, social interactions, relationships with the opposite sex, etc. We will be discussing behavior in these areas in order to help you develop more satisfying and appropriate ways of thinking, feeling, and acting, for our definition of behavior is broad and includes not only outward actions but thoughts, feelings, and emotions as well. The most important thing for you to realize, however, is that these principles and techniques which we will be discussing with you will work but to work, *they must be applied* in your own living situation and not merely discussed. When you first use the techniques they may seem rather artificial because of their newness, but as you continue to apply them they will become very natural and will aid you in modifying your eating patterns in a natural and comfortable manner. In fact, you should overdo the principles on a regular basis and after a few weeks you'll find that they will become habitual and spontaneous.

Each week we will introduce one or two new techniques which, if correctly applied, will help you overcome your weight problem. You are to try each new technique and, as time goes on. you naturally will be making the most use of the techniques you have found most helpful. Also each week we will review techniques we introduced in the past, particularly the ones introduced in the previous session. All of us together will serve to help each of you apply these techniques specifically to your individual circumstances. Group members are encouraged to help each other because helping and rewarding others facilitates learning in the trainer. By the sixth session, we will have introduced all the major techniques in the program. The last four sessions, then, will be used to review the techniques and to aid you further in correctly applying them. Are there any questions at this point? [The therapist should reemphasize the basic rationale of the treatment program from time to time throughout the other sessions.]

All the techniques to be used in this program are designed to help each person develop desirable habits concerning the *WHEN, WHAT,* and *HOW MUCH* of eating. You will learn to eat sensibly and really enjoy eating. By gradually learning to change your food habits, you won't feel deprived, but rather will find yourself eating less but enjoying it more. Developing self-control over the *WHEN, WHAT,* and *HOW MUCH* of eating doesn't mean that you will never have an in-between-meal snack, or never have a second helping. Rather, it means that, in general, you will be able to fit such eating occasions into an all-around pattern of appropriate eating habits which promote weight control and help you learn to really enjoy food, not just gulp it down. The goal of the program is not simply to aid you with weight reduction but to enable you to learn new eating patterns which will be lasting and satisfying habits. This program then does not prescribe a diet and you should not constantly talk with others about dieting since such conversation tends to make one feel deprived of eating pleasures and misses the real purpose of the present program — developing eating habits which fit into one's pattern of living and allow for weight loss and maintenance.

The therapist then uses the rest of the discussion phase to *present* and *discuss* technique No. 1 ("Building Positive Associations concerning Eating Control"); technique No. 2 ("Keeping Records of Eating Behavior"), at which time recording booklets are distributed to members; and technique No. 3 ("Shaping of Behavior"). It is imperative that in presenting the techniques the therapist encourage discussion aimed at helping each client work out ways in which she will implement the technique in her own life circumstances.

At the end of the discussion phase, the therapist presents a brief summary and encourages all clients to concentrate on implementing the techniques introduced, reminding them that he expects each of them to be at least 2 pounds lighter next week, but that they are to accomplish this by a shaping process.

Session Two

These techniques are introduced: No. 4, "Developing Appropriate Stimulus Control of Eating," and No. 5, "Manipulation of Deprivation and Satiation."

Session Three

These techniques are introduced: No. 6, "Rewarding Oneself for the Development of Self-control," and No. 7, "Development of Personally Meaningful Ultimate Aversive Consequences (UAC's) of Overeating."

Session Four

These techniques are introduced: No. 8, "Obtaining Reinforcers from Areas of Life Other than Eating," and No. 9, "Establishing Alternative Behaviors Incompatible with Eating."

Session Five

Technique No. 10 is introduced — "Utilization of Chaining."

Session Six

Technique No. 11 is introduced — "Supplementary Techniques."

Sessions Seven, Eight, and Nine

These sessions are devoted to detailed review of each member's utilization of techniques. Individuals are encouraged and helped in tailoring the techniques to their specific life situations so that maximum benefit can be obtained. Discussions should utilize the detailed records of eating behavior which each pariticpant has been encouraged to keep throughout treatment.

Session Ten

The therapist opens this session by presenting an overall summary statement and a parting message to motivate members to continue losing and maintaining their weight loss. The statement should be similar to the following:

Since this is our last meeting, we want to leave you with a parting message. Some of you may be pleased with your progress and others may feel somewhat discouraged. However, all of you have been given training in methods to modify your eating habits in such a way that you will lose weight. We've also pointed out how you can change your thoughts, feelings, and actions in other important areas so that you can achieve more satisfaction from other areas of your life and hence feel less need to overeat. Although our formal sessions are terminating, your progress should continue. In the final analysis only you can change yourself and by continuing to *put into practice what you've learned here*, you will continue to lose weight, maintain this loss, and become a happier person. You may slip up now and then, but don't let that discourage you. The minute you realize you have been slack, start *at that very moment* again, applying what you learned here. A steady, gradual weight loss is your best bet to take off pounds and stay slim. When you reach your desirable weight you can slowly increase your caloric intake while watching the scales. You'll find the number of calories you can consume to keep your weight constant. Then weigh yourself once a week. If you have gained, immediately take those extra pounds off before letting pound upon pound build up. Those of you who had much weight to lose should continue trying to lose at least 2 pounds a week. Just think, by such a rate, one can lose over 100 pounds in a year and can keep it off.

No magic formula exists to lose weight. No matter what causes contribute to your being overweight, the only reliable way to take pounds off and keep them off is to reduce caloric intake. The principles we discussed are among the most effective, efficient, and natural ways to lose weight that have been worked out. We believe that in general, individuals who have completed a program such as the one you have just completed should continue to reduce after the formal meetings have been discontinued. This should be true of fast-moving members as well as of more slowly progressing ones.

So remember that the techniques we've discussed are effective, but only *you* can apply them. Continue counting calories and continue eating well-balanced meals; make your daily caloric intake range between 1000 and 1500 calories. Regardless of the difficulty you've had, *you can* effectively and naturally change your eating habits to become slim and stay slim. Now let's spend the remainder of the discussion period by having each member discuss her progress and plans.'

The remainder of the session is spent helping each client review her progress and realistically planning how to continue losing weight, if such is indicated, and to maintain weight loss.

The therapist then closes the meeting by wishing the group luck and reminding them that they should and can continue to lose weight and maintain the loss. At this last meeting the therapist should make a point of giving a parting greeting and bit of encouragement to each participant as she leaves (e.g., "It was nice working with you, Mary, and keep using the techniques; you can achieve your desirable weight and I know you're the type of person who will, even when the going gets a bit hard" or "I've enjoyed knowing you, Jane; remember to keep using the principles and in a couple of months you'll have achieved your goal").

SPECIFIC TECHNIQUES

This section describes and explains the specific therapeutic techniques to be used in the cognitive-behavioral treatment for helping participants change their eating patterns so that they will lose weight. Once they reach their desired weight, they will have developed normal eating habits appropriate to maintaining their weight at this level. The techniques are described in the order in which they are to be introduced and implemented in the discussion phases of the separate therapy sessions. It is emphasized that, while these techniques have been designed to be maximally effective in aiding individuals to modify their eating behavior and consequently lose weight, they must be *applied* and *used* by individual members. Discussion alone will not bring about desirable results. The therapist's most important task is *to help each individual specifically implement these techniques* in a manner appropriate to the circumstances and situations arising in her particular mode of living.

When the techniques are first introduced, the therapist must take care to explain them well, defining terms as the need arises and eliciting feedback from the group to ensure that they understand precisely the way in which the technique must be implemented in order to be effective. Discussion should be elicited from the participants concerning the manner in which each member can implement the technique in her living pattern. The first half of the discussion phase in each session is to be spent checking on how each member has been implementing the techniques, with more attention devoted to the techniques introduced in the previous session, but with routine checking of all techniques introduced up to that point. Misunderstandings and errors in application should be corrected during the discussion phase, with the therapist himself providing support, encouragement, reinforcement, and persuasion, as well as eliciting these from the group.

It is to be expected that not all individuals will find all techniques equally effective, nor will individuals be equally disposed to implement and apply all techniques to the same degree. The therapist should encourage participants to try all techniques at least for the week following their initial introduction; then he can explain that the members may focus more upon those techniques which they have found most effective and which seem to be more applicable to their individual eating habits. However, should the client be omitting a technique that would seem very important in helping her to acquire more appropriate eating habits, the therapist must call this to her attention and try to persuade and encourage her to utilize the particular procedure.

In the course of treatment, participants may introduce ideas relating to techniques not yet formally introduced. When this occurs, instructions concerning the technique ought to be given to ensure that the participants will be applying it correctly. However, the technique should again be explained and discussed in the session designated for this. If a participant introduces a worthwhile technique not formally included in the treatment outline, it can be discussed if it seems to be of value to the individual. Again the purpose of the discussion would be to aid the participant in proper application. Techniques which participants introduce and which are poorly adapted to promoting appropriate eating habits should be identified as such, accompanied by an explanation of why they are likely to be ineffective.

An explanation of the techniques used in this treatment condition follows. The therapist is not merely to explain the techniques and encourage members to implement them; he should also elicit discussion and comments about the techniques from the group, getting members to talk specifically about how they can use the technique.

Building Positive Associations Concerning Eating Control

The therapist explains that the purpose of this program is neither to put participants on a diet nor to take away their eating pleasures. On the contrary, the program is designed to add to their pleasure of eating by teaching them to eat properly and to eat intentionally like a gourmet, one who really enjoys her food to the fullest with all of her senses (visual, olfactory, tactile, gustatory). One who eats indiscriminately just stuffs food hastily into her mouth without really enjoying the eating experience. By changing one's eating habits, one can eat less but enjoy it more. One can learn to enjoy food by looking at it — appreciating the coloring of the food and its arrangement — and by enjoying its aroma. Most importantly, one can learn to eat slowly and enjoy each *small* mouthful with her lips and teeth. The taste and texture of the food can be more fully enjoyed by chewing the food thoroughly, using the taste buds on the right side of the tongue, the left side, and then the back of the tongue before swallowing. To fully enjoy food this way, one must eat slowly and obtain more oral gratification with less food by using more lip and chewing movements. The purpose of this program, then, is not to deprive individuals of their pleasure but to increase those pleasures. By changing eating patterns to consume fewer calories, one can at the same time learn to enjoy eating more.

Participants, then, are to *EAT INTENTIONALLY*. When they are eating, they should do nothing else (no studying, no reading, no watching television). Eating is to be dissociated from other activites. When the individual eats, she should enjoy it to the fullest and let nothing distract her. By doing nothing else while eating, the participant can learn to enjoy eating more. Also stimuli from other activities lose their control in initiating the chain of behaviors and conditions that terminate in eating. When one eats intentionally, one should relish every mouthful. If she is going to eat, she should enjoy it. Such a procedure brings eating behavior under the control of one's intentions, helps break associations between eating and other behaviors, and slows the rate of eating.

Individuals should not consider themselves on a diet. By dieting we frequently mean eating only certain low-calorie foods in order to lose weight. Dieting and changing eating patterns are not the same thing. Participants should consider themselves not as dieting, but merely as changing their eating patterns so as to achieve weight reduction and to acquire eating habits that will later enable them to remain at their desired weight and still retain the pleasures that eating affords. Too many diets consist of crash programs. Although they may effect a rapid weight loss, such a weight loss increases a person's disposition to eat, and this disposition usually becomes strong enough to overcome the person's temporary motive concerning the desirability of weight loss. Many diets so severely limit the kind and amount of food a person may eat that the dieter begins to feel deprived and discouraged and finds herself breaking the diet and regaining the lost weight. A good many diets advocate foods which an individual can consume only for a limited time period (e.g., liquid diets, the grapefruit diet) and teach the person nothing about better eating habits. People lose weight — only to regain it when they attempt to return to a more normal eating plan. Such diets requiring specialized foods and situations are difficult to maintain; when eating circumstances return to normal, the individual finds herself returning to old habits and she puts on weight. Other diets such as the carbohydrate diet are based upon false nutritional assumptions. It has been demonstrated that the only reason people on carbohydrate diets lose weight is because, by limiting their intake of carbohydrates, they also decrease their caloric intake. Calories are still what really count. Furthermore, adhering to the carbohydrate diet for a long period of time can be definitely detrimental to one's health. Hence, group members are to keep in mind the fact that if they really want to lose weight and not regain it, they must change their eating habits in a sensible way. Developing effective self-control in the area of eating requires eating a nutritionally balanced diet daily and learning self-control under circumstances and with foods which are to be the individual's permanent eating pattern. Accomplishing this requires changing habits concerning when one eats, what one eats, and how much one eats. Well-balanced diets not only ensure good health but have the extra advantage that the individual will not have a strong craving for carbohydrates, sugars, and fats because, unlike dieting with specific foods, a well-balanced diet allows the person to eat an appropriate amount of these foods.

All the techniques to be used in this program are designed to help each person develop desirable habits concerning the WHEN, WHAT, and HOW MUCH of eating. Participants will learn to eat sensibly and really enjoy eating. By gradually learning to change their food habits, they will not feel deprived but rather will find themselves eating less but enjoying it more. Developing self-control over the WHEN, WHAT, and HOW MUCH of eating does not mean that the person will never have a second helping. Rather, it means that, in general, she will be able to fit such eating occasions into an all-around pattern of appropriate eating habits which promote weight control and help the subject learn really to enjoy food, not just gulp it down. The goal of the program is not simply to aid members with weight reduction but to enable them to learn new eating patterns which will be lasting and satisfying habits. This program, then, does not prescribe a diet, and participants should not constantly talk with others about dieting, as such conversation tends to make one feel deprived of eating pleasures and misses the purpose of the present program — developing new eating habits.

The importance of building positive associations concerning eating control cannot be overemphasized. The whole purpose of the technique is to help clients view their efforts in changing their eating habits as a program designed to increase their enjoyments rather than depriving them of their pleasures. The greatest contribution of this technique lies in engendering the client's motivation to actually implement a behavioral program and to continue to use behavioral techniques to control eating habits once formal treatment has terminated. Clinical and research experience strongly suggests that clients might be more motivated to undergo the hardships of caloric restriction if the therapist can aid them in critically examining their construals concerning excess weight, caloric restriction, modifying eating habits, and utilizing various behavioral techniques. Weight reduction is almost guaranteed if individuals will follow the behavioral program designed for them. The problem lies in motivating clients to implement the program and to stick to it. One handle on the motivational problem may well lie in examining what the client is telling herself about reducing her caloric intake and gradually modifying her eating patterns. Mahoney and Mahoney (1976) approach this task by encouraging the client to evaluate her cognitive ecology and clean up her cognitive pollutants. Is a client saying that she is really not too overweight? Is she telling herself she needs all those extra sweets? Does she believe that cutting down on food is too hard for her? Does the client view herself as deprived of pleasures while watching calories? These construals will be highly idiosyncratic for each individual, but they can profoundly affect the degree to which a client will be committed to a behavioral program of weight management. When a client can be helped to construe a weight management program in a more realistic and adaptable way, the task of employing weight management strategies can be rendered less difficult. It would seem that one of the most significant potential benefits that cognitive approaches have to offer weight management programs is a method of mustering the client's motivation for the difficult task of changing eating habits by helping her acquire more realistic and adaptive construals concerning weight loss and all it entails. This aspect of treatment is one which will require the therapist's continued attention throughout the duration of treatment if members are to be encouraged to implement other treatment techniques and to undergo the hardships of caloric restriction.

Keeping Records of Eating Behavior

Each participant should be given a small notebook which she can carry in her purse. In the notebook she is to record every day: the food eaten, the amount, the number of calories consumed, the occasion (e.g., breakfast, study break, after-dinner snack), what happened before eating, what happened after eating, any particular emotional feeling at the time (e.g., tense, blue, tired), and the total amount of calories consumed each day. Recording eating behavior is to be used as both an assessment and a treatment technique. As an assessment technique, the records should help identify the current discriminative, eliciting, and reinforcing stimuli associated with the eating behavior. Since from the first session the therapist will be asking participants to lose at least 2 pounds a week, participants should be instructed that for the first three weeks they should make records not only of the occurrence of eating, but also of times they were tempted to eat but did not because of their commitment to lose weight. In recording times they resisted eating, they should list: the food desired, the occasion, what happened before the temptation to eat, what they did instead of eating, what happened after resisting the temptation, and any emotional feeling experienced when tempted to eat. Records of actual eating behavior should be kept throughout the program and consulted at the beginning of each discussion period. The records will serve as a treatment technique since recording will aid participants in cutting down on food when they realize how much they actually eat. Such recording actually takes little time and, with moderate eating, such record keeping becomes very simple. The heavy eater and the frequent snacker will, of course, have to record more than the controlled eater. Most participants will find that, in order to lose weight, their total daily intake will need to be reduced to between 1000 and 1500 calories. One pound of fat is equivalent to approximately 3500 calories. Thus, in order to lose 2 pounds a week, an individual must reduce her weekly calorie consumption to 7000 calories below that needed to provide energy for normal activities while keeping body weight constant. A woman who is moderately active needs about 1800–2400 calories per day to sustain normal activity and body weight. Therefore, in order to lose 2 pounds a week, most women will have to decrease their intake to about 1000–1500 calories daily. Daily intakes above 1600 calories give such slow results in weight loss as to be too discouraging. Once a person achieves her desirable weight she can, of course, gradually increase daily caloric intake to the point where she observes that her weight remains constant.

Participants should learn an active verbal repertoire with which they can translate caloric intake into ultimate body fat. They should learn the caloric values of different kinds of foods. For example, an average piece of pie (approximately 275 calories) is equal to about one-tenth of a pound of fat. Pie has approximately the same number of calories as a baked potato with a pat of butter and a small serving of steak. Also, for example, two pieces of fudge (220 calories) are equivalent in calories to three medium-sized apples (225 calories). Such a procedure helps the participants become more calorie conscious. Keeping records of food intake helps them discriminate situations in which they tend to eat, helps them become more fully aware of their eating habits, and aids them in learning to eat on purpose.

Weight loss usually does not proceed evenly, and some weeks may show more loss than others even though the person is decreasing her caloric consumption by the same amount. In general, though, an average weight loss of 2 pounds per week can be steadily maintained.

The records will be discussed and evaluated during discussion periods, and suggestions appropriate to more desirable habits concerning the *WHEN, WHAT,* and *HOW MUCH* of eating will be made. Discussion will also revolve around the degree of hunger when the food was eaten, how satisfying the food was, the emotional feelings before eating, how easily one could have not eaten, and how this might have been successfully accomplished.

Shaping of Behavior

The members are to be instructed how to use a shaping procedure to modify their eating patterns. The importance of small steps and realistic goals in developing more appropriate eating behavior should be emphasized throughout *all* sessions. Developing more self-control of eating behavior is a gradual process involving the planning of goals which are limited enough to be realistic. Behavior should be changed gradually so that the changed behavior will be reinforced. Changed eating behavior should be planned for hierarchies of situations which gradually increase in difficulty within a framework of realistic goals and self-rewards. Some methods of shaping behavior follow:

1. Set goals only for each day and each moment (e.g., no snacks this morning; no eating in the living room).
2. List situations in which one eats most, and stop eating in some of these situations, first concentrating on situations in which it will be easiest not to eat.
3. Before attending social events, determine how much one will eat (e.g., only twelve peanuts and one slice of cake; only one piece of pizza).
4. Do something incompatible with eating when in a situation in which one tends to eat (e.g., file nails while watching television).
5. Use aids to help one not to eat. Smoke a cigarette, chew gum, have a noncaloric piece of candy.
6. List the situations in which one eats less, and further decrease and finally eliminate eating in these situations (e.g., no refreshments at movies or ball games).
7. Limit between-meal eating to certain specified foods. For example, after-work snacks can be limited to diet cola or coffee with an artificial sweetener. When going out to have a snack with a group, one can order a salad or a dish of fruit. If a fountain does not have diet cola, one can order a coke and drink only half of it. (Waste the money — that's better than acquiring fat!)
8. List the activities and situations in which one does not eat and then engage in those activities more often and enter those situations more frequently (e.g., study in the library where one cannot eat; if one does not eat while writing, start studying with a pencil in hand and write study notes).
9. Control between-meal snacking by gradually lengthening periods of abstention, working first with periods of the day that cause least difficulty in the temptation to overeat. When one has succeeded in abstaining a specified period of time, allow a highly rewarding food at the end of that time. However, the amount to be eaten should be determined beforehand.

The therapist should help individual members decide how best to start shaping their own eating behavior toward the establishment of appropriate eating habits. The emphasis should be on gradualness and realistic goals.

Developing Appropriate Stimulus Control of Eating Behavior

While this technique is given formal introduction in the second session, throughout remaining sessions participants should be aided in using shaping to narrow the range of stimuli which control eating.

Certain situations present the stimuli for a person's eating behavior. One can modify her eating patterns by either changing these stimuli or by changing the behavior that occurs in certain stimulus situations. Participants should be instructed to select carefully the stimuli that are to control their eating behavior. This can be accomplished in several ways.

Narrowing the Range of Stimuli Which Control Eating. People with weight problems frequently eat in a large variety of circumstances. One way to control eating is to limit the situations in which eating is allowed to occur. When the participant eats, she should do that and nothing else. The subject should not allow herself to engage in other activities (e.g., studying, reading, watching television while eating). At home, the person should see to it that eating can occur only in certain places, for example, at the kitchen table, or in the dorm lounge and not in the dorm room. Temporal control over eating can be developed by specifying a time for eating meals and sticking to that time. The client is not to skip meals but to eat them at a regular time. Following a strict temporal pattern for eating usually results in feelings of hunger disappearing except just before mealtime. Women having difficulty restricting their eating to meals should arrange a *routine* extra feeding, such as milk and crackers or vanilla wafers. These should always be taken at the same specified time, however.

The main goal in establishing appropriate stimulus control of eating is to bring eating under the control of stimuli that occur infrequently in the participant's normal activities. Hence, eating should be dissociated from the routine activities of the day. Each participant can discover the stimuli which mark the occasion for her eating and can change these stimuli. She may do this in many ways: seeing that snacks are not around; not walking home past the bakery; shopping only from a list which is prepared after a satisfying meal; not lingering at the table after a meal; going for a walk during a study break instead of making a trip to the snack-vending machines; working, studying, and relaxing in places where eating is not allowed or is less likely to occur; not carrying money for between-meal snacks; and, if a snack such as a candy bar is bought, breaking it into small pieces and placing it in an inconvenient location. The client should also gradually restrict the situations in which she allows herself to eat.

Highlighting the Stimuli Associated with Appropriate Eating. Clients are to be encouraged to allow eating to occur only in the presence of certain stimuli. Such stimuli can include a temporal pattern, a particular place, or particular items. For example, the client can specify that she will never snack till at least three hours after meals. She may make a rule never to eat unless she is sitting at a table. Individuals can decide to limit between-meal snacks only to specified foods such as apples, vanilla wafers, celery sticks, or carrot sticks. By specifying the stimuli under which she will allow herself to eat, the individual will find that she is less tempted to eat under other circumstances and that if she does eat in response to stimuli other than the ones she has designated as appropriate, she will feel guilty.

Manipulating Deprivation and Satiation

It is important that the client does not severely deprive herself but rather embarks upon a gradual program of weight reduction. Food intake should be planned to avoid long periods of deprivation and to help through difficult periods. Also keeping other needs satisfied will reduce hunger. Participants can also eat non-fattening foods (e.g., orange, apple, cracker) after brief periods of abstention. Participants can arrange to have highly desirable foods available only when hunger is low (e.g., encountering desserts only at the end of meals) and less desirable foods available when hunger is high (e.g., Rye-Krisp only for between-meal snacks). It may also be helpful to eat a bit of filling food just before entering a situation in which she will have a strong tendency to eat (e.g., 6 ounces of juice or milk just before mealtime or attendance at a party). Participants should be discouraged from losing weight too fast (e.g., more than 5 or 6 pounds per week) because a very rapid loss produces a level of deprivation and a disposition to eat which exceeds the existing self-control. Also participants are to be discouraged from limiting the diet to one specified food such as protein because such a diet will likely produce a heightened disposition to eat other food. A well-balanced diet will have an adequate satiety value. Most-liked foods should be eaten when deprivation is less, and less-satisfying but filling foods should be eaten when deprivation is higher. During a meal the participant can practice eating the least desirable foods first and the most desirable ones last.

Rewarding Oneself for the Development of Self-control

It is important that the participant reinforce herself for the development of self-control in the area of eating, or the developing self-control behavior will cease, especially since the reinforcing consequence of weight loss is accomplished slowly. Food itself is highly rewarding and it is mandatory that the participant find powerful rewards for her behavior of not eating. Members are to construct a list of ways by which they can reward themselves for not eating and to bring this list to the session for discussion. To reward herself for the development of self-control, the client should set limited and realistic goals and make a reward contract with herself for accomplishing the goal (e.g., "If I have a salad for lunch, I'll allow myself to read an interesting novel for one-half hour"; "If I eliminate all evening snacking this week, I'll treat myself to a movie Friday night"; "If I keep supper to 600 calories, I'll allow myself to watch a television program during a study break this evening"; "If I have a fruit salad for lunch, I'll allow myself a piece of pizza at the party tonight").

Another helpful procedure is to have the participant develop reinforcers that remove her from situations in which she is tempted to eat. For example, instead of stopping after class for a snack, she might go to her room and relax by listening to her stereo. If the participant tends to watch television and eat on Friday nights, she can arrange to attend a movie or play, having decided beforehand that she will not buy refreshments there.

A participant should also be encouraged to set up a self-reward system for long-term maintenance of self-control. For example, she can make a chart and give herself an X for each day she has limited her caloric intake to less than 1500 calories. For every ten X's she earns, she can buy a new stereo record. Or she might reward herself for every 5-pound loss by treating herself to a nice restaurant dinner (she should see to it that she has a small breakfast and lunch that day, however, so that her total caloric intake is not excessive). She may also place twenty-five or fifty cents in a jar for each day that she successfully limits her caloric intake, and use this money to purchase some desired object. The therapist should encourage group discussion of how each individual might establish an effective reward system for the development of self-control of eating behavior.

Developing Personally Meaningful Ultimate Aversive Consequences of Overeating

Each participant should develop and write out a rather long list (at least ten) of the ultimate aversive consequences (UAC's) of overeating and being fat. The trouble with overeating is that its undesirable consequences are far removed in time from the act of overeating. When a person is in a stimulus situation which tempts her to eat, she usually is not seriously contemplating the undesirable consequences that will later befall her because of her indiscriminate eating. However, if an individual can seriously contemplate and mentally rehearse these UAC's at the time a stimulus to eat inappropriately presents itself, these UAC's will serve to punish thoughts about overeating, and the actual behavior of overeating in such situations will be less likely to occur. Also if an individual actually has overeaten, immediate mental rehearsal and contemplation of the UAC's of this behavior will operate to make the individual feel guilty about overeating, so that it will be less likely to happen again. It is important that the client *not* rehearse the UAC's before actual appropriate eating because such a practice may invite adaptation to the aversive properties of the UAC's.

In composing her list, each member is to list UAC's which are specific and meaningful to her rather than generalized abstract statements (e.g., "Overweight women die younger"; "Overweight girls aren't popular dates"). Verbal descriptions of aversive consequences the members have actually experienced and are experiencing currently can be quite compelling (e.g., "Last summer some boys snickered at me when I appeared at the pool in my bathing suit"). Statements of actual or imagined social rejection, sarcastic treatment, critical references to bodily contours or proportions, extreme personal sensitivity over excess weight, demeaning inferences concerning professional incompetence or carelessness can all be effective (e.g., "When I wear shorts, my legs look like hams"; "That blind date never asked fat me out again"; "My mother-in-law's subtle sarcasm came through with 'You sure do love to eat, don't you, Betty?' "; "Because I choose to overeat, my Saturday night date is the TV set"; "My being overweight narrows my chances of getting married"; "People feel I'm sloppy because I'm overweight"; "Because I'm fat, my friends kid me about being carefree and irresponsible").

Participants are to memorize a large repertory of UAC's and to mentally rehearse them in situations in which they are tempted to eat or immediately after they have eaten inappropriately. They should carry the list and rehearse the UAC's frequently but should not rehearse them prior to appropriate eating.

Members should also be encouraged to keep an unflattering snapshot of themselves or of a very fat person in their purse and to view it often throughout the day, telling themselves that this is the high price they are paying for inappropriate eating. They should contemplate this picture when they encounter a situation in which they are tempted to eat inappropriately or immediately after indiscriminate eating.

The UAC's can thus serve as a punishment technique as the individual thinks of the ridicule, deprivation of sexual and social satisfactions, etc., resulting from excess weight. By verbal self-criticism in a situation in which she tends to eat inappropriately, she decreases the probability of her eating in such situations. Saying these self-criticisms immediately following indiscriminate eating serves to punish such behavior and reduce its future probability.

Obtaining Reinforcers from Areas of Life Other than Eating

While behavioral treatment is aimed directly at changing behavior, therapists must remember that behavior is to be broadly defined to include not only motoric behavior but verbal and emotional behavior as well. While much attention should be devoted to eating behavior per se, this does not mean that current behavior in other areas is to be ignored. Behavior therapy must be concerned with any behavior (or lack of it) that has a relationship to the eating behavior of the participants.

One of the most important things for the therapist and client to be aware of is that many people overeat because they are not receiving sufficient satisfaction from other areas of their life such as work, relationships with the opposite sex, companionship with one's own sex, recreation, leisure activities, etc. The therapist is to help each group member to survey major areas of her life, note where she is not gaining sufficient satisfaction, and help her (with the aid of the group) to develop behavior that will increase her satisfactions in these areas. Participants may have to be coached in ways to make themselves more attractive to men, ways to meet men, methods for obtaining better grades, procedures for being more popular with women, methods of meeting new friends, means by which they can develop more satisfying leisure activities, means for enjoying the nonacademic aspects of college, etc. The therapist may find a number of different techniques helpful here, such as role playing, examining irrational ideas, assertion training, coaching, and instructing participants in a hierarchy of desirable behaviors to be learned and practiced. Helping individual participants develop and maintain reinforcements from the major aspects of their lives will comprise one of the most important tasks of the treatment. To the extent that many participants can accomplish this, they will have less need to turn to overeating as one of the major pleasures in their living pattern.

Establishing Behaviors Incompatible with Eating

The disposition to eat can be lessened by supplanting it with other activities which are incompatible with eating. The behavioral repertoire in various situations should be developed so that activities incompatible with eating become strong and the eating behavior weakened. Whenever possible, these incompatible activities should be ones that the participant finds highly reinforcing. There are many ways in which participants can implement and apply this technique:

1. The client can save highly reinforcing activities for times when there is a tendency to eat (e.g., read a favorite magazine, read a newspaper, watch a television program, or perform other pleasant activities during work breaks).

2. When the client is tempted to eat, she can start highly reinforcing incompatible behaviors which will be aversive to interrupt (e.g., going for a walk, taking a bus ride, writing a letter, washing her hair).

3. The participant can develop reinforcing incompatible behaviors to perform in group situations when others are eating. When the other girls are sitting around, chatting and eating, she can polish her nails, smoke, or suck on a low-calorie piece of candy.

4. The participant can modify situations so that she would lose face by eating in these situations. For example, she will be less likely to eat dessert if she announces to her table companions, "I've given up all desserts this week." When offered a snack at a party she can respond, "No thank you, I've eliminated between-meal snacks this week." Such statements from the participant establish situations in which it would be incompatible for her to eat.

5. The participant can have a list of other activities she can substitute for eating. In the area of recreation, she can involve herself in a card game or engage in some sport (e.g., hiking) or competitive games (e.g., ping-pong). She can substitute work-related activities such as studying (having promised herself never to eat while studying), ironing, doing the laundry, or polishing shoes. She can choose social activities in which she will be less likely to eat, such as attending plays, movies, or concerts. She can keep her mouth busy by chewing gum, sucking dietetic hard candies, or smoking. Pleasures that are incompatible with eating but appropriate and available can be substituted (e.g., sexual activity).

6. One may eat to avoid other activities which have aversive aspects. In such situations the participant should be encouraged to rehearse the UAC's of eating and to perform some other reinforcing activity.

7. The participant can enlist friends to help her lose weight. She can go over her daily caloric intake with a friend whom she has asked to approve her successes and admonish her for her failures. She can also make bets with friends that she will lose so many pounds by a definite date.

8. It is important that the participant develop reinforcing incompatible responses which occur in response to various emotions that, in the past, have been followed by eating behavior. When depressed, she can phone a friend, go visiting, or force herself to watch a television program. When angered, she should learn to assert herself appropriately rather than to brood and eat. Engaging in physical exercise (e.g., swimming) can serve to combat both weight and tension.

9. The participant can respond to tension and anxiety by going through relaxation procedures (instead of eating) when she is in a situation where she can do this. After she relaxes, she can allow herself a short nap (setting the alarm to specify the length of her nap). Going through the relaxation procedure need not be confined to times when she is upset or anxious but can be used as a reinforcing break or activity to be substituted for eating, as in work breaks.

Utilizing Chaining

Chaining may be defined as a series of responses in which one response produces the stimuli for the next response. The frequency of the behavior that occurs at the end of a chain (in this case, eating) can be changed by altering the responses making up the chain. A chain can be broken or lengthened, or the consequences of certain responses in the chain can be manipulated so that the end behavior of eating will occur less frequently. Some ways in which participants may utilize chaining to make eating behavior less frequent follow.

Lengthening the Chain. The participants will tend to eat less but enjoy her food more if she takes small bites on the fork or spoon, does not start chewing till the fork is put down again near the plate, and does not put the next bite on the fork until the food in her mouth is chewed slowly, chewed well, and swallowed. While doing this, she should completely relish and enjoy her food as described in the first technique, "Building Positive Associations concerning Eating Control" (pp. 13–16). The participant can learn to slow her rate of eating (and thus decrease the amount she eats) by interrupting her eating behavior with conversation or holding the food on the fork for increasingly longer periods before placing it in her mouth. These interruption procedures can first be practiced near the end of a meal, when the participant is not so hungry, and gradually be moved toward the beginning of the meal. The participant can gradually learn to eat small amounts, slowly and with great pleasure. To be able to stop eating at any point, she can lengthen the chain of behaviors that would terminate in appropriate eating in many ways. The main goal is to have many steps in the sequence of actions which would have to occur between the desire to eat and the actual eating. The participant can make it inconvenient to eat inappropriately by refusing to carry money for snacks or change for vending machines. If she decides that she will do all of her snacking only at a fountain which is some distance from her home, she will be less likely to snack. The participant might allow only ten cents per day for snacks, thus forcing herself to save several days for a coke or even longer for a hamburger.

Learning to Eliminate Parts of a Chain. If the client refuses to have snacks around, she will not be able to engage in the behavior of swallowing food. If she carries only her checkbook with her and refuses to cash a check for food, she will be less likely to eat when she goes out. By walking a route where she cannot stop for food, she will not end up eating. By going with her friends to a movie instead of to a restaurant, she also reduces the probability of her eating.

Decreasing the Reinforcement for Individual Members of a Chain. When the participant first feels the desire to eat a snack, she should go over the UAC's or look at the picture of the fat lady or at an unattractive picture of herself; she can keep a list of the UAC's in her change purse and rehearse them when she starts to get change for food. At home, the participant can paste a picture of a fat lady on the door of the refrigerator. She can make it rewarding to resist the temptation to eat. Each time she refuses a snack, she can put a quarter in one section of her purse and use this money for other pleasures (e.g., records, new clothes).

Using Supplementary Aversive Conditioning Techniques

The techniques described here are to be employed in the situation where the participant is having difficulty abstaining from eating too much highly fattening food such as nuts, candy, pastry, starches, soft drinks. These techniques can be employed to reduce the intake of those foods. She should use these techniques only if she is eating too much of a particular fattening food and has not been able to limit eating this food by use of the other techniques. Some suggested techniques are:

1. The participant should think of this food very often (fifteen to twenty times per day) and imagine as vividly as she can that eating this food will make her extremely nauseous. She should associate this food with images of things that make her sick to her stomach. She should tell herself that that food will make her vomit if she eats it.

2. The participant can list the food on a card and carry it around with her. Several times each day she should take this card out (and possibly put it beside her "fat" picture) and tell herself that *this* food causes her to be fat and ugly.

3. The participant can consider the taste of this tempting food and imagine that the taste is so repulsive she cannot stand the flavor. She should vividly imagine the food tasting like something which she finds very unpleasant. She should try to convince herself that the particular food has this highly unpleasant taste. If, for example, the participant is fond of pizza, she can imagine pizza made with smelly spoiled sausage and modly bacteria-infested crust. She should tell herself the taste of pizza is unbearable and that eating it will make her vomit. She should go through the procedure several times daily, doing it first when she is not very hungry and when the temptation to eat this favorite food is low or nonexistent, and then gradually going through this imagining exercise when she is hungry and more tempted to eat the food.

THE PROBLEM OF CONTINUING LOSS AND MAINTENANCE

The ten-week program described herein has been demonstrated by controlled research (Hagen, 1974; Wollersheim, 1970, 1977a, 1977b) to be effective in promoting weight loss and to be adequate in teaching clients how to implement learning principles in changing their eating patterns. Nevertheless, depending upon their degree of obesity, a number of clients will have to continue weight loss after the formal treatment has terminated. Other clients will have to focus upon maintenance. Continued weight loss and/or maintenance are not easily accomplished after treatment as group reinforcement for weight loss terminates at this point. Some participants will not have lost enough of their excess weight to warrant enough reinforcement from their own appearance or from their family and friends to motivate them to endure the hardships of continued caloric restriction. It is important, therefore, in the last session to encourage members to continue setting realistic goals and pick themselves up immediately when they fall off their program of caloric restriction. Clients need to be reminded that once their desirable weight is reached, they can gradually increase and monitor their caloric intake to reach an amount that proves effective in keeping their weight constant. It is extremely helpful to encourage clients to monitor their weight weekly after they have reached their desirable weight and immediately to implement caloric restriction when they observe a weight gain of 2 pounds or more.

Clients who have a large number of pounds to lose can be further helped by attending booster sessions. The therapist can arrange for such clients to meet at regular intervals after the tenth session for 15–20 minutes to use the positive expectation-social pressure techniques and obtain encouragement to continue applying the learning principles which were detailed in the formal treatment program. After clients have lost a considerable and noticeable amount of their excess weight, natural reinforcements for such weight loss can be expected to occur in the ordinary living environment of the participants. Reinforcements from improved appearance, less fatigue, smaller clothing size, and positive comments from friends and family make it easier for clients to be less dependent on the reinforcement obtained during group meetings. The hardships of continued caloric restriction can then be more comfortably accomplished without the assistance of formally organized programs.

REFERENCE NOTE

1. Jeffrey, D. B. and Wollersheim, J. P. Cognitive theories: Applications and limitations in weight control. *Cognitive Processes and Problems in Weight Loss Management* (Thoresen, C. E., Chair). Symposium presented at the meeting of the American Psychological Association, Toronto, August 1978.

REFERENCES

Hagen, R. L. Group therapy versus bibliotherapy in weight reduction. *Behavior Therapy,* 1974, *5,* 222–234.

Mahoney, M. J. and Mahoney, K. *Permanent Weight Control: A Total Solution to the Dieter's Dilemma.* New York: Norton, 1976.

Wollersheim, J. P. The effectiveness of group therapy based upon learning principles in the treatment of overweight women. *Journal of Abnormal Psychology,* 1970, *76,* 462–474.

Wollersheim, J. P. Testing the efficacy of relaxation in a treatment package for obesity. *JSAS Catalogue of Selected Documents in Psychology,* 1977, *7,* 76 (Ms. No. 1531). (a)

Wollersheim, J. P. Follow-up of behavioral group therapy for obesity. *Behavior Therapy,* 1977, *8,* 996–998. (b)

13

Hypnotherapy in the Treatment of Obesity*

Milton V. Kline

Obesity, which has been a major area of concern to physicians, psychologists, and psychotherapists, continues to be a multidimensional problem from both an etiological and a treatment standpoint. By definition, obesity is a bodily state characterized by excessive collections of fatty tissue beneath the skin and within the tissue of organs of the body. In states of health, the skin is provided with a layer of fat which ordinarily increases and decreases as the state of health, the amount of food, and the amount of exercise vary. Obesity, however, can become a disease when the increase of fatty tissue interferes with the functions of the body and its various parts. The condition may be inherited or acquired. At the present time, both the means of inheritance and the dynamics or mechanisms of acquisition constitute intriguing and, at times, paradoxical and puzzling areas of investigation by scientists in many of the areas of behavioral investigation (Kline, Coleman, and Wick, 1976). The primary cause of most but by no means all cases of obesity is the ingestion of more food than is required by the body. Psychologists and psychotherapists probably confront more often than not, a condition in the past referred to as bulimia, now simply described as a feeding disturbance. The concept of feeding disturbance is a diagnostic entity and falls under the category of special symptoms.* This category is for the patient whose disturbance is manifest by a single specific symptom. Frequently, anorexia nervosa as well as obesity would be considered under feeding disturbance; they

---

*In some instances it may be secondary to more serious psychopathology.

fall in line with other special symptom disturbances such as speech problems, specific learning disturbances, psychomotor disorders, tics, disorders of sleep, enuresis, as well as a variety of less distinct, but equally disabling symptomatic problems. This category would not apply, however, if the symptom is an organic illness or in conjunction with a defect or a distinct mental disorder.

Needless to say, the problem of an eating or feeding disturbance is frequently overdetermined, and a simplistic solution from either a dietary or a psychotherapeutic point of view is not usually readily at hand. For this reason, a variety of therapeutic approaches have been developed, most of which are helpful to a percentage of patients suffering from feeding disturbances.* Thus, at the present time, we find that, like insomnia, obesity constitutes a symptomatic disturbance encountered in a very high percentage of the population, one that frequently creates frustration on the part of the patient, the physician, and the psychotherapist. Treatment results have generally been less than satisfactory and confirmation of this is to be found in the ever-expanding utilization of nonprofessional remedies, techniques, and approaches to the management of this disorder. In all fairness, it must be pointed out that while fad diets, pharmacologic therapies, and innovative psychotherapeutic approaches continue to evolve, no one specific approach, scientific or nonscientific in origin, has proved to be significantly helpful on a permanent basis to a vast percentage of individuals caught up in the dilemma of obesity.

Hypnotherapy, a specialized and selectively utilized treatment modality, constitutes an effective approach to the treatment of obesity either as a primary clinical entity or as a secondary syndrome in more serious emotional disorders.

GROUP HYPNOTHERAPY IN THE TREATMENT OF OBESITY

In recent years, the most strking evidence for the effective control and alteration of behavior has emerged from experimental investigations within the framework of learning theory and the extensive contributions of both clinical and experimental studies with hypnosis (Kline, 1971). The greatest significance of experimental work with hypnotherapy has been the indication of how behavior patterns can be altered and shaped through cognitively induced changes in perception, sensation, and the effective utilization of imagery (Kline, 1980). Although the use of highly specialized hypnotherapeutic procedures may not be indicated in all behavioral disturbances and is not readily available, the implications are that many of the mechanisms subject to alteration via hypnotic procedures are also accessible by directing other psychological approaches to the same learning modalities.

---

*A good account of this issue may be found in Andersen (1980).

It seems strongly indicated that many individuals, in the absence of severe psychopathology, are capable of altering patterns of disruptive, self-defeating, and frustrating behavior through the use of motivated cognition which places considerable emphasis upon the role of sensory and perceptual factors both in behavioral change and in the maintenance of this change. In this respect, the contributions of hypnosis and the state of homeostasis and spontaneous desensitization which ensues reflect the importance of reducing focal tension states which lead the individual to adopt a compensatory and frequently disruptive pattern of behavior (Kline, 1970a; Kline and Linder, 1969).

The treatment approach described here relates to those individuals whose obesity is intimately bound up with personality dynamics and for whom obesity is a disrupting, frustrating, and depressing element in their life patterns, but whose needs will best by met not by conventional psychotherapy, but rather by an effective program of therapeutic weight control. Previous investigations of the underlying mechanisms responsible for behavior change and particularly behavior alteration association with therapeutic gain in focally oriented hypnotherapy have emphasized the central role of desensitization and homeostasis (Kline, 1970b).

The selective and intensive use of hypnotherapy in the treatment of obesity has probably been as productive or more effective than other therapeutic approaches which exist at the present time. Nevertheless, the number of patients for whom hypnotherapy is an accessible treatment modality and who are in a position to obtain individual hypnotherapeutic care constitutes only a small minority of the obese population. The evidence that hypnosis as a technique can be useful in bringing about cognitive control over a wide variety of seemingly involuntary functions directly related to patterned or habitual behavior has been well documented in clinical investigations and reports (Kline, 1976, 1980).

There has been needed a therapeutic approach which might utilize the behavioral modification capabilities of hypnosis without the demand for high susceptibility levels and preferably in group form. Earlier reported work on the use of hypnosis in the treatment of cigarette habituation had revealed the fact that extended group sessions of five to ten hours within which hypnosis and group dynamics were combined, yielded a significantly higher rate of smoking control than any other reported method, and in a comparatively brief period of treatment. Self-hypnosis was an integral part of the treatment procedure (Kline, 1963, 1965, 1967, 1980).

The need to define, execute, and maintain effective control over deprivation behavior has been singled out as the major factor in the therapeutic success or failure in correcting or modifying habituation disorders. Feeding disturbances like cigarette smoking are closely bound up with deprivation mechanisms. The general dysphoria, irritability, depression, and even EEG changes noted in drug abusers undergoing initial deprivation have not been studied as well in obesity, nor is this behavior as simple to investigate although it appears to be similar.

Group hypnotherapy was utilized with a group of women who had repeatedly been able to lose weight under a group program of direct, diet-oriented motivation, only to regain the weight within a reasonable period of time, and thus were considered as treatment failures. The process was similar in its structural form to the operation of group therapy except for the fact that the group was instructed that there were to be only four group hypnotherapy sessions, each one month apart and each session would be five hours long.* Patients were further instructed that self-hypnosis would be a required part of the treatment between group sessions. The treatment orientation was explained within a framework of cognitive control of motivated behavior with an emphasis on concurrent issues in everyday life experience which created sufficient demand or stress to impair the voluntary capacity to control eating behavior while maintaining a low-calorie diet. The group action had little to do with dieting factors, but focused upon the stress situations in which these individuals lived and which produced for them varying degrees of tension that became linked with either feelings of hunger, visual preoccupation with food, or other sensory cues directly related to inappropriate and excessive eating behavior.

As part of the therapeutic approach, the group was impressed with the fact that voluntary control over eating behavior was possible and that the degree to which volitional behavior could be produced would depend on the ability to manage deprivation feelings. Deprivation behavior was described and defined as an emotional response to a feeling of inadequacy, frustration, irritability and, in general, a state of dysphoria. The reasons for these mood swings and attitudes were examined within the framework of the individual's everyday life patterns, both within the family and in other segments of the environment.

The group process permitted considerable ventilation and intensified interaction among the members of the group, and it continually focused and refocused upon individual patterns of deprivation behavior and the manner in which it would reflect itself in excessive eating patterns.

Hypnosis was induced initially during an individual clinical diagnostic session and again as part of a group induction. Group size was limited to a maximum of ten. The degree of hypnotic depth evidenced upon clinical examination was noted but was in no way used as a factor for inclusion in the treatment group.† The only patients excluded from this treatment program were patients with borderline diagnosis, in which the possibility of regression under stress existed,

---

*Cost effectiveness factors as well as treatment effectiveness were determinants of this format.
†Clinical depth proved to be insignificant in relation to initial treatment response.

and patients with a history of psychiatric hospitalization. Included were individuals with long-standing emotional disorders, previous periods of psychiatric or psychological therapy, and those still in treatment.

All patients were instructed early during the first group session in the induction of self-hypnosis. Group and individual induction techniques were employed with all group members. Group induction was also initiated by tape recording and reinforced by personal induction.* Clinically, it was noted that hypnotic depth tended to increase during the group experience, which had previously been noted in our work with cigarette and drug habituation. From the standpoint of therapeutic productivity, the most significant signs of increased hypnotic responsiveness resulting from one group experience were (1) increasing ease in developing visual imagery, (2) the production of bodily relaxation through self-hypnotic methods, and (3) the ability to induce affective states clearly recognized by the patient by virtue of subjective sensations. These states included for example, calmness, joy, energy, love, and strength. In an overall clinical assessment, it can be said that all patients in this program achieved a distinct level of hypnotic involvement by the end of the first five-hour group session. Though the range of depth was from very light to somnambulism, all could achieve self-hypnosis and evidenced developing ability to accommodate to the treatment conditions.

During the first session all patients were instructed in the development of relaxation through self-hypnosis, the relaxed state being defined subjectively by each patient himself. In addition, each group participant was given a small pack of seventeen cards upon which was lettered in bold print a word defining a particular affective state, which in an earlier psychosynthesis study (Assagioli, 1970) had been found to significantly enhance feelings of well-being. The patients in this treatment program selected as many affective or psychological conditions as they found desirable to induce via self-hypnosis. The words utilized in this study were *will, harmony, calm, energy, relax, wisdom, enthusiasm, goodness, joy, courage, love, silence, confidence, simplicity, serenity, gratitude,* and *patience*.

The procedure for utilizing the cards and inducing desired feelings was reinforced by individual tape recordings. After discussion and definition of deprivation in relation to food or eating, each patient organized a hierarchy of psychological conditions or states as described on the cards relative to what he felt would be most useful individually. Many thought that at different times, depending upon external as well as internal circumstances, different feelings and states of being would be most effective in combating the need to eat.

The states to be achieved were designated for use at peak or critical periods during the day in relation to maintaining diet control and deprivation management.

---

*Some advantages to this technique are evidenced in the use of self-hypnosis via tapes.

All patients were on a standard low-calorie weight control diet or one recommended by their personal physicians. At regular intervals during each day, determined in part by each person's daily routine and emotional reactions, they would induce self-hypnosis first for simple bodily relaxation. The period of relaxation recommended was ten minutes to be followed by five or more minutes of induced affective states chosen from the states described on the cards. The procedure for using the cards was as follows: following self-hypnosis and bodily relaxation with the eyes closed, each patient would continue the hypnosis but now with the eyes open. Concentration upon the chosen card for two or three minutes was recommended, to be followed by visual imagery of the printed word with eyes closed for at least five minutes, but longer if desired.

The general recommendations were for four self-hypnotic sessions per day, one in the morning, one in the afternoon, one after dinner, and one before retiring. The length was variable as described, but generally averaged about fifteen minutes per session. At times, more sessions were used and in some instances where deprivation reactions were intense, more periods of visual imagery for the words and induced states were recommended. The entire procedure was clearly defined during the first group session, and each patient practiced it until there was no question of technique. Questions regarding variations in the procedure, which might arise between the monthly group sessions, were handled by telephone conversations.

Each group session devoted some time to reinforcing the self-hypnotic procedures, intensifying the visual imagery, and assisting each patient to feel as completely as possible the induced states of well-being.

Assessment of the deprivation reduction system was evaluated in the second group session by subjective reports as well as by the use of an electronic pulsemeter and polygraphic responses indicative of respiratory patterns. Objective data were seen as a strong reinforcement to subjective awareness of deprivation reduction.

Part of the group sessions were devoted to training in self-hypnosis as described and to the integrated use of visual imagery and induced states of well-being in relation to the direct control of deprivation resulting from diet control. In addition, time was devoted to discussion and some evaluation of patterns of eating in relation to stress and tension stemming from family, work, and interpersonal relationships. Interaction within the group was utilized to dramatize the dynamics involved and to stimulate expression of those feelings most closely bound up with the desire for excessive eating. Hypnosis was used to stimulate a desire for particular foods not on the diet, and the attempt to create intense feelings of desire for such food objects was a primary function of each group session beyond the first. Following such stimulation, each patient would induce self-hypnosis and those states which reduced both the thought of, and drive for, food objects. Each patient was helped to create as intense a desire for a nondiet-food object as was possible, and in most instances, this was accomplished with much evidence of agitation, dysphoria, and anger in the face of the apparent frustration. It was at this point that the subjective value of tension deprivation reduction through the use of hypnotic methods became most apparent to each patient and created considerable confidence in the procedure and an emerging sense of self-mastery in relation to food deprivation and diet control.

The group also came to look upon the goal-directed weight loss as a group phenomenon and not just as an individual one. Aggregate weight loss for each group session became a focally determined goal, so that if an individual or several individuals in the group did not lose significant weight the fact that the total group weight might drop became a meaningful incentive and a measurable objective.

Individual methods of reducing stress or deprivation behavior at times when striving for food would become greatest were emphasized with a variety of psychological devices depending upon individual needs, characteristics, and the demand situation in which the individual functioned. Members of the group were encouraged to call each other when they felt inclined to move toward the food which they knew should voluntarily be eliminated. Self-directed thinking patterns and imagery activity designed to produce freedom from irritability, tension and, in general, a sense of deprivation were encouraged. This experimental program of group hypnosis, emphasizing the effectiveness of consciously directed efforts to alter drive and habituation elements in relation to food striving and food needs, met with initial success. All participants in this program* mailed in a weekly form to the therapist reporting two factors: (1) weekly weight loss and (2) a subjective checklist measuring the degree to which the prescribed diet had been followed. The results for the entire group were tabulated and mailed to each member. Weight loss was noticeable during the first week of the group's activity, and weight loss continued throughout the entire period of treatment. During this period, there were no dropouts.

A two-year follow-up indicated that 66 percent of the treatment population (350 patients) had lost and maintained a loss of 40 pounds or more. The remaining patients lost more than 15 pounds, but less than 25 pounds. After two years, 20 of the 23 patients in this study were still utilizing self-hypnosis, primarily for relaxation.

All the patients in this treatment program were able to follow the treatment procedures involving self-hypnosis and, in general, they deviated from the prescribed routine only under unusual circumstances. No significant variations can be reported. Most members of the group preferred to utilize one or two of the selected affective states, usually relying upon one, but at times working with another, depending on their personal feelings. All experimented with most of the

---

*Weight Control Treatment Program, The Institute for Research in Hypnosis and Psychology. New York, N. Y.

visually suggested states and tended to use those that were closest to their preferred feeling tones as well as most strongly experienced. After a while, most participants found they did not need the cards but could move right into the visual imagery. However, they did report that the cards were most useful in the beginning.

CASE ILLUSTRATIONS

A 56-year-old married woman, 32 pounds overweight, had sought medical help for many years in an attempt to lose weight. Previously, she had managed on a number of occasions to lose as much as 20 pounds, but could never maintain the loss for more than a month or two. She would always deviate from her diet by seeking ice cream and bread in excessive amounts. Other foods could be well controlled, but she could never maintain complete deprivation of these two. Without them, she would become irritable, depressed, and agitated. Through the use of self-hypnosis and the induction of a feeling of calmness as well as joy, she maintained her diet effectively and at the one-year follow-up level had lost 32 pounds, ate only moderate amount of bread, and had not had any ice cream since she entered the treatment program.

A 36-year-old woman, mother of three children, was seen during the first month of her fourth pregnancy. She weighed 193 pounds and was 5′ 4″ tall. She had been consistently overweight since adolescence and could only lose weight through large doses of amphetamines which had in the past produced only brief periods of weight loss, but resulted in severe depressive reactions and hysterical episodes which had required psychiatric treatment. Following the birth of each child, she experienced severe postpartum depression. She now not only desired to lose weight for the usual reasons, but was worried about the increased stress of pregnancy and the risks involved. She also felt that she would again become depressed if during this pregnancy she became still further overweight. This woman had always had moderate and diet-directed regular meals, but between meals she might consume several quarts of ice cream, pizzas, five or six hot dogs, and all varieties of cookies, cakes and candies. Upon entering the program, she evidenced initial resistance to the self-hypnotic procedures by forgetting to use them. At first, she deviated from the diet severely, but after the second group session, she began to consistently use the self-hypnosis, abandoned all her in-between meal eating and at the time she delivered a six-pound baby girl, she weighed 148 pounds.

One factor which appears most significant in relation to the effectiveness of this treatment method was the extent to which eating between meals was in many cases totally abolished and in others drastically curtailed. Our experience with most cases of obesity is that regular meals tend to be not any larger than for nonobese individuals, but that food intake between meals is excessive, compulsive, and the primary weight gaining device. The use of self-hypnosis, the management of food deprivation through a systematic method of self-mastery, and the motivating interaction of intensive group sessions during which deprivation control is acquired tend to abolish the habituation to in-between meal eating, eliminate obsessive concern with special foods, and lead to effective dietary management and weight control.

EMOTIONAL INTENSIFICATION AND EVOCATION IN HYPNOTHERAPY OF CHRONIC OBESITY IN PATTERNS WITH SEVERE EMOTIONAL DISORDERS: CLINICAL OBSERVATIONS

Emotional intensification and evocation constitute flooding procedures in relation to psychotherapy and have taken on a somewhat mixed and varied characteristic both in clinical reports and in experimental investigations. Frequently, flooding procedures are related to desensitization and, at times, implosive therapeutic techniques. There is, however, much modification of this, and some delimitation of the concept of flooding as a procedure in hypnotherapy is one of the purposes of this paper. Particularly, the use of hypnosis in relation to the elucidation of flooding responses and its integration into therapy in those instances where there are rather definitive indications for affective stimulation and experience prior to cognitive or lexical expression. Much of the research in this area has produced contradictory and, at times, confusing results (Kline, M. V., 1980).

The utilization of hypnotically induced flooding procedures in the treatment of chronic obesity in patients with severe emotional disorders wherein the obesity is a symptomatic component of the patient's illness has proved to be therapeutically effective.

Flooding procedures generally have been considered within the framework of behavior modification approaches and frequently have been aimed at the reduction or elimination of conditioned fear and avoidance behavior. It has also been clear that flooding may lead to a desensitization experience and, of course, this brings it into concomitant relationship with a variety of other therapeutic procedures, not all of which need necessarily be considered behavior modification in approach. Flooding would appear to parallel a variety of hypnotherapeutic procedures which produce either planned or spontaneous desensitization. The role of desensitization as a basic component of many aspects of hypnotherapy has been pointed out earlier (Kline, 1970a, 1976, 1980) and, in an experimental investigation, proved to be equally effective in the hands of more-skilled as well as less-skilled psychotherapists. It is of considerable importance to differentiate and evaluate therapeutic procedures in relation to both the efficacy of the results and the ease of implementation. If a particular therapeutic technique is tied exclusively or predominantly to a very high degree of therapeutic skill, then its applicability obviously will be limited.

Cobb, Ripley, and Jones (1973) have noted that during hypnosis, subjects tend to readily relive past experiences of strenuous exercise and have significant physiological alterations during the reliving of the past emotionally stressful situations. They further determined that the capacity to respond to suggestion was greater and more consistent during hypnosis than with intravenous sodium amytol.

The durability and the experiential quality or meaningfulness of a hypnotically elucidated response continue to be important elements in the use of this response within a therapeutic maneuver or treatment procedure. Those that can be more casually produced or those that can occur via suggestion without hypnotic transference involvement may constitute significant differences in the interacting experience for the patient and consequently lead to different responses or different results therapeutically. The need for flexibility and ingenuity in the treatment situation varies with the methodology of the laboratory and leads to equivocal and contradictory results. Nevertheless, I think we see that the role of hypnotic suggestion in being able to produce genuine affect and genuine recall, and in serving as a connecting link between cognitive and affective experience, is a central issue in any therapeutic approach which utilizes, either directly or indirectly, methods of desensitization and flooding. The viability of these clinical procedures within the framework of hypnotherapy requires us to define and assess the quality of the hypnosis and the experiences produced via the hypnotic situation and relationship.

Although the designation of therapeutic emotional flooding has in the recent clinical literature been related to behavior modification of primarily phobic reactions, it is clear that emotional flooding is operationally equivalent to older techniques of affect intensification, abreaction, and cathartic evocation — all of which are an integral part of the domain of hypnotherapy. The application of emotional flooding procedures through hypnotic intervention in psychotherapy with other than phobic patients has been reported by this author* and others (Morganstern, 1973). In relation to selected cases of obesity, it has proved to be an effective means of therapy and warrants further intensive clinical use.

SOME NOTATIONS REGARDING PSYCHOPHYSIOLOGIC ASPECTS OF EMOTIONAL FLOODING

There is evidence (Grossberg and Wilson, 1968) that skin resistance responses are more frequent during scene descriptions, while heart rate responses are more frequent during the actual image. Estimated vividness of the image was significantly correlated with heart rate, but not with skin resistance. Lang et al. (1970) found a similar relationship between vividness and both heart rate and skin

---

*Paper presented at the Scientific Meeting of the Society for Clinical and Experimental Hypnosis, Newport Beach, California, November, 1973, and the American Psychological Association, New York, 1979.

resistance response, although only heart rate correlated significantly with objective anxiety. One of the most consistent findings that has emerged from a review of psychophysiologic approaches to desensitization in the laboratory is that imagined phobic scenes as used in desensitization evoke large autonomic responses in scenes judged to be neutral and that, with repetition, these responses show a consistent decliment. This clinical observation has not generally been supported by psychophysiological evidence. Such a response increment does seem to be the exception rather than the rule and its occurrence may depend upon relatively high anxiety in a subject or on the frequent application of high-intensity stimulation. These conditions have been described as those which disrupt the usual process of habituation to repeat a stimuli and they lead to an upward spiral. This may be self-limiting and, in the end, will also lead to a reduction in autonomic anxiety responses. In reviewing a good deal of work reported to date, it would seem that, in the main, flooding appears to be somewhat superior to desensitization for the reduction of pathological fear (Morgenstein, 1973).

Hypnotic flooding is clearly not a technique to be applied to patients indiscriminately. It does cut down treatment time significantly, even for patients with other than anxiety reactions. It seems to be particularly effective in the management of a number of hysterical components within a broad range of emotional and behavior disorders. Prolonged flooding has been instrumental in reducing residual symptoms both of an obsessional nature and, in many instances, of somatic formation. Flooding, as a psychotherapeutic procedure, appears to be extremely promising as a technique not simply for the reduction of pathological fear but also for the treatment and management of a wide range of psychological and psychophysiological disorders.

The diagnostic labeling of neurotic disorders has many advantages and disadvantages. While we are familiar with the definitive considerations of hysterical disturbances and obsessional disorders, we are equally aware that the vast majority of severe neurotic disorders involves a combination of symptomatic configurations within which hysterical and obsessional features are frequently found.

Over the years, a number of specific hypnotherapeutic techniques have been found to be particularly successful in dealing with individuals whose emotional disturbances, among other things, include hysterical and/or obsessional features. Frequently, it is the hysterical or obsessional feature which becomes a symptomatic block in the patient's recovery, offers significant resistances to treatment procedure, and tends to become focalized on the patient's part in terms of seeking relief. Since the primary goal and purpose of psychotherapy is, in a pragmatic sense, to bring relief to a patient in distress, it is not unwarranted or without meaning to attempt to deal directly with those elements in emotional and behavioral disorders which may constitute the binding or blocking mechanism and frequently constitute the focal symptomatic problem. As therapists, we are well aware that other issues play predominant roles in the origin of the patient's difficulties and in working out of long-term solutions. On the other hand, the ability to relieve those hysterical and obsessional features which may be present has been found to offer an avenue to the spontaneous recovery in other areas of patient behavior.

The hysterical components of neuroses are generally characterized by involuntary psychogenic loss or disorder of function. This may vary in degree and kind. Symptoms frequently begin and end suddenly in emotionally charged situations. While some of these symptoms can be modified by suggestion alone, there are a number which tend to involve a mixture of conversion and dissociative reactions which do not respond readily to suggestive or supportive approaches.

With the presence of some degree of dissociation, there can be distinct but fluctuating states of alterations of consciousness or in identifying process, such as to produce symptoms which are in part related to alterations in memory including a tendency toward amnesia, some partial rather than complete degrees of somnambulism, aspects of fugue, and even personality alterations suggestive of, but not typical of, multiple personality (Kline, 1980).

Bulimia as a symptom is frequently tied in with significant secondary gains, displacement behavior, and evidence of regression to oral levels of instinctual functioning. As the dynamic mechanism of coping with regressive elements in characteriologic disorders, the feeding disturbance not only assumes aspects of an organ neurosis but is based upon clearly defined hysterical and obsessional elements in the patient's personality. The resulting obesity can be successfully treated only by gaining access to these components. The need to liberate the atavistic and primary process nucleus of a feeding disturbance symptom can frequently be best approached through hypnotic intervention and the use of emotional flooding procedures.

It is through the use of hypnosis as an exploratory and uncovering, as well as a sensing, device that one becomes more and more aware of the degree to which the hysterical components involve many or all of the features specified above. Sometimes, these exist in such subtle form as not to be present except inferentially, and are difficult to contact except at levels of therapeutic involvement which require the kind of unconscious participation that may be possible through intensive analytic work or, more specifically and directly, through briefer dynamically oriented hypnoanalytic procedures (Kline, 1968). Along with the hysterical features, the obsessive-compulsive characteristics involve the intrusion of a number of unwanted thoughts, urges, or actions with which the patient becomes preoccupied, but with which he is unable to deal. The cognitive disorders may range from those which involve actual concern with ruminating ideas or trains of thought to relatively subtle reversions to earlier experiences, concepts, and associations. While actions typically may involve a simple to complex ritualistic movement, the most typical to be encountered are those which are anxiety and distress oriented and in which the patient generally has the feeling of not experiencing a normal sense of self-mastery. Feeding disorders are most frequent symptoms of this level of psychodynamic conflict.

Emotional flooding in hypnotherapy is a means of directly encountering the hysterical and obsessional elements frequently found in mixed neurotic disturbances in which therapeutic progress has been stopped by the symptomatic distress usually unresponsive to a reasonable amount of psychotherapeutic work and frequently unresponsive to pharmacologic therapy. Obesity is typical of this circumstance. The utilization of hypnotic procedures with emotional flooding involving the integration of sensory and motor phenomena along with cognitive activity has been found in a number of instances of extremely refractory patients to bring about relatively rapid improvement, alleviation of distress, and the stimulation of an ability to deal with other psychological issues in the patient's life once the focalization process has been disrupted and a meaningful degree of symptomatic relief obtained. Most noticeable is the rapid emergence of an increased sense of self-mastery, particularly in relation to regressive function as may be found in eating compulsions.

Flooding is produced following the induction of hypnosis by utilizing sensory and motor responses that appear to be linked to conflict stimulation, as previously described (Kline, 1963), and somewhat related to fantasy evocation techniques. Concentration upon the focal aspects of presenting symptoms or already examined defensive characteristics are used in order to enlarge and create an expansive model for the imagery. Suggestions are usually in keeping with the patient's personality style and with the dynamics of therapy as it has thus far evolved. Intensification is brought about by direct suggestion of affect linked to imagery in some instances and, in others, by indications that what is being experienced will grow stronger or clearer or closer. Additional feelings and sensations usually emerge spontaneously and continue in intensity, in keeping with the patient's wish to experience that which is being explored.

Hypnotic intensification of sensations and images related to the patient's eating behavior, associations to oral experiences, and related imagery have proved most provocative in liberating the repressed primal sources of orally regressed eating symptoms and in their eventual integration into more voluntary, cognitively structural behavior.

Frequently, there is a rapid regression to more complete sensory and motor levels of behavior with vivid intensification of imagery. Verbalization is not encouraged until the patient reveals a wish to do so. At times, the flooding experience may proceed on a completely nonverbal level and become incorporated into nocturnal dreaming or, toward the end of the session, into verbal expression.

In considering much of the material that comes forth following intense emotional flooding with imagery, one aspect which is most striking is similar to what appears to be inner speech and thought. The articulation of feeling, the experience of thought that remains within the sensory order, becomes much more available to the patient and frequently is revealed either through activity of an affective nature, sensory response, or physiological activity. When this continues for sufficient time, and the time element is of considerable importance, it will then be reflected in cognitive activity and verbal expression. Observations to date with the use of flooding techniques in hypnotherapy suggest that what happens is a rapid intensification of speech impulses which then give rise after a period of time to mental operations which become articulated as speech and spontaneous thought. The system of externalized speech has, however, within it many of the characteristics of the internalized speech order, very much like some of the dynamisms of dream production. Thus, in terms of the speech patterning itself, or the stylizing of the speech as well as the lexical or linguistic structure, we are dealing with a different kind of expression, which can best be referred to as inner speech, and its organization into spontaneous and, at times, clearly regressive aspects of cognitive expression (Kline, 1971).

The process of emotional flooding is useful in dealing with patients, regardless of the type of pathology or disturbance presented, who have in common the problem of poorly organized and poorly operating communication systems within the self and a distinct gap or distance between inner speech, inner thought, and externalized speech and thought. The bridging and integrating of this process has proved to be an effective and at times rapid means of creating productive therapeutic progress and symptomatic improvement where the focal symptom, as in obesity, is the use of regression to satisfy instinctual needs deprived of adequate ventilation and fulfillment through interpersonal experience.

CASE HISTORIES

Case 1

This 21-year-old obese woman, married, divorced, and remarried, was admitted to the psychiatric section of a general hospital from the emergency room where she was brought after slashing her wrists superficially in an attempt to get herself admitted to the hospital. The patient had a long but intermittent psychiatric history since the age of fifteen when she began staying home from school, lying around the house or staying in bed, and spending most of the time masturbating. Since that time, she had been seen by a number of psychiatrists and psychologists. The patient was married at the age of seventeen, immediately following her high school graduation. Despite many absences from school, she was bright and did well.

From the age of sixteen on, she began to gain excessive weight through what she termed binging. She could consume three quarts of ice cream and pounds of cookies following her dinner. She frequently would carry a large jar of peanut butter and jelly in her handbag and would eat it throughout the day. Her eating habits were extreme, bizarre and, for her, depressing to the point of suicidal ideas.

All types of diets and diet therapies including "fat doctors" and pills were sought at various times, with initial success and rapid regression. She hated to look at her body when overweight and at times of extreme obesity would become a recluse. She could lose weight readily when free of her compulsive eating, but only for brief periods of time.

Immediately following her marriage, she became pregnant and then became so disturbed that a therapeutic abortion was performed on psychiatric recommendation. While in group therapy, she was divorced, met a man in the group, and married him. At the time that she was referred to the present therapist, she was married to this husband and weighed 260 pounds. Three months after this marriage, she had become pregnant upon her own wish, and both she and her husband looked forward to having the child. She began vaginal bleeding several weeks after learning of her pregnancy. The vaginal bleeding continued over the course of approximately two months, and she was on bed rest and in the hospital on two occasions. The patient was told she could not have relations with her husband unless the bleeding stopped for three days, but over the course of about a month and a half, there was always bleeding more frequently than for three days, so she had no relations with her husband during that time. The patient felt extremely frustrated sexually, and gradually became more and more annoyed over having to call her gynecologist. She had never been able to achieve orgasm by manual masturbation and had discovered that using a vibrating electric razor on her external genitalia did serve some form of sexual gratification. However, on the several occasions that she used this, bleeding would occur soon afterward and these two events were related in her mind. One night she said, "What the hell," and used the electric razor again. Following this, she stayed up most of the night waiting for what she felt would happen and, indeed, at 5 A.M. she began to bleed. She was admitted to the hospital, examined by the resident, and told that she was having a spontaneous abortion. While in the hospital, she began to feel extremely upset. She resumed psychiatric treatment following her discharge, becoming during the course of this treatment more and more irritable and depressed. Her psychiatrist admitted her to the hospital when she appeared suicidal in his office, and she remained in the hospital for seventeen days at which point she was discharged because her insurance had run out. The diagnosis at that time was depressive reaction and chronic undifferentiated schizophrenia.

At the time she was referred for hypnotherapy she had had several more psychiatric hospitalizations, including one state hospitalization because the psychiatric section of the general hospital found her unmanageable after she had started a fire in the kitchen of the hospital and thrown boiling water on a psychiatric resident. Following a period of several months at a state hospital, her parents and an attorney obtained her release and she was referred to the present therapist for continued help. At the time of her discharge, the psychiatric summary was as follows:

This obese twenty-one year old married woman with a marked psychiatric history has had many episodes of depression, hysterical and psychosomatic complaints and sadomasochistic perverse sexuality following what must have seemed to her, the self-induced abortion of a wanted child. Diagnosis: Hysterical personality with underlying chronic schizophrenic process.

When first seen, she appeared to be depressed, withdrawn, extremely childlike and defensive, but at the same time, reaching out for help. She was prone to move into long monologues essentially descriptive of turmoil, discomfort, and intermingling historical aspects of her life.

She responded well to hypnosis, achieving relatively deep involvement within a short time, and was able to relax completely and, at the same time, describe her ability to be aware of suggested sensory experiences and image formation.

Emotional flooding techniques were utilized primarily to amplify imagery related to reconstructed life situations, and it was suggested that she describe those situations to herself, mentally, rather than to the therapist. Eventually, she was encouraged to translate these experiences and to discuss them within the hypnotic situation.

During one hypnotic session, when emotional flooding had produced intense bodily reactions, the patient, after a short period of abreactive exhaustion said, "Let's talk."

This is a stream of ideas, uncensored and yet not unthought out, that I would like to put down. I have a desire to go back into my childhood and relive all those years with different patterns of doing, including those of eating. Habits form and are of long standing, and it is only by reliving them that I can be different. Not only eating, but reading, studying, playing, loving, and enjoying. In fact, all doing, revisited. That is really what I would like to have happen, and the moving of my head back and forth, as I did in the first two sessions, is a sign that I wanted to do that. I did it when may uncle hypnotized me, and I went back to a long-past experience.

My left hand wants to help, but it is only a part and has difficulty communicating with the whole. When it moves the fingers, as if it were playing the piano, it is agreeing and happy, but it's not very vocal and really has only a voice of agreement or disagreement. All week it has liked some ideas but lacked the enforcement.

At one point, I felt an electric shock. The legs moving, I feel now, though not then, were asserting that there was more to me than the left hand.

My throat hurt, and I wondered if you could cure it.

In a further session, the patient verbalized her experiences of flooding that had been directed to an area of identity conflict which emerged during the previous session. While the flooding was in progress, she expressed the following awareness:

I was aware of a rape fantasy going on and this seemed to follow childbirth. My abdomen then was opened and snakes were put in. They were trained to go up and down to the vagina and bite on any penis that might enter. They could also go up and come out my tits. I would like to have a hysterectomy performed though I might as well turn myself into a man, physically. Shrinking up into a little ball. Very strong clitoral stimulation. It's almost overwhelming, yet I want to go to sleep. I can "feel" my mother nursing my sister and the terrible anger that my mother expressed and the baby turning red and the eczema following the next day.

The patient then assumed a fetal-like position and entered what seemed to be a sleeping state. A few moments later, she said:

Now I want to have intercourse — the vaginal feeling all over — I feel different about it — I feel very sexual both clitorally and in conjunction with more of me. "That" would suffice — I want somebody not to play with me — I feel very oral — I want someone to kiss me and put their tongue in me — I feel like encompassing someone — I'd like to suck a cock.

I'm a little child petulant child in an ass with all the shit around me. I feel obstinate and stubborn — I'm sitting here — I won't get out — I'm in command. I do this with people all the time — it seems to be related to money — I hate to pay some people.

Imaginal activity typically revealed low tolerance for any kind of frustration. She would frequently exhibit an explosive volatile temperament at which time she would throw herself around on the couch, talk to herself, and become extremely negativistic and infantile. Her poorly controlled emotional outbursts appeared to have a large role-playing component, and she was encouraged to structure imagery in which she would act out these feelings. In talking to herself about her physical symptoms, they would appear to be bizarre and blood curdling and clearly self-induced. While acting out intense episodes in hypnosis, she eventually came to translate and discuss them outside the hypnosis. She would suddenly be capable of increasingly better control and would be rather good humored and reasonable, although very coy in a little-girl fashion. She began more and more to relate directly to the therapist. She was able after several weeks of this kind of experience to state that her dreams and magical expectations would never turn out the way she wanted them, and that if she were to persist in seeking this type of outcome in life, life would always be intolerable. Although extremely attractive, when asked to intensify the image of herself, she would describe herself as ugly and empty, and she related many scenes of abandoment and loss of love.

Emotional explosiveness disappeared rapidly. She began to use self-hypnosis to structure more and more desirable outcomes.

She began a carefully prescribed low-calorie diet and was able to maintain it without deviation during the duration of therapy. Weight loss was dramatic and consistent.

Six months after treatment, she and her husband moved several hundred miles away, where he had obtained a new job. She became pregnant and, during the first six months of the pregnancy, came in once a month and eventually had a healthy female child. The marriage relationship worked out well, and one year after the birth of her child, during which there had been communication with the therapist but no actual visits, she indicated that she had begun to attend a branch of the state university on a part time basis and was contemplating completing an undergraduate degree in preparation for being a teacher. She reported that she ate normally and now weighed 130 pounds.

Emotional flooding played an important role in permitting this patient to express impulses and infantile needs which up to that time she had been acting out. The abreactive aspect had a cathartic and desensitizing effect, as well as increasing her ability to relate to the therapist and her acceptance of the therapeutic relationship. The ability to "talk to herself" led to a greater understanding of herself in ways that before had not been present in her thinking. She could now express her ideas in a totally different context and could exercise judgment and reasonableness in a way that, on a voluntary level, had never been available to her. It is anticipated that this patient will continue to have some difficulties from time to time, but fundamentally, she will continue to make progress. The self-hypnotic experiences continue to be used both for relaxation and, obviously, although she does not emphasize it, to reinforce her ability to talk to herself.

Case 2

Another example of the use of emotional flooding is in the following case of a 48-year-old physician with a history of anxiety and depression and still suffering from impotence and obesity despite a number of years of analytic treatment. He sought hypnotherapy for some modification of these symptoms. Emotional flooding during hypnosis was directed toward his sensory experiences during the induction of hypnosis which had been verbalized spontaneously following eyelid closure as a "feeling of horror – very unpleasant – chills throughout all of me."

Suggestions for visualization and intensification of this experience produced the following description: "The scene is pulling in all directions. All the corners. Turmoil. Now it fades away. Shadows take over the screen." The patient then described the fact that his penis was shrinking and he expressed feelings of tremendous fear and impotence. Then, quite suddenly, he began to describe the recollection of a dream sometime back in which "I couldn't place things properly. I now remember the feeling. It must have been panic. That's what is was. I didn't know it then, but I know it now. And, that's what I've got now. Yes. I'm feeling extreme panic." He began to rub one finger over another and said, "It's as if it's not my skin. Touching something else, just as though these two pieces of skin are not both part of me. Touching something strange – stonelike, yet some warmth is there."

He then continued almost by way of self-interpretation to say, "I see this is related to a dream I had a couple of months ago. It was about [and here he used the name of a woman with whom he had been having an affair]. This woman had many qualities which were very male and I must have seen her as a male frequently. I'm suddenly aware that I have had homosexual feelings – not just homosexual ideas that I learned about in my analysis, but really homosexual feelings – and they're really not so bad, they're not frightening at all. In fact, they feel rather good and warm." The patient then began to put his two fingers together very strongly and said, "It's her body. It really is. It's her body."

In the following session, hypnosis was induced and the eyelids began to flutter a great deal. The face squirmed almost uncontrollably and then he began to relax – the eyelids still fluttering. The patient placed his hands over them to quiet and control them. Suggestions for the flooding experience were then introduced.

The patient experiences an apparent spontaneous regression during which there was a great deal of licking of the lips and sucking. He began to talk primarily to himself rather than to the therapist, describing the fact that he felt very hungry and experienced sensations of great dryness in his throat. He seemed to be distraught, agitated, and frustrated. The depth of hypnosis began to lift at this point and he said that he felt he was coming out of it. He said that the oral sensations had disappeared. Instructions were given for reintensification of the flooding procedure. The patient began to sigh deeply — tremendous sighs — and then began to roll back and forth in a rocking motion on the couch. He seemed again very distraught and agitated, saying:

All my thoughts are associated with my mother's breasts and I feel a stirring in my penis. It seems to go away however, as I talk about it. I think of my mother, not as today, but when I was a little boy. I feel like a baby at her breasts. I don't feel as though I received something. I don't feel the hunger or the parched feelings in my throat now. I feel as though I received something. My fingers and hands are cold now. You know, my mother is really very plastic — like clay to me — she's not real. That's it — she never was real. No love — love was only a form of protection — overprotection — clothing, shelter, food. She didn't want me — she wanted a girl. Perhaps I was a girl until my sister came along. There was no need to pretend. I felt crushed and abandoned like I feel now. I feel fat and ugly. What a thing to carry through life. I always wanted my mother's love. I never got it. Now I know — now I remember — there wasn't any to give. You know, I feel that I've grown up. I don't need her. For the first time, I realize this — but in a different way than I've ever known before — I don't need it any more. I think of all the damage I've done to myself, my family, because of it.

At this point, the patient went into an apparently very deep hypnosis and said, "I feel the depth in my eyes. I can see whatever I need to now. Whatever I need to — I know how to see." Diet control was manifest from this point on, and in four months the patient lost 50 pounds which he has still maintained two years later.

Case 3

A 44-year-old college professor experienced panic states during lectures at the university and increasing fear of colleagues' judgments. He was aware that he was becoming somewhat paranoid and fearful of not being able to maintain control of himself in the presence of others. He had always been concerned about his ability to compete professionally and had never accepted his accomplishments but only his limitations. Several years of psychoanalysis had created a buffer against some of the anxieties in everyday life, but had not permitted him to move ahead as he had wished to. At this point, he seemed to be experiencing a crisis both professionally and in his marriage and, once again, sought psychotherapy, this time with hypnosis. Obesity had been a problem for more than ten years and had been accepted as "incurable."

During the induction of hypnosis, he had become aware of some strange feeling in his hand, and emotional flooding was developed around the intensification of the sensations and the visual image of the hand. The patient then described the following awareness, "I don't want to have a hand like this." At this point, the patient threw himself on the floor, began to scream in anguish and gradually regressed to an infantile state during which he rolled over and over again and crossed the room back and forth, screaming in a childlike voice, but not very coherently. Then, suddenly he became quiet and said:

Self-awareness seems to begin at the shoulders. They feel full and strong and not without resemblance to the shoulders of an athlete. That's rather vain on my part, I guess. At any rate, the shoulders support a base that's a body. Although I do not feel the rest of my body as clearly, I have to imagine that with such a pair of shoulders, only a vibrant and strong body can be attached. Body – shoulders – and body again – the mind is silent – like someone who, having tried doing something and not having succeeded, will step aside and watch the next fellow take over – watch with interest how he does it and how he succeeds. It would be silly to talk of an angry separation of mind and body – the mind being somewhat disdainful. No. It is my body that has taken over and my mind, the very interested onlooker, watches.

A great fear may immobilize the person on the spot. Eyes closed, deaf and blind and mute, all the senses surrender their function and the body ceases to move. What use is there for such a body completely cut off from its environment? None. And, so far as it clings on to the mind, will reduce utterly the meaning of the body to the point where it can no without the body. Poor body! First immobilized – then loosening all its functions with the surroundings – then shrinking in size – then on the verge of complete disappearance – freedom – that's when fear dies. That's when something would give back to the body its lost attributes. The first thing the body would do coming out is like Sleeping Beauty from a deep and long-lasting slumber or like Lazarus coming out of death – the first thing the body would do coming out is MOVE – make a movement – perhaps a passionate movement. Something is going on inside me and I don't believe I have ever had such an experience. "Inside" would not mean in this instance my mind, but rather the flesh and bones of my body. Let's assume my body has a mode of knowledge all its own. It perceives, arranges perception, and acts upon them all by itself. It does not have to sum up signals to the mind and wait for answers before proceeding with the necessary steps. No. My body is fully organized – silently organized. Should I run screaming that my body is taking over and henceforth will lead my life? No. I feel no compulsion. The movements of the body are smooth, correspond totally to a given goal – nothing hectic, irrational, or hysterical.

The feeling of satisfaction borne in the body tends to communicate itself — to permeate — to enter and color the mind. Black Power. Black revolution to restore in the Black man his pride trampled underfoot for so long. Extinguish the deep-seated and devastating fear within. Indicate that this fear is not imbedded for all eternity and can be expulsed. Do not tackle the causes of fear but rather insist on the possibility of loosening it — freeing one's self. The body as a means of liberation, as a state of liberation, even if no explanation has been provided for the fear — bypass fear, so as to speak. That remains to be seen.

Following this flooding experience, the patient had a number of spontaneous dreams, many going back to childhood, dealing with and clarifying a number of conflicts that had occurred but had never been resolved. He made great use of silent articulation and when it was expressed verbally, filtered through sensory bodily experiences, it came through as meaningful, productive, well-organized thought. This thought exerted considerable influence upon him and he began to undertake writing courses which before had terrified him.

As part of an emerging clarification and commitment to the self, a rigorous diet and a regime of exercise were spontaneously undertaken. One year later the patient had maintained a normal pattern of eating, weighed 152 pounds, as compared to 201 pounds at the start of treatment, and now described himself as productive and free.

The use of hypontically induced emotional flooding in the treatment of obesity in patients with severe emotional disturbances can be effective and relatively brief. In these cases, hypnotherapy must be applied within a framework of dynamic psychotherapy which perceives the obesity as a symptom directly related to the regressive behavior of the patient and to the deprivation of instinctual needs through available life experiences. As part of an intensive psychotherapeutic approach, hypnotic emotional flooding can gain rapid access to areas of oral conflict and create more cognitive sources of behavior regulation. Obesity constitutes a distinct threat to one's health and is frequently associated with depressive reactions resulting from the increasing effects of obesity, both socially and psychodynamically. From every point of view, the need to mobilize all resources of research and treatment in order to combat this problem effectively is a most urgent one at the present time.

REFERENCES

Andersen, M. S. The treatment of obesity by hypnotherapy. Doctoral dissertation, The International Graduate School of Behavioral Sciences, 1980.

Assagioli, R. The Technique of Evocative Words. P.F.R. Issue No. 25, Psychosynthesis Research Foundation, 1970.

Baum, M. Entinction of avoidance responding through response prevention (flooding). *Psychiatric Bulletin*, 1970, *74*, 276-284.

Borkovec, T. D. Effects of expectancy on the outcome of systemic desensitization and implosive treatments for analogue anxiety. *Behavior Therapy*, 1972, *3*, 29-40.

Boulougouris, J. C. and Marks, I. M. Implosion (flooding): A new treatment for phobias. *Br. Med. J.*, 1962, *2*, 721-723.

Boulougouris, J. C., Marks, I. M., and Marset, P. Superiority of flooding (implosion) to desensitization for reducing pathological fear. *Behav. Rs. Ther.*, 1971, *9*, 7-16.

Calef, R. A. and Mac Lean, G. D. A comparison of reciprocal inhibition and reactive inhibition therapies in the treatment of speech anxiety. *Behavior Therapy*, 1970, *1*, 51-58.

Cobb, L. A., Ripley, H. S., and Jones, J. W. Free fatty acid mobilization during suggestion of exercise and stress using hypnosis and sodium amytal. *Psychosom. Med.*, 1973, *35*, (5).

DeMoor, W. Systemic desensitization versus prolonged high intensity stimulation (flooding). *Journal of Behavior Therapy and Experimental Psychiatry*, 1970, *1*, 45-52.

Grossberg, J. M. and Silson, H. K. Physiological changes accompanying the visualization of fearful and neutral situations. *J. Pers. Soc. Psychol.*, 1968, *10*, 124-133.

Kline, M. V. (Ed.). *Clinical Correlations of Experimental Hypnosis*. Springfield, Ill.: Thomas, 1963.

Kline, M. V. (Ed.). *Psychodynamics and Hypnosis: New Contributions to the Practice and Theory of Hypnotherapy*. Springfield, Ill.: Thomas, 1967.

Kline, M. V. Sensory hypnoanalysis. *Int. J. Clin. Exp. Hypn.*, 1968, *16* (2), 85-100.

Kline, M. V. The use of extended group hypnotherapy session in controlling cigarette habituation. *Int. J. Clin, Hypn.*, 1970, *18* (4), 270-282.

Kline, M. V. The role of desensitization and homeostasis in relation to the therapeutic gain derived from hypnotherapy. *Psychotherapy: Theory, Research and Practice*, 1970, *7* (4), 213-216. (b)

Kline, M. V. Research in hypnotherapy: Studies in behavior organization. *Beitrage zur Verhaltenforschung, Akt. Fragen. Psychia. Neurol.*, (Bilz, R., and Petrilowitsch, N., Eds.) Vol. 11. Basel: Karger, 1971.

Kline, M. V. Psychodynamic issues in The Treatment of Obesity By Hypnotherapy (in press) 1980.

Kline, M. V., Coleman, L. L., and Wiek, E. *Obesity, Etiology, Treatment and Management*. Springfield, Ill.: Thomas, 1976.

Kline, M. V. and Linder, M. Psychodymanic factors in the experimental investigation of hypnotically induced emotions with particular reference to blood glucose measurements. *J. Psychol.*, 1969, *71*, 21-25.

Lang, P. J., Lazovik, A. D., and Reynolds, D. J. Desensitization, suggestibility and pseudotherapy. *J. Abnorm. Psychol.*, 1965, *70*, 395-402.

Malleson, N. Panic and phobia: A possible method of treatment. *Lancet*, 1959, *1*, 225-227.

Morganstern, K. P. Implosive therapy and flooding procedures: A critical review. *Psychol. Bull.*, 1973, *9*, 318-334.

14

Exercise and Obesity

Allan Geliebter

As Americans become more health conscious, they are increasing their participation in physical activity. A recent Harris poll (1979) revealed that 59 percent of Americans over 18 were exercising for more than two and a half hours per week, with the most popular exercise being walking; a poll in 1961 showed only 24 percent of Americans exercised this much per week. It is too early to tell whether this increase in physical activity will eventually cause a decline in the incidence of obesity which has been steadily increasing since 1863 (Van Itallie, 1979).

For a long time,the emphasis in treating obesity has been on reducing food intake. But, food intake is only part of the picture. Obesity results when calorie intake exceeds energy expenditure. Energy expenditure, long neglected, is now being given more attention, in part because of the public's surging interest in exercise.

Two reasons often given to detract from the value of exercise in treating obesity are:

1. Exercise uses up relatively little energy. For example, to burn off a pound of fat, a person would have to walk for 14 hours.

2. Exercise automatically leads to an increase in appetite so that any benefits are automatically canceled by an increase in food intake.

To deal with the first objection, there is no reason why the weight must be taken off with a single bout of exercise. After all, obesity is a condition that has gradually developed over many years. By walking an extra 1 hour per day (provided food intake is constant), a person can lose a pound every 2 weeks and 25 pounds in a year.

EXERCISE AND APPETITE

The second objection can also be refuted. During 1954–56, Mayer and his associates conducted two elegant studies. Rats that had been accustomed to a sedentary existence in a cage were exercised on a treadmill for various durations, ranging from 20 minutes to 6 hours daily. Their spontaneous food intakes and body weights are shown in Figure 14-1. Rats exercised for short periods, 20 to 60 minutes, significantly decreased food intake and lost weight as compared to rats that remained sedentary. Above 1 hour, food intake increased proportionately so that weight was maintained. Above 6 hours, the rats became exhausted and rapidly lost weight.

To extend these findings to man, Mayer et al. (1956) studied 213 men in West Bengal who worked in a jute company. Their work was classified into five categories of physical activity, ranging from sedentary to extremely hard manual work. Food intakes were obtained by interview and body weights were measured. As can be seen in Figure 14-2, in the sedentary range both calorie intake and body weight increased. It is only within the more active range that food in-

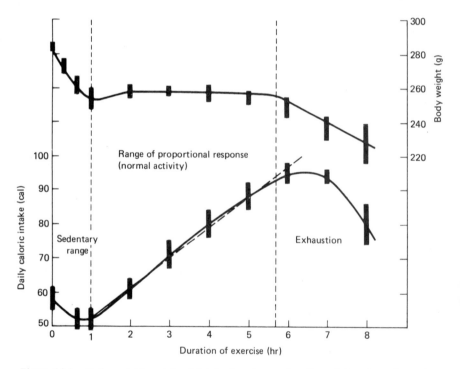

Figure 14-1. Body weight and food intake in rats as a function of duration of exercise. (Adapted from Mayer et al., 1954)

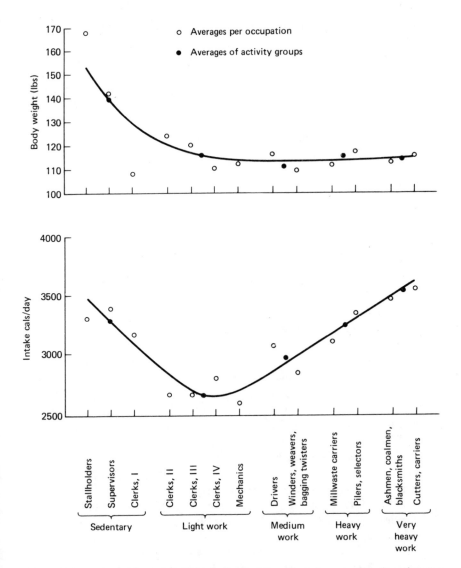

Figure 14-2. Body weight and food intake in West Bengal workers as a function of energy expended in occupation. (Adapted from Mayer et al., 1956)

take kept up with expenditure, while body weight remained unchanged at a normal level.

Additional data come from Keys (1970) who, as part of an epidemiological study on coronary artery disease, collected data on physical activity and weight of 12,770 male workers, aged 40 to 59, in seven countries. He found that the percentage of men in each country who were sedentary correlated highly with their relative weight.

Moreover, it is well known that spontaneous physical activity declines with age, so that by age 60 most people are 20 percent less active than at age 30 (Gwinup, 1974). Also with age, both body weight (Metropolitan Life Insurance Company, 1959) and body fat (Brozek, 1952) increase steadily. Even at the same body weight, on the average, a man of 60 contains almost twice as much fat as a man of 20.

These data on humans, although quite suggestive, are correlational in nature. A paper presented by Campbell and Becker in 1975 provides some experimental data. Five men of normal weight stayed in a hospital ward and obtained their only food from a liquid dispensing device which recorded intake without their knowledge. The subjects kept a record of their physical activity for estimation of energy expenditure. After an initial period of sedentary activity, subjects exercised on a treadmill for several days at levels of 13 to 27 percent and then at 32 percent above the sedentary level. At both exercise levels, subjects significantly increased their food intake. The caloric compensation was adequate to balance the extra energy expenditure. Weight data were not given.

In a recently completed dissertation project at St. Luke's Hospital, BasuRoy (1980) studied four obese men who stayed in the Metabolic Unit. They received three meals daily, with each menu item provided in several servings in large bowls, from which subjects took as much as they wanted. For periods of 7 to 10 days, subjects exercised by walking on a treadmill at levels of 20, 40, or 75 percent above their usual energy expenditure. These subjects did *not* increase their intake to compensate for the extra energy output.

From the above two studies, it seems that exercise is more likely to stimulate appetite in lean individuals than in obese ones. In a report by Boileau et al. (1971), 23 male college students were divided into an obese group (mean weight = 269 pounds) and a lean group (mean weight = 149 pounds). All participated in a physical conditioning program that involved walking or running for 1 hour a day, 5 days per week, for 9 weeks. Exercises were prescribed so that each subject expended 500 to 600 calories per day. Food intake was not restricted. Both groups lost weight, but only the obese group lost a significant amount, 7 pounds, versus 2.2 pounds for the lean group. The change in body composition for the obese subjects was greater than could be accounted for by the energy expended. It seems likely that the obese group reduced their food intake as a result of exercising.

Leon et al. (1979) had six sedentary obese men complete a 16-week program of vigorous walking for 90 minutes, 5 days per week. Subjects lost 12 1/2 pounds, which resulted from a combined loss of 13 pounds of fat and a gain of 1/2 pound of lean mass. Food intakes, which were recorded by the subjects, initially increased slightly and then decreased to below the level when subjects began the program.

Furthermore, Glick and Kaufmann (1976) observed three groups of Israeli recruits about to begin 6 weeks of intensive basic training. From the thickness of skinfolds at three sites of the body, the recruits were classified as small (n = 65), medium (n = 33), and large (n = 31). Food was eaten ad libitum. Table 14-1 shows how their weights changed during the training period. The small soldiers gained a significant amount of body weight as well as body fat as shown by an increase in skinfold thickness. The medium soldiers did not show a weight change but did show a reduced skinfold thickness. The large soldiers showed a significant decrease in both weight and skinfold thickness. It is likely that exercise had different effects on the food intake of the three groups.

An exception to the rule that exercise decreases food intake in the obese individual is found in some extremely obese persons with hyperplastic juvenile onset obesity who failed to lose weight after exercise (Sullivan, 1976), although some others of this group did lose weight (Bjorntorp, 1973).

By what mechanism could exercise decrease food intake? Exercise stimulates secretion of the catecholamines, adrenaline and noradrenaline. When adrenaline was injected into rats, they ate less food (Russek and Pina, 1962). Exercise also causes lactate levels to go up. Lactate injections depressed food intake in monkeys (Baile et al., 1970). Levels of lactate (Chlouverakis and Klocke, 1975) increased to a greater extent in the exercising obese individual than in the lean individual even when calorie expenditure was kept equal.

When Stevenson et al. (1966) exercised rats on certain days, the rats ate less food on those days but ate more on the days when they were rested, although not above the level that existed before the exercise program began. For maximal appetite suppression, it is therefore probably advantageous for exercise to occur frequently. When human subjects exercised only twice a week, no weight or body fat was lost (Pollock et al., 1969).

Exercise may also be more effective when it occurs shortly before the usual mealtime. When exercise was scheduled just before a lunch period, school children ate less than when the exercise was scheduled at other times (Epstein et al., 1978).

Aerobic exercises of moderate intensity may cause a greater reduction in food intake than strenuous exercises that are partly anaerobic (Swenson and Conlee, 1979). Aerobic exercises are also more likely to use fat as a substrate for oxidation than are anaerobic exercises that rely on the anaerobic process of glycolysis (Girandola, 1976).

TABLE 14-1. Weight and Skinfold Thickness, Before and After Training.*†

Group	n		Weight (kg)	Relative Weight (%)	Triceps Skinfold (mm)	Subscapular Skinfold (mm)	Abdomen Skinfold (mm)	Sum of Skinfold Thickness (mm)
Small SSFT‡ (S)	65	Before training	54.1 ± 6.6	90 ± 8	4.4 ± 1.0	6.4 ± 1.1	6.1 ± 1.3	16.9 ± 2.2
		After training	55.2 ± 6.6		4.7 ± 1.1	6.6 ± 1.0	6.8 ± 1.6	18.1 ± 2.6
		Difference	+1.1		+0.3	+0.2	+0.7	+12
		P	<0.001		<0.01	<0.05	<0.001	<0.01
Medium SSFT (M)	33	Before training	61.8 ± 7.4	104 ± 6	7.8 ± 1.9	9.8 ± 1.9	12.3 ± 2.3	29.9 ± 3.2
		After training	62.2 ± 7.4		7.0 ± 1.4	9.4 ± 1.9	11.5 ± 3.3	28.9 ± 4.5
		Difference	+0.4		-0.8	-0.4	-0.8	-20
		P	N.S.		0.01	N.S.	N.S.	<0.02
Large SSFT (L)	31	Before training	86.8 ± 11.2	135 ± 18	14.5 ± 5.0	23.8 ± 7.1	26.7 ± 5.2	65.0 ± 13.6
		After training	83.9 ± 10.8		12.2 ± 3.9	19.6 ± 6.0	22.6 ± 5.3	54.4 ± 12.2
		Difference	-2.9		-2.3	-4.2	-4.1	-10.6
		P	<0.001		<0.001	<0.001	<0.001	<0.001

* From Glick and Kaufman (1976).

† Data are means ± S.D.

‡ SSFT = sum of skinfold thickness values.

OBESITY AND INACTIVITY

Added impetus for using exercise to treat obesity would be provided by studies showing that obese people were generally more inactive than normal people. After examining the case records of 154 obese persons, Greene (1939) traced the onset of obesity in 104 cases to a period of inactivity resulting from illness, disability, or convalescence. Bruch (1940) studied the case histories of 140 obese children that were based on information derived from both parent and child, as well as from direct observation during interviews. Bruch classified 72 percent of these children as less active than normal. According to Bruch, most obese children are inactive and overeat. For these children, "food has an exaggerated value and stands for love, security, and satisfaction; muscular activity is associated with the concept of danger, threat, and insecurity." Because food and muscular activity have opposite emotional values, Bruch finds plausible the increased food intake in association with the decreased activity.

Johnson et al. (1956) interviewed 28 obese high school girls and 28 matched controls to determine daily calorie intake and physical activity. Activities were divided into classes according to approximate energy expenditure. The amount of time spent on each activity, as determined by interview, was recorded for each subject. For the class "active sports and other strenuous acts," obese girls spent 4 hours per week as compared to 11 hours per week for the normal girls. The obese girls also consumed fewer calories per day than the normals.

In a study of 14 pairs of obese and normal weight boys attending camp, Stefanik et al. (1959) found no significant differences in physical activity between the two groups, although the head counselor rated the obese boys as more likely to prefer sedentary activities. Again, the obese boys ate less than the lean boys.

Bullen et al. (1964) analyzed 27,211 motion picture frames of obese and lean girls participating in swimming, volleyball, and tennis. During each activity, the obese girls spent less time being physically active. For example, during a swimming period, only 9 percent of the obese girls were actually observed to be swimming as compared to 55 percent of the normal weight girls. Figure 14-3 shows the results for tennis.

While Mayer's group (Bullen et al., 1964; Johnson et al., 1956; Stefanik et al., 1959) was observing obese adolescents, Stunkard and his associates began studying the physical activity of obese adults by means of a pedometer. (A pedometer, worn suspended from the waist, registers every step a person takes while walking. The error for distance walked is less than 15 percent (Stunkard, 1960)). In a study of 15 obese women and 15 controls, Dorris and Stunkard (1957) found that the obese women walked an average of 2 miles per day as compared to 4.9 miles per day for the controls. Similarly, Chirico and Stunkard (1960) found

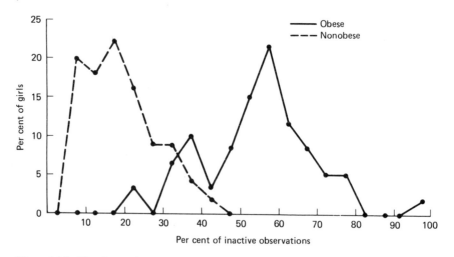

Figure 14-3. Time-lapse photography of obese and lean girls playing tennis. A much greater percentage of obese girls were observed to be inactive. (Adapted from Bullen et al., 1964)

that 25 obese men walked an average of 3.7 miles per day as compared to 6 miles per day for the 25 nonobese controls.

Results were not as clearcut when Stunkard and Pestka (1962) observed 12- to 13-year old girls during the last two weeks of camp and during a week at home. Although the obese girls walked slightly less than the normal weight girls, the differences were not significant.

Numerous studies (Bloom and Eidex, 1967; Corbin and Pletcher, 1968; Craddock, 1969; Dean and Garabedian, 1979; Durnin, 1966; Hutson et al., 1965; Rose and Mayer, 1968; Thomson et al., 1961) have supported the general conclusion that obese people tend to be less active. There have, however, been a good number of reports finding no difference (Lincoln, 1972; Maxfield and Konishi, 1966; McCarthy, 1966; Waxman and Stunkard, 1980; Wilkinson et al., 1977). For example, McCarthy (1966) obtained 24-hour recalls of physical activity from 63 obese Trinidad women and 26 normal weight women. There were no differences in the amount of time spent lying down, sitting, doing light exercises, or doing moderate to heavy exercises.

Few authors have actually estimated caloric expenditure during activity, which would take into account the extra energy necessary for an obese person to move around a larger mass. From among the studies described above, Bullen et al. (1964) estimated that obese girls expended less energy than normal weight girls during camp activities. Dorris and Stunkard (1957) also found that obese women expended less energy than normal women. In contrast, although obese men walked less than normal men, Stunkard and Chirico (1960) calculated that the obese men expended the same energy. Among obese girls, Stunkard and Pestka (1962) calculated that although the obese girls walked less, they actually expended more energy than the normal girls. Using heart rate as a measure of energy expenditure, Bradfield et al. (1971) found no difference between six pairs of obese and nonobese high school girls. Bradfield et al., concluded that because the obese girls weighed more, they had to be less physically active in order to expend the same amount of energy. Thus, although many obese persons are more sedentary than normal, their tendency to expend less energy than normal is not established.

What happens to the activity level of the obese person after weight reduction? Stunkard (1960) observed that after weight loss, his patients increased their walking distance. Bradfield and Jourdan (1972) found no change in energy expended as measured by heart rate when obese patients reduced their weight. This result suggests that such patients actually become more active, because now being lighter they have to move around more to achieve the same energy expenditure.

TREATMENT OF OBESITY WITH EXERCISE

Given that inactivity is as much a characteristic of obesity as is overeating, it makes sense to use exercise in the treatment of obesity. There are only three possible ways to treat obesity: reducing food intake, increasing energy expenditure, or a combination of both. It is widely accepted that reducing intake alone has not been very effective in the treatment of obesity (Stunkard and McLaren-Hume, 1959). After losing weight by dieting, the great majority of obese patients put it back on (Stunkard, 1977). For this reason, many treatment programs are turning to exercise alone or, more commonly, exercise in combination with dieting. For example, Weight Watchers has recently introduced an exercise protocol into their program.

Exercise Alone

For obese patients who have repeatedly failed to lose weight by dieting, exercise alone may be indicated. Weight loss can be expected to be steady but slow. Oscai and Williams (1968) conducted a training program for five overweight sedentary males ranging in age from 35 to 46 years. The subjects exercised three times a week for 16 weeks. Initially, the program consisted of 15 to 30 minutes of intermittent walking and jogging and progressed until each subject ran continuously for 30 minutes and covered at least 3 miles. Heart rate during training ranged from 155 to 170 beats per minute. Although food intake was ad libitum, the subjects lost 10 pounds (of which 8 pounds consisted of fat) and were satisfied with their rate of weight loss.

More recently, Gwinup (1975) recruited obese patients who had previously failed to maintain weight loss after dieting. Patients chose a form of exercise in which they could engage on a daily basis. Most chose walking. The length of the exercise period was increased by 1 minute per day until it reached a minimum of 30 minutes. Only those subjects who walked for 30 minutes or more daily lost weight. Eleven women, all of whom chose walking, maintained the minimum daily amount of exercise for a year, during which period they lost a mean of 20 pounds. Most had by this time increased their walking periods to 2 hours per day. At this level of exercise, the subjects believed they were consuming more food than they had before, although by not nearly enough to cancel out the benefits of the exercise. The two most obese women weighing 210 pounds and 215 pounds, also lost the most weight, a mean of 40 pounds in 80 weeks.

Zuti and Golding (1976) conducted a 16-week study of 25 women who were 20 to 40 pounds overweight. They were randomly assigned to one of three conditions – diet alone, diet in combination with exercise, and exercise alone. In the diet condition, the women reduced calorie intake by 500 calories per day; in the exercise condition they expended 500 calories during a supervised one-hour exercise program and by additional walking; in the combination condition, they reduced calorie intake by 250 calories and increased energy expenditure by 250 calories. The calorie deficit for the three groups was therefore identical. Figure 14-4 shows that the three groups lost 11.7, 12.0, and 10.6 pounds, amounts which were not significantly different. However, only the combination group and the exercise group, as compared to the diet-only group, significantly increased body density as a result of losing fat and gaining lean tissue.

Exercise and Diet

The loss of less than 1 pound per week as in the previous study may be discouragingly slow to a number of obese persons. For this reason, exercise has been used in combination with more restrictive diets. Strong et al. (1958) showed that obese patients could maintain up to 4 hours of walking outdoors while on a 400-calorie diet. Patients lost 4.7 to 6.0 pounds per week.

Buskirk et al. (1963) observed that obese patients who walked 7.5 miles per day, in addition to dieting, lost more weight than by dieting alone. In general, the less restrictive the diet, the more of an increment in weight loss the exercise program made.

Kenrick et al. (1972) compared two groups of extremely obese patients, only one of whom had an exercise protocol added to a diet providing 1000 to 1500 calories per day. The exercises consisted of 30 minutes per day of treadmill walk-

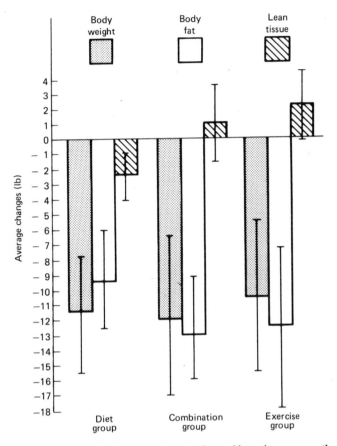

Figure 14-4. Average changes in body weight, body fat, and lean tissue among three groups: diet alone, combination of diet and exercise, and exercise alone, with each group expending 500 calories per day. The combination group and exercise group significantly increased body density by losing fat and gaining lean tissue. (Adapted from Zuti and Golding, 1976)

ing and calisthenics. After 6 months, the exercised group lost 14 pounds more than the nonexercised group. Since this report, Foss and his associates (1975, 1976, 1980) have developed individualized protocols for exercising extremely obese patients (mean weight = 380 pounds) in conjunction with a 600-calorie diet. Initially, such patients were unable to walk half a mile on the average. By the end of the 3-, 5-, or 7-week physical training program (depending on the initial work tolerance of the patient), all were able to walk 2 miles continuously. Calorie expenditure per mile did not change much during the program and remained about 185 calories despite the improvement in physical conditioning.

Problems in exercising obese patients especially the extremely obese include maintaining motivation, preventing dropouts, and successfully encouraging subjects to continue exercising when they leave the program. Early enthusiasm by very obese patients for an exercise program that consisted of treadmill walking and calisthenics waned after a few months (Wunderlich et al., 1973), and the physical therapists were subjected to increasing hostility by patients who were becoming reluctant to exercise. Foss et al. (1976) who exercised obese patients on an indoor track for up to 7 weeks, experienced less resistance by patients, but they note that such very obese patients "require more attention, encouragement, and often stern direction from the therapist than would comparable groups of overweight or nonobese adults." No resistance was encountered in a walking-jogging calisthenics program with moderately overweight women (Lewis et al., 1976). Many of these women remained enthusiastic throughout. Thus, the more overweight the subjects, the more difficult it usually is to sustain enthusiasm for physical training.

In an 18-month follow-up of obese and normal weight women who had participated in a 12-week, 4 days per week, jogging program, only 40 percent of the normal women and 33 percent of the obese were still engaged in jogging (MacKeen et al., 1978). When the program had just ended, 80 percent of the normal weight and 78 percent of the obese women had said they would continue jogging.

Behavior Modification

Recent reports of behavior modification programs that incorporate physical training stand out because of their relatively low dropout rate and high success after follow-up.

Harris and Hallbauer (1973) described the results of including an exercise protocol in a behavior modification program. They divided their subjects into three groups that focused on (1) eating behavior only, (2) eating behavior and physical activity, and (3) neither behavior (control group). Group 2 was told to choose a daily exercise program that would be enjoyable but not so strenuous that it would cause exhaustion. Besides this regular exercise program, subjects were told to increase calorie expenditure as part of daily life, for example, by parking the car several blocks away from one's destination, by getting off the bus a few stops in advance, by taking the stairs rather than the elevator or escalator.

After 12 weeks, the eating behavior group lost a mean of 6.9 pounds and the combination group lost 9.1 pounds, an insignificant difference. After a 7-month follow-up, however, the combination group lost 13.1 pounds which was significantly more than the 8.8 pounds lost by the eating group.

In 1979, Dahlkoetter et al., also using a behavior modification approach, compared the effect of (1) increasing physical activity alone, (2) decreasing calorie intake, and (3) using a combination of both. In the exercise groups, each member chose a partner with whom to exercise. During the group meetings, the last half of each session was used to demonstrate and practice new exercises. All groups met once a week for 8 weeks. None of the subjects dropped out. At the conclusion of the program, the combination group lost more weight, 13.3 pounds, than either the eating, 7.0 pounds, or the exercise group, 6.1 pounds. The difference between the latter two groups was not significant. At 6-month follow-up, only the combination group continued to lose weight, an additional 3 pounds, whereas the eating group regained 2 pounds and the exercised group showed no change. Not surprisingly, on measures of physical fitness such as the Harvard Step Test, the exercised groups showed the most improvement.

BENEFITS OF EXERCISE

Besides weight reduction, regular exercise provides psychological and physiological benefits. Hanson and Nedde (1974) administered the Self-concept Scale Tests to a group of eight sedentary women who were somewhat overweight, before and after an 8-month physical training program. Significant improvements were found in measures of self-satisfaction, self-acceptance, and sense of personal worth.

Among 216 persons, Carter (1977) found a significant correlation between a person's happiness and degree of physical activity. According to the Harris poll of 1979, physically active people reported more self-confidence, better self-image, and greater psychological well being than inactive people. Psychiatrists have recently used running as therapy to improve the mood of normal and depressed individuals (Brown et al., 1978; Greist et al., 1978).

The overweight subject who exercises as part of a reducing regimen does not have to endure the privation of a very low-calorie diet that also may not supply adequate amounts of essential nutrients. Exercise may be psychologically easier to accept than dieting because it represents a positive approach to controlling weight — one must do something. This is in contrast to dieting which is a negative approach — one must not do something.

Especially for sedentary obese subjects who often tire and get out of breath from moving around a large mass, regular exercise reduces the incidence of fatigue. By adapting to more strenuous activities, the body more easily copes with the lesser strains of everyday life. Muscle strength and stamina are both enhanced by exercise.

Exercise also lowers insulin levels especially in the obese who often have elevated levels (Bjorntorp et al., 1970). Exercise probably also causes an increase in the ratio of high-density lipoprotein (HDL) to low-density lipoprotein (LDL) (Leon et al., 1979). A relatively high ratio of HDL/LDL has been postulated to protect against coronary artery disease (Miller and Miller, 1975). Indeed several epidemiological studies have implicated inactivity as a risk factor for heart disease (Morris et al., 1977; Paffenbarger et al., 1978). Inactivity leads to an increase in both the incidence of myocardial infarction and the likelihood that the infarction will prove fatal (Shapiro et al., 1969).

Aerobic exercises, which are also the type of exercises likely to cause weight and fat loss (Pollock, 1978), provide cardiovascular and respiratory benefits. The heart and lungs adapt to the extra demands of exercise. The heart develops an enhanced capacity to pump large amounts of blood, hence a decline in resting heart rate. The lungs increase their ability to extract oxygen during each inhalation which leads to an increase in the maximum oxygen consumption.

Walking and running are good aerobic exercises, but sprinting is not. Weight lifting programs produce large increments in muscular strength, but little improvement in cardiovascular-respiratory fitness (Pollock, 1978).

Aerobic exercises should be strenuous enough to substantially raise heart rate and breathing rate without causing exhaustion. Although there are no firm guidelines on the desirable range for heart rate, a range between 70 and 85 percent of maximum is widely accepted. Figure 14-5 shows the desirable range and is adjusted for age. Roughly speaking, the age-adjusted maximum can be calculated as 220 minus age in years.

Pollock et al. (1975) compared running, walking, and bicycling at the same frequency (3 days per week) and duration (30 minutes), with heart rate kept equal. To increase the intensity of walking, the treadmill had to be raised to an angle of 10°. Increases in aerobic capacity and changes in body composition were comparable. Thus mode of training does not appear to be important. For obese persons, because of the additional mass, a heart rate high enough to produce cardiovascular fitness can generally be produced by vigorous walking on level ground.

Pollock et al. (1969) showed that a minimum exercise frequency of three times per week is generally necessary to cause significant weight and fat loss in sedentary individuals. Both the training effect and weight loss increase in direct proportion to the duration of the exercise with a minimum of 10 to 15 minutes per training session usually regarded as necessary (Milesis, et al., 1973; Morehouse and Gross, 1974).

The greater the intensity, frequency, and duration of the exercise, the greater is the calorie expenditure. Therefore to get the same expenditure as from running 10 miles per hour for 1 hour, a person would have to walk 4 miles per

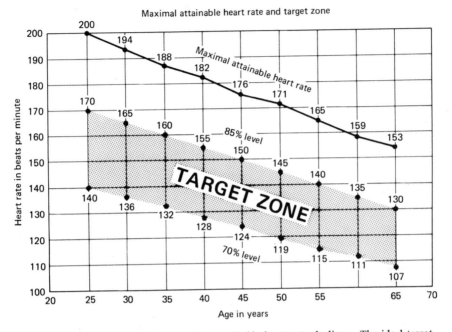

Figure 14-5. As people age, the maximal attainable heart rate declines. The ideal target zone for aerobic exercises is between 70-85% of this maximal heart rate. (Adapted from Zohman, 1979)

hour for 4.1 hours (see Table 14-2); running a mile consumes somewhat more energy than walking a mile.

To calculate expected weight loss in pounds, one should divide the total calorie expenditure by 3500 calories, which is roughly the energy in a pound of adipose tissue (Keys and Brozek, 1953). For example, suppose a person weighing 210 pounds walks 4 miles per hour for 2 hours, 5 times a week. The calorie expenditure would be 324 calories X 2 X 5 per week or an expected weight loss of almost 1 pound per week, if food intake was constant.

An increase in expenditure of 250 to 500 calories per day is a reasonable goal. At 250 calories per day, weight loss would be about 1/2 pound per week; at 500 calories per day, it would be about 1 pound per week.

Morehouse and Gross (1974) recommend a combination of 350 calories expended by exercise and a reduction in intake of 250 calories for a total daily reduction of 600 calories. With this reducing regimen, weight loss would proceed at an average of 1.2 pounds per week.

In any exercise program, it is wise for the individual to progress slowly. A running program should begin with walking, then with intermittent walking

TABLE 14-2. Caloric Cost of Physical Activity.*

Type of Activity	Body Weight (lb)					
	120	150	180	210	240	270
Lying still	6	7	8	10	11	12
Sitting quietly	22	27	32	39	44	49
Standing	27	35	41	48	54	60
Ironing clothes	54	66	84	96	108	120
Walking (3 mph)	108	138	162	192	216	246
Carpentry	126	156	186	222	252	272
Cycling (moderate)	138	168	204	240	276	306
Dancing	162	204	246	288	324	365
Walking (4 mph)	187	229	277	324	374	414
Skating	192	240	288	336	384	427
Sawing wood	312	384	453	547	624	697
Swimming (2 mph)	426	533	642	758	852	968
Boxing	619	775	930	1085	1238	1390
Running (10 mph)	770	960	1160	1350	1540	1740
Rowing in race	870	1090	1300	1520	1740	1960

* Values in table: calories expended for one hour of activity (above basal metabolic level).

Table is from Antonelli, V., *The Computer Diet.* New York: Evans, 1973, p. 5.

and running, and finally with continuous running (see Cooper, 1970, and More-house and Gross, 1974, for more details). Time should be allowed for warm-up and stretching exercises before and after a training period. Whenever pain, fatigue, weakness, or dizziness occur, a person should stop exercising. During exercise, one should be able to maintain a conversation; if not, the exercise is probably no longer aerobic.

An exercise program should be designed to sustain interest. For instance, walking outdoors is usually more enjoyable than walking on a treadmill. Providing feedback to the subject indicating the progress made in physical conditioning is desirable. It is also helpful to have subjects exercise with a partner or a group.

With each additional decade, it takes about 40 percent longer to achieve the same conditioning effect, starting from the sedentary level. Therefore, older individuals should expect to progress more slowly. Although physical fitness generally declines with age, a group of 45-year-old men who continued training for 10 years showed no decrement in aerobic capacity or body composition (Pollock, 1978).

Before beginning an exercise program, it is prudent for the subject to have a thorough physical examination. Above the age of 30, a resting EKG should be included. Above 40 and at any age when obesity is manifest, an exercise stress EKG should be added (Cooper, 1970; Devore and Nemiro, 1980).

Specific exercise programs for obese individuals may be found in Morehouse and Gross (1974) and for extremely obese individuals in Foss et al. (1976). The recent shift in treatment methods toward increasing energy expenditure makes good sense. As we have seen, reduced activity is as much or more a characteristic of obesity as is overeating. Furthermore, increasing the energy expenditure of the obese person can itself cause food intake to decrease. An increased activity level may be more tolerable, even enjoyable, than perpetual dieting, and may more easily become a way of life. That is certainly suggested by the Harris poll (1979) referred to earlier.

The current increase in exercise participation may represent the first reversal in the process begun with the Industrial Revolution by which people have been gradually relinquishing their own muscular energy for the energy provided by machines. The physical expenditure of energy that people once obtained from the tasks of daily living and work, is now being sought during leisure time. If the present trend continues, we may soon see a downturn in the incidence of obesity.

REFERENCES

Baile, C. A., Zinn, W. M., and Mayer, J. Effects of lactate and other metabolites on food intake of monkeys. *American Journal of Physiology*, 1970, *219*, 1606–1613.

BasuRoy, S. Effect of increased exercise on spontaneous food intake in moderately obese sedentary individuals. Doctoral dissertation, Columbia University, 1980.

Bjorntorp, P., de Jounge, K., Krotkiewski, M., Sullivan, L., Sjostrom, L., and Stenberg, J. Physical training in human obesity. III. Effects of long-term physical training on body composition. *Metabolism*, 1973, *22*, 1467.

Bjorntorp, P., de Jounge, K., Sjostrom, L., and Sullivan, L. The effect of physical training on insulin production in obesity. *Metabolism*, 1970, *19*, 631.

Bloom, W. L. and Eidex, M. F. Inactivity as a major factor in adult obesity. *Metabolism*, 1967, *16*, 679–684.

Boileau, R. A., Buskirk, E. R., Horstman, D. H., Mendez, J., and Nicholas, W. C. Body composition changes in obese and lean men during physical conditioning. *Medicine and Science in Sports*, 1971, *4*, 183–189.

Bradfield, R. B. and Jourdan, M. Energy expenditure of obese women during weight loss. *American Journal of Clinical Nutrition*, 1972, *25*, 971–975.

Bradfield, R. B., Paulos, J., and Grossman, L. Energy expenditure and heart rate of obese high school girls. *American Journal of Clinical Nutrition*, 1971, *24*, 1482–1488.

Brown, R. S., Ramirez, D. E., and Taub, J. M. The prescription of exercise for depression. *Physician and Sportsmedicine*, 1978, *6*, 35–45.

Brozek, J. Changes in body composition in man during maturity and their nutritional implications. *Federation Proceedings*, 1952, *11*, 784–793.

Bruch, H. Obesity in childhood. IV. Energy expenditure of obese children. *American Journal of Diseases of Children*, 1940, *60*, 1082–1109.

Bullen, B. A., Reed, R. B., and Mayer, J. Physical activity of obese and non-obese adolescent girls, appraised by motion picture sampling. *American Journal of Clinical Nutrition,* 1964, *14*, 211–223.

Buskirk, E. R., Thompson, R. H., Lutwak, L., and Whedon, G. D., Energy balance of obese patients during weight reduction: Influence of diet restriction and exercise. *Annals of the New York Academy of Sciences,* 1963, *110*, 918–940.

Campbell, R. and Becker, E. Effects of exercise on meal taking in man. Paper presented at Eastern Psychological Association, April 1975.

Carter, R. Exercise and happiness. *Journal of Sports Medicine,* 1977, *17*, 307–313.

Chirico, A. M. and Stunkard, A. J. Physical activity and human obesity. *New England Journal of Medicine,* 1960, *263*, 935–940.

Chlouverakis, C. and Klocke, R. A. Metabolic effects of exercise in human obesity. *Recent Advances in Obesity Research* (Howard, A., Ed.), Vol. I. London: Newman, 1975.

Cooper, K. H. Guidelines in the management of the exercising patient. *Journal of the American Medical Association,* 1970, *211*, 1663–1667.

Corbin, C. B. and Pletcher, P. Diet and physical activity patterns of obese and non-obese elementary school children. *Research Quarterly,* 1968, *39*, 922–928.

Craddock, D. *Obesity and Its Management.* London: Livingstone, 1969.

Dahlkoetter, J., Callahan, E. J., and Linton, J. Obesity and the unbalanced energy equation. *Journal of Clinical and Consulting Psychology,* 1979, *47*, 898–905.

Dean, R. S. and Garabedian, A. A. Obesity and level of activity. *Perceptual Motor Skills,* 1979, *49*, 690.

Devore, P. A. and Nemiro, D. D. Exercise testing of obese subjects. *Physician and Sportsmedicine,* 1980, *8*, No. 4, 47–54.

Dorris, R. J. and Stunkard, A. J. Physical activity: Performance and attitudes of a group of obese women. *American Journal of the Medical Sciences,* 1957, *233*, 622–628.

Durnin, J. V. G. A. Age, physical activity and energy expenditure. *Proceedings of the Society of Nutrition,* 1966, *25*, 107–113.

Epstein, L. H., Mosek, B., and Marshall, W. Pre-lunch exercise and lunch-time caloric intake. *Behavior Therapist,* 1978, *1*, 15.

Foss, M. L., Lampman, R. M., and Schteingart, D. E. Physical training program for rehabilitating extremely obese patients. *Archives of Physical Medicine,* 1976, *57*, 425–429.

Foss, M. L., Lampman, R. M., and Schteingart, D. E. Extremely obese patients: Improvements in exercise tolerance with physical training and weight loss. *Archives of Physical Medicine and Rehabilitation,* 1980, *61*, 119–124.

Foss, M. L., Lampman, R. M., Watt, E., and Schteingart, D. E. Initial work tolerance of extremely obese patients. *Archives of Physical Medicine and Rehabilitation,* 1975, *56*, 63–67.

Glick, Z. and Kaufmann, N. A. Weight and skinfold thickness changes during a physical training course. *Medicine and Science in Sports,* 1976, *8*, 109–112.

Girandola, R. N. Body composition changes in women: Effects of high and low exercise intensity. *Archives of Physical Medicine and Rehabilitation,* 1976, *57*, 297–300.

Greene, J. A. Clinical study of the etiology of obesity. *Annals of Internal Medicine,* 1939, *12*, 1797–1803.

Greist, J. H., Klein, M. H., Eischens, R. R., and Faris, J. T. Running out of depression. *Physician and Sportsmedicine,* 1978, *6*, 49–56.

Gwinup, G. Effects of diet and exercise in the treatment of obesity. *Treatment and Management of Obesity* (Bray, G. A., and Bethune, J. E., Eds.). New York: Harper and Row, 1974.

Gwinup, G. Effects of exercise alone on the weight of obese women. *Archives of Internal Medicine*, 1975, *135*, 676-680.

Hanson, J. S. and Nedde, W. H. Long-term physical training effect on sedentary females. *Journal of Applied Physiology*, 1974, *37*, 112-116.

Harris, Louis and Associates, *The Perrier Study: Fitness in America*. Conn.: Great Waters of France, 1979.

Harris, M. B. and Hallbauer, E. S. Self-directed weight control through eating and exercise. *Behavior Research and Therapy*, 1973, *11*, 523-529.

Hutson, E. M., Cohen, N. L., Kunkel, N. D., Steinkamp, R. C., Rourke, M. H., and Walsh, H. E. Measures of body fat and related factors in normal adults. *Journal of the American Dietetic Association*, 1965, *47*, 179-186.

Johnson, M. L., Burke, B. S., and Mayer, J. Relative importance of inactivity and overeating in the energy balance of obese high school girls. *American Journal of Clinical Nutrition*, 1956, *4*, 37-44.

Katsch, F. I. and McArdle, W. D. *Nutrition, Weight Control, and Exercise*. Boston: Houghton Mifflin, 1977.

Kenrick, M. M., Ball, M. F., and Canary, J. J. Exercise and weight reduction in obesity. *Archives of Physical Medicine and Rehabilitation*, 1972, *53*, 323-327.

Keys, A. Coronary heart disease in seven countries. *Circulation*, 1970, *41* (Supplement I), 1-211.

Keys, A. and Brozek, J. Body fat in adult men. *Physiological Reviews*, 1953, *33*, 245-325.

Leon, A. S., Conrad, J., Hunninghake, D. B. and Serfass, R. Effects of a vigorous walking program on body composition and carbohydrate and lipid metabolism of obese young men. *American Journal of Clinical Nutrition*, 1979, *33*, 1776-1787.

Lewis, S. Haskell, W. L., Wood, P. D., Manoogian, N., Bailey, J. E., and Pereira, M. B. Effects of physical activity on weight reduction in obese middle-aged women. *American Journal of Clinical Nutrition*, 1976, *29*, 151-156.

Lincoln, J. E. Calorie intake, obesity, and physical activity. *American Journal of Clinical Nutrition*, 1972, *25*, 390-394.

MacKeen, P. C., Franklin, B. A., and Buskirk, E. R. Eighteen-month follow-up of participants in a physical conditioning program for middle-aged women. *Medicine and Science in Sports*, 1978, *10*, 52.

Maxfield, E. and Konishi, F. Patterns of food intake and physical activity in obesity. *Journal of the American Dietetic Association*, 1966, *49*, 406-408.

Mayer, J., Marshall, N. B., Vitale, J. J., Christensen, J. H., Mashayekhi, M. B., and Stare, F. J. Exercise, food intake, and body weight in normal rats and genetically obese adult mice. *American Journal of Physiology*, 1954, *177*, 544-548.

Mayer, J., Roy, P., and Mitra, K. P. Relation between caloric intake, body weight, and physical work: Studies in an industrial male population in West Bengal. *American Journal of Clinical Nutrition*, 1956, *4*, 169-175.

McCarthy, M. C. Dieting and activity patterns of obese women in Trinidad. *Journal of the American Dietetic Association*, 1966, *48*, 33-37.

Metropolitan LIfe Insurance Company. New weight standards for men and women. *Statistical Bulletin*, 1959, *40*, 1-4.

Milesis, C. A., Pollock, M. L., Bah, M. D., Ayres, J. J., and Linnerud, A. C. Effects of different durations of physical training on cardio-respiratory function, body composition, and serum lipids. *Research Quarterly*, 1973, *47*, 716-725.

Miller, G. J. and Miller, N. E. Plasma-high-density-lipoprotein concentration and development of ischaemic heart disease. *Lancet*, 1975, *1*, 16-19.

Morehouse, L. E. and Gross, L. *Total Fitness in 30 Minutes a Week*. New York: Simon and Schuster, 1975.

Morris, J. N., Marr, J. W., and Clayton, D. G. Diet and Heart: A postscript. *British Medical Journal,* 1977, *2,* 1307-1314.

Oscai, L. B. and Williams, B. T. Effect of exercise on overweight middle-aged males. *Journal of the American Geriatrics Society,* 1968, *16,* 794-797.

Paffenbarger, R. S., Wing, A. L., and Hyde, R. T. Physical activity as an index of heart attack risk in college alumni. *Journal of Epidemiology,* 1978, *108,* 161-175.

Pollock, M. L. How much exercise is engouh? *Physician and Sportsmedicine,* 1978, June, 50-74.

Pollock, M. L., Cureton, T. K., and Gereninger, L. Effects of frequency of training on working capacity, cardiovascular function, and body composition of adult men. *Medicine and Science in Sports,* 1969, *1,* 70-74.

Pollock, M. L., Dimmick, J., Miller, H. S., Kendrick, Z., and Linnerud, A. C. Effects of mode of training on cardiovascular function and body composition of adult men. *Medicine and Science in Sports,* 1975, *7,* 139-145.

Rose, H. E. and Mayer, J. Activity, caloric intake, fat storage and energy balance of infants. *Pediatrics,* 1968, *41,* 18-29.

Russek, M. and Pina, S. Conditioning of adrenalin anorexia. *Nature,* 1962, *193,* 1296-1297.

Shapiro, S., Weinblatt, E., Frank C. W., and Sager, R. V. Incidence of coronary heart disease in a population insured for medical care (HIP). *American Journal of Public Health,* 1969, *59,* 1-101.

Stefanik, P. A., Heald, F. P., and Mayer J. Caloric intake in relation to energy output of obese and non-obese adolescent boys. *American Journal of Clinical Nutrition,* 1959, *7,* 55-62.

Stevenson, J. A. F., Box, B. M., Feleki, V., and Beaton, J. R. Bouts of exercise and food intake in the rat. *Journal of Applied Physiology,* 1966, *21,* 118-122.

Strong, J. A., Passmore, R., and Ritchie, F. J. Clinical observations on obese patients during a strict reducing regimen. *British Journal of Nutrition,* 1958, *12,* 105-112.

Stunkard, A. J. and McLaren-Hume, M. The results of treatment of obesity. A review of the literature and report of a series. *Archives of Internal Medicine,* 1959, *103,* 79-85.

Stunkard, A. J. Behavioral treatment for obesity: Failure to maintain weight loss. *Behavioral Self Control,* (Stuart, R. B., Ed.), pp. 317-350. New York: Bruner/Mazel, 1977.

Stunkard, A. J. and McLaren-Hume, . The results of treatment of obesity. A review of the literature and report of a series. *Archives of Internal Medicine,* 1959, *103,* 79-85.

Stunkard, A. J. and Pestka, J. The physical activity of obese girls. *American Journal of Diseases of Children,* 1962, *103,* 812-817.

Sullivan, L. Metabolic and physiologic effects of physical training in hyperplastic obesity. *Scandinavian Journal of Rehabilitation Medicine,* 1976, Supplement *5,* 1-38.

Swenson, E. J. and Conlee, R. K. Effects of exercise intensity on body composition in adult males. *Journal of Sports Medicine,* 1979, *19,* 323-326.

Thomson, A. M., Billewicz, W. Z., and Passmore, R. The relation between calorie intake and body weight in man. *Lancet,* 1961, *1,* 1027-1028.

Van Itallie, T. B. Obesity: The American disease. *Food Technology,* December 1979, 43-47.

Waxman, M. and Stunkard, A. J. Caloric intake and expenditure of obese boys. *Pediatrics,* 1980, *96,* 187-193.

Wilkinson, P. W., Parkin, J. M., Pearlson, G., Strong, H., and Sykes, P. Energy intake and physical activity in obese children. *British Journal of Medicine,* 1977, *1,* 756.

Wunderlich, R. A., Kenrick, M., Pearce, M., Lozes, J., and Ball, M. F. Psychologic considerations in physical therapy for obese patients. *Physical Therapy,* 1973, *53,* 757-761.

Zohman, L. R. Beyond diet: Exercise your way to fitness and health. *CPC International,* 1979.

Zuti, W. B. and Golding, L. A. Comparing diet and exercise as weight reduction tools. *Physician and Sportsmedicine,* 1976, *4,* 49-53.

Author Index

Abe, R., 160
Abraham, K., 91, 96
Abraham, S., 147, 154
Abrahms, J. L., 208
Abramson, E. E., 207, 208
Adler, A., 92, 96, 119, 121
Adler, K., 97
Ahern, J. K., 160
Aldebaran, V., 199
Alexander, F. A., 15, 88, 193
Allen, G. J., 208
Anderson, C. F., 157
Aragona, J., 214, 215
Ashby, W. A., 219, 236
Assagioli, R., 272
Atkinson, R. M., 88, 95

Back, K. W., 19, 130, 147, 148, 149, 154
Baile, C. A., 295
Baker, E., 140
Banks, R., 19
Bass, A., 219
Basuroy, S., 293
Beck, S. B., 151
Becker, D., 91, 95
Becker, E., 293
Becker, M. H., 157
Bellack, A. S., 207
Beller, A. S., 152
Bemis, K., 19
Beneke, W. M., 218, 219
Berblinger, L. G., 116

Bibring, E., 88
Birky, H. J., 25
Bjerkedal, T., 158
Bjorntorp, P., 295
Blackburn, G. L., 21
Bloom, W. L., 298
Bogdonoff, M. D., 157
Boileau, R. A., 293
Borden, B. L., 225, 226
Borhani, R. O., 158
Bosin, H. W., 88
Boudewyns, P. A., 209
Bowlby, J., 97
Bradfield, R. B., 211, 299
Brandt, E. N., 160
Bray, G. A., 23, 24
Breslow, L., 158
Breytspraak, L. M., 157
Brightwell, D. R., 218
Brown, R. S., 303
Brownell, K., 212, 213
Browning, S., 147
Brozek, J., 293, 305
Bruch, H., 16, 18, 20, 88, 91, 95, 96, 107, 110, 112, 113, 115, 154, 166, 167, 188, 190, 193, 297
Bruner, C. G., 233
Bryans, A. M., 162
Buchanan, J. R., 130
Buchwald, H., 19, 22, 23, 24
Bullen, B. A., 110, 115, 298, 299
Burchinal, L. G., 116

Burt, V., 19
Buskirk, E. R., 301
Bychowski, G., 88, 91, 177, 190

Cahnman, W. J., 130, 133, 163
Callahan, D. J., 211
Campbell, C. H., 161
Campbell, I. W., 161
Campbell, M. M., 19
Campbell, R., 293
Campbell, V. A., 19
Canning, H., 19, 136, 137, 214
Cappon, D., 19
Carrera, R., 110, 111
Carter, R., 303
Cassady, J., 214
Cautela, J. R., 226, 228, 230, 236
Chamberlain, K., 17
Chirico, A. M., 299
Chlouverakis, C., 295
Christ, M., 211
Christensen, A., 218, 233
Clifford, E., 150
Cobb, L. A., 277
Cohen, E. A., 217
Coleman, 238, 268
Coll, M., 162
Collins, A., 25
Colwick, J., 214
Combrinck-Graham, L. A., 215
Conger, J. C., 157
Conlee, R. K., 297
Cooke, C. J., 220
Cooper, K. H., 306
Copley, D., 22
Corbin, C. R., 298
Craddock, D., 298
Craft, C. A., 131
Craighead, W. E., 25
Crisp, A. H., 18, 22, 23
Cunningham, S., 19
Currey, H., 161
Currey, H. S., 209, 213

Dahlkoetter, J., 211, 303
d'Aquili, E., 153
Davis, B., 17, 156, 212, 215
Dean, R. S., 298
DeJong, W., 131
Devore, P. A., 306
Diament, C., 226
Dinoff, M., 214
Dodd, D. K., 25, 217
Dornbusch, S. M., 147
Dorris, R. J., 298, 299

Douglas, J. W. B., 18
Douty, H. I., 151
Drabman, R. S., 214
Dreikurs, R., 121
Drenick, E. J., 138
Drummond, T., 215
Durnin, J. V. G. A., 298
Dwyer, J. T., 133, 150, 151, 152, 165
Dyrenforth, S. R., 131, 149, 161, 167

Eckert, E. D., 19, 23
Edwards, K. A., 214, 217
Eickwort, K. R., 137, 138
Eid, E. E., 18
Eidex, M. F., 298
Elman, D., 17
Eppright, E. S., 116
Epstein, L. H., 216, 297
Espmark, S., 23

Feinstein, A., 162
Feinstein, A. R., 238
Feldman, J. J., 133, 150, 151
Fenichel, O., 16, 88
Ferguson, J. M., 22
Ferster, C. B., 17, 207, 225, 228
Filion, R., 225
Filion, R. D. L., 153
Finlay, J., 157
Fixx, J., 291
Flagg, G. W., 15, 88
Foreyt, J. P., 226, 232, 236
Foss, M. L., 301, 302
Fox, S., 153, 225
Franzini, L. R., 217
Fremouw, W. J., 213
French, T. M., 195
Freud, S., 88, 91, 179
Frohwirth, R. A., 208
Fromm-Reichman, F., 97

Galper, R. E., 147
Garabedian, A. A., 298
Gareis, F. J., 19
Garfinkel, P. E., 19
Garner, D. M., 19
Garrow, J., 162, 163
Gastineau, C. F., 21
Gaul, D. J., 25
Gazet, J. C., 23
Gelfand, D. M., 217
Gellert, E., 19, 25
Ginsberg-Fellner, F., 214
Girandola, R. N., 297

Glucksman, M. L., 20, 188
Goldberg, P. S., 25
Goldberg, S. C., 19
Goldblatt, P. B., 88, 95, 152, 153, 182
Golding, L. A., 300
Goldman, N., 133
Goodlin, R. C., 160
Goodman, N., 147
Gordon, A., 133
Gordon, J. B., 136
Gotestam, K. G., 218
Graff, H., 22
Greenacre, P., 88
Greenberg, I., 21
Greene, J. A., 297
Greist, J. H., 303
Grimes, W. B., 217
Grinker, J., 20
Gross, L., 304-307
Gross, L. P., 133
Grossberg, J. M., 277
Gwinup, G., 300

Haber, L. D., 138
Hager, R. L., 242, 266
Hall, R. G., 225, 226
Hall, S. M., 219, 225
Hallbauer, E. S., 302
Halmi, K. A., 19
Halverson, J. D., 177
Hamberg, D. A., 182
Hammar, S. L., 19, 112
Hampton, M. C., 18
Hanson, J. S., 303
Hanson, R. W., 225, 226
Harris, L., 307
Harris, M. B., 233, 302
Hartford, D., 151
Hastorf, A. H., 147
Hayes, S. C., 212
Hechter, H. H., 158
Heckerman, C. L., 212
Herman, C. P., 25
Herman, M. W., 152, 163
Hibscher, J. A., 163
Hirsch, A. A., 213
Hirsch, J., 20
Holfing, C. K., 118
Holland, J., 22
Homme, L. E., 233
Horan, J. J., 226
Horney, K., 92
Huston, E. M., 298
Hvenemann, R. L., 18, 21

Ingram, D. H., 157, 166
Innes, J. A., 161
Isreal, A. C., 212, 213

Jacobsen, E., 88
Janda, H. L., 226
Jeffrey, D. B., 242
Jeffrey, R. W., 161, 208, 212, 218, 225, 226
Jensen, J., 217
Johnson, M. L., 297
Johnson, R. G., 226
Johnson, S. F., 21
Johnson, W. G., 211, 217
Jones, D., 208
Jones, E., 15
Jones, J. W., 277
Jordan, H. A., 162, 207
Jordan, M., 211
Jourard, S. M., 151
Jourdan, M., 299

Kalisch, B. J., 131, 151
Kalucy, R. S., 23
Kaplan, D., 210
Kaplan, H. I., 119, 177, 181
Kaplan, H. S., 177, 181
Karabenick, O. S., 147
Kastenbaum, R. P., 228
Kenrick, M. M., 301
Keys, A., 293, 305
Kingsley, R. G., 215, 218
Kissileff, K., 162
Kline, M. V., 238, 268
Klocke, R. A., 295
Knittle, J. L., 214
Koch, C., 95
Kolotkin, R., 25
Konishi, F., 299
Korgeski, G., 25
Korn, S. J., 146
Krauss, B. J., 196
Krauss, H. H., 196
Kroeger, W. S., 226, 227
Kuldau, J. M., 182
Kurland, H., 88, 100, 166
Kurtz, R. M., 151

Lang, P. J., 277
Larkin, J. E., 138
Lascelles, B. D., 22
Laslett, B., 148
Lazarus, A. A., 226, 227, 230, 236
LeBow, L. D., 211
LeBow, M. D., 25

Leon, G. R., 192, 207, 209, 225, 226, 294
Lerner, R. M., 19, 146
Levin, B., 20
Levitt, E. B., 17
Levitt, E. G., 207, 225, 226
Levitz, L., 162
Levitz, L. S., 207
Liederman, V. R., 19, 130, 147, 148, 149, 154, 156
Lincoln, J. E., 299
Linder, M., 270
Linton, J., 211
Lloyd, J. K., 18
Locas, B., 19
Louderback, L., 139, 140
Lutz, R. N., 218
Lyman, S., 135, 136

MacCuish, A. C., 161
Mack, D., 25
Mac Keen, P. C., 302
Maddox, G. L., 19, 130, 147, 148, 149, 154, 156, 157
Mahoney, K., 212, 220, 256
Mahoney, M. J., 25, 207, 210, 220, 225, 226, 238, 256
Maiman, L. A., 157
Malcolm, R., 161, 209, 213
Mann, G. V., 158
Marshall, W. R., 216
Masling, J., 22
Masseck, B. J., 216
Mathews, V., 149
May, R., 92
Mayer, J., 18, 19, 95, 133, 136, 137, 140, 151, 159, 163, 164, 165, 193, 214, 292, 298
Maxfield, E., 299
McCarthy, M. C., 299
McClelland, D. C., 92
McCoy, J. F., 216
McGee, G., 216
McGee, J., 157
McGuiness, B., 22
McLaren-Hume, M., 157, 161, 207, 299
McLear, P. M., 151
McReynolds, W. G., 218
McReynolds, W. T., 212, 213
McSweeney, F. K., 25
Meedle, A. L., 161
Meisels, M., 147
Meland, M., 19
Mendelson, M., 19, 22, 113
Meyer, J., 162
Meyers, A., 220

Michaels, S., 148
Milesis, C. A., 304
Miller, G. J., 304
Miller, N. E., 304
Millman, M., 133, 141, 149, 150, 158
Mitchell, B. W., 18
Moldofsky, H., 19
Monello, L. F., 133
Monroe, J., 219
Monti, P. N., 212
Moore, J. B., 151
Moore, M. E., 152, 153, 157
Moores, N. L., 19
Morehouse, L. E., 304-307
Morgenstein, K. P., 78
Morris, J. N., 304
Morrow, J., 160
Mulligan, R., 226
Munro, J. F., 161
Musante, G. J., 209

Nedde, W. H., 303
Nemiro, D. D., 306
Nikelly, A. G., 127
Nisbett, R. E., 88
Nornberger, J. I., 17, 207, 225
Nussbaum, D., 19
Nylander, I., 18

O'Neil, P. M., 213
Orbach, S., 155
Oscai, L. B., 300

Paffenbarger, R. S., 304
Parker, L., 216
Passmore, R., 162
Paulsen, B., 218, 219
Penick, S. B., 178, 225
Pestka, J., 299
Pilkington, T. R. E., 23
Pines, H. A., 138
Pletcher, P., 298
Polivy, J., 25
Pollock, M. L., 297, 304
Pomerantz, A. S., 21
Pool, K., 146
Powdermaker, H., 155

Rand, C. S. W., 177, 178, 181, 182
Reading, J. C., 22
Reichman, F., 88, 95
Richardson, S. A., 147
Rickard, H. C., 214
Riddle, E., 161
Riddle, F. E., 213

Rimm, A. A., 159
Rimm, D. C., 226
Ringuette, E., 88, 95
Ripley, H. S., 277
Rivinus, T. M., 215
Robinson, S., 192
Rodin, J., 16, 17, 133, 147
Roe, D. A., 137, 138
Romanczyk, R. G., 225, 226
Rose, H. E., 298
Rosenthal, B., 25
Ross, J. M., 18
Roth, L., 17, 19, 21, 209
Rothman, M., 91, 95
Rubin, T. I., 130, 158
Rudofsky, B., 154
Rush, J., 22
Russek, M., 295

Saccone, A. J., 212, 213
Sallade, J., 214
Sareen, C., 19
Schachter, S., 16, 88, 95, 99, 133, 161, 209
Schell, R. E., 19
Schonfeld, W. A., 19
Schroeder, C., 146
Schroeder, H. E., 17
Schwartz, M. F., 17
Schwartz, M. Z., 22
Sconbuch, S. S., 19
Secord, P. R., 151
Seltzer, C. C., 150, 163, 164
Sexauer, J. B., 213
Shapiro, L. R., 18
Shapiro, S., 304
Sicuranza, B. J., 160
Silverstone, J. T., 21, 22
Simonson, M., 157
Sjostrom, L., 18
Sloan, C. H., 218
Slochower, J., 17, 147
Spitz, R., 92, 96
Srole, L., 153
Staffieri, J. R., 146
Stalling, R. B., 25
Stalonas, P. M., 211, 217
Stancer, H. C., 19
Stefanik, P. A., 297, 298
Stevenson, J. A. F., 295
Stollack, G. E., 223
Stonehill, E., 18
Stout, C., 160
Strasser, A. L., 138
Straus, R., 132
Strong, J. A., 300

Stuart, R., 17, 156, 207, 209, 212, 215, 225, 226, 230, 232, 233
Stunkard, A., 19, 22, 88, 93, 95, 96, 113, 119, 130, 152, 153, 156, 157, 159, 161, 162, 177, 178, 181, 192, 193, 207, 210, 225, 226, 238, 298, 299
Sullivan, H. S., 92
Sullivan, L., 295
Swenson, E. J., 297
Swenson, W. M., 21
Szasz, T., 148

Taylor, C. B., 22
Taylor, C. I., 213
Teed, D., 19, 23
Thompson, A. M., 298
Thompson, P. D., 208
Thorn, M. E., 209
Thorpe, G. L., 225, 226
Tipton, R. M., 147
Tisdall, L. H., 160
Tobias, A. L., 136
Touraine, G., 126
Tracy, D. A., 225, 226
Tucker, D. H., 133, 134, 140, 143, 145, 161
Turner, C., 217

Van Itallie, T. B., 291
Varco, R. L., 23
Vender, M., 218

Wagner, M. G., 155
Walen, W. S., 18
Wang, V. L., 157
Ward-Hull, C. I., 151
Warren, C. A., 148
Weber, J. J., 182
Weiss, A. R., 215, 220
Weiss, E., 147
Werner, L. H., 159
Westie, C., 149
Westlake, R. J., 212
Whatley, J. L., 157
Wick, E. E., 227, 238, 268
Wilson, G. T., 212, 218, 219, 225, 226, 236, 238
Wing, R. R., 161, 208, 218, 225, 226
Winnik, H. S., 192
Wolf, S., 160
Wolff, O. H., 18
Wollersheim, J., 209
Wooley, S. C., 131, 132, 149, 159, 161, 162, 163, 167, 227

Wooley, O. W., 131, 132, 149, 159, 161,
162, 163, 167
Wunderlich, R. A., 302

Yserloo, B. V., 159

Zimbardo, P. G., 128
Zuti, W. B., 300
Zitter, R. E., 213

Subject Index

Addictive personality, 26
Alienation, 100
Amino acids, 78
Aminostatic hypothesis, 4
Anxiety, 40, 41
Appetite, 292-293
Attrition, 242, 243

Binging, 125
Biological "set point," 60
Body image, 18-21, 112-115
Booster sessions, 219, 238
Boredom, 54-56
Brown fat, 104
Bulimia, 279

Catecholamines, 44, 67, 295
Childhood obesity, 214-217
Cholecystokinin, 78
Cortisol, 6, 10, 12
Cultural factors, 104, 105, 153-156

Development obesity, 16
Discrimination, 131-139, 143-145
Discrimination and the medical profession,
    156-158

Eating patterns, 162, 163, 226, 227, 233
Environmental factors, 25

External responsiveness, 16, 17, 51-53, 57,
    58, 62, 63, 65, 71-73, 133-135

Family relationships, 115-117
Fat-thin syndrome, 20
Food logs, 228
Free fatty acids, 4, 7

Genetic factors, 18, 32, 46, 47
Glucagon, 10
Glucostatic hypothesis, 4
Glycerol, 4
Group hypnotherapy, 269-275
Growth hormone, 10

High-density lipoprotein, 304
Hypothalamus, 3, 4, 66, 67, 68, 76

Illness, 158-161, 166, 293, 304
Inactivity, 37, 297, 299
Inferiority complex, 119, 121
Insulin regulation, 5, 6, 7, 8, 9, 35, 36,
    68-71, 304
Internal regulatory cues, 63, 65

Jejunoileal bypass surgery, 22-24

Learning theory, 17-18
Legal issues, 142-145

Lipogenesis, 7
Lipostatic hypothesis, 4
Love, 98, 99
Low-density lipoprotein, 304

Metabolic factors, 34-36
Mood changes, 22
Morality, 148, 149
Morbidity, 158-161

Neurological mechanism, 67, 68, 75-79

Obesity and age, 59, 60
Obesity and drive for power, 91-93,
    120-123
Obesity and manic-depressive disorders,
    97, 98
Obesity and schizophrenia, 99, 100
Obesity and self-defeat, 100
Obesity and women, 149-152
Obesity
    biopsychosocial model, 31, 32
    cellular development, 2
    consequences of, 45, 46
    definition of, 1, 32, 33, 111, 112, 164,
        165, 268
    difference between normals and obese,
        5, 10-12
    hyperplastic, 1, 2
    hypertrophic, 1, 2, 7
    psychoanalytic theories, 90, 91, 183-189

psychodynamic theories, 15-16, 110,
    111, 193-195
    regulation of, 2-5, 10-12
Overfeeding, 73-75

Parent-child relationships, 95, 96
Prolactin, 10
Psychological characteristics, 21-22

Reactive obesity, 16, 118
Restrained eaters, 25, 45
Revenge motive, 123-125

Sexuality, 108, 186, 187
Socioeconomic factors, 48, 49, 59, 60, 88,
    89, 152-154
Stress, 40, 41

Taste, 4, 61, 62, 65
The National Association to Aid Fat
    Americans, 140-142
Thermostatic hypothesis, 4
TOPS (Take Off Pounds Sensibly), 244

Unrestrained eaters, 26, 45

Ventromedial nucleus, 3
Visual cues, 50, 52
Vocation, 109

Weight stability, 58, 59

RAMSEY CAMPBELL

THIRTEEN DAYS BY SUNSET BEACH

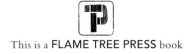

This is a **FLAME TREE PRESS** book

Text copyright © 2018 Ramsey Campbell

FLAME TREE PRESS
6 Melbray Mews, London, SW6 3NS, UK
flametreepress.com

Distribution and warehouse:
Baker & Taylor Publisher Services (BTPS)
30 Amberwood Parkway, Ashland, OH 44805
btpubservices.com

Publisher's Note: This is a work of fiction. Names, characters, places, and incidents are a product of the author's imagination. Locales and public names are sometimes used for atmospheric purposes. Any resemblance to actual people, living or dead, or to businesses, companies, events, institutions, or locales is completely coincidental.

Thanks to the Flame Tree Press team, including:
Taylor Bentley, Frances Bodiam, Federica Ciaravella, Don D'Auria,
Chris Herbert, Matteo Middlemiss, Josie Mitchell, Mike Spender,
Cat Taylor, Maria Tissot, Nick Wells, Gillian Whitaker.

The cover is created by Flame Tree Studio with
thanks to Nik Keevil and Shutterstock.com.
The font families used are Avenir and Bembo.

Flame Tree Press is an imprint of Flame Tree Publishing Ltd
flametreepublishing.com

A copy of the CIP data for this book is available from the British Library
and the Library of Congress.

HB ISBN: 978-1-78758-033-6
PB ISBN: 978-1-78758-031-2
ebook ISBN: 978-1-78758-034-3
Also available in FLAME TREE AUDIO

Printed in the US at Bookmasters, Ashland, Ohio

RAMSEY CAMPBELL

THIRTEEN DAYS BY
SUNSET BEACH

FLAME TREE PRESS
London & New York

For Gary and Emily –
an old man's tale…

THE FIRST DAY
20 AUGUST

"Don't joke about it, Ray. I gave you my passport before we got on the plane."

"Sandra, I'm not joking." Once he might have, but no longer. "You didn't give it me," he said, "the last time we had to show them."

When he reached for her capacious tapestry shoulder-bag she swung it and herself away from him. "Just let me have a chance to see."

Beyond her all three queues for the immigration desks were shrinking fast, but he managed not to urge her to be quick, even when she searched the bag a second time. "See, it isn't here," she said, surely not in triumph. "You must have it, Ray."

"I promise you I haven't," he protested, digging in the bag he'd used for carrying his laptop when he had one, and fished out the travel wallet that the agency provided. "You know I always keep them in here. There's just mine, look."

"Don't say we've left it on the plane."

"Wait here." At least this interrupted the panic that seldom left him alone any more. "Row nineteen. Seat D, weren't you? D for, yes, that was you," he said and limped fast to the doors, praying she'd missed some of his utterance.

A blaze of Greek air met him. A planeload of holidaymakers was crowding into the airport terminal with a rumble of wheeled cases just small enough to be stuffed into an overhead locker. Across the tarmac his and Sandra's plane was already swallowing trolleyloads of luggage while departing tourists clambered up the steps to the doors, and Ray hastened back to her. "They mightn't let me on," he panted. "Let me just check your bag."

"I know what's in my own bag," she complained but shrugged it off her shoulder. When he parted the frayed mouth it let out a faint musty perfume. He felt not just intrusive but shamefully condescending as he groped among the contents – the wallet full of bank cards and plastic memberships, not to mention miniature photographs of the children and grandchildren; a tube of lip balm instead of the pink lipstick she used to wear; a comb stuck in a brush along with several grey hairs; a mirror so small it suggested she didn't much care for it, especially since it was smeared with powder... As he moved aside a tarnished powder compact he'd bought her many years ago in Venice Sandra said "What's there?"

"Where?" His nerves didn't let him sound gentle. "Where do you mean?"

She reached a shaky hand to pinch the side of the bag between fingers and thumb, emphasising a rectangular outline through the canvas. The item must be inside the lining, and Ray was dismayed to think he might have to damage a favourite possession of hers – but she thrust her fingers into a gap and retrieved the passport. "I'm sorry, Ray," she murmured. "I didn't know I'd sprung a hole."

"Good lord above, nobody's to blame. I'll buy you a new bag if you like." This revived thoughts he didn't want to have. "Let's hurry or we'll miss the boat," he said, only to realise that now the lines for immigration stretched back almost to the doors. It took him and Sandra several minutes to shuffle halfway to a booth, at which point the man behind it stood up, indicating that his queue should use the other booths. A chorus of amiable murmurs and mutterings of resignation provoked Ray to blurt "If we don't catch the ferry to Vasilema I don't know where we'll be until tomorrow."

He hadn't realised he'd spoken so loud or seemed so vulnerable, unless it was Sandra who did. Several people gestured them to overtake the queue they'd had to join, and they were making to comply when the man inside the booth ahead knocked on the glass. "Back," he urged. "Back."

A minute took them closer, and another did. In two more they were at the window, where the immigration officer stared at their faces and then at their passports without disclosing an expression. "Vasilema," he said.

"That's if we ever get there." In the hope of speeding up the interview Ray said "Do you know when the last ferry is?"

"No boats out or coming here after dark. Vasilema," the man said again. "You are going back?"

"It's our first time," Sandra said and grasped Ray's arm.

"You leave it late." As Ray refrained from retorting that they were being delayed further, the official closed the passports. He slid them under the window of the booth, murmuring "Long life."

Sandra gripped Ray's arm harder. "Let's find our cases," she said.

He returned the passports to the wallet in his bag as he followed her into the arrival hall. "Which is it?" she said. "Can you see them?"

He heard her attempting to suppress the disquiet he was trying not to find a reason for. None of the luggage carousels was in motion, and he couldn't see a single case. While the further carousel was surrounded by holidaymakers, the flight number on the sign was disconcertingly unfamiliar. "Excuse me," he called as he limped ahead of Sandra. "Is this the Manchester flight as well?"

Half a dozen people turned and shrugged or shook their heads. "That's finished, hon," said a woman who'd tried to make way for him and Sandra at immigration. "They've all took their bags and gone."

"We haven't," Sandra protested.

"They've never lost your bags for you," the woman cried and poked her husband with a fist. "You two sit down and Jack will see what he can do. What's your luggage look like?"

"That's very kind," Ray said, "but there's no need, honestly. Let's see if they come round again."

"Jack, go and find someone who knows what's going on. And you two tell me what to look for. What'll your name be?"

"Really," Sandra said, "you mustn't go to so much trouble." When the woman made to disagree she added "Please don't fuss."

"Suit yourself." As Sandra headed for a gap in the crowd around the carousel the woman said "Is she always like that, hon?"

"No," Ray said as an alarm seemed to voice his state of mind. It was announcing luggage, though the belt took quite a time to start its crawl. Most of its length made a circuit before the leader of the procession – a pink suitcase painted with greenery – butted the plastic strips at the entrance to the carousel aside. That wasn't Ray's case or Sandra's, and nothing on the belt was. The carousel was almost empty by the time another parade edged into the open, led by a large black suitcase rendered individual by a cross of grey tape. Sandra squeezed Ray's arm, only to bruise it as a man on the far side of the carousel swung the case off the belt. "Excuse me," Ray shouted and had to clear his throat just as loud. "I think that's ours."

The man spent some moments in deciding he had been addressed. "You think wrong," he said and strode away, towing the suitcase.

Ray was about to chase him when Sandra caught his arm again. For a disoriented moment he thought she was so desperate for peace that she would even give up their luggage, and then he saw that two more cases marked with crosses had emerged from hiding. They weren't quite as black as the one he and Sandra had misidentified. "Sorry," he called after the man, "just an old fool," which earned a look from the determinedly helpful woman. He hauled one suitcase off the belt and would have hastened to prevent Sandra from lifting its twin, but the man called Jack did. "Have yourself a time," Jack said. "Try and not lose anything else."

"Just don't lose each other," said his wife.

Ray didn't look at Sandra, because they had to find the travel representative. He put on all the speed he could with the heavier case and tramped into the airport concourse. At least a dozen people were brandishing clipboards with names or messages, but for long enough to let panic regather in his guts he could see nothing he recognised. Surely their contact hadn't given up on them, and at last Ray caught sight of the Frugogo uniform, an orange T-shirt with the syllables stacked on it, the lower pair overlapping. The girl was matching new arrivals with names on a list, and renewed her polished smile for Ray and Sandra. "Where are we taking you?" she said.

"Vasilema," Sandra said.

"Mr and Mrs Thornton. You're the last ones for the island." She crossed them out before saying "I'm afraid I've had to let the coach go. He did wait as long as he could."

Ray found he was bruising his fingers on the handle of his suitcase. "We were delayed. What are we supposed to do now?"

"Take a taxi," the girl said and glanced at her watch. "If you hurry you should still make the connection."

"Could you get it for us?" Sandra said.

"I still have all these people," the girl said with a smile at the gathering queue. "Just get a receipt and give it to your rep on the island."

Ray thought she might have asked if they had Greek money, which they had. He made for the exit as fast as Sandra could keep up with him. Beyond the glass doors his breath tasted hot at once, and he might have proposed covering their heads if the hats hadn't been in the suitcases. The handle of the case grew clammy in his grasp as he hauled it past the airport building to a rank of cars in various stages of dustiness. All the drivers were leaning against the wall of the terminal, but as soon as Ray lifted a hand one of them strode to him. "Where for you?"

"We need to catch the ferry," Sandra said.

"Must be quick." The swarthy moustached man seized both cases and sped them to the foremost car, then opened the door wide. "Sit quick."

Once Sandra was seated she set about hitching herself across the hot upholstery until he thumped on the roof. "No time," he shouted as he slammed the boot, "other side," and Ray had barely limped around the car and climbed in beside Sandra when the driver sent the taxi forward. By the time the Thorntons managed to persuade the tags on their seatbelts to reach the sockets and fit into the slits, the car had left the airport and was racing down a dusty road between fields of grass gilded by the low sunlight. "Which boat for you?" the driver said.

It seemed to be Ray's turn to say "Vasilema."

The rosary that dangled from the driving mirror appeared to describe a sign in the air as the taxi swung around a bend. "Not Sunset Beach," the driver said.

"Too lively for us. That's for the young folk. We're just along the coast at Teleftaiafos."

The driver's eyes gleamed, perhaps with the low sun. "I find you room here."

"No need, thank you. We're all booked."

"Very nice room in town. Very clean."

"As I say, we're going to the island. It's all paid for, the ferry too. It's a package."

"Why you not on coach?"

"It left without us. Now if you don't mind – "

"Why they don't pay for me?"

"They will." Absurdly, Ray felt implicated if not accused. "They'll reimburse us," he said, "if you give us a receipt when we get to the ferry."

"Maybe they have to pay for room in town."

"Is it someone you know?" Sandra said with a forgiving laugh.

"Brother." The man plainly failed to find this humorous. "If you stay one night," he said, "maybe you like."

"It's all right," Ray said, though his tone was at odds with the words. This was among the elements of travelling abroad he welcomed least – having to refuse an offer again and again. From feeling embarrassed he'd grown used to saying no as soon as anybody accosted him, but he could do without it on this trip. "I'm sure it's splendid," he said, "but we're expected on the island."

"All our family is coming," Sandra said. "They're meeting us over there."

As Ray glimpsed the sleepily glittering sea across a field the driver said "How much family?"

"Our children and their partners and the grandchildren as well," Ray told him. "The youngest will be very disappointed if we don't show up. I'm sure they all will."

The driver peered at him in the mirror. "Some are young."

"That's what I said."

"You look after them."

It might have been a query or an admonition. "Of course we shall," Ray said.

This seemed to lend the taxi more speed. "Look to sun," the driver said. "Watch what sun does."

Perhaps he meant how the shadows of a line of poplars striped the road ahead. As a breeze set the shadows groping for the car, Ray decided that the driver had been talking about sunburn or sunstroke. He refrained from answering in case that slowed the taxi down, and held Sandra's hand, which felt like sharing too many unspoken thoughts. He let go when at last they saw a ship's funnel ahead.

By the time they reached the port he'd sorted out cash for the taxi and the voucher for the ferry. The driver had to slow down for a crowd on the dock, beside which the vessels looked massively weightless as clouds. Beyond several of these was a boat less than a quarter of their size. The driver honked the horn at it as he came alongside, though passengers were still boarding. Indeed, others hadn't finished disembarking – dull-eyed young couples so encumbered by their backpacks that just one girl raised a hand to greet the incomers, a feeble gesture that might almost have been trying to convey a different message. Ray would have said they needed a holiday to get over the one they'd just had. "Too much night life," he remarked instead as the driver parked in the middle of the road.

Sandra was out of the taxi before Ray succeeded in releasing his seatbelt. "I'll make sure they don't go without us," she said and made for the ferry, tugging her suitcase.

The man heaved the second case out of the boot and gazed at it while Ray paid him. "You use cross."

"It's a way of distinguishing our luggage." Ray felt oddly abashed by explaining "It isn't religious."

"No good."

"Well, they're some use. You've seen other people with the same idea, you mean," Ray said as Sandra joined the queue at the gangplank. "Forgive my hurrying you, but could you – "

The driver wrote the date and time and payment on a notepad with a stubby pencil whose thick lead was worn down almost to the wood, and eventually handed Ray the slip, which at least bore the details of the taxi firm. Ray was pulling up the handle of his case when the driver said "Look after lady too."

Ray felt as if the man had somehow gleaned too much. "What do you mean?"

"Bring her back."

As Ray opened his mouth Sandra called "They need the voucher."

"I'm coming now," he shouted, and the driver turned away as though he'd been rebuffed. Ray made for the ferry as fast as the suitcase allowed, dragging at his arm like a reluctant child. He was halfway to the gangplank when a sailor came to snatch the voucher. "Go on," the sailor said, not much like a welcome at all.

Sandra had dragged her case on board. When Ray followed her he found the deck was trembling with the impatience of the engines. Beyond a muster of luggage several dozen passengers sat on plastic bucket seats in a lounge overlooked by a small rudimentary bar bereft of staff. Sandra trundled her case to the nearest trio of seats and waited for Ray to bring his. "What was he saying to you?" she said.

"Just how he didn't think these crosses would be much use."

The engines began throbbing like Ray's insistent pulse, and the ferry edged away from the dock. As the vessels moored alongside shrank to fit the windows of the lounge Sandra clasped his arm in both hands. "Nearly there," she said with a surge of the excitement holidays had always prompted, "and soon everyone will be."

All summer he'd had the unhappy impression that her eyes had faded like her close-cropped hair, no longer glossy black, and her small face that oughtn't to have room for so many lines, but now her eyes seemed to have regained a brighter blue. While her lips were still pale, she could still smile, and she even wrinkled her long slim nose in the old amused way he'd been in danger of forgetting. She didn't relinquish his arm until he managed to smile, and then he turned quickly to the window. The sun was hovering above the horizon, from which it laid a path of amber light for the boat to follow. Otherwise there was only water as still as the cloudless sky except around the vessel, and Ray didn't know he'd abandoned the view until his head jerked up. "Sorry," he mumbled.

"Why, Ray? You've earned a rest. You drove us to the airport when you should have been asleep."

"I don't want to leave you alone."

"You won't, will you? I'll know you're here."

For years he hadn't slept much in the weeks before a holiday – every night his mind would run through all the tasks and items he had to remember, not to mention all the apparently innumerable things that could go wrong – but by now he'd forgotten how it felt to sleep all night or even for a few unbroken hours. "Say you'll wake me if you need me," he said.

"I always need you, but if I need to wake you I will."

Instead a dull impact wakened him. How badly had she hurt herself by slipping off the plastic chair? At least people were hurrying to help, except that when Ray widened his shamefully reluctant eyes he saw all the young holidaymakers heading for their luggage. He'd felt the ferry bump against a jetty, and Sandra was upright on the seat beside him.

At first he thought Vasilema Town had been illuminated to welcome the newcomers. A multitude of white buildings tinged with red clung to a hill as haphazardly as shells on a rock, and window after window shone crimson. As he and Sandra hauled their cases onto the dockside the lowest windows darkened, and before Ray could take much of a breath the next highest row of lights went out. He saw the light retreating from him and Sandra, and glanced behind him to confirm that it was just the sunset, the horizon having sliced the red orb in half.

The darkness crept uphill as they followed their fellow passengers along the wharf to a coach attended by a girl in a Frugogo uniform. "Take your time," she called. "You're important to us."

The driver seized each case and swung it into the compartment full of luggage while the cigarette between his lips kept hold of at least an inch of ash. Ray cupped Sandra's elbow to help her up the steps and felt how thin her arm had grown. She scrambled onto the seat immediately behind the driver's not unlike an excited youngster. As soon as he joined her Ray tugged the belt across himself to encourage her to be equally safe. He was trying to riddle the mechanism that would lock the arm of the seat in position when a young man leaned across the aisle to fix it by raising it above the horizontal and easing it down. "No probs," he said, and Ray felt mean for reflecting that the generation to which all the passengers except him and Sandra belonged seemed increasingly to speak in the language of their text messages. He'd often said so to his pupils at school, but the thought left him feeling even more out of date.

The driver took a last drag at his cigarette and squashed it out between a finger and thumb varnished with nicotine as he climbed aboard. While he eased the coach forward the Frugogo girl picked up a microphone and stood with her back to the windscreen, beneath an icon of a Greek saint with a spear in his hand. "Kali mera," she said and, having explained that it meant good evening, repeated it until the passengers echoed it loud enough to suit her. "I'm Sam, and welcome to our island. Who hasn't been before?"

"We haven't," Sandra murmured.

"I'm promising some of you will be back. Lots of our guests say they've had the best nights of their lives." The travel representative blinked at Ray and Sandra as though she'd almost overlooked them, but her broad roundish suntanned face stayed placid. "If you've come for a rest," she said, "you'll get that too."

She handed out envelopes that contained invitations to tomorrow's welcome meeting, together with an island map that Ray thought could have been more detailed. By now the coach was speeding along the coast road, beside which a ruddy afterglow was sinking into the ocean. Sam returned to the microphone to mention local drawbacks – mosquitoes, bathroom plumbing – which were so familiar from previous Greek holidays that Ray stopped hearing them. She'd said he could rest, and Sandra had as well.

This time light and uproar wakened him. The coach was at a standstill and almost empty too. Both sides of the teeming street blazed with colours he might have expected to find in a nursery or else a cocktail. A neon jester pranced above a bar while a neon cat leapt back and forth across the entrance to another, as though it kept losing if not playing with some invisible prey. All the bars and clubs seemed determined to blot out whatever music their neighbours were emitting. Ray could see nobody older than the passengers Sam was ushering to an apartment block beside the coach. The driver had one foot on the lowest step while he sucked at another cigarette. "Soon be quiet," he said.

"It's Sunset Beach," Sandra told Ray. "I wouldn't like to try to sleep here."

"They don't," the driver said mostly to himself, "when it's dark."

Ray wondered if the resort ever was, except out of season. He'd resumed nodding before Sam reappeared. The turmoil of light and noise took some time to fall behind, giving way to a deserted road where moths fluttered into the headlamp beams. In a few minutes the beams found a sign for Teleftaiafos, and then the village itself. Beyond a handful of tavernas the coach halted outside a stone arch overgrown with flowering vines. "Sunny View," Sam announced.

As Ray stepped down into the hot night he heard the distant pulse of Sunset Beach, reduced to a single insistent repetitive beat. He was taking Sandra's arm to help her down the steps when a woman bustled out of a house across the marble courtyard beyond the arch and practically ran to the coach. "Here you are at last," she cried. "Mr and Mrs Thornton."

"This is Evadne." Although Sam was presumably used to the spectacle, she seemed a little overwhelmed. "She'll look after you," she said.

The large woman embraced Sandra like an old friend and gave Ray an equally vigorous hug, not so much patting as thumping his back. A wide smile dug creases into her loosely lined brown face. "What shall I call you?" she was eager to establish.

"Ray," he said or at any rate gasped.

"Sandra," Sandra said, having regained her breath.

"You must call Evadne if you need anything at all. If ever I am not here, call Stavros."

As if she'd given him his cue a man even brawnier than Evadne crossed the courtyard to engulf the handles of the cases in his extravagantly hairy hands. A cat fled not much more loudly than its shadow across the marble flagstones and hid behind a pot of purple blossom while Evadne led the Thorntons into the house. Except for a counter and the pigeonholes behind it, the office just within the doorway might have been a parlour. As Evadne lifted a key off a hook Ray said "Do you want our passports?"

"Give them tomorrow. You can't go anywhere, can you? Now we take you to your room."

Behind the house four white two-storey apartment blocks boxed in a swimming pool. A gap through the middle of the left-hand block led to three further sets of apartments surrounding a play area, where rotund faces painted on the swings and slides and roundabouts displayed toothy grins to welcome children. "Your young ones come tomorrow," Evadne said.

"Only one of them is this young," Sandra said as a shadow leapt off a swing – another cat, Ray saw.

"We could not put you all together. You all have the view, but you are at the top and the rest are down below," Evadne said and gave her a concerned look. "Both of you are good for climbing up, yes?"

"I've a bit of life in me yet."

Ray had to swallow as an aid to saying "And I'm fine."

Stavros was waiting with the luggage by a flight of marble steps, and the Greek couple tramped up to the balcony alongside the top floor with a suitcase each. By the time Ray and Sandra caught up with them Evadne had unlocked an apartment and inserted the key fob in a socket to rouse the lights in a large white room. It contained a double bed, a wardrobe and a dressing-table attended by a sketchy chair, a hob and a microwave beside a sink at the far end of the room, where a refrigerator burbled to itself. Whoever made the beds had left a flower on each pillow. "They're lovely," Sandra said as Ray was put in mind of laying down a flower.

While Stavros wheeled the cases in Evadne crossed the room and slid the floor-length window open. Beyond a balcony on which a pair of chairs matched a round white plastic table, the hem of the dark sea drifted back and forth across a dim beach planted with drooping umbrellas. The distant lights of Sunset Beach seemed to be keeping time with a disco beat. The blurred sound was no louder than the sea, but Sandra said "Does that go on all night?"

"They sleep in the day. It is such a place." Evadne sounded apologetic, and Ray had the odd idea that her animation was designed to compensate. "You should not let them trouble you," she said.

"I was only wondering if we could have kept it up, even at their age."

"They take life from the night."

"That's one way to put it," Sandra said, switching on the bathroom light. "Oh, isn't there a mirror?"

Above the sink opposite the toilet and beside a shower was a human frieze – a photograph of dancers with their arms on one another's shoulders. "Nobody will mind how you look on holiday," Evadne said.

"I'd still like a mirror, and I'm sure Ray would for shaving."

"I can bring one," Evadne said, though not before she'd gazed at both of them. "Will you want air conditioning? It is five euros every day, but your safe, that is free."

She seemed more apologetic than ever. "At that price we'll have air conditioning," Ray said.

"I will bring you control." Evadne paused in the doorway to add "Any of us who want to come in, we knock twice and wait for you to answer."

Sandra unzipped her case, and Ray set about unpacking his. "I'm already glad we came, aren't you?" she said.

"In that case I couldn't be gladder."

He didn't know how much he was playing with words. Sandra opened the wardrobe, revealing the safe and a hidden chest of drawers. She was transferring dresses onto hangers when somebody knocked at the door. "Come in," Ray called.

"No."

Evadne sounded more admonitory than he understood. She knocked again, and Sandra called "Come in."

"That is right," Evadne said and opened the door. "We knock twice and then you say."

She switched on the box on the ceiling opposite the beds, and metal slats rattled apart to fan out a chill. She showed the Thorntons how to operate the remote control and then substituted the mirror she'd laid on a bed for the photograph in the bathroom. "May the night bless you," she said.

Once she'd gone Sandra gave Ray her wide-eyed bemused look. "Do we think that's a local tradition?"

"Blessing your guests, you mean."

"That too, but I was thinking of the routine with the knocks."

"Maybe now we know one Doug and Pris won't have heard of."

Sandra found plates and glasses and utensils in a cupboard under the sink, and then opened the refrigerator, where a three-litre bottle of water was growing misty with condensation. "Well, nobody's going thirsty here," she said and filled two glasses. "Shall we sit out before we go to bed?"

When they sat on their balcony the dividing wall blocked out the muffled thudding of percussion and the neon glow of Sunset Beach. Before long Ray saw the sky retreat from the sea, hinting at a vaster darkness. A star seemed to conjure forth a dozen, and then many more began to glimmer as if they were being silently born from the dark. Ray saw how intent on them Sandra had grown, and how they were bestowing some kind of peace. He could only try to count them, but he had no idea what total he'd reached when his head lurched up from nodding. "You go and catch up on your sleep," Sandra said. "I won't stay out much longer."

"Are you sure you don't mind?" This was just a way to postpone asking "How do you feel?"

"Honestly," she said with some surprise, "I feel better than I have for weeks. I wish it could always be like this."

Ray thought she meant not just herself but the night as well. He planted a hand on the slippery table to help himself up and squeezed her thin shoulder, then stooped to leave her a dry kiss. As he turned away he caught sight of a distant figure on the beach. He was glad to conclude that the sand must be firm – he'd never cared for walking on soft sand even when he was considerably fitter – since the silhouette against the neon glow was approaching at quite a pace.

He left the window open while he went into the bathroom, where he couldn't help reflecting that he could have done without the mirror or at any rate the sight of himself. Age was dangling an unreasonable amount of his face beneath the chin, dragging down his features – the baggy eyes, the wrinkled lips he had to keep remembering to hitch up at the corners, even the broad nose in which hairs too often lurked – as well as draining colour from them and his previously auburn hair. He brushed his teeth and washed his face in reluctantly lukewarm water, and then he went to the window. "I'll have to shut this," he murmured, "or the air conditioning won't work."

"I'll know you're there. Close the curtains too."

"Good night then."

"It is."

He couldn't think of any response that wouldn't betray he was loitering. He found his way to bed by the glow from the lamps in the play area, but switched on Sandra's bedside light to help her when she came in. He slipped beneath the thin quilt to discover that it hid a pair of single beds pushed together, suggesting a separation that made him unhappier than he wanted to comprehend. He thought the light would keep him awake to wait for Sandra, but it went out almost instantly, or he did.

It wakened him as well. He blinked his sticky eyes wide to find he was alone in bed. He fumbled at the bedside table, only just saving his watch from falling to the floor. When he managed to capture it he found that he hadn't seen Sandra for nearly an hour. At once his mouth was dry as sand, and yet he felt unexpectedly resigned, a preamble to all the feelings he would have to experience. He levered himself up on his shaky arms and floundered off the bed to trudge across the chill marble floor to the window.

Sandra was lolling half off the plastic chair. Her head was on one side and propped on the back of the chair, turning her face to the stars. Ray threw the curtain out of the way and hauled the window open. "Are you all right?" he pleaded.

Her head took some moments to wobble erect. "You woke me," she protested. "I was having such a dream."

"You don't want to stay out here all night, do you? I went in an hour ago. What were you dreaming?"

"It's gone." Not much less peevishly she said "All right, I'm coming in."

She relented as he shut the window. "You must have been worried," she said. "I'm here now." She used the bathroom and then joined Ray in bed, capturing his hand to draw it around her bony waist. As she switched off her light she murmured "That was it. The dark."

"What was?" Ray felt oddly reluctant to ask.

"My dream." As if trying to summon it back she said "It was dark, but there was some kind of light, and it went on for ever."

THE SECOND DAY
21 AUGUST

"I wouldn't want a different life."

Sandra's voice wakened him. She was talking to the walker Ray had seen last night, who had sprung onto the balcony as easily as he'd come along the beach. Of course he hadn't, though Ray felt as if he was remembering it, presumably from a dream. Had the family arrived? He untangled himself from the quilt to reach for his watch. While they weren't due for hours yet, he was dismayed to find that it was nearly noon. How long had Sandra been up without him? He threw off the quilt and hurried to the bathroom.

He could hear Sandra and their neighbour through the small high window above the shower stall. Sandra was recalling how she and Ray had met at teacher training college, where they'd been involved with other people but had always come back together; how they'd almost parted for good over whether Ray should move to Coventry to live with her or she should join him in York; how they'd compromised on Manchester when they'd both found jobs there; how they'd been heads of departments by the time they retired, Sandra running English while Ray took care of Mathematics... He didn't care to think how much this resembled an obituary, though at least her account was livelier. He tramped back to the bedside table for his morning medication, swallowing pill after pill, not to mention tablets. Once he'd pulled long-legged swimming trunks over his bulbous greying stomach he went to find Sandra. "Here's the sleeping beauty," a woman said.

She was plump and, to judge from the locks that had escaped from the towel around her head, generously red-haired. Her bare arms rested on the dividing wall, hands clasped as if in a casual prayer. "There's just one beauty at this table, and it isn't me," Ray said.

Sandra was wearing her new green one-piece swimsuit, and he was unhappy to think that by sleeping he'd kept her from venturing out of the shade on the balcony, since the sunlight was almost everywhere else. "I'm for the pool," their neighbour said. "Don't forget to see to that bite, Sandra."

As the woman started or perhaps resumed a hearty conversation in the next apartment Ray said "What bite?"

"Something must have got me when I was asleep out here last night." Sandra pointed to a red mark on the side of her neck. "It doesn't hurt," she said. "I hadn't even noticed till Jane, you just met her, told me it was there."

Peering closer, Ray saw that the mark was swollen around a hole somewhat larger than a pinprick. "We'd better put something on it all the same."

"I was going to." As she made for the apartment Sandra said "Jane was saying which tavernas they recommend."

"Are you hungry?" Ray was able to hope.

"Do you know, I think I could be. I'm thirsty, I can tell you that." Sandra drained her bedside glass of water and fetched a tube of ointment from the chest of drawers. As Ray rubbed ointment on the bite as gently as he could and winced on her behalf, she said "Let's find a supermarket too."

She donned a long dress over her swimsuit and planted her hat firmly on her head while Ray hid some of his less appealing aspects with a shirt and retrieved his own hat from its perch on top of the safe. She put on her sunglasses as he opened the door. The play area was deserted, but several children organised by a girl wearing a Sunny View cap were playing ball in the pool, around which older folk lay on loungers, reading electronic texts or books. A truck piled with vegetables was coasting through the village while the driver advertised his produce with a microphone, and the Thorntons followed in the dusty wake. Among the tavernas and small shops between the Sunny View and the village square they came upon the Superber supermarket. "Is that a word?" Sandra said.

Outside the entrance a wire stand displayed English newspapers, days old. They might have been trying to cling to the past, Ray thought, to postpone some disaster. Another stand held paperbacks so faded the covers were ghosts of themselves, with pages brown as parched grass. Beyond the glass doors the air was several degrees cooler than the street, and Sandra gave a tiny sigh. A defiantly moustached old woman in black watched from behind the till as Ray followed Sandra from shelf to shelf. Each item she placed in his wire basket – a plastic bottle of retsina, a packet of olives, a hunk of feta cheese – felt like a token of her old self. "Look, there's a bakery," she said, "we can get fresh bread in the mornings," and he saw a renewed light in her eyes. "And here's a bucket and spade for William."

When she made to pick up a bundle of six bottles of water he grabbed it with his free hand, barely managing to cross the shop before he had to dump the bottles on the counter. The old woman didn't glance at it or the basket he planted next to it, but pointed at the beach toys Sandra was carrying. "You have young," she said.

"We've had a couple," Sandra said, suppressing her amusement. "We have a little grandson now."

"Here."

Presumably this did duty as a question. "He should be on the ferry at this moment," Ray said.

"Coming here." Her next question sounded somewhat more like one. "Where you are?"

"Staying, do you mean? The Sunny View."

"You stay home."

Ray was too bewildered not to ask "Why should we have done that? We like what we've seen so far."

"Home." As if she was sharing an unfavourable view of men and their comprehension she told Sandra "Home at Sunny View."

"Well, I think we'll be having some days out," Sandra said. "We'd like to explore your island."

"Not all." The old woman shut her wrinkled eyelids while she said "Not Sunset Beach."

"I shouldn't think we're tempted," Ray said, "but why not there?"

"Not for you."

"I think we rather had that impression," Sandra said.

Her hint of humour seemed to provoke the old woman, who made a visible bid to marshal her language. "They not like us."

"They aren't so very different from how we were at their age."

"And it wasn't very long ago," Ray said, "that we were teaching people just like them when they weren't much younger."

The old woman abandoned trying to communicate. She didn't so much plant each item on the counter as thump it with them. She let Sandra fumble over opening a carrier bag, and Ray had the impression that she regarded visitors as more necessary than welcome. He hoisted the bottles against his chest, and as soon as he emerged from the supermarket the heat seemed to weigh on them. The Sunny View was less than a quarter of a mile away, but his forearms began to ache before he'd trudged half the distance. They were throbbing by the time he reached the viny arch. As he stumbled across the courtyard Evadne looked out of the office and then ran to him. "You must not carry those," she cried. "Next time call Stavros."

She seized the six-pack and marched ahead, jogging up the steps to the apartment. She was still holding the bottles when Ray arrived with the bag he'd taken from Sandra, who unlocked the door to reveal the apartment had been serviced. Even the flowers on the pillows had been renewed. "Thank you for everything," Ray said.

"It is only little," Evadne said. "We value what guests bring."

She stood the bottles on top of the refrigerator and closed the apartment door so gently that she might have been quitting a sickroom. As Sandra unloaded her bag into the refrigerator she said "Are you hungry?"

Ray tried not to sound too urgent. "Are you?"

"I feel as if I need to eat. I'll have a bite."

"Would olives and cheese do the job?"

"Or we could go out for lunch. We can try somewhere close so we'll see when everyone arrives."

Ray tried to keep surprise out of his voice. "Let's do that by all means."

They were making for the door when Sandra laid a not entirely steady hand on his arm. "Remember, we mustn't give them any reason to suspect. As far as they're concerned nothing's wrong."

"We'll keep them all happy. We're a team," Ray said, but he'd been reminded how hard the next thirteen days might be.

★   ★   ★

The nearest taverna was across the road, in sight of the Sunny View. Beyond a low white wall draped with a mass of sapphire flowers, Chloe's Garden contained a dozen tables among pots of basil, while as many tables surrounded a bar and kitchen under a roof. As Ray and Sandra took their places by the wall a slim long-faced young woman with glossy amber skin brought them menus. "You will have wine."

It scarcely bothered sounding like a question. "How did you know?" Sandra said.

"You bought some before."

"Small place, hey? Nothing goes unnoticed." Ray wasn't

certain whether to be disconcerted or amused. "We'll have a litre of your white wine from the barrel."

"And one of water too, please," Sandra said.

By the time the waitress brought this in a bottle and the wine in a red clay jug, the Thorntons had made their selection: calamari, whitebait, beans the menu called gigantic, pork in wine. "Yammas," the waitress wished them, and they raised their glasses in response. "Yammas," Ray said to Sandra, and was reminded that the word meant health.

He was watching her sip her wine more minutely than she used to when the waitress returned with plates and a basket of bread. "Do you mind if we sit somewhere a bit shadier?" Sandra said. "We'll still see the coach."

She dropped her hat on an empty chair once they were seated in the shadow of a pine. "At least my wife won't get bitten here," Ray said.

"I pray not," the waitress said quite like a prayer. "Why do you say?"

"You're keeping off the insects." He pointed at the pot of basil behind Sandra and then at her neck. "Would that have been a mosquito?"

"None here."

"That's what I said. There must have been one on our balcony last night, though."

"There should not be that. You should not go out there again."

"I expect we'll be all right," Ray said. "We'll use a spray."

A handbell jangled in the kitchen, where a short plump woman was placing dishes on a tray. The waitress served them to the Thorntons and said "Yammas" once again, and might have been about to say more if the older woman hadn't called "Daphne." As Daphne returned to the kitchen Ray picked up the serving spoon from the dish of jumbo beans in sauce. "Would you like some?" he prompted Sandra.

"You take yours and I'll get my own."

He sensed that she was stopping barely short of telling him not to fuss. Watching her eat could be construed that way, but he risked saying "It's good, isn't it?" since the dishes were, and didn't think her agreement was just meant to reassure him. Having waited until she'd had a mouthful of every item, he was heartened to see her take another of each. Was Daphne arguing with the woman he'd deduced was Chloe, her mother? Between Greeks a chat about the weather could sound fierce enough for a declaration of war, but he wondered why both women kept glancing towards him and Sandra. While he didn't understand a word, he saw Chloe reach a decision, folding her arms as she stepped out of the kitchen. At that moment Sandra cried "Is this them?"

A bus was approaching along the road from Sunset Beach. Sandra took off her sunglasses and craned over the wall. When the bus halted in front of the Sunny View she backed out of the sunlight, shading her eyes with her free hand. The door of the bus folded open, and she squeezed Ray's arm. Did she mean to convey that the deception was about to begin? Perhaps that wasn't on her mind, since she said eagerly "It is."

She began to wave as soon as the first passenger stepped down, and Ray saw Chloe retreat with a shrug into the kitchen. Doug was leading the way off the bus, followed by Pris and their son Tim. They all had their habitual contentedly dishevelled look, as if they were windblown and ready for more. "Mum, dad," Doug shouted, which seemed faintly to pain Natalie's partner Julian, who was busy giving the village a critical look. Natalie's daughter Jonquil was behind him, although not too close, and shook a hand at Ray and Sandra in her teenage version of a wave. Last came five-year-old William with Natalie at his back. She raised a hand to greet her parents while blinking not entirely favourably at the apartments and tavernas. "It's grandma and grandad," William shouted and made to run to them.

One long step took Julian in front of him. "What have we discussed about behaviour on the road?"

"But there isn't any traffic, daddy."

"We aren't talking about traffic. What did we agree?"

"Not to run out on it." Inspiration widened William's eyes as he said "But we're on it, so – "

"I'm not about to argue with you, William. We never run on the road, and we never cross it by ourselves."

"I'll take him over, Julian," Jonquil said.

"Your mother and I would prefer you to deal with your luggage. Please check while you're unpacking that all your things and William's are numbered."

That didn't mean counted, Ray knew. Julian had introduced the principle that any items even slightly likely to be lost should bear his and Natalie's phone numbers. "Is all the family here?" Evadne called as she and Stavros crossed the courtyard. "You leave your bags with us. We will put them in your rooms."

"Thank you very much," Natalie said, "but we'll see to them. Come along, William. You carry on with your meal," she told her parents, "and we'll say hello properly soon."

"Some of us will now," Doug declared, striding to embrace Sandra and then Ray. He swept his hair back from his high forehead as if to tug more eagerness into his elongated wide-eyed face, where the nose and chin competed for largeness and prominence. "How's Pris's choice and mine so far?" he said.

"We wouldn't ask for better," Sandra said.

"Then here's hoping you both have the time you deserve."

Ray was aware that Sandra wasn't speaking, and he found he couldn't either. "And let's hope the quiet will do for Nat and Jules," Doug said, "though it can't be as quiet as Sunset Beach."

"You'll be joking, will you?" Ray assumed.

"When we came through there just now we didn't see a living soul except for the ones who got off the bus."

"They'll all be in bed with hangovers," Sandra said. "You had a few of those at their age."

"I wasn't quite that bad, was I? Our driver didn't seem to think too much of them. They get used up at night, he said."

"So does their money," Ray observed. "I should think the locals don't mind that, or ours either."

"We got the feeling he was glad to have them on the island but didn't want to be." Doug frowned as if his brows might squeeze the notion into focus, then abandoned the task. "I'll go and see how the others are doing," he said. "We want it to be good for everyone."

Sandra watched him cross the road and the marble courtyard before she took another mouthful from her plate, and Ray replenished her wineglass by way of encouragement. Once he'd cleared his own plate he eyed the Sunny View until Sandra said "Have some more. Don't wait for me."

"I don't mind waiting," he said, a tame version of the truth. Suppose sensing that he hoped she would eat more only made her stubborn? He helped himself to a small portion from each dish, and was lingering over them so as not to finish before Sandra when he heard footsteps approaching the courtyard.

As Jonquil and William came in sight he was ashamed to feel he wouldn't mind if they were on their own, and did his best to be equally pleased to see not just their mother but William's father behind them. "Be careful on the road," Natalie said.

"You heard mum," Jonquil said as though to demonstrate she hadn't been addressed as well.

She took the boy's hand to lead him to the taverna, letting go a few yards short of the wall, an act that plainly failed to please his parents. He dashed to hug Sandra and then Ray, and Jonquil followed with not much less of an embrace. Natalie outdid it for vigour — Ray felt some of her bones creak — after which Julian shook his hand, having clasped Sandra's shoulders. "I'm sorry if we seemed at all abrupt when we arrived," Julian said. "We wouldn't want you to assume we weren't glad to see you."

"We're just as happy to see you, aren't we, Sandra?" Ray said.

"Then everybody's satisfied." Julian straightened his prominent lips as if to underline his sharp nose and turned not quite towards the younger members of the family. "Now I believe someone has some words for their grandparents."

William marched forward, hands behind his back. His face was a miniature edition of his father's, and the pale blue eyes looked even bigger for their setting. "'m sorry – "

"You can speak more clearly than that, William," Natalie said.

"I'm sorry I caused trouble on the road."

"That's the fellow," Julian said. "I don't know if anyone else feels they ought to speak."

He hadn't changed his stance. Jonquil's face grew blank – the deep brown eyes and broad snub nose that recalled her father's, as the expansiveness of her pink lips did, and even her soft short reddish hair. When he didn't hear from her Julian's pout grew less inadvertent. "Was your insurance all it should be, Raymond?" he said.

"It's everything we asked for," Ray said.

As he saw Sandra relax, having shared the thought he'd kept unspoken, Daphne came over. "Welcome to our garden. Will you join your friends?"

"Our family." Julian gazed at her as if this ought to have been obvious. "We had a sandwich on the ferry, thank you," he said. "Just a bottle of water for us."

"Be together," Daphne urged.

With his help she shoved the nearest table against Ray's and Sandra's, and then she headed for the bar. "How's your accommodation?" Sandra said.

"Jonquil's sleeping in my room," William announced.

"I think we should say it's both yours and hers," Natalie said.

"I'm sure Doug booked the best he could for us."

"He didn't say who had which room, did he?" Jonquil said.

"You won't expect William to share ours at his age," Julian retorted. "And I can't image you would want to, not that there's any question."

"Did Uncle Doug say how many rooms we had to have?"

"No, the man who paid did. You might have had a say if you were contributing."

"We're roughing it as well, Jonquil," her mother said. "We're here to have a good time with your grandparents, so let's try."

Ray attempted but failed not to ask her "What's the matter with your room?"

Natalie widened her eyes and seemed to gaze inwards, an expression he'd known ever since she was a child. Her face was a composite of Sandra's and his own, small and delicate except for the nose he was responsible for, as brightly blue-eyed as her mother used to be, pinkly thin-lipped. "We're supposed to have a suite," Julian said, "so we would have expected at the very least a bathroom."

"With a mirror in," Jonquil said.

Daphne was setting glasses on the table. Ray thought she was about to speak, but once she'd poured the water she went back to the kitchen. "Just let Evadne know you want a mirror," he said.

"She ought to know without having to be told. Too many people are like that these days." Perhaps Julian was looking not at but past Jonquil. "Well," he said, "here's the organiser."

Pris and Tim as well as Doug were crossing the Sunny View courtyard. Pris had tugged her long blonde hair into a pony-tail, which made her broad large-featured face look even more primed for excitement. She hugged Ray and Sandra, and then fifteen-year-old Tim had a turn, leaning down from the height that seemed increasingly to embarrass him. His face was mostly Doug's but more inclined to blush. "We were just discussing the mirror situation," Julian told Doug.

"You haven't got one either, then. Even we thought that was odd."

"Maybe it's a religious issue," Pris said, "and they don't want people to be vain."

"It's not their place to dictate how their customers behave," Julian said. "That isn't to say there aren't people who could be less concerned about themselves."

Ray was relieved to see Evadne approaching. "We'll have a jug of wine," Doug said. "Three glasses for us, and anyone else?"

Julian gave fifteen-year-old Jonquil a sharp glance. "Just your three," he said.

"Fair enough, save yourselves for dinner. And mum and dad, don't let us interrupt your lunch."

"I think I've finished," Sandra said, laying her utensils to rest.

Apparently Julian had been waiting for Evadne to depart before he enquired "And what's this business about knocking twice?"

"You find that all over Greece," Pris said. "It's to do with the vrykolakas."

"What's one of those?" Tim said and sent Jonquil an anticipatory grin.

"The local style of spirit. If you don't invite them the first time they'll find someone else."

"What's local about them?" Jonquil said. "I mean, what's special?"

"Some of us don't need to know," her mother interrupted, twitching her head to indicate William. "Remember we said we'd see everyone has a nice time."

"Yes, Jonquil," Julian said, "that's quite enough," and Ray was grateful yet again for Daphne's reappearance. As Daphne brought the tray over he saw Jonquil's face revert to introverted blankness even though Tim had sent her a sympathetic wink. Ray felt for her too, though he wasn't sorry that the subject had been suppressed. Where the family was concerned, far worse was being left unspoken.

★   ★   ★

Ray was watching Tim and Jonquil spin William on the grinning roundabout beyond the gap in the apartment block when Evadne came to find the family by the pool. "Your ride is here," she said.

"Not ours," Julian said before anyone else could speak.

"Yes, to go to Sunset Beach."

"Then it's certainly not ours. We've no intention of going anywhere near such a place."

"Sam from your travel will meet you there."

Doug took the invitation out of the envelope. "This says we're to wait here."

"Yes, to be taken."

"She said nothing about that to us," Julian objected. "And it's emphatically not somewhere we want our son to be."

"There won't be too much activity this early in the evening, do you think?" Natalie said.

"I believe I've made my view clear."

"I will tell the driver you are talking," Evadne said and left them.

"I could stay with William," Sandra said. "If there are any trips you think I'd like, Ray, you can book them."

"I was going to propose we vote," Julian said, "once we've heard the options."

"Do we need to?" Pris wondered. "If there's something some of us aren't up for, they can do something else."

"I understood the aim was to keep the family together." As Pris looked more abashed than Ray thought she had any reason to feel, Julian said "In the interests of fairness, everyone should choose what we do for a day."

"How," Doug said, "if mum isn't there?"

"You can phone William and me when you know what's on offer," Sandra said. "I'd like to sit him while I have the chance."

She pushed herself off the lounger and made for the play area, calling "I'm going to play with you now, William."

"We were looking after him," Jonquil protested.

"You were, and very well too, but the welcome meeting won't be any fun for him."

As the teenagers sauntered to the poolside Julian said "Quickly and quietly, please." Presumably he was ensuring William didn't realise they were going elsewhere, but Ray had the impression that he wasn't just addressing Tim and Jonquil.

A minibus was parked outside the courtyard. The driver, a slow bulky man with not much less hair blackening his arms than topped his squarish head, slid the door shut once everyone had clambered in. As the vehicle moved off, Natalie said "Can you tell us where we're going, driver?"

Ray tried not to mind how she increasingly sounded like her husband. "Sunset Beach," the driver said.

"My wife is asking exactly where."

"Bright Nights."

"Is that a bar? We don't want to be surrounded by rowdies." When the driver gave him an uncomprehending look in the mirror Julian said "People who don't behave as they should."

The driver gave a grunt or possibly a laugh. "In the day you are safe."

The road had wandered away from the coast, but the pallid sandy beach was visible beyond an elongated field of grass. A swollen orange sun hovered above the sea and paced the minibus. Sunset Beach cut off the sunlight as the resort closed around the road, the sparsely populated pavements bordered by dormant neon. "At least some people have got up," Pris said.

"More come out soon," said the driver.

Ray assumed he was seeing recent arrivals, since they all looked in need of a tan. The minibus pulled up in front of the Bright Nights, where drinkers sat beneath the red-tiled roof of an extensive bar. If Ray's professional eye hadn't deserted him, quite a few weren't much older than Tim and Jonquil. Sam from the travel company came to meet the Thornton party, and Ray gave her the receipt for the taxi fare. "You nearly didn't see some of us," he said. "This chap wanted to keep us on his island."

"Welcome to Sunset Beach," Sam said before her broad tanned face grew a little less placid. "Weren't there more of you?"

"Just the youngest," Ray said, "and the oldest apart from me."

"We knew the venue wouldn't be appropriate for our son," Julian said.

"Too young, you think," Sam said and perhaps agreed. "Sit anywhere you like and Nikos will bring drinks."

"One soft, thank you," Julian said, "or is anybody besides Jonquil not having alcohol?"

"Not in this family," Doug said.

As Ray hoped Julian hadn't taken this for a gibe at him Natalie said "May we know why you've held the meeting here?"

"Because all our other guests at this end of the island are in Sunset Beach."

"You didn't plan to try to sell the place to us," Julian said. "There are people here for whom it's wholly inappropriate."

"I don't really know what you mean," Sam said and went to stand beside a large map of Vasilema. "Welcome again, everyone," she said as the barman brought the Thornton party a trayful of drinks. "I expect I'll be saying that to some of you next year."

She hadn't much to say about the island's history, though perhaps as much as some of her audience might have the patience for. The island had originally been called Iliovasilema, which meant a sunset. Lord Byron had once said it had "the finest sunsets in this world or any other." During the Second World War Italians occupied the island and shortened its name. Until the present century it hadn't attracted many tourists, but

Greece's economic troubles persuaded the islanders to develop holiday resorts, Sunset Beach in particular. "But there's plenty for everyone," Sam said with a glance at Julian, and used a pointer like a thin stake to indicate places on the map while she described them along with tours that were listed in a brochure. "If anyone's interested in any day trips," she said with less conviction than Ray would have expected, "let me know."

"Don't you do tours off the island?" Pris said.

"Not too many people go on those." Ray could have thought she resented the question on Vasilema's behalf. "We can book you one," she said.

"How about trips to your monastery?" Doug said.

"Which one is that?"

"St Titus's, who else? He's your patron saint," Doug seemed surprised to have to tell her. "He drove the Arabs out of Crete and here and made your island Christian."

"There isn't much left of the monastery. I think you'd be wasting your time."

"That's not how it sounds in our book," Pris said.

"The book must be out of date. Is there anything else I can set up for you?"

"We'll let you know in a few minutes," Julian said.

"Don't be too long, will you? I expect your driver would like to get away."

"I imagine he can wait until we're ready. We didn't ask for him in the first place."

Ray glanced towards the minibus. The driver was gazing at the icon that was set above the mirror – St Titus brandishing his spear – but Ray couldn't tell if he was praying. The twilit street had grown a little busier, and beyond a gap between a supermarket and a bar he saw a few people beneath the extravagantly wide umbrellas that sprouted from the beach. As Sam went to a couple who had beckoned her over Julian said "Does anybody want to state a preference?"

"We usually like to explore a new place as soon as we can," Ray said.

"We'll put that down as your day, shall we?" Julian said and took out his mobile to make notes. "Who's next? Priscilla?"

"Definitely the monastery. It can't be all that ruined when it was carved out of the rock."

"I'll have the cruise around the island," Doug said.

Julian noted those and said "Natalie, my love."

"I wouldn't mind seeing other islands. Don't take that personally, Doug."

"Timothy?"

When Tim didn't answer, Pris nudged Doug. The boy was gazing at the street with a smile that looked at the very least inviting. "Someone's made a conquest," his mother murmured.

A girl was silhouetted against the crimson sky above the stretch of beach the buildings framed. Her pale elongated Grecian face and especially her large eyes reminded Ray of a statue, though the rest of her rather undermined the image. The arms the long white dress exposed were thinner than seemed healthy. Of course these days many girls of her age were, except how old was that? Ray was failing to guess – he'd always been able when he was a teacher, and he was unexpectedly dismayed to have lost the skill – when she looked away from Tim and saw the other watchers. She passed a hand over her face from the high domed forehead to the long chin as though slipping off a mask and at once, with a fluid movement that her dress concealed, was out of sight. "Sorry, Tim," Doug said, though with some amusement. "We didn't mean to scare her off."

"Doesn't matter," Tim mumbled, blushing.

"So may we hear your thoughts, Timothy?" Julian said.

Tim seemed to have to recapture his wits before saying "I'd like the drive off the road."

"The off-road tour for Timothy." As Julian tapped the tiny

keyboard he said "Natalie tells me you and Sandra used to like cycling on holiday, Raymond. Do you still?"

"I'll ask her." In an attempt to deflect any speculation about her Ray said "What about William?"

"Some cycles have child seats at the rear. Well, that's my choice for now," Julian said with just a hint of petulance. "I thought it might be good for all concerned."

"I think you've left somebody out of the choosing," Natalie said.

"Not at all, my love. Let's be hearing from you, Jonquil, before we speak to your grandmother." Without a pause he said twice as sharply "Jonquil."

Ray was close to pointing out that she'd had no time to answer when he saw her face. She was smiling at someone on the street, and for an unsettling moment he thought the girl who had taken Tim's fancy was back. Certainly the boy watching Jonquil was just as thin, and the little that Ray could distinguish of the long face against the sky from which the crimson had begun to drain reminded him of the Greek girl's face. As Jonquil parted her lips Julian held up an open hand to the newcomer. "Nothing here for you," he called. "Kindly move on."

Several people stared at him from the darkening street as the boy turned away. In a moment Ray couldn't see him for the crowd. "We ought to tell you that's quite rude, Jules," Doug said, "holding up your hand like that to anyone in Greece."

"There's been rudeness, I agree. Did you have something to say, Jonquil?"

"Make your day an ace one," Tim said.

This seemed to hearten her or at any rate to head off some words she didn't utter. "We haven't got any days on the beach," she said.

"I assume we'll be filling in with those." Julian poised a finger above his mobile and then erased an inadvertent B it had summoned up. "Is that really all that comes into your mind?"

"I'd like to go where she said it's best for shopping."

"Where Samantha said." When looking hard at Jonquil failed to make her say the name, Julian began to type. "I should think the rest of us will find more than that to do there," he said. "Will you be calling Sandra now, Raymond?"

Ray found his phone and brought up her number. He touched the call icon so gently he felt timid, and couldn't help counting as the bell rang. He'd heard twelve shrill notes in pairs when Sandra said "It's all right, I'm here."

He turned on the loudspeaker and laid the phone on the table. "How's everyone?"

"We've been having a lovely swing, but someone's getting hungry. Shall we wait for you?"

"We won't be long now, William," Natalie called. "Just be good for grandma."

"Evadne was saying there's a saint's day celebration," Sandra said, "so we can make that my day if everybody likes. That's still nobody, William. Just a shadow."

"What is?" Natalie demanded.

"He keeps thinking someone's in our room, Ray. It's just from the last of the sun."

"What did we say, William?" Julian said as he typed Sandra's choice. "Behave yourself for your grandmother and don't play tricks on her. Now, what kind of a day would you like?"

"Stay at the hotel. There's a lady who'll play with me."

"It isn't really a hotel, is it?" Julian said, glancing not quite at Pris and Doug. "I wonder what there would be for the rest of us."

"I don't mind a day by the pool," Jonquil said.

"You've already been given a day, Jonquil."

"While Will has his, she means," Tim said. "By the pool's okay with me."

When his parents and grandparents agreed William risked a cheer. "And look," Sandra said, "the shadow's gone."

"We'll see you very soon," Ray told her and followed Julian over to Sam. Places were available on all the tours, and tomorrow's was the cruise around the island. Sam took payments from the credit cards so speedily that she almost tore the vouchers in the machine. She handed back the cards and gave Julian the tickets, which appeared to placate him in some way. "I'll keep these in the safe," he said, "so we'll know where they are."

Ray might have objected to the assumption of authority if he hadn't remembered the passport episode. "If it keeps you happy, Jules," Doug said.

"I think your driver wants to be off," Sam said.

"He's not alone," Julian said. "I don't think any of us will be coming back here."

"It isn't to your taste, then."

Could Sam be hoping so? She'd glanced towards the street, where more than one pair of eyes gleamed red with neon, but Ray took her to be concerned with the driver. Ray made for the minibus to encourage everyone to do so, and the driver climbed out at once to slide the door back. "Sorry for the wait," Ray said when everyone was seated.

The driver sent the minibus forward. "Doesn't matter now," he said and returned his gaze to the crowded road so immediately that Ray couldn't tell who he'd been watching in the mirror.

◀

THE THIRD DAY
22 AUGUST

Ray could only think he had been dreaming. He wasn't even certain whether a knock had wakened him. Perhaps a guest at the Sunny View had come back late or was looking for a friend's room, since the next noise was even more distant and so discreet it sounded close to insubstantial, if he was hearing it at all. While he didn't think anyone opened a door, he heard no other sound, not even footsteps, though he didn't recall hearing any of those in the first place. What suggested that some if not all of this had been a dream was that as he reached across the conjoined beds to reassure himself about Sandra, he had an impression of somebody stealing out of the room.

Since it wasn't Sandra, it couldn't have been real. Just the same, as Ray clasped her waist he tried to focus the dim room. It resembled a charcoal sketch of itself, and it was as still as the hour – nearly three in the morning – ought to be. Sandra stirred beneath the quilt and murmured a few indistinct words about feeling, unless he'd misheard her. "Are you feeling all right?" he whispered despite hoping not to interrupt her sleep. He was happy to take her silence for assent, even for a kind of contentment, which he did his best to reinforce with not too fierce an embrace.

He thought she'd enjoyed last night's family dinner, even if at times it had felt carefully polite rather than entirely convivial. He'd caught Julian and Doug avoiding areas of disagreement for her sake rather than risk another argument such as they'd had at Christmas. They'd seemed close to quarrelling when Julian had started to dissect the bill with the precision he boasted of applying to insurance claims, but then Doug had made a joke of it – almost too much of one for Julian's taste. "Always look after your money and anyone else's you're responsible for," he'd counselled William, and Ray had seen Doug resist taking this as a gibe about how he tried never to deny payments to clients at the unemployment centre, just like Pris. At least the muted confrontation came too late to interfere with Sandra's appetite. She might almost have been eating for two people, and Ray only wished her waist weren't still so thin.

If the Greek sun was bringing her back to herself, he prayed it would continue its work. He hugged her as if this might help to preserve her state; he squeezed her waist so hard that it grew fluid, practically shapeless. The sensation shocked him awake, and he clutched at the boneless mass next to him in bed, only to discover that he was alone except for the quilt he was struggling to embrace. As he tried to shove himself upright, all the pains of age seemed to gather in his shaky arm. His shoulder thumped the concrete wall, and Sandra slid the window open. "I was just coming to find you," she said. "I've got bread for everyone. Come and have some before it's time for the boat."

His watch gave them almost forty minutes. Once he'd finished in the bathroom he joined Sandra on the balcony. Doug and his family were breakfasting below and to his right, while Natalie's were on the next balcony along. "Sorry I'm belated," Ray called down to them all.

"You're on holiday, dad," Doug told him. "Some of our younger members weren't too eager to greet the sun either."

"I was," William protested.

"And didn't you let everyone know," Jonquil said.

"I was up before it was," Sandra said, "me and the baker."

As Ray sat down he glanced towards Sunset Beach. He couldn't see if anyone was under the outsize umbrellas, but he wondered if their size was meant to tempt people from the neighbouring resorts. Or perhaps anybody staying in Sunset Beach wouldn't welcome too much sunshine after a night on the town. Sandra had put out salt and olive oil for the bread, and he was heartened to see crumbs already on her plate. When he took a chunky slice of the remains of the loaf she did as well. He was savouring a mouthful while he listened to the musing of the sea when the idyll was undermined by the offstage flushing of a toilet and an outburst of giggling from William. "What do you think of our special plumbing, Will?" Doug said.

"What's special?"

"Putting paper in the bin instead of down the loo, your uncle means," Pris said.

"Shall we find a better subject for discussion over breakfast?" Julian said.

Perhaps William didn't think he meant immediately. "Mummy says we haven't got to because it's unhygienical."

As Ray made to put Sandra's frown into words, their red-haired neighbour Jane did. "Everybody needs to use the bins, otherwise the pipes get clogged."

"I don't think it can be quite that bad," Natalie said.

"I'm telling you it is, and I'm a plumber."

There was silence while she returned to her apartment, and then Natalie said "Well, thank you so much for showing me up."

"Don't be like that, sis," Doug said. "When did you stop mucking in? You always used to when we went away with mum and dad."

"Maybe I didn't have a choice." Perhaps because she realised this would upset them, Natalie was quick to add "Or maybe it's different now I have a little boy to look after."

"Then you should have said before I booked for everyone."

"Stop it now, you two," Sandra called. "They've always been like this," she told whoever needed to be told.

"In that case," Julian said, "Natalie can't have changed that much."

"Nobody was blaming you, Julian," Pris said.

"I wouldn't have assumed it. You might want to say what there is for anyone to be blamed for."

"Mum was saying she didn't."

"That's very loyal of you, Timothy, but please consider the example you're setting."

"Tim, we think you're a credit," Sandra said.

Ray felt impelled to break the silence in which the waves on the beach seemed to have grown nervously shrill. "I was going to ask," he called, "if anybody tried to get into your rooms last night."

"Are you saying there are thieves about?" Julian demanded.

"I'm not at all. I just wasn't sure if I heard someone knocking on a door or two."

"I'm sure they didn't knock on ours," Sandra said.

"We didn't hear anything," Doug said.

"Nor did we," Julian said. "What is it, William?"

"I thought I did, but you're not supposed to answer."

"Then I hope you didn't. Good boy." Less enthusiastically his mother said "I hope you weren't thinking of that silly story of your uncle's."

"I didn't make it up, Nat."

"I don't care who did. We don't want that kind of thing keeping anyone awake."

"I went back to sleep," William said. "It didn't even really wake me up. It was too soggy."

"Well, that's the first time I've ever heard about a soggy knock," Sandra said. "Are we all finishing our breakfasts? We don't want to miss the pickup."

★   ★   ★

As everybody crossed the courtyard a coach slowed to a halt beyond the arch, and a chubby young man with a shock of unmistakably bleached hair pranced down the steps. His badge named him Jamie, and his gestures were graceful enough for a dancer. "Good morning, all you lively people," he cried, waving extravagantly as well.

William giggled before Natalie could hush him. Ray helped Sandra up the steps and kissed her hand. They and their party were the first passengers on the coach. "You have the front seat, William," Sandra said.

"Just you thank grandma," Natalie said as he made to do so. They took the seat while Julian sat opposite, and she murmured "Don't be rude again, William."

"I said thank you."

"You know perfectly well what your mother means," Julian said, and Ray wondered if he was annoyed because Jonquil hadn't sat with him. "We don't laugh at anyone. We've told you, other people make different choices about the kind of life they live."

Though he wasn't looking at Jamie the guide said "That's if you think everybody has a choice."

"I do, yes. Otherwise we'd have no morals."

"Some of the folk here might give you an argument."

"We're aware the economy has problems. That doesn't mean they can't choose how to solve them."

"They have," Jamie said, picking up a clipboard to plant crosses next to names. "Elysian Apartments next, Alexandros."

The bus was speeding along the deserted dusty road to Sunset Beach when Pris said "What's with the musical chairs, you two?"

Ray glanced back to see Tim and Jonquil moving to his side of the aisle. Although like their grandmother they were wearing hats and sunglasses, Tim said "Too sunny over there."

"You aren't still determined not to get a tan," Doug protested.

"That's how some people like to look these days," Natalie said. "Remember when we used to fight over who had the best one?"

"I'm glad you've calmed down, then," Julian said. "All the same, it's a pity to spend money on the sun if it won't be put to use."

The road through Sunset Beach looked as dead as all the signs. The electric jester was arrested with one bent leg in the air, while the neon cat would be poised all day at the start of a leap. A few of the locals were cleaning or tidying bars and tavernas at a sleepy pace that struck Ray as typically Greek. The coach halted in front of an apartment complex, outside which a young couple sat in the shade of a trellis so laden with vines that the tendrils appeared not just to be growing on the grey wood but feeding on it. "Good morning, lively folk," Jamie cried, and they blinked at him.

Two of the accommodations where the coach stopped didn't yield up any customers. "You'd wonder why anyone would bother booking," Sandra commented, "if they aren't going to put in an appearance."

"They should have got someone to give them a knock," Doug said.

"Do you have to keep talking about that?" Jonquil complained.

"No need for impoliteness," Julian said, "even if you're trying to protect William."

"Can't I do anything right?"

"A great many things," Sandra told her. "And we like how you look after your brother. Our two did for each other."

Ray wondered if she meant they'd stopped, because he didn't think they entirely had. As Jamie returned to the coach by himself again Pris said "Why would anyone come all this way to your island and then miss a day like today?"

"Something brings them," Jamie said. "They keep coming back."

Once the coach left Sunset Beach behind, the hills that formed the spine of Vasilema rose on the inland horizon. More passengers boarded in resorts that Ray had previously slept through – fishing villages colonised by apartments and hotels – and then the port appeared, its bony buildings swarming uphill while the bay brandished masts at the increasingly overcast sky. "Everybody follow me when we leave the bus," Jamie said. "If I lost anyone it'd break my heart."

When William made a small anxious sound Natalie said "I'm sure you never have."

"I'm sad to say we lost a visitor just last week."

"How did you manage that?" Doug said.

"Not on any excursion of ours. The gentleman went off by himself," Jamie said, waving to mime carelessness. "He had a room not far from where you're staying."

"I take it you'll have tracked him down," Julian said.

"I wish I could tell you that. He disappeared last week and nobody's found him." As Natalie began to interrupt, Jamie raised his voice. "He was talking to the lady at his digs about visiting the mainland," he said. "Somebody here at the harbour said they thought they saw him take the ferry, so we think that's where he must have wandered off to."

Sandra was speaking at the very least for Ray as she said "How long has he left of his holiday?"

"That's what has people worried. He should have gone home days ago, but he couldn't have without his passport." Jamie moved to the top of the steps as the coach reached the harbour. "The police have that," he said and gazed at William. "What do you think is the moral of the story, sunbeam?"

William giggled at the nickname before saying gravely "Don't lose your passport?"

"That's wise advice, but I'll tell you what I meant — never go anywhere by yourself without letting somebody know where you'll be. Best of all," Jamie said and raised his eyes to include every passenger, "just don't go anywhere by yourself."

★　　★　　★

"Won't that be too spicy for you, William?" his mother said. "We don't want you wandering about in the night."

"Nobody was," Jonquil said.

"I wasn't saying you were, Jonquil. We don't want him being kept awake, that's all."

"I didn't wake him." More urgently than Ray would have thought was called for, the girl said "Did I, William?"

"This isn't about you, Jonquil," Julian said. "Quite a few things aren't, young lady."

"You don't need to tell me."

Ray suspected Pris meant to head off any further confrontation by saying "I don't think anything's too spicy here."

They were in Chloe's Garden, where Doug had suggested everybody at the table share their dinner. "Just have a little taste of anything you like the look of, William," Natalie said as if she were doing someone else a favour.

Ray was more concerned to see Sandra sample everything, which she more than did. She appreciated it aloud as well, though he wasn't sure how much this was designed to encourage William. The boy set about competing with her expressions of pleasure, to nearly everyone's amusement. "So do you like the tabepna, Will?" Tim said.

The boy giggled so vigorously that he had to wipe his mouth. "Use your serviette, William," Julian said.

Before he'd finished dabbing with the paper napkin William said "That isn't what it's called."

"It's the polite name for it, William," Natalie said.

As Ray saw Sandra reflect that they'd never used the word, William giggled again. "Not what you said, daddy. What Tim did."

"See what the sign says, William," Jonquil said and grinned at her cousin.

"Could you refrain from trying to confuse your brother," Julian said with no hint of a question. "If you want to be involved with him, please set your standards higher."

As Jonquil's grin collapsed, Tim sent her a wink. Ray saw Pris and Doug exchange a glance, but it was William who spoke. "It does say that, daddy, look."

"You know perfectly well this is a taverna, William," Julian said and glared at Jonquil. "Greek people use a different alphabet, that's all."

"I can't see why they don't get rid of it," Natalie said, "if they're so eager for tourists."

"Maybe Greeks come here for a holiday as well," Doug said.

"That isn't how the driver from the airport made it sound. He was saying people here aren't like other Greeks."

"That's what Greeks say about Crete," Pris said. "Doug and I thought we all might like somewhere tourists hadn't taken over."

Natalie looked stubbornly unpersuaded, an attitude Ray recalled from her teens. "Can I just say something to everyone?" Sandra said.

Perhaps she meant to quell any argument, but Ray felt as if her words had pierced his guts. Had she thought better of keeping the secret? "Why," Natalie said, "what's wrong?"

"Nothing whatsoever with my holiday. I was only wondering if anyone would mind if I had a different day."

For a shaky breath Ray was furious that she'd made him panic. In a bid to leave his shameful reaction behind he said "Different how?"

"I wouldn't mind finding that little beach with the cave. I don't think it's too far from a bus stop."

He knew where she was thinking of – a secluded sandy beach the cruise had passed, at the foot of a cliff about halfway between Sunset Beach and Vasilema Town. A grassy section of the cliff sloped down to one end, while at the other an inlet vanished into a cave where the light from ripples lapped the walls and the equally spiky roof. She'd wakened just in time to see all this, having dozed beneath the awning of the boat throughout much of Jamie's commentary, which Ray had found somewhat relentless and bereft of detail. "You can have my day if you like, gran," Tim said. "I don't mind going there."

He and Jonquil had roused themselves at the sight of the beach or the cave. They'd been almost as sleepy in the shade as their grandmother. "We can put your day and mine together, Tim," Pris said. "The monastery is off the road. I'd still love to do your saint's day, Sandra."

"Are there any more changes of plan?" Julian said without encouraging.

"Don't let it throw you, Jules," Doug said. "Let's just all have a good time."

Julian let everybody see him taking out his phone. "The way to make sure of that is to be organised."

"Then let's organise the beach tomorrow," Ray said and was aware of a disagreement in the kitchen. Whatever Chloe and her daughter were murmuring about, the mother won. As Ray watched her approach, asking other diners on the way how their meals were, he had an odd sense that she was readying herself. She reached the table at last and gave the depleted dishes an approving nod. "How is all?" she said.

"Delicious," Sandra said with sufficient gusto for the whole party.

"That is good," Chloe said and met her eyes. "Bitten," she said, touching her own unmarked neck.

"I was the other night. I've been more careful since."

Chloe shook her head. "Never once."

"Some people seem to attract them, don't they?" Pris said. "They aren't bothered about us."

"We've put repellent in the room," Ray said.

"No good," Chloe told him.

"It's worked wherever else we've found mosquitoes. If there's a local secret I hope you'll share it with us."

Chloe was pursing her lips when Natalie said "Could I just ask if we really need to have cats around the table while we're eating?"

"You'll have noticed we're English," Julian said. "It wouldn't be allowed in any restaurant at home."

"I don't think they're doing any harm, are they?" Doug said. "Now dad was asking – "

"It's a question of cleanliness, Douglas. I believe you'll agree we've already lowered our standards to save trouble."

As Doug visibly withheld a response Chloe said "That is life here. All feed."

"Well, they won't be feeding from us," Julian said and held up a hand to fend off any rejoinder.

Chloe stared at the hand before closing her eyes as a preamble to stalking away. "Do pardon me," Julian called after her, but she didn't turn. "I'd forgotten we aren't allowed to do that. As I say, we're English."

"There goes mum's chance of not getting bitten," Doug said.

"I don't think she was going to tell us," Sandra said. "And I don't even notice it's there any more."

Perhaps she'd forgotten how a twinge had wakened her on the cruise, where she'd fingered her neck as the boat came abreast of the cave. As Ray peered at the mark – the dimness left him unsure whether it had faded – William said "Jonquil got bitten too."

"Where?" Natalie said. "Let me see."

The bite on her forearm was very like Sandra's but redder. "Is that on the vein?" Natalie cried. "Why didn't you ask for some ointment?"

"I'm afraid someone needs to be more open with us," Julian said.

"I forgot about it," Jonquil told her mother. "That's how much it hurts."

Natalie was looking not just unconvinced but rejected when Tim said "I've got one as well."

"There's another secretive teen for you," Doug said as Tim displayed his upturned arm. "Any more casualties? Just mum and the young ones, then."

"I haven't got one," William protested.

"Well, don't invite it," Pris said. "Not that I'm saying anyone else did."

Ray didn't know why he should feel that her words were

loitering in the dark beyond the streetlamps, but they seemed to hover in the air until Sandra said "So long as we've an adventure tomorrow I think I'm off to bed."

Jonquil nodded and then Tim did, so that Ray could have fancied they were miming slumber. "You said I could stay up late on holiday," William objected to his parents.

"You already have, William," Natalie said. "Really quite late. You can't mind going to bed when your big sister is."

Ray thought the boy was about to disagree, though he couldn't see why William should, until Julian waved before beckoning Daphne over. How much was being left unsaid around the table? As Julian took out his phone and brought up the calculator Ray saw Pris put a quick finger to her lips, hushing Doug in advance, and felt as if a clutch of unaddressed subjects had gathered in the sultry windless dark. Then Daphne brought the bill along with glasses of liqueur, and he lost whatever thoughts he might have been close to grasping. That was how his mind worked now, or rather didn't work. That was growing old.

THE FOURTH DAY
23 AUGUST

"I had my dream again last night."

"Which one was that, Sandra?" Pris said.

"It was dark." As though she had to find her words in it Sandra added "It was the darkest place I've ever seen."

Ray didn't know why he felt prompted to grope for a joke. "You could see that, anyway."

"There was some kind of light far away."

"Well then," Ray said with more relief than he could have explained, "it wasn't really dark."

"I don't think I saw it, just knew it was there. I felt – "

They were in the Superber supermarket, where Tim and Jonquil were trying to find hats wide enough to suit them. While they'd each brought one to the island, perhaps this was the latest fashion or, Ray thought, envy of Sandra's broad Mexican headgear. As a frown found more wrinkles on her brow Sandra said "I felt as if it would take me all my life to reach it."

Ray was searching for a safe response when Tim said "I had a dream like that last night as well."

"Must be in the blood," Doug said. "What's your version, Tim?"

"I was in this huge place with no light and I didn't want to see. Something sounded…" Tim might have been suppressing a word before he said "Huge."

Jonquil tugged her latest hat down as if she wouldn't mind hiding beneath the brim. "That's like my dream."

"All right, Jonquil, no need to compete," Julian said. "Or least make sure the competition's worthwhile."

As Ray saw Pris and Doug refrain from taking this as an insult to their son, Jonquil said "I'm just telling them. I was in a dark place too, and there was something living in it that was that big."

Ray wasn't sure if Tim was reluctant to ask "What was, Jonk?"

"I only heard it. Maybe William made me. It sounded like he said the knock he heard did."

"Soggy," William was delighted to contribute.

"Kindly don't bring William into it."

"Yes, don't start giving him your dreams," Natalie said. "Have you finished shopping?"

"I just want to get some more water."

"I will too," said Tim.

"Then three of us are thirsty," Sandra said. "Anybody else? I'll buy."

As Ray took three plastic bottles to the desk the moustached old woman in black stared past him. "Never dream dark."

"Jonquil, will you take William to find the bus stop," Julian said. "I'll pay for your hat and you can settle with me later."

When Jonquil closed her hand around his the boy seemed about to demur, presumably feeling too old to be led. As soon as the two of them had left the shop, Julian rounded on the shopkeeper. "Pardon me, what were you saying?"

"Never dream dark." Ignoring Julian, she stared at Tim. "You bring it here," she said.

"I don't think anyone can do that just by dreaming," Pris said.

This time she responded, but in Greek. "Did anybody understand that?" Natalie said, more a protest than a question.

"Something like – " Pris tapped her forehead with a fingertip, which put Ray in mind of touching an onscreen icon to summon information. "People who want the sunset," she suggested, "invite the dark."

The old woman gave that a single vigorous nod. "Friends of dark."

Ray was trying to decide whether this was agreement or a correction when Julian said "Speaking of nonsense, may we ask you all to keep it away from William."

"What sort of thing would that be, Jules?"

"Bad dreams. Unpleasant legends. You've already had him imagining knocks in the night with that tale of yours, Douglas."

Before Ray could take responsibility Tim said "My dream didn't feel exactly bad."

"I think it's time to move on," Julian said at once.

As he and the Thorntons left the supermarket they heard a bus approaching. Ray took Sandra's hand as they jogged after long-legged Tim, subsiding to a trot when they reached a bend in the road. Tim was already with Jonquil and William by the bus at the stop, and dabbing at his forehead while he sucked on a bottle of water. The first few rows of seats were occupied by local folk, and as the Thornton party made their way along the aisle several women in black gave them a sign of the cross, pointing with the finger. "Thank you," Sandra said more than once, an example Tim and Jonquil followed.

Nobody boarded the bus at Sunset Beach. When it passed a loiterer in a shady side road blinking at the sunlight, the women in black covered their eyes with a hand. "Is that another tradition?" Natalie murmured.

"Looks as if it's religious," Pris said.

"Maybe they aren't supposed to look at sinners," Doug said, "which could mean anyone at Sunset Beach."

Ray thought this might be so, since they left their eyes uncovered when the bus reached the next village, where a good many people were to be seen. After that the road wound between fields not too far from the sea and past the occasional lonely bus shelter, until Doug craned forward and then poked the bellpush on the nearest metal pole. "We're here," he said.

He might have been telling the driver, who seemed in no hurry to brake. As Doug led the procession up the aisle the bus slowed, halting with an exhausted gasp some yards past a rudimentary stone shelter. The doors stayed shut as the driver turned to him. "Where you want?"

"We're off to the beach."

The man's eyebrows, outposts of his shaggy black moustache, seemed to darken his eyes. "Sunset is better."

"You're saying we should see it there?" Pris said.

The driver's eyebrows hunched lower. "Where you came from."

"We'll be back there for the sunset," Doug said.

The driver might have been shrugging as he released the doors, which parted with a sigh that could almost have denoted resignation. All the women in black made the sign again while the party left the bus. "Well, we're nothing if not blessed," Sandra said as Ray took her hand to help her down.

The doors thumped shut and the bus rumbled away, disgorging an oily grey cloud. Julian planted his hands on his hips and watched the bus vanish around a bend before he said "You're sure this is the right place, Douglas."

"A bit late to ask if it's not, don't you think?" As Natalie met this with her incredulous face – Ray remembered how often they'd performed such a routine when they were Tim's and Jonquil's age – Doug added "It's the only stop with a shrine by it, and I found it on the map."

The roadside shrine might have been marking or guarding the start of the path that led across a grassy field. It was the kind of memorial Ray and Sandra had often seen in Greece, a small glass-fronted wooden hutch standing on four stilts. Whoever it commemorated, their curled-up photograph had fallen on its face beside the extinguished stub of a candle in a tin holder. A grim-lipped icon of St Titus stood above the photograph, flourishing a lance. "What's he doing?" William said.

"It's a way of remembering where someone died, Will."

Natalie gave Doug a censorious look. "It's showing respect, William."

"Yes, but what's the man doing? Why is he waving his spear?"

This brought Sandra and the teenagers out of the bus shelter. Was the icon lenticular? Certainly the shaft of the lance appeared to be somehow unstable. Doug stooped close and then straightened up not much less than hastily. "Something's alive in there, Will."

The lance was split, Ray saw. A white mass bulged out of it like stuffing from a damaged toy. The mass was a cocoon from which dozens of tiny pale spiders were swarming. Natalie clutched William's shoulders to move him aside and leaned her hands on the frame of the window, only to recoil with a cry. Spiders were streaming through a crack beneath the pane and down the left front leg of the shrine. "Stay well away, William," she urged. "They could be anywhere."

"It's just life, Will," Pris said to reassure him. "It grows anywhere it can."

Tim crouched lower at the shrine than his father had and nudged Jonquil. "Being a saint didn't do him much good."

"That's no excuse for not behaving properly," Julian said.

"Nobody isn't that I can see," Doug said and turned to the overgrown path.

A hot breeze came to meet them all. It rattled through the parched brown calf-high grass beside the narrow path like a flight of creatures lying low, and Ray saw Natalie pretend not to notice. A few solitary trees shrilling with cicadas punctuated the track. William struggled through the grass to overtake Doug and ran to the first tree, but as he looked for the insects the incessant sound dodged to the next one. "You won't see them, William," Sandra called, "unless they want you to."

When he dashed to the second tree it fell silent while the noise recommenced at the first one. The game seemed to frustrate him as much as it amused him, and he clenched his fists as he sprinted to the third tree. "Don't go too far ahead, William," Natalie shouted.

Though her voice was dwarfed by the huge blue sky, it appeared to halt the boy. Ray thought he'd found a cicada on the tree until they reached it. While William was gazing at the scaly trunk, there was no insect, just an image someone had carved. "It's him again," William said.

It was indeed St Titus, so crudely outlined that only the upthrust lance made him unmistakable. Ray glanced back at Sandra, but she and the teenagers were lingering under the last tree. How could he have been so thoughtless that he'd gone ahead? "Are you all right?" Pris called.

"They're just keeping me company," Sandra said and advanced along the path.

Everyone apart from William waited for the stragglers. As he reached the next tree, displacing the screech of cicadas, the boy shouted "He's here as well."

Ray let Sandra and the teenagers go ahead, since they seemed eager to reach the tree. "He's poking something," William announced.

"William," Natalie said in case his observation called for a rebuke.

Once Ray was close enough he saw another carving. This one was cruder still and possibly unfinished, since the opponent the figure had pierced with his lance was too shapeless to identify. Had there been carvings on the trees nearest the road? William was already dashing to the next one, silencing its stridulation. "I've found him," he cried.

"Don't go any further, William," his father called. "You're nearly at the cliff."

In fact the edge was several hundred yards beyond the tree, on which another image had been hacked out of the wood. The foe skewered by the lance looked as unsure of its own shape as a cloud, and the saint wasn't much clearer. William hopped from foot to impatient foot while he waited for someone to head for the cliff, and followed Doug so closely that he might have been tempted to slip past him. Doug caught hold of his hand as they left the path, and leaned over the edge of the cliff. "Here's your beach, mum," he called, "and your cave."

Ray took a step along the path and glanced back. "No need to wait for us," Sandra said more sharply than he thought was called for. "We're coming."

Doug waved to her and the teenagers under the tree. "Plenty of shade down there."

"I thought we were here for the sun," Julian said and strode towards the slope down to the beach. "Come along, William."

Ray found Natalie waiting for him at the end of the path. "Don't think too badly of Julian, will you?" she murmured while nobody else could hear. "He needs a holiday if any of us do. They've cut back at the company and he's doing two people's jobs. Tell mum when you're alone, could you?"

In that moment he was close to telling Natalie a great deal. Then she hurried to catch up with her husband and son, and Ray watched Sandra and her young companions advance along the path. He felt he'd overlooked something, but try as he might he couldn't bring it to mind. Was this yet another unhappy symptom of age? He gave up when Sandra reached him, and took her hand to usher her to the beach. As long as they were on the wide gentle slope he was able to imagine he could keep her safe.

⋆　⋆　⋆

"I think he's finished, William," Jonquil said. "What are you going to call him?"

The boy was scooping up sand with his hands to replenish the face of the supine figure he and Jonquil had built in the shadow of the cliff, a shadow that had merged with the beach since the sky had clouded over. Whenever William succeeded in shaping the features the hot breeze erased them, which no longer amused him as much as it had. "I thought he was going to be the man in the box," he said.

"We call that a shrine," Sandra said before Julian could. "And he's called St Titus."

"If that's who he is, William," Jonquil said, "we ought to find him a spear."

The boy surveyed the beach, which offered only sand and pebbles polished by the waves. "What's he got to fight, then?" he was eager to hear.

"I don't think that's necessary," his father said and gazed at Jonquil. "No good comes of bringing badness."

William made a last attempt to consolidate the rudimentary upturned face but gave up once the eyeholes he'd poked began to crumble. "Thank you for helping me make him, Jonquil," he said.

"I wanted to show you. My daddy used to make them with me."

As William's father conveyed how quiet he was remaining, Sandra said "I don't know what's the matter with my brain today. It must be too much sun."

She added a weak smile as though she'd made a joke she didn't fully understand. "Why," Ray had to ask, "what's wrong?"

"We should have bought somebody some beach toys when we were in the supermarket. I'd like to while I have the chance."

"I'm certain you've plenty of time left," Julian said.

Ray felt as if the response he and Sandra were withholding had stolen his breath. He was searching for words to say before the silence tarried too long when William said "Can I go for a swim now?"

"Please may you?" Once he'd heard the required phrase Julian said "I expect your lunch will have gone down by now. Swim out to your mother."

"I'll come with you, William," Jonquil said at once.

"Are you coming too, grandad? We'll teach you how to swim."

"I don't think even you can do that for me, William. Maybe I'll brave the water in a while."

The boy dashed into the shallow waves as though to demonstrate how it was done and threw himself flat as soon as the sea grew deeper. As Jonquil set about racing him to their mother, Julian said "If you'll excuse me I'll join them."

"Do you mind if I go out too, Ray?"

"How could I mind?" Ray said and clasped Sandra's hand, barely refraining from squeezing too hard. "You enjoy everything you can."

As Julian strode into the water she limped after him. Ray was watching her venture deeper when she stumbled, falling full length. He lurched helplessly to his feet and was about to yell to somebody to go to her – Tim was closest, and had left his awkwardness behind the moment he'd immersed himself – when she regained her old grace and surged forward through the water. He could have thought she'd grown almost as fluid as the waves. He mustn't panic just because he couldn't follow, not when she had the family around her, but he was dismayed to think she was out of his reach.

He did his best to relish the pleasure she was taking in the swim, but found he couldn't bear to watch her growing more remote. There wasn't much to distract him on the beach. Apart from clothes and backpacks abandoned on towels he was alone except for the figure made of sand. Most of both the holes it had for eyes had gone, and the nose had collapsed, while the mouth dwindled as he watched. As it vanished from the left side of the face he heard William call "Please may I go in the cave?"

"Just give me a few minutes," Julian said, "and I'll see if it's safe for you."

Ray saw how he could be some use to everyone. "I'll go and look," he shouted.

"Will you be all right by yourself, dad?" Doug called.

"I'm not past it quite yet. I'll be fine," Ray told anyone who was concerned, and sat forward with a groan he hoped nobody heard. At least the arthritic twinge that made him flinch distracted him from taking his son's words as an omen. Once he'd fastened the straps of his sandals he had to kneel in order to struggle to his feet and plod along the beach.

The pale sand gave way to ribbed slabs of rock a few hundred yards from the cave. At first Ray was able to stride across the grey rock, but then waves rose to meet him. He had to take so much care on the increasingly slippery surface that he felt barely competent to walk. He wished he'd worn his trainers, which would have lent him more confidence. He inched across the rock to plant a hand against the stony cliff, and hoped none of the swimmers noticed his difficulties. The support of the cliff let him feel not quite so vulnerable, capable of moving less like a geriatric. When he reached the cave he leaned on a projecting rock beside the mouth and peered in.

While the mouth was wide and high enough for a ferry to enter, the clear water was so shallow that he could see the stony floor. From this side of the entrance it looked possible for even Ray to clamber along the rocks above the water to a bend in the cave. He'd undertaken to look out for William, and perhaps he'd meant to give Julian a break. He let go of the handhold and grabbed the next one, and stepped into the cave.

A stony chill closed around him at once, and so did the sound of water. A hollow echo multiplied the lapping of ripples, which sent up light to drift over the ridges of the walls and roof. The seaweed that bordered the rocks underfoot was borrowing restlessness from the waves. The slimy growths gave him yet another reason to take his time, along with the need to keep waiting for his vision to catch up with the dimness so that he could search for footholds on the uneven narrow ridge. He had only started to make headway around the bend when the ridge sloped downwards, vanishing underwater a few yards ahead.

Ray was clutching at the wall with both hands by the time he reached the last unsubmerged inches of the ridge. Water slopped over his sandals to drench his ankles, and he couldn't see how far the ridge extended underwater, let alone whether it offered him any footing. Even if he didn't feel safe, he needed to go further to see what lay around the bend. At least he had his swimming trunks on — trunks for walking in the sea, in his case. He took a breath that roused a faint echo, and then he crouched on all fours to grip the ridge with his shivery fingers and let himself down into the water.

While the waves had chilled his feet, he wasn't prepared for how cold an immersion would be. An icy ache raced up his legs and seemed to clench around his stomach. Wasn't this enough to warn William against? But the boy and the rest of them could well be used to the temperature of the sea by now, which meant just Ray was weak. The toes of his sandals scrabbled at the submerged wall, and he couldn't judge how deep the water might be. He bruised his fingers on the ridge as he lowered himself, not fast but excessively fast. When the water clamped his hips he felt his penis shrivel, and his gasp echoed through the cave. He twisted around in a flurry of water to see if he'd alarmed anyone, only to find that the bend had already blocked his view out of the cave. All the dim light came from reflections on the nervous waves. The loss of his family — even of the sight of them — disconcerted him so much that he didn't immediately grasp that his feet had found the cave floor.

It felt no more secure to walk on than the ridge had. Ray kept one hand on the ridge as he ventured forward until the arm was submerged up to the wrist, forcing him to stoop sideways, and then he groped for handholds higher up the wall. The ripples he was making surrounded him with echoes that seemed to render distance audible – the remoteness of the beach. Just enough light reached around the bend to let him make out some of the way ahead.

Beyond the bend the cave grew several times as wide and extended further than he could be sure of. Traces of light almost too feeble for the name fluttered under the roof, and some faint illumination must be reaching the far end of the cavern, if that was the end. Certainly Ray thought he saw movement there, an extensive whitish glimpse that immediately withdrew into the dark. A high-pitched giggle distracted him, a sound that seemed more senile than he wanted ever to be, but of course it was one of the watery echoes that were lending the cave a kind of life. As his vision started to cope with the dark he became aware of a pale shape in the water to his left, against the wall he was following. It was a tangle of vegetation, which meant he needn't have recoiled, sending dim ripples into the cave. While the clump of pallid weeds did resemble the top half of a scrawny figure with its hands raised, it was stirring only with the movement of the water. As it bobbed up and down it put him in mind of somebody eager to catch a ball, and he wondered how it would look to William.

He had a feeling that Natalie and Julian mightn't like the similarity. Perhaps even William wouldn't if it or his parents made him nervous. His grandfather was meant to be seeing the place was safe, and Ray supposed this ought to include establishing exactly what the object was. Sliding his hand along the rough wall, he shuffled inch by inch through the dark water.

He was advancing into blackness. Such illumination as there was – more like a memory of light than any aid to seeing – fell short of this stretch of the wall. He could have used the flashlight on his mobile, but however waterproof the phone was claimed to be, he didn't want to test that more than was essential. He groped along the wall and edged his feet over slippery submerged rock. Seaweed fingered his shivering legs, and once a pebbly protrusion sprouted limbs beneath his hand before scuttling down the wall to plop into the water. The object he was trying to discern kept nodding what would have been its head as though to encourage his approach. He'd inched within a few yards of it, and was starting to marvel at how nearly human its shape remained even at this distance, when it spoke his name.

Ray stumbled backwards, and his feet skidded from under him. His fall would break some of his bones, if he didn't drown from panicking in the dark. He sprawled on his back in the water, which surged into his eyes and filled his nostrils, denying him any breath. He threw out a hand under the water, stubbing his fingers on the jagged wall. He managed to grab the rock despite the throbbing of his fingers and hauled himself to his feet. As he struggled to stand on his tremulous legs while he spat and spluttered and fought for breath, ripples and their giggling echoes swarmed away from him. His ears were so waterlogged that at first he wasn't sure he heard the voice repeat his name.

He was even more uncertain where it was in the echoing dark. As he poked at his ears and tried to shake them clear of water it said "Can you hear me? Are you in difficulties?"

By now he couldn't mistake Julian. He turned in the water as fast as he dared and saw a succession of ripples precede the swimmer into the larger cavern. "I'm quite all right," he felt bound to declare.

"I thought it would be best to see for myself," Julian said, presumably not about Ray, and jerked his head up. "What's that behind you?"

"I was just about to look," Ray said, peeling open his hip pocket to take out the phone. He shook every drop of water off it before wakening the screen and touching the flashlight icon. While he took care not to swing around too fast the beam trailed across the water. It barely reached the limit of the cave, but he was able to make out a gap several feet wide in the rear wall. No doubt the movement he'd glimpsed there earlier had been a stray reflection that had outlined the gap, appearing to fill it. The light grew more concentrated as it glided towards him over the wall, so that by the time it reached the bobbing object it was a white glare. For just a moment Ray was loath to aim the beam directly at the object – he thought he'd already seen too much – and then the light caught it. "Good God," Julian said, and in case this failed to convey his shock "Good God."

The shape had once been much more human, but now it seemed to sum up age and decay. It looked as withered and contorted as the husk of a spider's victim. The man's head was thrown back as if it had been paralysed in the act of uttering a final cry, which had shrunk the lips back from the teeth in a tortured grimace. The hands might have been lifted to fend off or deny his fate, unless a convulsion had raised them. Although Ray had no means of judging how long the corpse had been in the water, perhaps the immersion went some way towards explaining its state, because the flesh that dangled from its bones resembled perished rubber. He was staring at it in helpless dismay – he felt unable to move the light until he or Julian managed to deduce what had happened to the man – when the corpse winked at him.

He saw it take a breath as well. No, the reflections of the ripples that were wagging its hands and nodding its withered head were at play among the shadows of its ribs, enlivening the collapsed bare chest as the beam shook in Ray's hand. But the drooping eyelid had certainly stirred, although only because a crab had emerged, bearing off a prize. "Come away, Raymond," Julian said as though rebuking a child. "We've seen quite enough. We need to make sure nobody sees who oughtn't to."

It took Ray some moments and a good deal of resolution to turn his back on the restless corpse, though he'd looked away quickly from the sight of the crab crawling askew down the ravaged pallid face. Julian was treading water where the cave narrowed. "Will you be all right to make your way out," he said, "while I go and deal with the others?"

Ray saw this was scarcely a question. As he mumbled a reluctant assent Julian struck out for the sea, and in seconds only his wake remained. Ray kept the flashlight on as far as the exit from the inner cavern, but he didn't want to run the battery down. He switched off the phone and stowed it in his pocket, and was leaving the darkness behind as swiftly as he dared to shuffle through the water when a cluster of ripples caught up with him.

The corpse hadn't made them. The pallid husk wasn't creeping after him in the dark, teeth bared, hands raised to seize him. In fact, he had a sense that the ripples were coming from the far end of the cavern. Those Julian had sent back must have rebounded there, and they would be the source of the shrill echoes Ray could hear, however much those resembled senile mirth. Just the same, he was glad when the activity subsided, and even more relieved to be able at last to clamber onto the ridge above the water.

He limped along it, clutching at the wall with both hands, until he could see out of the cave. Julian was standing guard in the waves outside the entrance, and glanced back at him. "Here he is now. As I told you, he's fine."

Sandra stood up, shading her eyes, though the sun was still behind the clouds. "Be careful on the rocks," she called. "Ray, are you going to tell us what's wrong?"

"As I've said, the place isn't safe." Julian turned his back on her, perhaps only to face Ray, and waited until he didn't need to raise his voice. "Will you call the authorities, Raymond?"

"The police, you mean." When Julian frowned and pinched his lips together, Ray said even lower "Do we know their number here?"

"Look it up," Julian barely pronounced.

Perhaps the cave had amplified their voices. "Why do you need the police?" Sandra called.

Julian threw up his hands as if he was flinging all responsibility to her and Ray. "Somebody's drowned," Ray mouthed at her.

All the family gazed at him, and Sandra's puzzlement overcame her silence. "Down…"

"Drowned." Even more vigorously Ray mouthed "Dead."

"Drowned dead, grandad's saying," William informed her.

"Well, now you know it all, William," his father said, though not only to him, "and I hope you're the better for knowing."

As the boy looked abashed Ray tried to divert attention away from him. "Does anyone have the number?"

"One one two will get them," Jonquil said. "It's the number you can call from anywhere."

"Thank you, Jonquil," Julian said. "That's a good point, Raymond. There's no need to call from here."

Ray had left the cave by now and was watching his unsteady step on the rocks. "Why, where do you think I should call from?"

"Not until we're on our way back to the accommodation. It's not as if there can be any urgency. Go and dry yourself and get dressed, William. Jonquil too, please."

"It's gran's day," the boy protested. "It's her beach."

"That's very thoughtful, but your grandmother didn't know what was here. Quickly now, please. I'm sure everybody will be coming with you."

As William tramped splashily towards the beach, miming enough frustration for several people, Ray said "I wonder if the police mightn't want us to wait here."

"They certainly aren't going to want William. I'm not disparaging you, son. Who do you suppose they would want, Raymond?"

"Me, since I found what I found. Maybe you as well, since you saw," Ray said and took out his phone, on which a single bar warned of the barest connection. As the swimmers waded to the beach he typed the emergency number. Listening seemed to draw a shrill whisper out of the cave – the secret chatter of the ripples

– and then a woman's voice said something he didn't understand. "Police?" he hoped aloud.

"This is emergency. Where is it, please?"

"Vasilema, do you mean?"

"Stay there." Presumably she was telling him to hold on, which he did for several breaths before a man said "Police."

"I want to report – " Ray faltered as Julian not merely held up a hand but thrust it at him. "What is it, Julian?"

Julian kept that to himself until he was close enough to mutter "What made you say the fellow was drowned?"

"I didn't want to speculate in front of William. Besides, what else – "

As Julian opened his mouth, the phone provided a voice. "You say someone is drowned."

"He looked as if he'd been underwater for some time," Ray said and was overtaken by a shudder.

"Say where that is."

"He's in a cave by a beach. It's near the only bus stop with a shrine by it, I believe."

Jonquil's tousled head emerged from the dress she was pulling on. "It's stop number eleven."

"Well spotted, Jonquil," Ray said and told the phone "Eleven is the closest stop."

"You are there. At the beach."

"We're still there, but – What is it now, Julian?"

"I'll speak," Julian said and leaned towards the phone. "We've a five-year-old boy in our party. You won't want us to loiter, I suppose."

"What is your name?"

Ray had to assume this was addressed to him. "Ray Thornton."

Julian took this to indicate that he could shepherd everybody off the beach. "You can talk while you're walking, Raymond."

Ray felt as if the official voice had seized him by the ear. "Did you find the victim?"

"I did, yes," Ray said and tried not to remember the incomplete face.

"Who else has seen him?"

"Just the gentleman you were hearing from before."

As Julian turned at the foot of the slope up the cliff to stare at Ray the policeman said "His name."

"Julian Banks."

Perhaps just the stare made Ray feel he might regret having said so. "Where do you stay?" the policeman was asking.

"We're going back there now." When he heard no interdiction Ray said "The Sunny View in Teleftaiafos."

"How long?"

"A fortnight." As Ray trudged uphill after Julian he said "Ten days, I mean."

"Ten days." After a pause that Ray couldn't help finding ominous the man said "What is your number there?"

"It's my number anywhere." Perhaps he shouldn't have risked a quip, but Ray was distracted by the sight of Tim and Jonquil helping Sandra up the slope, where he could almost have thought they were sharing her energy rather than lending her theirs. "It's a mobile," he said and gave the number.

"You will be at your apartments if we want you."

"We'll be out most days. I'll take the phone with me."

"There are places it will not work."

Ray waited to be told where, only to realise that the call had been cut off. Presumably this was no fault of the coverage, since the onscreen symbol had turned into three upright stakes. Sandra and the teenagers had reached the cliff top and were putting on speed towards the nearest tree, though they could no longer walk abreast. "That's the spirit," Julian said. "Best foot forward, everyone."

"I think we've left it far enough behind," Doug said, "what you two saw."

Ray wondered if his son resented the exclusion, and Pris seemed to think he did. "I shouldn't think anyone would have wanted to see it," she murmured.

"I'm simply trying to make sure," Julian said, "that nobody misses the bus."

William dashed through the grass beside the path and was first to the tree. He barely waited for Sandra and the cousins to join him before he sprinted to the next tree while they guzzled water. "Don't go on the road, William," Julian shouted.

"But if the bus is coming," Doug called, "wave it down."

Natalie turned on him. "Didn't you hear what his father just said?"

"No need for the nerves, Nat. All right, I'll catch up with him."

Ray examined the trees as he passed them. He'd overlooked carvings on those nearest the road, which didn't give the saint's foe any more of a shape. As he waited for Sandra and the teenagers under the last tree but one he saw headlights jittering between the twigs of a hedge beside the road. He thought the police had arrived until a higher stretch of road let him see the bus. William waved a frantic semaphore with both arms while his uncle kept hold of his shoulder, and then the boy jumped on board to detain the bus as the family hurried or trotted or limped along the path. "Thank you, William," Julian said but frowned at Doug for letting go of him.

As the bus left the stop Ray saw headlamps flash in the driver's mirror beneath yet another icon of St Titus. He looked back to see a police car swing off the road and speed past the shrine, widening the path. He had to admit he was grateful that Julian had saved the family from any need to meet the police. The car had halted at the top of the slope to the beach when William said "I know what he was killing."

"What are you talking about, William?" Natalie demanded. "Who?"

"The man on all the trees."

Ray wasn't sure that he wanted to ask, and saw the boy's parents weren't anxious to. It was Sandra who said "Tell us then, William."

"Spiders."

Julian gave a laugh or at any rate a summary of one. "I don't think so, son."

"I think they were. Like the ones that were eating his spear in the shrine. They were in a bag like that," William said with untypical defiance, and Ray tried not to recall how shrivelled the husk of the man in the cave had been – how like a spider's victim.

THE FIFTH DAY
24 AUGUST

Ray thought that Sandra was standing by the bed, and then he recognised the corpse from the cave. It was leaning towards her, and he took it to be weeping for her until he saw it was blind, not to mention far from tearful. The bulging white eyes were cocoons from which spiders streamed down the loose withered cheeks. At least Ray was able to realise it was a dream, and now he grasped that the visitor wasn't the carcass he'd found but some other creature animated by a parody of life. For some reason this disturbed him more, and it took him far too long to struggle awake.

The room was grey with dawn. Sandra was lying beside him, resting her head on one arm on the thin pillow. In the dim light he could just distinguish the mark on her upturned neck. Was that how she'd lain in his dream? He didn't know why it seemed important to remember. He slipped an arm around her waist and then inched his hand over her ribs as though groping for her breath. When he felt her chest rise and fall he managed to relax before his embrace could waken her. He ought to let her rest – stay peaceful while she had the chance – though he had to fend off the phrase his thoughts suggested. For a while he watched her shape grow almost imperceptibly brighter as the light in the room became less subdued, and then he edged out of bed.

When he emerged from the bathroom Sandra still wasn't awake. He needn't rouse her, since over dinner everyone had agreed to spend today on the beach by the Sunny View. He was on the balcony, watching small waves snatch at the sunlight, when he heard William protesting down below. Once the boy raised his voice Ray was able to make out the words. "I thought he came to see Jonquil."

"You were dreaming, William."

"No call to be so fierce about it, Jonquil," Julian said. "We know it had to be a dream."

"So long as he does."

"You're trying to buck him up, aren't you," Natalie said. "Just forget about it now, William."

"I want to. It was somebody I couldn't see, but I think they came out of that cave."

Ray was disconcerted by the resemblance to his own dream until he saw that they both must have had the cave on their minds. "Nobody's going to come out of there, William," he called. "We'll have a better time on this beach."

Sandra hauled the window open and blinked with a wince at the day. "Are we all going down now?"

"We're nowhere near going," Doug assured her. "Tim isn't even with us yet."

"I am now," Tim only just pronounced.

"Well, there's a miracle," Pris said. "You looked like you were sleeping the sleep of the, as if you were very asleep."

"I know what he was," William informed her. "Like the dead. Like Jonquil."

"I'd like to know what you mean by that, William."

"Kindly leave it, Jonquil," Julian said. "You were certainly fast asleep. I hope you're more refreshed than you look."

Ray might have observed that Sandra didn't seem to have benefitted much from sleeping in, but doing so would have dismayed him. He made coffee and had set out breakfast on the balcony by the time she joined him. She was wearing a sundress together with her hat and sunglasses even though the balcony would be shaded for hours. As she saw off a second glass of orange juice somebody knocked at a door. "Yes, who is it?" Julian called.

"You aren't supposed to answer first time," Jonquil said in a tone Ray wasn't sure of.

"Don't talk nonsense, girl. Take no notice, William." Julian's voice was receding through the apartment towards another knock. "I said who's there?" he urged.

Ray heard the door open, and Evadne in the distance. "The car is here for you," she said.

"I'm afraid you're mistaken. We've ordered no car."

"No, it is the police. They will take you and Mr Thornton."

"Then they should have given us some warning. As you see, I'm hardly even dressed."

"They say you know."

"In my case they're misinformed. Please come through." As Julian's voice spilled onto the lower balcony he demanded "Are you hearing what I'm being told, Raymond? Did you know about this?"

"No more than you did," Ray said less sharply than he might have. Peering at his mobile let him add "Nobody's been in touch that I can see."

Julian craned out to meet his eyes. "What do you propose doing?"

"We may as well get it over with, do you think?"

He was consulting Sandra too, but Julian was gone at once. "Please advise them we'll be along shortly," he said.

"I'll take them all down to the beach," Sandra told Ray, who saw her playing her old self. Perhaps so far as the family was concerned, she could. "Honestly," she said and gripped his hand, "you go and I'll be fine."

He was holding on as if he'd forgotten how to let go of her when Doug called "Jules, you might want to take a bit of care how you talk."

"I wasn't aware I was rude."

"Where you're going, I mean. It's not a good idea to get on the wrong side of the authorities in this part of the world. I'm saying don't peeve the police."

"I really can't imagine what you have in mind."

"Uncle Doug's saying don't pee off the police."

"William," Natalie cried, though Ray couldn't judge whether the boy meant to translate or to relish the usage. "Wherever did you learn that? Certainly not from either of your parents."

"They say it at school."

"I'm quite sure your teachers don't," Julian said.

"They do, daddy, and they say – "

"Never mind, William," Natalie said. "We don't want to hear, and we don't want you ever to say anything like that again. Bad words bring bad things."

"What do they bring, mummy?"

"We won't talk about it. I'm positive nobody would use language like that when your grandparents were teaching." As Ray grasped that her pause might have been inviting confirmation she said "And we definitely don't around the children I look after."

"That's a nursery. They're littler than me."

"It doesn't matter how old you are, William," his father said. "You should always be careful what you say."

"You've got it, Jules," Doug said.

While the silence seemed to grow increasingly expressive, Ray kissed Sandra's hand and released it at last. "I'm coming now, Julian," he called.

He was waiting outside the Banks apartment – wondering if anyone would respond if he knocked just once – when Julian appeared, buttoning a moderately colourful short-sleeved shirt over his shorts. As the men passed Evadne's office a young woman in a blue police uniform marched across the courtyard. "Banks," she said. "Thornton."

"I'm Mr Banks," Julian said, "and this is Mr Thornton."

Ray hoped the policewoman didn't find this as reproving as it sounded. She said nothing while she led the way to a car parked across the entrance to the courtyard as though to hinder anyone's escape. She watched her passengers take their seats and then sat behind the wheel, locking all the doors with a decisive multiple click. In moments the car was speeding away from the village. "May we know where we're going?" Julian said before Ray had a chance to speak.

The policewoman glanced at him in the mirror beneath the apparently inevitable icon of St Titus. "Sunset Beach."

"I expect you find plenty to occupy you there."

This time her glance was sharper. "You say…"

"Drunken people misbehaving. Drugs too, I shouldn't wonder."

"You know about drugs."

"I've no experience of them whatsoever. I imagine you might, though." Presumably Julian saw this was a careless choice of words. "Investigating them, that is," he said without much patience. "Whatever makes the people how they are."

Her gaze found him in the mirror. "Who do you say?"

"The crowd who come out at night." When her gaze didn't let him alone Julian said "People unlike us."

"People from our country," Ray contributed. "I feel as though I should apologise for some of them."

"We can thank them. Without them we don't live how we should."

"Well, that's generous of you," Julian said, and when she stared at him "Very understanding."

The car slowed as it reached Sunset Beach, where a solitary figure dodged off the road bordered with slumbering neon into a lane. "There's one," Julian said, which put Ray in mind of a schoolboy telling tales. "He didn't look too eager to be seen."

"He will be," the policewoman said as she turned the car along a street between a taverna and a nightclub.

The street led between apartments to a crossroads with a police station on one corner, a single-storey building that stretched along two streets at right angles to its entrance tower. Like the police vehicles lined up alongside, the building was white trimmed with blue. It might have looked welcoming, Ray thought, if blue shutters hadn't covered every window. The driver released the doors and opened Ray's for him. "Come," she said.

An archway in the tower let them into a white lobby where two policemen watched Ray and Julian from behind a counter. Six bare straight chairs stood against one wall outside a corridor. The policewoman indicated the chairs with a hand before turning to her colleagues, and Ray was failing to understand or even identify a single word of theirs when Julian said "Perhaps we should have brought Douglas."

The policewoman swung around at once. "Please stay," she said and marched along the corridor.

Ray hoped Julian didn't think they were being addressed too much like dogs. "Why are you missing Doug?"

"In case we want a translator."

Julian was staring at the posters on the wall behind the counter. All the writing on them was in Greek, and several included photographs of young men and women who looked neither criminal nor local. "I expect we'll be interviewed in English," Ray said.

"I shan't have a great deal to say otherwise."

Ray did his best not to think how desirable this might be. Perhaps his silence was eloquent enough, because Julian lowered his head as if his pouting lips had dragged it down, so that Ray felt compelled to speak. "I hear you're having to deal with some problems at work."

"I'm facing challenges, if that's what you mean to say."

"I just wanted you to know we appreciate you may be under some strain."

"Has Natalie been feeling she has to apologise for me?"

"Not at all. She simply wanted me to know how hard you're working for the family."

"No harder than she does at her nursery, I should think." As Ray prepared to make the most of this rapport Julian said "Still, I'm glad if you appreciate my efforts."

"I expect everybody does," Ray said in the hope of convincing him.

"You're an optimistic fellow, Raymond. I've often noticed that you look for the positive in any situation. That's no bad way to live your life, especially at your age and Sandra's."

Ray found he had to look elsewhere, meeting the eyes of the posters, flattened eyes drained of colour above captions in a language he didn't understand. "But I wonder if you realise," Julian was saying, "what a job it is to take over someone else's child."

"Maybe you shouldn't try and take her over quite so much, do you think?" Having blurted this, Ray saw no reason not to add "We all need to be ourselves."

"Assuming that's acceptable." Before Ray could declare that Jonquil was, Julian said "I take it that's how you and Sandra raised your own children."

"It is, and we're proud of them both. And all the grandchildren."

"I won't argue with you. It's obvious neither of you likes me correcting Jonquil. I've let plenty slide, believe me. I shouldn't like anyone to see how she'd present herself if her mother didn't take a stand. You'd think the girl had taken a positive dislike to mirrors."

"Tim's been a bit like that too, hasn't he? Maybe it's a teenage trait these days." As he saw this fail to find acceptance Ray said "Sandra was a bit dishevelled at breakfast as well. It's feeling free when you're on holiday, that's all."

"There's far too much indulgence in the name of freedom these days. You understand I don't mean Sandra when I say I shouldn't like to think that staying here brings out the worst." Though Julian was staring at the men behind the counter Ray didn't expect him to speak to them, let alone demand "Is there some issue? Are we not allowed to talk?"

As both men scowled in response Ray told them "We aren't trying to get our story straight and we aren't maligning your island." This didn't seem to please them, any more than "We're just glad we didn't stay in Sunset Beach."

One policeman made a comment to the other, and Ray did his best to fix the sounds in his mind in case Doug could translate. When Julian opened his mouth Ray was afraid he was about to call for a translation, but Julian said "I wonder if you think anyone else should be making an effort."

Rather than admit how much he was Ray said "At what?"

"To ensure everybody has a decent time. Perhaps Douglas mightn't keep amusing himself quite so much at our expense."

"He's always teased his sister, and she used to tease him. It's just how he is. You shouldn't mind."

"In that case I'd welcome any tips on fitting in."

"I'm not sure what you – "

"Passing for one of the family. I'm well aware I've taken someone else's place."

"We really don't feel that about you, Julian."

"Is that a way of saying there's no place for me?"

"Not by any means." If Julian was revealing a hidden self at last, Ray thought he could have chosen somewhere more appropriate. Perhaps the stares of the policemen were making him defiant, even reckless. "If you'd like my advice – " Ray said and no more, because the burlier of the policemen was striding towards them.

The flap in the counter slammed behind him like a lid, and Ray couldn't tell how ominous his tread was meant to sound. He met Ray's eyes and then Julian's, and beckoned as he turned his back. "Come now," he said.

He led them along the corridor, where the white glare of the walls was relieved only by doors bearing plaques etched with words in Greek. As the man knocked at a door, Ray deduced that the phone call he'd been peripherally aware of must have been internal. He was distracted by observing that nobody responded until the policeman knocked a second time. "Go in," the policeman said.

Julian was between Ray and the door, and stared at their escort until he opened it for them, scowling afresh. Beyond it was a white room so bare it struck Ray as close to monastic. Although the slats of the shutter at the window were only slightly parted, a stark light had gathered in the room. Below the window a slim but hardly slight man sat behind a heavy desk. His dark blue jacket bore a vertical trio of stars and several medals on ribbons. His mop of curly black hair seemed incongruous, and his thin face looked set to counteract any impression of the kind, though Ray imagined Julian deploring the unruliness. The man rose not quite to his feet as their escort shut the door, and Ray took the outstretched unapologetically hairy hand to be offering a handshake until its twin indicated the second of the chairs before the desk. "Please take a seat," the man said.

Julian waited for Ray to sit down before he did. Presumably he meant to ingratiate them both by saying "Thank you, Inspector."

The man resumed his seat without haste. "Captain Apostolides," he said.

"Our apologies. An easy mistake to make, I'm sure you'll agree. We aren't too familiar with your local ways." When none of this earned any perceptible reaction Julian pointed several fingers at the dangling badges. "We can see you've had quite a career."

"I have served my island." While he said so Apostolides looked as solemn as the photograph of some venerable dignitary on the wall to the left of the desk. "Now," he said, "you are…"

"Julian Banks, and this is my – "

"There is no haste, please." Once a pause had underscored this, Apostolides said "I thought you would be Mr Banks."

"May I know why?"

"You are the one that talks."

"If you mean when we reported the incident, it was Mr Thornton here who contacted you."

"Ray Thornton, yes." Without having looked away from Julian, Apostolides said "You are the one who wanted to be gone."

"Was there anyone who didn't, Raymond? I didn't need to ask my son's mother if she did."

"Why did she?" Apostolides said.

"He's five years old. Didn't whoever Raymond spoke to tell you that?"

The policeman left the question unacknowledged. "What did you fear for your son?"

"We didn't want him seeing what was there. Would you like your young children to know about that kind of thing?"

"Nothing else."

"I should think that's quite enough to keep from him."

"Here nothing comes that is not called for."

Ray supposed this was meant as reassurance if not a declaration on behalf of the island, but Julian retorted "I shouldn't think the fellow in the cave would agree with you."

At once the policeman's gaze seemed as keen as the rays of sunlight through the shutter. "Who in the cave?"

"The man you've brought us here to talk about. Why else have we had to come?" When the scrutiny didn't relent, Julian said "You can scarcely expect us to know his name."

Apostolides looked away at last, to fix his gaze on Ray. "You have your passports."

"Not on me. Have you brought yours, Julian?"

"Nobody advised us that we should," Julian made sure the policeman appreciated. "None of your people was in touch."

"All right, Julian, I'll see to it." Ray thought it best to show Apostolides his phone, only to find a belated report of a missed call. "It looks as if someone did try to get me," he admitted.

"We will wait," Apostolides said, folding his muscular arms on the desk.

The sense of retrieving the call from a number in England made Ray feel unexpectedly isolated, cut off from home. That was just a few hours away if Sandra needed to return, but why did he have to think about that now? The call had indeed been from the police. "I'm sorry," he said. "They did give us the pickup time and ask us to bring our passports."

"Things can interfere with your reception on our island," Apostolides said and breathed out just as hard as in. "Well, so I must write your details."

As the desk expressed the tedium with a creak of the drawer he dragged out, Julian said "Don't you delegate tasks like that? It's hardly worth having subordinates otherwise."

While Ray saw he was trying to engage with the policeman, he was afraid Apostolides mightn't realise. "Mind you," Julian said as Apostolides found a pad of printed forms, "I know what a chore it can be when you're lacking staff. When you're promoted you don't expect it to bring you more work and less sleep."

Ray couldn't help blurting "You didn't say it was that serious."

With enough resentment to be directing much of it at the policeman Julian said "I've had to say it now."

"When you are ready." Apostolides was poising a ballpoint over the topmost form. "Mr Thornton will come first," he said.

The blades of light through the shutter had swung close to Ray by the time the policeman completed the form, which entailed minutely inking words in narrow rectangles and crosses in boxes before poring over the results. At last Apostolides raised his head to ask or to warn "You teach the right way."

"I hope I did. As I said, I've retired from teaching, like my wife."

"Are you looking for a new life now?"

Before he could hold back Ray said "Coming here seems to have given her one."

"Would you say?" Julian said. "I haven't noticed any difference since we saw you at Christmas."

"Mr Banks," Apostolides said, for which Ray was painfully grateful.

Where Ray had answered all the questions as amiably as he could manage, Julian was curter. Perhaps Apostolides was growing more deliberate by contrast if not as a reprimand. At last the form was filled in and examined, which apparently required a punch line. "You think everything should be insured."

"I think it's wise to keep yourself as safe as possible."

"That is your safety." Apostolides was aligning the forms on his desk with the hairy edges of his hands, and his eyes didn't signify how much of a question he'd intended. He lifted his head but not his gaze as he said "Now we shall talk about why you were sent for."

"I don't know what more we can be expected to contribute," Julian said.

"You are here for examination." Once his eyes had made this plain Apostolides turned them on Ray. "Tell me why you were there," he said.

"On that beach? My wife liked the look."

"The look," Apostolides said and intensified his own.

"Yes, of the place. She thought it would be quieter than the other beaches. Well," Ray said with a sally at a laugh, "it was."

"How did she know it was there?"

The question seemed more searching than Ray understood, unless he was confusing it with the glare through the shutter. "The cruise around the island took us," he said.

"You say the boat went to the beach."

"Just past it," Ray said and had an odd sense of defending the boatman. "We didn't stop."

"Did nobody tell you about it?"

"What would there have been to tell?" When Apostolides let the question loiter Ray said "The guide didn't have anything to say about it, no."

"If I may interrupt," Julian said, "may we know what use this is? It's keeping us away from our families when we're supposed to be here on holiday."

"We are building up your picture." Apostolides didn't bother glancing at him. "How did you find the way?" he said.

Ray too had begun to feel the questions were excessively trivial. "My son figured it out," he said.

"This is not your son."

"I'm not," Julian said, "but may I ask why you think it's so obvious?"

Apostolides gave him a glance so terse it barely qualified as one. "Your name."

"That's what betrayed me, is it? Regrettably I've no control over that."

He sounded so bitter that Ray might have responded if Apostolides hadn't said "How did you go to the beach?"

"We took the bus," Ray said, "and then we went along the path with the carvings on the trees."

Apostolides raised his face an inch while holding Ray's gaze with his own, so that Ray wondered what he'd provoked until the policeman said "Well, so you are at the beach. Why did you go into the cave?"

"I was seeing whether it was safe for our grandson, that's Julian's son."

"The boy again. You thought it may be safe in there for him."

Ray felt unfairly criticised. "I should think Greek boys like exploring caves, don't they, even at his age?"

"Some they do."

"If you don't like people going down there," Julian objected, "perhaps you ought to put a warning on the path. And those things on the trees can't be much help. They're more liable to tempt people to see what's along there than keep them away."

"They were meant to guard the way." Apostolides was still watching Ray. "What did you see?" he said.

"In the cave? That poor man."

"That is all. A poor man."

"I'd say he was, yes." Having grasped that he was being prompted to say more, Ray said "He'd drowned and ended up lodged in the rocks, had he? Or did he have a heart attack because he'd trapped himself somehow? Have you established how he died?"

"You did not touch him."

Ray would have much preferred an answer instead of this suggestion. "I couldn't have," he said, shivering despite the rays that had found him through the shutter.

"You saw no more to tell me." When Ray shook his head, which failed to dislodge the memory of the perished whitish corpse, Apostolides said "Mr Banks, it is your turn to speak."

"Have you identified the gentleman?"

"We have done that."

"Are you going to say who he was?"

"He was like you." As Ray hoped Julian wouldn't take any exception to this the policeman said "A tourist from your country staying in Teleftaiafos."

"Was he the fellow who was supposed to have vanished after he went to the mainland?"

"That will be the person. Now, Mr Banks – "

"In that case I don't understand."

Apostolides took a breath that stirred the badges on his chest. "What is not clear?"

"If the gentleman died last week I don't see how the body could have ended up in that state so soon."

"No, he was reported last month."

"The guide on the cruise said he went missing last week. You'll confirm that, Raymond."

"I'm sure the police know better than he did if he didn't mean to say last month."

Ray was afraid that Julian would argue, and not just with him, until Apostolides intervened. "What state are you speaking of?"

"The fellow looked diseased to me. I didn't go as close as Raymond did, but I could see that much."

As the light probed Ray's eyes Apostolides said "Is that all?"

"I think it's quite enough to need investigating."

"That has been done." The policeman's gaze veered between Julian and Ray while he said "You may tell your families that he had a seizure and drowned. He was underwater for some weeks and then the tide took him into the cave, where as Mr Thornton says he was trapped in the rocks."

"They don't need to hear all that." Just as unenthusiastically Julian said "And how was he identified?"

"His passport was at his apartment."

"I was thinking of his family. Did he have any children? They'd be something like my age, of course, or older."

"Family, yes. They were not required."

"You wouldn't want them to see him like that. Will you be warning them?"

Apostolides gazed at him before saying "Warning them of what, Mr Banks?"

"What they'll find if they should want to see him. I take it he'll be sent home for a proper funeral."

"His ashes will go back."

Ray sensed Julian's dissatisfaction and tried to head it off. "I expect under the circumstances – "

"You know that was his wish, do you?" Julian was still interrogating the policeman. "Or has the family asked for it?"

"It is our decision, Mr Banks."

"Perhaps you should wait and see what they say." Since staring hard at Apostolides failed to provoke an answer, Julian said "Have you even consulted them?"

"It is already done."

"You're telling us you've had their authorisation."

"He has been cremated. They would not have liked to see the head."

"The face, you mean." When Apostolides answered only with a frown that clenched his eyes Julian persisted "Why are you saying the head?"

Apostolides plainly regretted having let himself be goaded, but he said close to carelessly "He was not together. It was apart."

"Good God, man, what are you telling us now?" Julian seemed about to lurch to his feet until Ray seized his arm. "All right, Raymond, I haven't lost control," Julian said but confronted the policeman. "When did that happen," he demanded, "and how? Even in his condition I don't see how it could."

"It is a police matter."

"You need to know he wasn't mutilated like that when we found him. Who could have done such a thing?" When the policeman failed to display outrage Julian said "It wouldn't be one of your traditions, would it? Is that why you're taking it for granted?"

"The police have to get used to such things, Julian," Ray tried to intervene. "They must have to deal with worse."

"There isn't much that's worse than desecrating the dead." Julian hadn't looked away from the policeman. "I'd like to know when it was done," he insisted. "We reported what we'd found and we saw your people arrive as we were leaving. How did somebody get to the beach in the meantime?"

Apostolides held up his hands on either side of his face and parted all the fingers. As the sunlight streamed between them he put Ray in mind of a saint delivering a benediction – some religious gesture, at any rate. Ray wasn't sure whether it was the light or the policeman's gaze that felt as though it was reaching deep into his skull, but one or both of them illuminated his thoughts. "I think we'd better leave it, Julian," he said. "Captain, we've told you everything we know."

"I have learned what I need." Just the same, Apostolides watched them for some seconds before rising not entirely to his feet. "I hope you enjoy the rest of your stay on our island," he said. "It will help to forget what you have seen and heard."

"Let's hurry back to everyone, Julian," Ray said, not least to quash whatever response his companion had been about to make.

The police driver met them at the end of the corridor. As she drove them through Sunset Beach, Ray saw Julian prepare to speak. Ray was afraid he meant to discuss Apostolides while the driver could hear, but Julian said "I know what you can do for me, Raymond, if you will."

"I'll do my best if it'll help."

"Then forget my outburst earlier. I can only apologise for my lack of control. I shouldn't like Natalie to hear of it."

"It wasn't much of an outburst," Ray said but shook the awkward hand that Julian thrust at him. So even his agreement not to speak had to be left unrevealed. He felt shut in by unmentioned issues, trapped inside himself by them. Until the car left Sunset Beach behind, the deceptively empty streets reminded him of his brain, so that he could have imagined they were hiding away just as much.

★　　★　　★

"Come on, Jules, just split the bill. You aren't trying to cut down someone's claim."

"Doug," Ray felt compelled to protest, "I don't think that's quite fair."

"I'd simply like to be sure we're only being charged for what we've had," Julian said.

"If there's anything else you want us to translate," Doug said, "just ask."

"Let me see," Julian said but glanced at the rest of the party. "Why don't you all take William to find the lights while we settle this."

They were in the Old Bridge, a taverna at the far end of the village from the Sunny View. A moon-faced road train – another treat that William was promised now – grinned at them across the village square. Beyond a low wall draped with white blossom a stream meandered under a stone bridge to the sea. Across the bridge the road led past the outlying houses into the dark, where dozens of lights flickered in the distance. "What are you saying you're going to settle?" Ray was anxious to be told.

"Not our differences, Raymond. Just the bill."

"Maybe you should settle those too."

"Come along, everyone," Sandra said. "The sooner we see what's out there, the sooner some of us can get to bed."

Presumably she meant William, though Ray was surprised to see both the teenagers nod as if they were anticipating slumber. "We'll catch you up," he said.

How much peace would he need to keep between the men? Julian continued squinting at the bill while the women and the youngsters crossed the bridge, and then he looked up. "I hope you didn't think I was being typical," he said. "We'll split it by all means. I was only making sure nobody hears who shouldn't."

Ray was disconcerted by having to glance about at the dark even though he'd grasped that Julian had William in mind. Perhaps Julian wasn't behaving as untypically as he believed, since he'd taken out his phone to use the calculator. "Hears what?" Doug said.

Julian made a barely patient gesture before fingering numbers on the screen. Once he'd shown Ray and Doug what they owed he counted his contribution onto the table. At last he said "I wanted to ask you something, Douglas. I expect Raymond can guess."

"I don't know if I can," Ray said, feeling apprehensive too.

"First let me say we appreciate your local knowledge, Douglas, and Priscilla's. I wonder if you might be able to explain what we heard at the police station."

"I knew it. I could see you two were keeping something back."

"There's a good deal we don't want the younger ones to know."

"You aren't including Tim, are you? He can cope."

Julian held up a hand, beckoning the waitress but at least not displaying the palm. "If that's your choice for him," he said, "but can we all keep quiet about it in front of William."

"Tim's pretty good at keeping stuff to himself. He's a teenager."

The idea or its implications seemed to displease Julian, who said nothing more until the waitress collected their payment. "Please don't trouble about change," he said, not that there would be much, and lowered his voice. "So, Douglas. I think the police would rather we hadn't learned this, but after we found the body it was mutilated."

"Well," Ray demurred, "mutilated. I don't believe – "

"The head had been removed. What else would you call it, for heaven's sake?"

"I think the policeman just said it was, how can we put it, unattached. Lord, what a thing to have to talk about."

"And just how else do you imagine that could have happened?"

"Do we really need to go into it?" Apparently they did, and Ray had to swallow first. "You didn't see the state the man was in," he said to Doug. "He must have been underwater for weeks. Maybe when they tried to move him he, oh lord, came to bits."

"I suppose that could have been the case," Julian said. "Thank you for bringing reason to bear."

"At least he couldn't wander," Doug said.

Ray heard ripples lapping under the bridge. They reminded him of the ripples that had seemed to follow him out of the depths of the cave, and he could have fancied they sounded as if some creature were assuaging its thirst in the dark. When Julian thrust out his lips to fend off Doug's comment, Ray felt delegated to speak. "What do you mean?"

"That's one way they're supposed to stop the dead going for a walk, cutting off the head."

"Who would do that?" With mounting outrage Julian said "Not the police."

"Whoever believes in that sort of thing, Jules. I don't know if they do round here."

"You can't be telling us that's how they treat their dead in this day and age."

"They used to in some parts of Europe. Anyone who died in a way that means they won't stay dead."

Julian ensured the others saw how absurd it was to ask "What way?"

"It depends where you are, I think. Suicide's a favourite, as I recall. And of course the obvious one – "

Julian didn't merely raise a hand, he thrust it up in front of Doug's face. For a moment Ray thought Julian was refusing to hear any more, and then he realised Julian was listening to Natalie. "Don't go scampering off," she called, somewhere out of sight across the bridge. "Jonquil, stay with him."

Julian shoved back his chair and stood up. "Let's deal with something that warrants our attention, shall we?"

Ray saw Doug make the effort not to feel disparaged. As they followed Julian across the bridge, the liquid monologue of the stream dwindled to a secretive whisper. A bat fluttered across a wall, or rather the shadow of a large moth circling a streetlamp did. A cat as black and noiseless as the shadow vanished into a garden full of drowsy flowers. In the darkness of a house beside the road a clutch of faces flickered into shape, lit by a television on which John Wayne was addressing a posse of cowboys in Greek. As Ray passed a solitary car parked by the road he saw the glass of the wing mirror begin to twitch. No, the reflection of a spider in its web that spanned the mirror had, and there was no reason to be unnerved by the creature's doubled hunger.

Beyond the last houses, all of which were silent and unlit, the road led past a high white wall. Through a gateway where a pair of wrought-iron gates were bolted open, Ray saw dozens of restless lights. As he limped closer they appeared to draw words and numbers out of the darkness – names and dates. They were flames inside lanterns in front of engraved stones, and the place was a graveyard, presumably the reason why Julian planted his hands on his hips and swung around to confront Doug. "Is this another one of your traditions?"

"Putting lamps on graves?" Ray said. "It's pretty common all over Greece, isn't it, Doug?"

"In that case it's regrettable that someone didn't say so sooner."

"We didn't know what they were then," Doug protested as Julian turned his back on him and marched towards the gateway. He gave his father a wide-eyed grimace, and Ray felt furtive if not partisan for returning a version of the look.

Beyond the gates a broad gravel path led into the depths of the graveyard, which extended so far that the most distant flames looked like stars fallen to earth. Ray had to think the place served more than the village, since it was so large. Sandra and Natalie were just inside the gates, and Julian was staring at his wife. "Why are you waiting here? What have you done with William?"

"We were waiting so you could see where we were," Sandra said.

"Thank you, Sandra, but we're talking about William."

"He's with Jonquil and Tim," Natalie said, "and Pris has gone after them."

"You think he should be at large in a place like this."

"Nobody's going to harm him, are they?" Sandra said. "It's the last place."

"And we thought it might be good for him," Natalie said.

"Please do define what on earth you mean by good."

"To help him get used to the idea of people dying," Sandra said. "That it's natural, not like the man you found."

"You genuinely believe that's required at William's age."

"I think it may be before very long, yes."

Julian gazed at her, and Ray wondered how much he'd understood. He was bracing himself in case she'd decided to make herself clearer when Jonquil called "Where are you, William?"

"I thought he was being looked after," Julian told whoever was to blame, and raised his voice. "Go to Timothy and your sister, William."

Ray heard the boy's giggle a good way ahead. Somewhere to its left Tim called "Go to her, Will."

"Why aren't you two staying together, Tim?" Pris called, which let Ray locate her in the dimness far along the path.

"Because we're trying to find William," Jonquil said, and Ray saw her in the distance beyond Pris.

"Stop playing, William," Natalie shouted. "Go to Jonquil now."

The boy giggled again, and Ray thought he heard a hint of nervousness. "Which one's Jonquil?"

"I'm here, William. Look, on the path."

"Shall we try and make less noise?" Perhaps Julian's frown acknowledged that he wasn't doing so. "Remember where we are," he said. "It's not a place for games."

Perhaps William took at least some of this to heart, since he was silent. "William?" Pris said as she went to Jonquil.

Ray didn't understand why there should be so much confusion, and he couldn't bear it any longer. "I'll go and help," he said.

Sharp pebbles gnashed beneath his sandals until he stepped off the path onto the grass. The gravel had started to bruise his toes, and in any case this was the most direct route to where he'd last heard William. There was more light among the graves than on the path. The grass yielded underfoot, and he thought the ground did as he made his way between stones that appeared to be captioning the unsteady flames with words he couldn't read. Dim figures stood over some of the graves, living up to Julian's appeal for silence. As Ray limped past one still figure he slipped on a moist patch of grass and had to clutch at an arm, dislodging a soft clammy handful – part of a sleeve of moss. He was recovering his balance and the breath he'd lost to a gasp when Pris and Jonquil called not quite in unison "William."

If the boy answered, it was covered up by a clamour of gravel. Julian and Doug and Natalie were tramping along the path, while Sandra followed not too far behind. Ray waited to be sure she wasn't having difficulties, since she was intent on the path – too preoccupied to notice him. Once she came abreast of him he turned away to look for William, only to see a face watching her from the dark.

He would have taken it for a memorial if it hadn't moved. It looked dauntingly ancient and yet as smooth as marble. The large heavy-lidded eyes and thin lips weren't much less pallid than the high bald cranium and long hollow cheeks and incongruously small nose, which seemed like an unsuccessful bid to lend the features some humanity. In a moment Ray saw that it wasn't moving as a face should. The flesh, such as it was, had begun to shift like water, rippling as if it couldn't stay entirely still. Were the pale empty eyes keeping Sandra in sight? Ray twisted around to see if she was aware of the watcher, but she already had her back to him and his uninvited companion. With a good deal of reluctance he turned to confront the figure – to see more than just the face.

There was no tall thin figure. Between Ray and the spot where he was sure it had been standing, a headstone was wobbling as though the occupant of the grave had grown tired of lying still. Ray couldn't breathe until he realised that the lid of the lantern on the grave was open, and only the heat from the flame had made the stone appear to waver. Behind the stone was an angel missing most of both wings, which had to be the figure he'd seen, even if he recalled it as having been closer. He was trying to recapture the sight of its face – presumably having looked directly at the flame had dimmed his night vision, such as it was – when he heard Julian. "Even if we're on holiday, William, that's no excuse for playing hide and seek in here."

"I wasn't."

"Then why did you go wandering off?" Natalie said.

"I was reading all the names over there."

As Ray returned to the path and saw the boy surrounded by the family ahead, Julian declared "I hardly think so, William. You can't decipher the language any more than I can."

"I could read those ones. They're all English."

"We won't argue about it," Julian said with enough finality to be addressing everyone. "There's no question you were hiding from Timothy and Jonquil."

"Daddy, I wasn't."

"William." When this rebuke didn't prompt a confession Natalie said "What do you think you were doing, then?"

"You said to go to Jonquil and I told you, I didn't know which she was."

Both his parents made to speak, but Jonquil was too quick for them. "Which what?"

"Which girl."

Though nobody seemed eager to respond, Julian said "You need to explain yourself, William."

"There was another one over there," William said and pointed at the dark between the twitching lights. "I thought she was Jonquil and I started going to her, then I saw she was looking for Tim."

"Don't say that, Will," Tim protested. "There wasn't anyone like that."

As Tim rubbed his arm hard enough to be trying to erase the bite Ray said "I think I know what you saw, William. I saw something like it too."

"What?" the boy said, not as if he was especially anxious to know.

"There are statues all around us, aren't there? And the lights make them seem to move. I thought one did just now. I'll bet that's the kind of thing you saw."

William looked stubborn. "She was watching Tim."

For a moment he made Ray feel as if not all the pallid figures among the graves might be composed of stone, and then Julian intervened. "I think we've had enough adventures before bed, William."

He led the way out of the graveyard, and Ray took Sandra's hand, not least to prevent her from rubbing the side of her neck. "It doesn't bother me," she insisted when he tried to ask about the bite. Once they were through the gates Natalie captured William's hand while Julian hung back to murmur to everyone else "We've had our fill of death now. I'll ask you not to bring it up again."

Sandra gripped Ray's hand, but he couldn't risk looking at her. As they headed for the Sunny View he saw a dark shape flutter across the road. It was the shadow of a moth, but what did it suggest to him? He glanced back at the graveyard, where nothing except lights appeared to move, and then he realised what was on his mind — a thought as useless as it was irrationally unsettling. The moth had reminded him how lights lured nocturnal creatures out of the dark.

THE SAINT'S DAY 25 AUGUST

"Well, that wasn't our best night," Natalie said. "I don't think we would have minded lying in."

Pris turned away from watching for the bus. "Sorry if I woke anyone too soon. I just thought we'd planned so much today I'd give everyone a shout."

"No need to blame yourself, Priscilla," Julian said. "Someone had already wakened us."

"I was only telling William to let me sleep," Jonquil protested.

"Perhaps you could have shown a little more consideration for your brother, since you knew he'd had a bad night."

Ray thought Sandra meant to rescue Jonquil by asking "What were you dreaming, William?"

"I thought a man got in the room."

Ray felt close to recalling a dream of his own until Sandra said "That doesn't sound like much of a dream."

"Well, it emphatically was one," Julian told William. "You said he went away without opening the door."

"I wonder if you might feel a bit responsible," Natalie said.

"Why on earth should I feel anything of the kind?" When she didn't answer Julian demanded "For what, for heaven's sake?"

"For working William up before he went to bed. Maybe for going on so much about things we won't mention instead of letting him come to terms with them."

"I think I'm exactly the wrong person to accuse of that."

As Natalie made to respond he said "And I wonder what you imagine you'll achieve by discussing this in front of him."

Ray would have liked the sound of a bus to break the ensuing silence, but it was Julian who did. "I appreciate you felt you had to defend your mother. Forgive me, Sandra, if I was abrupt."

"You're forgiven," Sandra said as they heard a bus approaching from the direction of the graveyard.

The driver stared so hard at her and the teenagers that he might almost have expected them to remove their hats and sunglasses when they stepped on board. Several women blessed them as they filed to their seats, and Julian seemed near to demanding why. He was silent until the bus reached Sunset Beach. "Don't bother looking, Jonquil," he said then. "We won't be wasting any more time here."

"What are you looking for, Sandra?" Ray said loud enough for Julian to hear.

"Just looking. Can't I look?"

Her reaction was fiercer than he understood. He was distracted by the women in the front seats, who were covering their eyes whenever someone came in sight ahead. Sandra peered at every solitary figure the bus passed, and he could have imagined she was searching for a face. She appeared not to recognise them any more than Ray did, and he told himself that it was comical to fancy either of them could.

The bus had passed through several villages by the time it reached the path that led to the beach with the cave. As it came abreast of the shrine Ray saw a large white butterfly fluttering its wings on the glass. He was about to draw William's attention to the resemblance to an angel when he realised that the butterfly was struggling in a cobweb. He glimpsed legs twitching into view around the window-frame before a massive spider darted out to seize its victim. He hoped the boy hadn't seen, and looked for sights to point out to him – a herd of goats fleeing up a slope bedside the road, an eagle hovering above the inland hills, the familiar Greek spectacle of uncompleted houses sprouting rusty metal rods where a roof should be. "That's one way of getting some sun," he said.

The comment would have been more appropriate if the sky hadn't started to grow overcast. "Sorry about the clouds," Doug said. "We only just read there's more here than anywhere else in Greece."

Masts appeared to be trying to poke holes in the sky above the harbour of Vasilema Town. A few passengers were disembarking from a ferry while a busload of homegoing tourists collected their luggage from the bowels of the bus. Most of them wore hats and sunglasses, and looked paler than their stay ought to have left them. They seemed weary too, but perhaps the holiday representative was urging them to be quick. As the sun found a gap in the overcast they hurried to the ferry with a thunderous rumble of luggage.

Beyond the harbour a side street led to the bus terminal – a square in which a line of shelters stood in front of a ticket office and a waiting-room. Once the family had stepped down Julian lingered to ask the driver "What time is the last bus back, please?"

The man jerked his hand at the windscreen, presumably gesturing at the ticket office rather than the sets of blind eyes that twitched above the mirror – the zeros of a defunct digital clock. "Most helpful," Julian said and marched over to the booth, where he planted his elbows on the window ledge until the woman at the counter looked up. "How late do you go to, you'll forgive me if I can't pronounce it. How late do you go through Sunset Beach."

She nodded at the waiting-room. "On board."

Ray might almost have imagined she was advising them to return to the bus, except that he saw she was indicating a timetable. As Julian made to retort Ray remembered Doug's warning not to antagonise anyone official. "It's not important,

Julian," he murmured. "We won't be going back that late."

"I prefer to have information before it's needed," Julian said but followed him as he made for the toilets off the waiting-room. Tim was peering at his reflection in a mirror that spanned the wall above the sinks. As soon as the men appeared behind him he dodged out of the tiled room so fast that his reflection was a blur. Ray wasn't surprised if Tim had found it hard to see himself; the glass was splintered in several places as though somebody had tried to smash the entire mirror, and Tim's sunglasses could hardly have made his view clearer. Ray used a urinal while Julian bolted a cubicle door and coughed immoderately to cover up the sounds he had to make. Once he'd washed his hands Ray dried them beneath a blower so fierce that it sent ripples through the loose flesh of his arms, a sight that reminded him of the face he'd imagined he was seeing in the graveyard. "I'll be outside," he called, which elicited a louder cough.

The family was waiting on a corner of the square, outside a tourist shop that displayed considerably fewer bottles of sun cream than of artificial tan. "Maybe you'd need that if you lived here," Doug said, and Ray saw he had the narrow streets in mind. Perhaps they were too narrow to receive direct sunlight even when the sky was cloudless, although had there been less sun cream than fake tan in the supermarket by the Sunny View? "We're over here, Jules," Pris called, "nobody's hiding from you," which drove the question out of Ray's mind.

The street that led uphill was too narrow for him to hold Sandra's hand in the crowd. Few of the tourists looked as if they came from Sunset Beach, even though some were as young. Ray assumed one of their generation was responsible for graffiti at the far end of a side street, where a name was sprayed on an otherwise unblemished white wall – RYK. Or had letters been erased on either side of those? He hadn't time to be sure before he followed Doug and Pris uphill.

Quite a few of the streets that climbed or crossed the hill were roofed with awnings overgrown by vines, which provided so much shade that Sandra and the teenagers took off their hats. Shops clustered together as if seeking the company of their own kind, so that one street sold only clothes and shoes, while another was devoted to herbs and oils and other Greek fare. Here was a street pale with embroidery – hanging tablecloths and doilies and place mats – while the next was ruddy with leather goods. Souvenir shops swarmed with images of the local saint, not just wooden icons but pottery bearing his likeness and even jewellery borrowing his shape. As Doug lingered in front of a window full of St Titus painted in a variety of styles, the proprietor waddled out to him. "Special price today," she said.

"Just looking, thanks. This chap gets everywhere, doesn't he?"

The woman folded her arms, which flattened her ageing breasts. "He is history."

"He's yours, you mean. Your island's." Since she seemed unaware that her words were ambiguous, Doug let them go. "I wasn't disrespecting him," he said.

The woman was examining the family. "Where do you stay?"

"Just along from Sunset Beach," Sandra said.

"I see it."

The woman's lined face darkened as she withdrew into the shop. "Actually," Pris called after her, "maybe you could tell us – "

The woman halted between two paintings of St Titus flourishing his spear, and Ray had the odd sense that she welcomed their protection. "What can I tell?"

"What's your saint supposed to fight? We've seen some images of him where he's fighting something, but we couldn't make out what it's meant to be."

"He did not fight. It was people's wish he did."

"In that case," Natalie said somewhere between patience and

amusement, "what didn't he fight that you wanted him to?"

"What came after."

"After his death, you mean." When the woman didn't contradict this Ray felt driven to prompt "And that was…"

"He was meant to keep island holy. Monks thought he would."

Ray wondered if the unholiness she had in mind might be represented by the likes of Sunset Beach. Apparently she'd said all she cared to, and was retreating between the saintly canvases when Julian commented "Someone needs to rethink their sales pitch. That didn't make the fellow sound much use at all."

The woman turned, though her resentment looked like unwillingness. "Maybe he helps you remember."

"Remember your island, you mean?" Pris said. "I'm sure we will."

"Some will."

Ray couldn't tell who she was staring at, let alone the reason behind her frown. "Who won't?" he blurted. "Why shouldn't they?"

The woman was already disappearing into a back room. "They come back and remember."

"Did anybody understand what that was all about?" Julian demanded, and not quietly either. "Doesn't anyone round here speak proper English?"

"They speak it better than most of us speak Greek," Pris said just as loud.

"They're pretty new to tourism," Doug pointed out. "I'd say they've made us welcome."

Sandra was making her way uphill as if the woman's frown had sent her onwards. Ray limped after her, ready to support her if she found the climb too much of a task. The street felt increasingly steep to him, though the gradient hadn't changed. How long had it been since he wouldn't have thought twice of such a climb? Remembering felt like trying to clutch at a past that was out of reach, but the present was all that should matter to him. Just now Sandra was all that should.

The way ahead was narrowed by a stall selling henna tattoos. Among the stick-on flowers and snakes and names he was unsurprised to see images of St Titus with his lance. Tim pointed at a troop of them. "We could get sainted," he told Jonquil.

"Don't so much as think of disfiguring yourself, Jonquil," Julian said. "We don't want to be seen with anyone who cares so little for herself. And the same applies to you, William."

The young woman seated on a folding chair beside the stall blinked fast and then more slowly at the teenagers. "Too late," she said.

"How's that?" Doug said as if he hoped she was joking.

"They are no good now."

"Is that another local custom, talking down your merchandise?" When she only blinked at Julian he said "I think I was perfectly clear."

"Sorry." Pris might have been apologising to the vendor on his behalf. "What are you saying about your tattoos?" she said.

"The boy said they would make them like the saint. Pictures can do nothing."

"I was kidding," Tim protested. "I won't have one if Jonk isn't."

"Please don't try to alter my decision," Julian said. "In every way that's inappropriate."

"I think Tim's just supporting his cousin, Jules," Doug said.

"I don't see why that's called for. We apologise for wasting your time," Julian told the young woman and strode uphill.

When Natalie followed him, the others did. As they crossed a lane Ray noticed more graffiti on a wall. The letters could have been advertising a local version of a worldwide drink – KOLA – or were they flanked by faint traces of more? He hadn't time to dawdle, since Sandra looked determined not to falter before reaching the top of the hill. At least he was able to take her hand, though he scarcely knew which of them might be sustaining the other, when they emerged into a square in front of a church.

The square gave them a view across the sea. Small curved waves reminiscent of fingernails clawed at a beach to the left of the harbour. The ferry that the bus had passed was sinking over the horizon, where the clouds fell short of a larger island, letting the sunlight brighten all its colours like a concentration of summer. A plane passed overhead, descending towards the distant island, and Ray and Sandra said "Casablanca" in unison as they always did. As slow protracted thunder trailed the plane across the sky Pris said "Shall we look in the church?"

The interior was brighter than the square. Hundreds of thin white candles flamed in holders along the walls and before the altar. At first Ray could hardly see, so that the figures with upraised hands seemed to form out of the distance beyond the flames. They were saints, and their gestures were blessings, though Ray could easily have felt admonished by the stern-faced golden frescoes and their stained-glass brethren. He was trying to decide which if any of the saints was Titus when Doug said "We aren't supposed to do that, Jules."

"There's a notice by the door," Pris said.

"For the love of all that's holy, what else aren't we allowed to do?" Julian demanded and continued photographing frescoes with his mobile. "It strikes me that they tell their visitors one thing and themselves another. If we aren't meant to hold our hands up, why are these fellows doing it?"

"Maybe there are some things only saints can do."

"I didn't know you were a believer, Jonquil."

"There's a whole lot you don't know about me."

Ray wondered whether this was a boast or a complaint if not both. He saw Julian preparing to reply, but as the flash made a saint gleam gold a man came out of a room near the altar and shouted in Greek. Ray thought he was rebuking Julian until he saw that the man was facing a side entrance to the church. The door had swung open, and the flames of all the nearest candles crouched low as if they were trying to flee the intrusion. "It's him," William cried. "It's the man in my dream."

Ray peered towards the door to see that several newcomers had entered the church. Through the unsteady haze of the dozens of flames that had sprung up once more, he could scarcely make the faces out or even count them. There were three of them, and they appeared to be not merely wavering but merging together. It reminded him of the sight of something underwater, except that they could have been composed of the restless liquid. He was wondering if he should recognise one or more of them when he found he was gazing at the vibrant air above the flames and nothing else. He limped fast to the side door, which was opposite a lane that led so steeply downhill it needed a stepped pavement and a handrail. The lane was deserted, though he couldn't see along the cross streets, except for a section of wall along which a blurred shadow vanished like a drying stain.

In the church the man was haranguing Julian. "No camera," he said and gestured at the frescoes. "Holy. Fade."

Ray was afraid that Julian might criticise the rudimentary language, but he slipped the phone into his shirt pocket. "Excuse me," Ray said as the man turned his back, "could I ask what you said to those people?"

Perhaps the man didn't hear him. He stumped into the side room, shutting the door with an emphatic thud that echoed through the church as the flames shivered. "Did you understand him, Doug?"

"Pris and I were trying to figure out what we heard. Something about feeding, we think."

"Maybe they were beggars," Pris said, "which means he wasn't being very Christian."

"He said something else, though," Doug told Ray. "As near as we could tell it was about some kind of transfer."

"Not those wretched tattoos again," Julian objected.

"No, Doug," Pris said. "I think I've got it now. Not a transfer, a transfusion."

If this was a clarification, Ray couldn't see what it made clear. "Now, William," Natalie said, "what was all that silliness about a dream? What did you think you saw?"

"That's how his face went in my dream." With even more defiance William said "Soggy."

"Then that proves it was a dream, doesn't it? I think you've just found a new favourite word," Sandra said. "I'm feeling a bit watery after all that walking. When everyone's seen what they want to see in here I wouldn't mind some lunch."

★   ★   ★

As the bus left the family behind, William said "Why is he up there?"

At the far end of a street that led from the main road, lengths of wood were piled at least twenty feet high in the middle of a village square. The figure perched on top wore a black robe with a cowl that hid its face. It was silhouetted against clouds stained red by the sun that had sunk beyond the unseen sea. "He looks like he's looking for someone," William said.

"He's just for people to look at," Jonquil told him. "Let's go and see."

"Stay out of the road," Natalie called after them.

The street was free of traffic, but William stayed on the pavement that the clustered houses had for doorsteps. Some of it was marble and some was red clay, not to mention patches of lumpy pimpled concrete. "Hold your sister's hand, William," Julian called.

Had the boy discovered rebelliousness? All he did was look askance at Jonquil. "Go on, William," Ray shouted. "Grandma's holding mine."

Her hand felt colder than he liked. He might even have found it less substantial than he wanted it to be. He squeezed it harder than he meant to and managed to relax his grip as William poked out a hand for Jonquil to take. By now Ray could see that the elevated figure was enthroned at the peak of the heap of wood. At least, he realised as the family reached the square, the effigy was tied by its arms and legs to the rickety wooden seat, which didn't look much like a throne. The head inside the cowl was a featureless white bag, and Ray would have preferred not to be reminded of the spider's cocoon in the roadside shrine. "Well, he doesn't look too saintly," Pris said and turned to a man who had picked up a stray branch to fling on the pile. "Kali nichta. Can you tell us about this?"

The man shrugged and held out his hands once they were empty of the branch. When Pris pointed to the effigy he said a word or two before ambling towards a corner of the square occupied by a makeshift stage. "So, Priscilla?" Julian said.

"The old man, I think. The old one."

"Not just old, Pris," Doug said. "The oldest. The ancient."

"Is that supposed to tell us something?"

Presumably Julian was finding fault with their informant rather than the translators, but Ray thought Doug was going to respond in kind until William said "Look, there's, you know. Look, she's there."

"Don't start seeing things again, William," Natalie said. "Just try and forget your dreams and then you won't have any more."

"Not my dream. That was a man. I'm saying the lady that was waiting for us."

He wasn't quite pointing, no doubt because he'd been told it was rude, at a taverna on the corner of the square opposite the stage. For a moment Ray thought he meant the dumpy woman who was leaving trinkets on the tables, having shown the diners a laminated card that signified she was dumb, and then he noticed a young woman in a dress printed with dark green vines – Sam from the travel firm. "She can let us know what's happening," he said.

She was alone at a small table with a glass of Mythos beer. As Ray went over she raised the glass to her lips and saw him. She took an appreciable swig before setting down the drink. "Mr Thornton, isn't it," she said. "Are you all having a good time? I'm just waiting for my friend."

Ray could have thought she was making sure none of them joined her, but Doug sat at the next table. "Drinks on Pris and me. Will you have one, Sam?"

"Thanks anyway. As I say, I won't be here long."

"I'll just sit with Sam for a minute," Ray said and did so in order to lower his voice. "I don't know if you'll have heard, but we found the gentleman your colleague said was missing."

"We both did," Julian said, squatting down between them.

"I hope it won't spoil your holiday too much."

"His was spoiled considerably more," Julian said. "What was his name, by the way? We weren't even told."

"Oh, his name." As Julian opened his impatient lips Sam said "Mr Ditton."

"And just remind us when he was discovered to be missing."

"Weeks ago," Sam said and took another gulp of beer. "Last month."

"We thought Jamie told us it was last week," Ray murmured.

"That's Jamie for you. Half the time he doesn't know what day it is. He's a lot of fun, but you wouldn't go to him for facts."

Perhaps Julian found the denigration unprofessional. He stared at her as a preamble to saying "Where was it he said Mr Ditton was staying?"

"I don't know what he said." As Julian's stare lost any patience it had contained, while Ray reflected that Jamie hadn't offered the information, Sam downed another mouthful. After that it seemed she couldn't delay saying "The Paradise Apartments."

"Thank you," Julian said but saved most of his effort for standing up.

"Have you finished your conference?" Doug called. "Sam, can you tell us what's going on?"

Sam lifted her glass and held it close to her mouth. As Ray found a seat at the family table she said "I don't know what you mean."

"Why's he on top of the pile over there? We didn't know St Titus was a monk."

"That isn't him."

The vendor of trinkets had left some of her wares in front of William, who was plainly taken with a cross that lit up colour after colour. "Would you like that, William?" Sandra said.

"We'll buy it for you," Ray told him as Pris asked Sam "Who is he, then?"

Sam seemed to wish she had more of a drink to linger over. "Someone he was supposed to stop," she said.

"There you go, Will. That's who St Titus had to fight."

William shook his head at the figure tied to the chair. "He isn't spiders."

"Don't be childish, William," Julian said.

As Ray laid his hand on the cross to identify the purchase to the vendor Sam said "He didn't fight him."

The vendor made a praying gesture, apparently in gratitude for the amount Ray handed her. "So what did St Titus do?" Pris said.

"People prayed to him. That's what they do here. That's what I meant. They did when the island was invaded in the war as well."

"Thank you, grandad. Thank you, grandma."

"Our pleasure, William," Sandra said as Doug waited to speak. "You still haven't said who that's meant to be," he reminded Sam, "and is that going to be a bonfire?"

"Yes."

Before Doug could prompt Sam yet again Natalie said "Don't

say any more if you think it'll be too much for little ears to hear."

Sam looked grateful. "It might be."

"Then just say as much as you think you can," Doug said.

Sam glanced around the square, but Ray gathered that she couldn't see her friend. She fixed her eyes on William and eventually said "He was the opposite of a saint, William. That's why the people prayed about him."

"Who was he?"

"We don't need to go saying his name, do we? He lived a long time ago. He was born centuries before your grandma and grandad."

"He must have died a long time ago too."

"I wish you'd stop thinking so much about death," Natalie said. "It isn't healthy for a little boy of your age."

For some reason Ray felt Sam welcomed the interruption, but William wouldn't be hushed. "What did he do?" he said with a hint of defiance, laying down his luminous cross.

"People took him in because he said he wanted to live like them, but then he lived off them instead."

As William looked unhappy with her vagueness Pris said "Can we guess they were monks?"

"That's what they were. They have to give shelter to anyone who asks. All the monks in Greece, I mean."

"When you say he lived off them you mean he exploited them."

"Drained them dry," Sam immediately seemed to regret saying. "I don't mean literally, William."

"I still can't see," Pris said, "why people thought they had to pray about him."

"Because of what he brought."

"You'll have to tell us now," Doug said. "Does Will need to cover his ears?"

"They said – " She didn't seem to want the rest to be heard. Perhaps she was mumbling for William's sake, and as soon as she'd finished she jumped up. "There he is," she said. "Enjoy the show. Have a good dance."

Ray saw her wave to Jamie, who was hurrying across the square. He could have thought her gesture ended by waving her colleague away – halting him, at any rate. "I wouldn't mind a word with him," Julian said.

"If it's about what I think it is," Natalie said, tilting her head to indicate William, "don't have it here."

As Julian rose from his seat Sam grabbed Jamie's elbow to steer him away. Perhaps she was anxious to catch some event, and they vanished beyond the dormant bonfire. "Well," Julian said, "she could hardly have been less helpful. You'd think living here had robbed her of her grasp of English."

"I think that was Nat," Doug told him, "making her watch what she said."

"A bit more than careful," Pris protested. "Did anybody catch what she was supposed to be telling Doug?"

"I thought she said the angry dog," Natalie said. "That's all, William, just a dog from a long long time ago."

The boy giggled. "She didn't say that, mummy."

"What do you think it was, William?" Sandra said.

"The hungry dark."

His words seemed to darken the square, which Ray thought had suddenly grown crowded. Perhaps the phrase simply made him aware how dark the place was, now that the red glow had sunk beyond the roofs like the last of a transfusion. "Why would she say a silly thing like that?" Natalie said with rather too deliberate a laugh.

"That's what that man brought the monks," William said and peered at the hooded figure, at its cocoon of a face. "The hungry dark."

"All right, you've said it now. No need to keep on. It doesn't make any sense, William, and besides it doesn't matter."

As the boy's face made his disagreement clear Julian said "I hope you've got what you wanted, Douglas."

Ray didn't know how his son might have responded if a waiter hadn't arrived with a trayful of drinks. The man frowned at the table Sam had vacated. "Your friend?"

"I expect she thought we were buying," Doug said. "Here's for hers as well."

"Look, William, they're starting," Jonquil said.

Musicians with stringed instruments had taken their places on the stage, and now a woman in an ankle-length white dress moved in front of them. As four men with flaming torches converged on the bonfire from the corners of the square, she began to sing, accompanied by a slow march of plucked strings and the wailing of a violin. "I like the howly music," William said.

"You mean holy, William," said his mother.

Ray wasn't sure whether she was wrong. He watched the men thrust the torches so deep into the foundations of the bonfire that they might have been ensuring any denizens were driven out or else trapped until they were consumed. As flames sprouted from the bonfire the march grew more solemn, but Ray couldn't tell if the singer was lamenting or celebrating; he could have fancied that nobody was meant to know. Sandra looked at William while she said "Are we going to want to know what she's singing?"

"Something about finding light in the dark," Pris said.

"And about the dark where there isn't any light," Doug added.

"I think that's probably enough," Julian told them. "William, look over there."

At the far end of a street off the square a figure at least as tall as the bonfire was rising into view. No, Ray thought: not rising to its feet but filling with light. It was an image of St Titus with his lance in the stained-glass window of a church. The saint's face remained in shadow, and the rest of him began to lose illumination as a procession bearing lit candles started to emerge from the church. The procession advanced at the pace of the musicians' march two abreast up the street to the square, and paraded around the bonfire while the flames snatched at the robed effigy. Ray could almost have imagined that the bound figure was struggling to writhe out of reach of the fire, but the chair was simply tilting as a section of the bonfire collapsed under one leg. All at once the figure burst into flame accompanied by oily smoke, and the bearers of the candles threw them high on the bonfire. The music speeded up and ceased to march, and as the singer grew more joyful the members of the procession linked hands to dance around the pyre. Once the circle parted, people in the crowd joined in the celebration. "I'm going to dance," Jonquil said. "Are you coming, Tim?"

Ray saw how standing up reminded Tim of his height, but he followed her not too awkwardly. "Stay in the square," Natalie called after them.

While they set about performing a version of the dance – arms stretched wide as if bound to a cross or just released from one, high stiff kicks – Pris glanced at Doug. "The light will come back?"

"That's what it sounds like to me."

"You mean that's what she's singing now." When they confirmed this Natalie said "Remember that, William. It always does."

Ray was watching Tim and Jonquil, whose dance had turned more English or at any rate American, when Sandra murmured "Aren't you going to ask me to dance?"

He wasn't much more skilled in this regard than at swimming, but he couldn't refuse her now. "Please may I have this dance?" he said.

He took her hand to help her up and led her into the square. The heat of the pyre met them as the blazing chair lurched further sideways and the smouldering cowl fell back to expose the misshapen faceless head. If blackened features seemed to writhe on it, they were only smoke. Around the pyre faces fluttered with the agitated light, which brought its own rhythms to the dance. "Never mind anybody else," Sandra whispered. "Just be with me."

When Ray made to let go of her hand she held on. She mustn't want to join in the celebratory dance, which would separate them. He slipped his other hand around her waist and tried not to be too aware of the bones of her spine. He'd begun to turn slowly in what he assumed to be some species of waltz, and was busy ensuring he didn't tread on her bare toes, when she murmured "Don't try so hard. Let me."

This meant holding his hand so lightly it came near to stealing his awareness that she was. In a moment she began to turn them both in the opposite direction from the one he'd led. At first it felt so odd that he was afraid of stumbling, and then her confidence infected him. She felt not just lithe but more youthful than he could recall her ever feeling when they'd danced together. If their dance seemed wholly unrelated to the music, why should that matter? Her face flickered like a recollection, and he was close to seeing their dance as a memory he would keep for the rest of his life, but he mustn't distance it that way when she only wanted him to be with her. He clasped her waist, not too hard, and gazed so deep into her eyes that he could hope he was reviving all the life they'd spent together. He thought he was seeing it in hers, distilled into a wordless look. He'd started to forget not just the dancers all around them but his own clumsiness – it seemed to have left him, though he didn't think he would be able to move as fluidly as Sandra was dancing – when he heard Julian. "It's you again, is it? What do you mean by following our daughter?"

Ray peered over Sandra's shoulder. The flames of the bonfire plucked at his vision, so that by the time he located Julian and Jonquil he had little more than a glimpse of whoever was being addressed – a thin retreating figure with a long face that the light appeared to render less distinct than everyone's around him. "That's right, stay away," Julian shouted, "and that applies to your friends as well."

The offender had been joined by two companions not unlike him, Ray saw. "Who is that?" he blurted.

He wasn't expecting Sandra to respond, but a nearby dancer did. "They come tonight too," he said and added a Greek word.

As Sandra turned to look the figures withdrew into the dimness beyond the firelight. In moments they were indistinguishable from the dark along a street leading to the beach. "What's wrong?" Sandra said. "I didn't see."

"We'd better find out," Ray said, though as he released her waist he felt as if he might be letting go of moments they would never regain.

With his fingers gripping his hips Julian looked like the antithesis of a dancer or else a Greek sculpture rendered russet by the flames. "How long were you dancing with that boy?" he demanded.

"I don't know." Perhaps just his tone made Jonquil frown, not her lack of knowledge. "He only came for a dance," she said.

"You know perfectly well that he wasn't approved. You gave us to understand you would be dancing with your cousin."

"I don't think Jonk said that," Tim objected as he joined them. "She never told me."

"Shall we all sit down?" Sandra said. "No need to have a scene out here."

Ray saw she hoped this would end the argument, but as they trooped back to the taverna Julian said "What did that boy say to you?"

"Nothing. We didn't need to talk."

"You must have given him some kind of sign."

"I didn't. He was just there when I looked." When Julian

made his dissatisfaction plain Jonquil said "Tell him yours was there as well, Tim."

"What's your secret, Tim?" Pris said with the start of a laugh.

"Just I was dancing with that girl you saw at Sunset Beach."

"We said you'd found yourself an admirer," Doug said. "You don't look too delighted, Jules."

"I'm not if the children are being stalked, and I'm surprised if you are. Weren't those people at the church today as well?"

"So were we," Sandra pointed out.

"That's by no means the same thing. They were told to leave even though they're local."

"Somebody said something about them just now," Ray remembered. "What was it, Sandra?"

"Vella, was it? Something along those lines."

"That'd be a parasite," Doug said.

"More like a leech," Pris told him.

"Well, I hope you'll both take notice of the people who should know." At first it wasn't clear that Julian was addressing Tim and Jonquil. "Even their own countrymen don't like your dancing partners," he said. "They're the kind who live off other people who can't see what they are."

"They haven't got much out of these two," Pris said.

"Shall we make sure as a family that they don't? If either of you should see them again, please let an adult know."

"And I will."

"That's very helpful of you, William," Julian said, though Natalie seemed not quite so taken with the proposition. "I think the subject can be closed now. Please don't let it put anybody off the dance."

Ray didn't think he was inviting anyone to join it, and nobody did. If Sandra had suggested returning to the dance Ray would have been on his feet at once, but he didn't want to risk detracting from the memory they already had. Suppose his clumsiness returned? Even the notion threatened to bring it back. Instead he watched the celebration, only to be distracted by thoughts about the day's events. Leeches, transfusions – did those fit together somehow? Perhaps the three were beggars who made some money by giving their blood, and the man at the church disapproved of the practice. Was Ray seeing figures beyond the reach of the firelight, on the road to the beach? The flames made the thin shapes seem to shift like mist, but whenever he strained to distinguish the trio he saw nothing in that street except the dark.

The pyre took a while to collapse into ash. While it did, the music trailed away and the dancers began to disperse. "I think someone's overdue for bed," Natalie announced, and William lifted his sleepy head. "I'm not," he protested despite the effort the words took.

He stumbled as they left the taverna, and Julian lifted him onto his shoulders. As Sandra passed some of the people who'd danced, one of them spoke to her in Greek. "What was that?" Ray asked Doug and Pris.

"Grow old in peace," Doug translated.

"Or maybe grow old and peaceful," Pris said.

"I don't see the difference."

Neither did Ray, and he had an odd sense of preferring not to. He was ushering Sandra towards the main road when he heard Pris murmur "You know, I don't think we got it quite right. I think she said grow old but peaceful."

He couldn't tell whether the ensuing silence signified agreement or unwillingness to talk. He didn't know if Sandra had heard, and he thought it best not to ask or to ponder the translation. He was glad to see the bus approaching as they came to the end of the road.

The last of the light from Sunset Beach glided through the vehicle, lengthening the shadows within, and then there were only the headlamp beams poking at the dark. Soon enough they found the entrance to the Sunny View. The bus stopped around the bend, outside the Paradise Apartments. As the rear lights disappeared over the bridge and the low note of the wheels gave way to the whisper of ripples, Julian said "I'll be along shortly. I want a word with someone."

"I'll come with you," Ray said at once.

He did his best to overtake Julian in the entrance courtyard of the Paradise Apartments, but Julian didn't stand aside to let him into the boxy concrete office, where a small stocky woman stood behind a counter. A patchwork of family photographs and a latticework of pigeonholes covered the wall at her back. She raised a wide smile, which didn't falter as Julian strode at her. "Yes, mister," she said.

"This is where the late Mr Ditton was staying, we believe. We're the people who found him."

"Yes, mister. Poor Mr Ditton," she said and let half her smile sag.

"Oh, quite. A dismal business." After an instant's rather than a minute's silence Julian said "We were wondering how long it has been since you saw him."

The woman let down the rest of her smile. "Not long."

Ray sensed Julian's impatience with her attempt to communicate. "Could you say about how long?" Ray said. "Weeks? A month?"

"Last week, mister."

"I knew I couldn't have been mistaken," Julian declared. "Someone owes us an explanation."

He turned towards the door as if he meant to find an informant at once, and then he faced the woman. "For the record," he said, "how old was Mr Ditton?"

The woman rested a hand at the edge of the pigeonholes. "As old as him."

"Not too old, then," Ray said.

Did she think he was boasting? He was simply disconcerted by how much older the corpse had looked. "Not old, mister," she said.

"Well, that's very kind of you."

She responded with a puzzled smile and then a broader one. "Not you, mister," she said and moved her hand. "Him."

For a moment Ray took her to be saying Ditton had been Julian's age, and then he saw the truth was worse. She wasn't merely resting her hand on the wall. She had been indicating one of the photographs, and now that she'd laid her fingertips on it there could be no mistake. The boy in the photograph was just a few years older than Jonquil and Tim.

THE SEVENTH DAY
26 AUGUST

"Will you be much longer up there?" Julian called. "Everyone is ready here."

Sandra finished a last bite of yesterday's bread and picked up her mug. "Shall we go and see what it's all about? We can take our coffee with us."

"So long as you aren't feeling rushed."

"You could have wakened me sooner. I'm not here to sleep all day."

"I wouldn't have let you," Ray said, though he hadn't liked to rouse her while she'd seemed so peaceful, even if he'd had to reassure himself more than once that she was breathing. "Let's find out why he's calling a conference."

Coffee slopped over the rim of his mug as he followed her down the marble steps with one hand on the rail. He was ashamed of making more work for the staff, and could have fancied that the faces on the play equipment were grinning at his clumsiness. Beyond the apartments across the deserted play area he heard splashes from the swimming pool. Sandra tapped on the door of the Banks apartment with the back of her wedding ring. "It's only us," she called.

"That's who it is," Ray said and couldn't help adding a knock.

"No need to say so." Obviously Julian had no time for the local custom. "Please come through," he said.

Ray was disconcerted by how tidy the rooms were, not least the one Jonquil shared with William. If it hadn't been for the laundered bear on the boy's pillow Ray might have wondered if it was their room. There wasn't a hint of the cheerful chaos he recalled from when Natalie and Doug had been either of their ages, not to mention the years between. Jonquil's room had been happily disarrayed while her father was married to Natalie, but then that had been true of their lives until those grew unhappily disorganised. It was pointless to recall how much he'd liked Jonquil's father except for the man's chronic aversion to criticism. "I apologise if we've taken you away from your breakfast," Julian said. "I just want to get this settled while we won't be overheard."

Doug and Pris were with Natalie on the balcony, where they'd brought extra chairs from next door. "Where are the young ones?" Sandra seemed anxious to learn.

"If they aren't in the play area they'll be at the pool," Natalie said. "I expect that'll help to wake them up."

"Tim was a sleepyhead as well," Pris said.

"I'm afraid our two were a bit more than that. I hope nobody else was disturbed."

"William had to be told nobody had got into his room," Julian complained. "I'd like to ask you all not to give him ideas he doesn't need."

"Maybe you should ask yourself," Natalie said.

"Remind me why I should be singled out."

"You made enough of a fuss about that boy at the dance, didn't you? I don't want him near my daughter either, but you shouldn't be surprised if William dreamed about him."

"All the more reason to make sure he doesn't hear what we have to discuss. Raymond, I've spoken to Evadne about Mr Ditton."

"What about him?" Sandra said, peering through her sunglasses from the shade of her hat. "What did you find out last night?"

Ray hadn't told her then, since he'd found her already asleep. "You'll agree with me, Raymond," Julian said. "Whatever killed him, it was a good deal worse than drowning."

"It turns out he was a lot younger than he looked when we found him," Ray admitted.

"Considerably too young to have had the seizure the police want us to believe he had. And he didn't just look a lot older than, you'll forgive me, either of you. How else would you say he looked, Raymond?"

"I don't know." Since this was plainly insufficient, Ray said "Diseased?"

"Exactly the word I would have used," Julian said by no means unlike a teacher encouraging a pupil. "We questioned the manager of his accommodation last night, Sandra, and Raymond will tell you how evasive she was. I'm afraid Evadne was just as unhelpful, but she's not the first person to learn they can't hide the truth from me."

As Ray sensed how Sandra was refraining from looking at him Pris said "What do you think she was trying to hide?"

"I asked her if there have been any other cases on the island. I put her on her honour and she said she was sure there haven't, but I'm very much of the opinion that she wasn't being honest with me."

Doug visibly struggled but failed to keep quiet. "You put her on her honour."

"I most certainly did, yes. Do you have some objection? Don't tell me I've offended against the local ways again."

"I think you might have done something like that, Jules."

"Perhaps you should be offended by their ways instead. Especially if it involves hiding some kind of epidemic from potential victims."

"Now where has that come from, Julian?" Pris said. "All we really know – "

"Kindly trust my judgement on this. I promise you Evadne was keeping quiet about the truth. I want us to consider our options, but as far as I'm concerned – "

For a moment Ray thought a pout had silenced Julian, but he was pressing his lips together as a preamble to saying "Not now, William. You were asked not to come till you were called, the three of you."

Ray turned to see William running past the balconies ahead of Tim and Jonquil. "And you really didn't need to go out looking like that, Jonquil," Natalie said.

Such of the girl's hair that wasn't tucked under her hat did look uncombed. "You wanted us out of the way," she said, blinking through her sunglasses.

"I expect I'm looking just as windblown," Sandra said.

The interruptions hadn't improved Julian's temper. "If you knew you weren't wanted, why did you come back?"

"Jonquil took some pictures to show you."

"We can see them later, William." When the boy grimaced with frustration Natalie said "What are they of?"

"The stones I said I saw and daddy didn't think I did. The names on them."

Julian lost any expression as he stared at the teenagers and William. "You've been to the graveyard."

Ray thought the boy meant to defend Jonquil by insisting "I wanted you to see."

"May I do so, then."

It wasn't a request or even a question, and Ray wasn't sure why it made his innards tighten. Julian held out an upturned hand until Jonquil produced her mobile and brought up her photograph album. As soon as she passed it over the balcony wall Julian moved out of her reach, and she leaned across the wall to see what he was doing. "That's the wrong one," she said as he tapped a command. "That's delete."

"Which is precisely what I intend to do."

"Don't," Jonquil cried. "You'll lose all my photos."

"I hope that will remind you that when you're told to do

something I mean what I say. You knew perfectly well that we don't want William anywhere near that place, and your instructions were to stay in the play area or the pool."

"I made her go," William protested. "And Tim."

"They were in charge of you, not the other way around. If they let you have the opposite impression that's another mark against them."

As Julian held up the phone for Jonquil to watch, Ray saw her face crumple and felt as though his innards had. She lurched across the wall to grab the phone, but Julian stepped back. "Stop it, Julian," Ray said.

"Kindly don't interfere. I'm dealing with the matter."

Ray hadn't known he meant to speak, and he was just as unprepared to spring to his feet and seize Julian's wrist, pulling the hand away from Jonquil's phone before he could confirm the deletion. "You mustn't do that," he said low.

"Please let go of me at once." Julian's lips had drawn inwards, restricting his voice. "This is wholly inappropriate," he said.

"Don't you realise Jonquil has pictures of Sandra on there? You'd be deleting them."

"The girl can take more if she behaves herself," Julian said and strained a finger towards the phone. "Now may we have an end to this ridiculous scene. Everyone is watching."

"Can't you see taking more won't be the same, you damned bloody idiot? Sorry," Ray added at once but didn't release Julian's wrist. "You have to understand every one of them is precious."

"I've no idea how valuable they may be to the girl, but I'm sure she has a long time yet to photograph her grandmother. Now for the last time – "

"You mustn't say that, Julian," Sandra said.

"I'm sure we've no reason to suppose you won't be with us for a good while yet, Sandra. Now will you please ask your husband – "

"I'm asking you not to say that."

"Why not?" The prohibition appeared to infuriate Julian as much as Ray's grip on his wrist. "Is it another of these wretched superstitions we seem to be surrounded by?"

"No." Ray thought Sandra might manage to leave it at that, since the solitary word felt like a burden that was constricting his heart, until she said "It's the truth."

"What is? All I said – "

"For God's sake, Julian." Natalie snatched the phone out of his hand and gave it back to Jonquil. "Promise you won't do anything else wrong," she said and without giving Jonquil time to speak "You two take William to play and don't go out of the accommodation. I'll come and find you when we're ready."

Ray saw that not only the teenagers understood how grave the situation might be. "We can go on the swings if you like," William said.

Nobody spoke until he'd led Tim and Jonquil out of sight, and then nobody appeared to want to be the first to speak. Ray had begun to hope the silence might quieten everybody's speculations when Doug said "You shouldn't think the worst either, mum."

"I can't say I wasn't."

"Then you're as bad as you were telling Jules he was. I don't mean bad," Doug said as Julian remained sullen. "You both know what I mean."

"And now you can stop thinking it, mum," Natalie said, "since you can't know."

Sandra took a breath as loud as words. Ray thought she was using it to keep some of those unspoken, but she said "Natalie, it's the truth."

Ray saw Julian make the effort to join in, and wished he'd found a different occasion. "What is, Sandra?"

Perhaps it was his tone – the way a patient adult might have spoken to an unreasonable youngster – that made Sandra press her lips together, only to say "I'm not expected to see Christmas."

Somebody gasped, but Ray didn't think it was him, although one of his feelings was a species of relief – a release from the dogged performance he had been maintaining for so long that it hardly felt like a choice, from having to keep so much not just unsaid but unsuspected. Everyone had frozen into a silent tableau with Sandra as its focus, where she seemed determined to fend off any sense that she was vulnerable or inviting sympathy – if anything, she looked angry with herself for having been provoked to speak. He didn't know how long the silence paralysed them all before Natalie demanded "Who says you aren't?" fiercely enough for a confrontation with the perpetrator.

"The hospital." Sandra sounded close to apologetic. "The specialists," she said.

Doug made to speak and had to clear his throat. "What kind?"

"The favourite," Sandra said with a wry smile too brief to convey much. "When my grandmother had it I used to call it canker. That's what I thought it was called, because my parents always spelled it out if I could hear. It can still do for a name."

"What treatment are you having, Sandra?" Pris seemed to find it hard to ask.

"I'm not." To a chorus of murmurs Sandra said "I saw what it does to people who are as far gone as I am. It may give them a few extra months, it might even add on a year, but I don't think the way they are is living. I'd rather not spend whatever time I have left in that state."

"But – " Ray thought Natalie hadn't set out to say "But how do you feel?"

"Since we've come here, better than I have for quite a long time, so thank you all for making it that way."

"We're glad if you're happy," Doug said, "but I think Nat was asking – "

"Not just happy. More like revived." Sandra pondered and said

"As if I've had some kind of transfusion. I actually feel younger than I did."

"I expect that's the sun," Pris said.

Ray saw she was trying to share Sandra's optimism, but the bid seemed to fall short of its goal. With a frown at the clouds Sandra said "Maybe it's the air."

"So long as whatever it is does you good," Natalie said not quite steadily, and gazed out to sea.

"You all are, and I don't want any of you feeling too sad for me." When this brought about another silence Sandra said "Including like that. Let's carry on with what we've planned, and don't go thinking you need to make any allowances. Just let's make sure the young ones don't find out about me. The last thing I want to do is spoil this holiday for them."

As Ray realised that he would have to keep the pretence up after all, Julian said "May we ask when you both knew about the situation?"

"After Doug booked us all in here," Ray said. "We thought of letting everyone know at the time, but I hope you understand why we didn't."

"Was it also after I arranged everyone's insurance?"

"I'm afraid it wasn't," Sandra said. "We couldn't very well let you know and expect you to keep it from everyone else."

"It needed to be taken into account, all the same."

"It'll only affect my insurance, won't it?"

"Not with the family package I bought, no."

"Then I'm sorry, everyone. I ought to have asked how it worked."

She looked sadder than she had over letting her secret be known. "There's no reason to suppose we'll need to claim, is there?" Ray said despite feeling that the discussion had turned insultingly banal. "We'll make sure there's no need."

"You look as if you think there might be," Sandra told Julian.

"Whatever I was thinking can't be allowed to matter now."

"It was why you wanted us all here, wasn't it? We haven't finished talking about that. Were you going to suggest we should go home?"

"Some of us won't be," Doug said at once.

"I'm simply concerned for others," Julian said. "In particular William and now you, Sandra."

"This disease you think is around here, you mean."

"You mightn't dismiss it if you'd seen the effects, Sandra."

"I saw as well," Ray reminded him.

"Then surely you don't want to contradict me."

"I went a lot closer than you did, but I don't seem to be infected, do I? And I don't believe we've seen anyone else in anything approaching that state."

"Perhaps we don't know what to look for. Or perhaps other victims are being hidden away. I've told you the people round here are hiding the truth."

"Can you blame them? We found one body and you're talking about an epidemic. If you were them, wouldn't you do everything you could to avoid that kind of panic? It could ruin their livelihood if people like us stayed away."

"I'd be sad if you took William home," Sandra said, "but I'd understand."

"I'll be staying with my mother," Natalie told Julian.

"That's two of us," said Doug.

"Count me in as well," Pris said.

"I gather I'm voted down."

"Jules, it's not a vote. You do what you feel you have to, because we are."

"Julian?" Before he could reply Sandra said "Will you be satisfied if we all watch out for any signs? Of this disease you think is about, I mean? And we'll all take special care of William."

"That's very thoughtful of you in the circumstances." Just the same, Julian made his pause count before he said "I'll trust you all to do as she suggests."

Sandra reached to squeeze his arm, a gesture that appeared to startle him. As he withdrew to a distance he seemed to find safer Natalie hugged her mother, and then Doug and Pris did. Sandra patted their hands as she said "Do you know what I'd like to do now?"

"Whatever you like," Doug said somewhat indistinctly.

"Go for a ride on the road train with William and everyone," Sandra said, and Ray welcomed the proposal with all the enthusiasm he could find in him. He would have felt more eager if he hadn't had to start pretending once again that all was well. He could only hope that the four who shared the secret now would give as convincing a performance.

THE EIGHTH DAY
27 AUGUST

"I'm sorry we had to send you three away like that. It was just your granny being silly, William. I won't do it again."

"How were you being silly, gran?"

"It was like your daddy said, just a superstition. We can't make things happen by thinking them. Not things we don't want to happen or things we want either."

They had all been on the road train when Sandra told him so, on their stately way through a village in the hills. Ray had felt as though by proposing the ride on the train, which resembled an escapee from a fairground, she'd been trying to recapture childhood by sharing William's – trying to consolidate the youthfulness she claimed to have found on the island. "We can't make things happen by thinking them…" Ray hadn't dared to yield to his emotions while she was speaking to William, but now he did as he lay beside her in the dark.

It felt like dissolving into grief. He was quivering so much with silent sobs that he had to ease his arm away from her waist for fear of waking her. For an immeasurable time he couldn't think for weeping, as if the flood had purified him of thoughts. It wasn't just that her words to William had overwhelmed him; letting the family into the truth had broken down the dam of his emotions, though it had still needed to hold until he was alone or at least unobserved. He had to quell his shaking, because he was afraid of transmitting it to the bed. When he managed to relax his body it renewed the storm of tears, until his pillow grew so sodden that he thought he felt it squelch beneath his cheek.

The sensation brought him back to himself – to the knowledge that his grief changed nothing. It was just a rehearsal for worse, and he was dismayed by how much it felt like wishing for the end. He could almost hear his own pathetic voice practicing the words that he would have to say to everyone – worst of all, to William. His body dragged him back from indulging in the future; his head pounded in the rhythm of his violent heartbeat, his eyes stung like wounds, his nose was clogged with catarrh. He was clumsily solid again, not lifted up by grief at all, and how much worse did he imagine Sandra felt when she pushed away a practically untouched meal or squeezed her eyes tight shut and dug her fingernails into the arms of her chair?

At least he hadn't seen her do any of those things since they'd come to Vasilema. He crept to the bathroom to blow his nose as surreptitiously as he could, and had an unexpected impulse to switch on a light, even though that might waken Sandra. There was nothing he needed to see in the room; the whisper of movement he'd seemed to hear as he left the bed had most likely been a wave on the beach, unless Sandra had stirred without waking. She was quiet now, and once he'd reassured himself that she was breathing he kept his arm around her while he tried to join her in sleep.

He thought he'd failed until a knock at the door roused him. As he floundered out of bed he heard another muted knock. He had a confused sense of obeying the tradition that prohibited answering first time. He fumbled the door open just enough to peer around it and saw the sun between Doug and Julian. "No panic, dad," Doug said. "There's been a change of plan."

Ray kept his voice low to indicate they should as well. "What's changed?"

"We've decided against bicycles," Julian said with a frown instead of a murmur. "We're hiring transport for the day."

Ray heard Sandra struggling awake to call "Don't change it on my behalf."

"We were thinking of William," Julian said. "His mother and I don't think he can be expected to travel like that as far as some of us are proposing."

"It's gone down well with the teens," Doug said. "It's the popular vote."

"We're going to pick up the vehicles now. If you two can be ready when we come back, that would be ideal."

"Well, that's us organised," Sandra said once Ray had shut the door, and then she grew serious. "I shouldn't have let it out, Ray."

He couldn't have said why her words seemed ominous. "What?"

"What else is there? The truth. I shouldn't have let Julian provoke me."

"I think it's right for Doug and Natalie to know."

She seemed unsure whether to believe this, and Ray was less than certain that he did. "I didn't just tell them," she said.

"Then they've got support if they need it, haven't they?" When he saw this fall short of reassuring her Ray said in some desperation "I hope I don't sound selfish, but I'm glad I'm not alone with it any more."

"I didn't realise you felt that way. How couldn't I have? I shouldn't be concerned just with myself."

Ray sat by her on the bed as she took hold of his pillow to prop behind her shoulders against the wall. "What's happened to this?" she protested. "It's damp."

"Just your disgusting husband. Sweat if it isn't drool."

"You'll never disgust me." She rested a hand on the pillow and gazed at him. "Oh, Ray," she said. "I can see from your eyes what it was."

"Never mind me, except how in Christ's name could I think I wasn't selfish? It's you that mustn't be alone with it, and you mustn't feel you are."

Sandra found his hands with hers and leaned against him. "I don't like to think you will be," she said. "Alone."

"I'll have the children, won't I? And nobody knows what happens after. Maybe it won't keep us apart very long."

Might this sound as if he was proposing to follow her by doing away with himself? He was only trying to conjure up their notion of an afterlife. It was less a belief than a hope too vague to bear examination, but it seemed to revive Sandra. "Nothing must," she declared forcefully enough to be addressing someone else besides him.

She clung to him until he felt she was trying to keep hold of the moment for ever, and then she let go of his hands. "We'd better get moving before we're told off," she said.

By the time he finished in the bathroom she'd made coffee and set out breakfast on the balcony. He'd drunk half his mugful and was counting empty loungers beneath the cloudy sky at Sunset Beach — even at that distance he thought most of them were unoccupied — when Sandra emerged. "Do I look all right?" she said. "I don't think I can tell."

"You look fine to me," Ray said despite suspecting that under the hat her hair might be somewhat dishevelled, given the visible strands. "You will to everyone."

"That's a promise, Sandra," Pris called from her balcony.

"We'll all second that," Natalie contributed.

Ray was afraid it would be obvious that their determination had no bearing on how Sandra actually looked. In a bid to distract her he called "So where are we bound today?"

"Wherever you two would like to go," Natalie said.

"I just like being driven," Sandra said. "That's always part of the holiday for me."

"We'll leave it to the researchers," Ray said. "Show us things we haven't seen."

"I've got one," Pris said.

Ray had an uneasy sense of having been too careless. "Which is that, Pris?"

"My monastery at last. We'll have cars that can go off the road."

Ray couldn't help thinking of the effigy tied to the chair on the bonfire, the blank whitish bag of a face lolling out of the monkish cowl. For an instant he was tempted to use William as an excuse to avoid the monastery – to suggest that it might somehow be unsuitable for his grandson – but what reason could he have to spoil the day? "I've been looking forward to it," Sandra called, and he put his qualms out of his head.

★   ★   ★

"I can't see where we are," Jonquil said.

Ray might have fancied that the sun was in her eyes if it hadn't been masked by the midday clouds. In any case she was still wearing her sunglasses, just like Tim and Sandra. Julian halted the leading vehicle and held out a hand without looking back at her. "Let me see."

Jonquil turned her phone towards him but held it out of reach. "I'm showing you."

Natalie twisted around to peer at the miniature screen. "There's no road on it, Julian."

Ray thought the rough track through the forest might not be called a road. Countless pines as silent as the clouds shut it in, and apart from the Thornton party it had been deserted since they'd left the main road. Tim leaned across William to examine the screen. "It's just a blur," he said.

"Some of my photos are blurred as well," Jonquil said.

"I trust I won't be blamed in any way for that," Julian said, having taken his hand back.

"I'm just saying something's wrong with my phone."

"It's your responsibility to take care of it."

"Julian," Natalie said as if she didn't want someone in the other car to hear her. "Jonquil."

Doug had halted it behind Julian's, and now he took out his own mobile. "It isn't just yours, Jonquil," he called. "Mine's lost the way as well."

Ray craned forward to see that the map on Doug's phone had turned an unrelieved green, a good deal paler than the trees. When Doug pinched the image between finger and thumb it stayed the same, and the opposite gesture left it just as vague. "There can't be much coverage," Doug said. "It isn't even showing the road we came from."

Over the chugging of engines Sandra said "We were going the right way, weren't we?"

"If you'd like to go on, Sandra," Julian said, "then of course we will. And I hope you can pardon the squabble."

Ray thought he was apologising more for Jonquil than, if at all, for himself. Julian eased his car forward, and Doug followed around the next bend. Ray was starting to find the sight of pines in every direction monotonous – his troubled sleep had begun to catch up with him – when he noticed that the faint piny scent that filled the air had changed. It was giving way to another smell, a dry odour that put him in mind of dust, though not the dust the roofless vehicles were raising from the track. He was trying to identify the dead smell when William pushed himself almost to his feet. "What's all that black?"

"Sit down, William," Julian said at once. "Will you two kindly make sure he stays seated and keeps his safety belt on."

As the teenagers reached for the boy Ray could have thought William shrank away from them, but surely that was just a moment of defiance. Once William resumed his seat Julian said "I'm afraid it looks as though there are vandals even here."

Both cars had rounded another bend, and Ray understood the smell. A few hundred yards ahead the trees were a mass of blackness. Beyond the charred timbers the road ended at the foot of a blackened ridge bare of vegetation. "Shall we see what's there?" Pris said.

When Doug drove past the point where the green trees turned black Ray felt as though darkness had gathered around him, oppressive and chill. Sandra shivered, and he put an arm around her while he tried to grasp what he'd just seen. What kind of fire could do that? The innermost ranks of green trees were blackened in patches on the side nearest the dead pines, but if this was as far as the blaze had spread, what had stopped it so abruptly? Surely forest fires usually spread until they were balked by trees they couldn't reach. He was about to remark on the anomaly when William cried "Auntie Pris, is that your monstery?"

Julian rewarded him with an indulgent laugh. "It's a monastery, William."

"It looks kind of monstrous as well," Tim said.

"Please be careful what you say, Timothy."

Ray refrained from agreeing aloud with Tim. Above the shrivelled treetops he'd seen holes in the blackened rock, and now he realised they were too regularly spaced and shaped for caves. They were the unglazed windows of a building that had the crest of the ridge for its roof. As the car followed Julian's out of the forest he saw an entrance midway between the dozens of windows, a tall wide pointed arch. A steep flight of high steps led to it, and an uneven path started where they did, doubling back to the arch from the outer side of the monastery – the side that didn't merge with the rock. "That's it, Will," Pris said. "It'd take more than a fire to destroy it."

"You think someone tried," Ray said.

"Why should anyone? More like someone dropped a cigarette."

Ray had a pointlessly random thought: the pyre in the village hadn't done away with the monkish figure either, it had just been a token destruction. As Julian and Doug parked near the steps, he saw how black the ridge and the building carved out of it were – even blacker than the nearby trees and the bare earth in which their roots were clenched like a symptom of a convulsion. "That's another reason smoking is bad for everyone, William," Natalie said.

The boy scampered up the steps as Ray helped Sandra out of the car. "Stay outside till we're there, William," Julian called and frowned at Jonquil, who was taking the easier path with Tim instead of following William. The teenagers halted at the bend, and Ray was dismayed to think they had to rest after so little exercise until he saw they were gazing around the end of the ridge. "Look where we've come back to," Tim said.

Jonquil pushed up the brim of her hat as if greeting the sight. "I never saw that on my map."

William ran to them along the upper stretch of path as Ray followed Sandra up the lower half. When Ray saw why the cousins were surprised he wasn't sure how the sight made him feel. The bend in the path overlooked a distant section of the coast road – a location he recognised. There was the shrine beside the bus stop and the path leading to the beach with the cave. "So much for your navigation, Jonquil," Julian complained. "We could have driven here in a fraction of the time."

"We used my phone as well," Doug reminded him and clambered along the side of the ridge away from the path. "We'd never have got here that way," he called. "There's heaps of rubble and undergrowth all the way to the coast road."

"Don't ever do what your uncle's doing, William," Natalie said. "Climbing on rocks is dangerous."

"Yes, come back, Doug," Pris called as if Natalie had let her admit to nervousness. "I want to look inside."

When Ray turned his back on the view, having waited for his son to scramble back to the path, he felt as if the blackness of the ridge had recaptured him. On the way to the entrance he saw the remnant of a chapel through the first window, and then a succession of monastic cells as unadorned as caves. They looked even blacker than the exterior, and he was trying to find some appeal in them when Julian said "Leave that alone, William."

He was too late. Fragments of a door were propped inside the entrance, and the boy had picked up a chunk. Ray didn't know if it was Julian's rebuke that made William drop the piece of blackened wood with a startled laugh that could have used more mirth. The wood had crumbled in his grasp like a lump of dirt, and when it struck the floor it broke asunder, not so much splintering apart as scattering wide. Even the dull thump didn't sound too wooden. "Look at your hand, William," Natalie cried. "Excuse him, everyone. Just you come outside."

She spilled water from a bottle over his stained hand before rubbing it furiously with her handkerchief. "We'll be going ahead, Natalie," Pris said.

Ray found he'd welcomed the deferral. When he stepped through the arch the walls of bare black rock closed around him, beneath a ceiling he could have touched with his fingertips. He suspected that a coalmine deep beneath the earth would feel very much like this. He had a sense of darkness awaiting the night, an impression that the muffled daylight only helped. Pris turned right at the end of the passage, away from the outermost side of the monastery, and led the way into the first cell.

There was barely room for everyone. Inside was nothing but a knee-high ledge carved out of one wall and the remains of a door strewn beside the doorway. Tim was last into the cell, and had to stoop. Perhaps he meant to leave self-consciousness behind by saying "There's your bed, Will."

"Of course it's not," Natalie said. "Don't listen, William."

"Someone had to sleep there, though," Pris told him. "It was supposed to make them holy."

"Am I holy, mummy?"

"I'm sure you are. Just see you keep that way."

"I expect I will if I keep going to grandma's and grandad's."

Before the silence could persist too long Sandra said "That's very sweet of you, William. What makes you say it?"

"I expect that bed's as hard as my one at your house."

As Doug risked a laugh Sandra protested "William, you should have told us. I'll see it never is again."

This time Ray could have thought the silence had borrowed darkness from the cell. While he tried not to imagine what several of the party might be leaving unexpressed, Pris said rather too hastily "Let's see what else there is."

The corridor led to cell after cell, each furnished with a stone bunk and scattered with the wreckage of a door. Had someone indeed tried to set the place on fire? The vandalism would have been mindless, since it took no thought to grasp that rock wouldn't burn, and yet Ray had to wonder how the forest fire had reached inside the monastery – how it had managed when the nearest trees were at least a hundred yards away from the ridge. As he glanced into the last cell Pris advanced along the corridor, beyond the dim glow that spilled out of the room. "Has everyone got a flashlight on their phones?" she said. "I'd like to see what's down here."

Ray had to give his eyes quite a time to adjust before he saw that the corridor hadn't come to a dead end. It continued steeply downwards, providing rough steps but no handrail, just jagged projections of rock. As he went closer he heard echoes of his movements, unnecessarily suggestive of someone retreating into the subterranean darkness. While the rest of the party approached the steps the echoes multiplied in the dark, so that Ray could have thought it hid a swarm of denizens. "Don't you want to see the chapel?" Natalie said.

"We can look there first if you like," Pris said.

Ray saw that Natalie had meant it as an alternative, not just a preference. She led the procession past the entrance and another series of empty cells, beyond which was a larger room – a kitchen, to judge by the rounded aperture in the roof. The adjacent room, with which it shared a doorway, was several times the size and absolutely bare except for bits of doors. "Do we think they could make it into more of an attraction?" Sandra said.

"Sorry, Sandra," Pris said more gently than Ray thought the question warranted. "Who could what?"

"The islanders. If they want to attract tourists, mightn't they restore this place and maybe hire a guide?"

"Maybe they don't want people coming here," Jonquil said.

Natalie frowned at her but stopped short of arguing, and made for the furthermost room – the chapel. Apart from the altar, which was carved out of the rock, it was as devoid of even the remains of furniture as the dining hall. The altar was an empty unadorned slab, a mute reproof to any kind of luxury. Once the walls must have been populated with painted icons, but not much was left of them. The faces and robed bodies had mostly flaked away, and their actions were beyond guessing, unless the figure that had managed to retain a tarnished quarter of its halo had been meant to bless the congregation with an upraised hand that had lost its fingers long ago. When the sun had shone into the chapel the undamaged icons must have shone like light rendered solid, but the traces were reduced to a glimmer that might have been struggling not to yield to the blackness of the walls. As Ray realised that he couldn't tell which or how many of the figures would have represented St Titus, Sandra said "Translation, anyone?"

She was gazing at a motto that surmounted the entrance to the chapel. The Greek letters were intact, having been incised in the rock. "Embrace eternity," Doug said after pondering, "and eternity will embrace you."

"More like immortality," Pris said, "don't you think?"

"Could be, or infinity." Doug tapped his forehead like a keyboard. "Or," he said, "I don't know, deathlessness."

"We never think to use our phones for translations."

"We don't usually need them, do we? They mightn't work here either." Nevertheless Doug took out his mobile and fingered a command. "Maybe she's here," he said.

He held the phone in front of his face and read the motto above the entrance so loud and slowly that Ray heard an echo somewhere along the corridor, almost catching up with Doug's voice. As the distant repetition fell silent the mobile acknowledged Doug's words with an electronic note, and then a woman's bright artificial voice said "Feed on everlasting, everlasting feeds on you."

"Maybe I didn't say it right," Doug said.

"Or she hasn't got as much of a vocabulary as we have," Pris suggested.

Ray had found the whole performance disconcerting – the remote imitation of Doug's words, the female voice that seemed intrusive, too bright for the gloom that had gathered in the chapel – and now he saw that it had prevented him from wondering why the motto was inside the doorway rather than outside, as though it denoted the entrance to somewhere other than the chapel. He was on the edge of raising the question when Julian said "Perhaps you can't expect your phone to speak better English than the natives do."

"Don't call them that," Natalie said. "Say local people, William."

"So who's coming downstairs with me?" Pris said.

William glanced at his parents, but before they could speak he said "Who's living down there?"

"Nobody lives here," Natalie said. "I'm surprised anybody ever did."

"Someone does, mummy. I heard them."

"William, please don't continue with this nonsense," Julian said. "What did you imagine you heard?"

"They ran away down there when we all went to look."

"I thought I heard that too. Give me a moment, Julian," Ray

said as the boy's father parted his displeased lips. "I was going to say, William, that was just us making a noise. There are lots of echoes here."

"So who's in the exploration party?" Pris said.

"I shall be," Julian said. "I'd like to see exactly what's there."

"Can I come, daddy?"

"As long as you stay with me I think you should."

"Then I will too," Natalie said.

"Anybody not?" Doug said. "Remember however far down it goes, that's how far we'll have to climb back up."

Ray could have imagined Sandra had been waiting for the excuse. "I'll sit this out if everybody doesn't mind."

Over a supportive murmur Jonquil said "I'll stay with you, gran."

"I will too," said Tim.

Ray had been about to offer, but the cousins seemed anxious to remain. "I'll have a look," he told Sandra. "If there's anything you would have liked I'll bring you back a photograph."

Pris and Doug were already leading everybody else to the far end of the corridor. As he followed them Ray had a sense of advancing into darkness – because the view beyond the windows off the corridor was as black as the walls, he told himself. Julian switched on his flashlight before Pris activated hers. "Stay behind me, William," he said, "and watch where I step."

As Pris and Doug started downwards the steps and walls and sharply sloping roof framed them with light. It seemed not to reach very far. Ray could have thought the darkness was absorbing some of it, or the rock was. Julian's flashlight beam jerked after it, intermittently overlapping it without appearing to increase the brightness. Two lights should be enough for now, and Ray resolved to conserve his. When Natalie followed William, one hand hovering close to his shoulder in case she needed to steady him, Ray stepped down into the dark.

He felt as if blackness hadn't merely closed around him but was weighing on him. The lights lurched ahead of him, and he had to remind himself that the passage wasn't as unstable as it looked, even if he might easily be. At every step the low roof shuddered while the walls wobbled from side to side, which made them seem close to collapsing, and Ray clutched at spiky lumps of wall, bruising his hands. His ankles had begun to ache from stepping down and further down by the time Pris's flashlight beam grew steadier. "Well," she said, "maybe upstairs was too comfy for them."

She'd reached a corridor hacked out of the rock. On both sides were narrow archways, crudely formed and unevenly spaced. As everyone else descended into the corridor she shone her flashlight through the nearest arch. "Maybe these were for meditating."

The hollow that had been carved out of the rock, if it hadn't just been broken into from the corridor, didn't have much of a shape. Except for the ledge chipped out of one wall, Ray mightn't have taken it for a cell. "Maybe you were meant to come down here if you were feeling sinful," Doug said.

Ray saw the corridor sloped downwards, as if the builders had been seeking the depths of the darkness. It seemed clear that they'd incorporated spaces already present in the rock. Beyond a line of cells, none of which appeared ever to have had doors, a hollow several times the size of any of them was littered with remnants of wood. Had the monks brought down furniture from the dining hall? As Ray tried to identify the blackened debris Julian's light swung towards William. "What's that mean?" the boy had said.

Pris was illuminating words scraped on the wall of a cramped cell across the corridor. Doug stepped through the lopsided archway for a closer look and then a frown. With deliberation not unlike reluctance he said "We feed him."

"Is that it, Doug?" Pris said. "I thought – "

"Surely not another argument," Julian complained. "Can't you two agree before you tell the rest of us?"

"We aren't machines, Jules. You're getting the personal touch. What were you going to say it was, Pris?"

"We feed for him."

"Now you say, it could mean either."

"They were religious people, William," Natalie said. "They must have believed they fed God with their prayers, and I expect they gave people food on God's behalf."

Ray thought this was at odds with the way the monks appeared to have retreated into the dark. The lights were moving onwards, and he limped rapidly after them. Presumably the monks had carried torches – the members of the order would have died long before electricity was harnessed, let alone brought here – though he'd seen nothing like a bracket on any of the walls. Pris shone her flashlight into the next cell and halted in the doorway. "Poor feller, whoever he was," Doug said. "His life must have felt like a sentence."

Ray peered between the two of them to see that the far wall of the windowless cell was covered with scratches – upright lines in groups of four, crossed out by a fifth. "What are they, Uncle Doug?" William said.

"They're how people mark the time off." At once Doug added "Mark the days."

"But in Greece do they count – " Having glanced at her brother's face, Natalie said "No, you're right. I see."

Ray had to step into the cell before he grasped what they'd left unremarked. For some reason the occupant had counted days in hundreds, adding an extra horizontal line whenever one came to an end. Three of those were followed by several smaller groups. The lines highest on the wall, and indeed for some way down it, looked disconcertingly faint with age. Pris moved onwards, but Ray was still searching for an explanation when Julian said from the corridor "Will you use your own light there, Raymond? I need to keep up with my son."

Ray couldn't have explained why he preferred not to be left behind. At least walking helped fend off the stony subterranean chill. Pris was sending her flashlight beam into cell after anonymous cell, and Julian's confirmed that there was nothing to be seen in them except inhospitable bare rock. The supine shape that reared up from slumbering in a cell was just the shadow of the ledge that would once have held a mattress – at least, Ray hoped so. How far did Pris mean to venture into the depths? His eyesight and even the air he was breathing seemed clogged with darkness. While the explorers had almost reached the end of the corridor, he was troubled to see that it wasn't a dead end. Beyond it the slope of the roof grew steeper, and as Ray peered between Doug and Pris he thought he glimpsed something else that unsettled him – marks on the floor. Could they be footprints leading further downwards? He was making for them when William said "Daddy, that's what I heard."

Julian held up a hand peremptory enough to halt Ray. "I'm hearing nothing, William."

As the boy sidled between his aunt and uncle Natalie hastened to capture his hand. Before Ray could protest they'd scuffed away any marks he might have seen. "Now then," Natalie said, "what are we supposed to hear?"

Beyond the corridor rough steps descended further than both flashlight beams could reach. Natalie was holding William back from leaning too far towards the dark when he cried "There it is."

Ray saw a dark form leap up the steps towards the boy. It was William's shadow, jerking at his cry as his aunt's flashlight had. As Ray's heartbeat set about calming down, Julian said "That's just water, William."

Now that it had been put into words Ray heard a faint sound

of lapping in the depths. "I think this as far as we should go," Natalie said.

"I wouldn't mind seeing what's down there," Pris said.

"I'll come with you," Doug said.

"Then somebody ought to wait here," Natalie said without enthusiasm, "in case anyone's needed."

Ray saw she was concerned about her brother. Perhaps she meant Julian to stay while she took their son back to the daylight, but Julian was busy saying "Are you satisfied now, William? As your mother told you, nobody lives here any more."

"Suppose."

"If you've any reason to disagree then please let us hear. Otherwise you really must accept that people who are older than you know best."

Ray was holding back from mentioning the tracks he thought he'd seen. He could have felt addressed as Julian said "Nothing more to say? Then let's mark the subject dealt with and shut the drawer."

Doug was already following Pris and her flashlight beam into the depths. Ray watched their silhouettes and the frame of illuminated rock shrink downwards step by tentative step, and then the light jerked askew and vanished. He was on the edge of calling out when he grasped that Pris and Doug had disappeared around a bend in the sloping passage. The darkness engulfed their cautious footsteps, after which Ray could hear nothing except a restless movement somewhere behind him. Perhaps he'd heard William, since the boy was gazing back along the corridor.

Voices rose from the depths beyond Julian's flashlight – Doug and Pris in some discussion, so muffled that Ray would have found them no less comprehensible if they had been talking Greek. Some development was growing close to visible down there, a shifting of the rock or some other activity. That was an effect of the light that was groping upwards around the bend. A shape as black as the walls climbed ahead of it and spoke. "Looks like it's just caves now," Doug said. "That's why we could hear water."

"They must have tunnelled down to them," Pris said, appearing at his back. "We don't know if they meant to."

Ray wondered what the builders might have hoped to find. "We'll see you in the open," Natalie said. "Come and get some fresh air, William."

Ray stood aside for Pris before trailing her and Doug up the corridor. Her flashlight beam snagged on the entrance to each cell, releasing a shadow that fled into its lair. Shadows swarmed away like vermin from the debris in the largest space, and at last the beam reached the foot of the steps, up which Natalie was urging William after Julian. As Pris began to climb, Ray switched on his own flashlight for a last look along the corridor. He hadn't turned when he heard movement behind him – the restlessness he'd heard earlier. He swung around to see a shape emerging from the furthest cell.

The legs came first – eight of them creeping around the far edge of the entrance to the cell. In a moment, though by no means a reassuring one, Ray saw they weren't legs at all; they were scrawny fingers clutching at the rock. As he struggled to breathe they brought their owner forth into the corridor. It was bent low with age or stealth, and entirely bald. Although it was naked, the whitish body was so withered that he couldn't guess at its sex. It twisted its thin head towards the light, and Ray glimpsed a face like a flimsy paper mask moulded to a skull. Were the eyes as entirely black as the rock? Even so, they gleamed with a life so fierce that it seemed to be concentrated in them, draining the ribbed torso of substance, shrivelling the crippled limbs. It bared its teeth at the light and stayed in its spidery crouch as it scuttled on all fours to the steps beyond the corridor. Before Ray could suck in a laboured breath it vanished into the dark.

He staggered around to find he was alone in the corridor. Even the other lights were no longer to be seen. He was shivering from head to foot, and not just with the underground chill. As he fought to recapture enough breath to call out or to set about climbing the steps he heard Doug, altogether too far away. "Is my dad behind you?"

"I don't see him," Pris said as a faint glow found a single step high above.

"Dad, are you all right down there?"

"Where are you, grandad?" William contributed.

While the voices were closer than Ray had feared, that meant William was too close for Ray to mention what he'd seen. Surely it had only been someone who had taken refuge. Wasn't that what even derelict monasteries were for? "I'm coming," he managed to gasp.

He didn't switch the flashlight off until he'd toiled more than halfway up the steps, where he had to rest while the pounding of his heart relented somewhat and the aches in his legs grew dormant. He shone the beam downwards as long as he stayed there, to convince himself that he wasn't being followed out of the dark. When at last he stumbled into the upper corridor he saw Sandra and the teenagers emerging from the chapel, a sight that left him more confused than ever. "Haven't you been outside?"

"It got a bit much for us," Sandra said. "Too much blackness, so we came back in."

How did this make sense? It was blacker still inside the monastery. Ray could only think one or more of them hadn't liked the sight of so many dead trees, but his thoughts troubled him as everyone made for the cars. Of course it was darkest underground, but even at ground level the interior seemed darker than the surrounding devastation. It was as though rather than reaching the monastery from the trees, the blackness had spread from it to the forest like a stain. "Shall we go somewhere brighter now?" Natalie said, and the image of voracious darkness was just one of the thoughts Ray was glad to leave behind.

★   ★   ★

"Was that worth waiting for, William?" Sandra said.

"It was good." Apparently in case he seemed ungrateful the boy added "It was best."

"We say it was the best, William," Natalie said.

"Did you and daddy think it was as well?"

Ray didn't think the boy meant this as a joke, but Julian seemed to suspect he did. To forestall any rebuke Ray said "Now you know why they call it Sunset Beach."

The family was seated at a table in a beach taverna near the Sunny View. The sky at the horizon had turned crimson almost half an hour ago, tinting the giant umbrellas along the coast a florid red. Now the sky above the sunken sun was turning dull, as if the vital colour was draining into the night that loomed over it. Traces lingered on the waves, which seemed bent on bearing them to Sunset Beach. Ray saw the resort was living up to the name; its beach had started growing crowded as soon as the sun touched the horizon. "What does our beach mean?" William said.

"Everybody's holiday together," Natalie said and seemed unable to take her eyes off him.

"I meant what it's called, mummy."

"That's a cue for the translators," Julian said. "Preferably just one."

"We know what it means," Pris told him.

"Teleftaiafos means Last Light, Will."

For once Ray wished Doug had disagreed with Pris. He squeezed Sandra's hand, only to fear that he'd drawn too much attention to Doug's words. Natalie and Doug and their partners looked away as if the gesture conveyed more than they could deal with, but while the cousins seemed embarrassed William ignored it. "There's the lady again," he said.

Julian fixed him with his gaze. "Which lady? What are you saying now?"

"The lady who brought my cross."

As Ray located the vendor distributing trinkets from her capacious shoulder-bag he wasn't certain whether he'd seen Tim relax. Some of the diners made it plain that they found her unwelcome, but at least she wasn't homeless, as Ray had decided the person he'd glimpsed in the monastery must have been. When her tour of the taverna brought her over William told her "I put the cross by my bed at night."

She passed her fingertips back and forth in front of her lips, which left Ray wondering if this indicated muteness or an ability to read what people said. When she reached in her bag he assumed she was offering trinkets again, but she only produced a book, which she planted next to Ray's plate and then shoved towards him. "For me?" Ray said and took out his wad of Greek cash. "How much?"

She waved it away so vigorously that the flame in the lantern on the table fluttered, and then she put her hands together to indicate the book. Ray couldn't see why she would be praying, but perhaps the gesture conveyed gratitude for how much he'd paid for William's cross. She watched him put away the money, and looked ready to watch him read. "Thank you very much for that," he said and turned the book to face him.

The large thin paperback had an aerial view of a group of islands on the cover, an image so generic that it could have been found online. Much of it was obscured by blocky lettering – HISTORY OF GREECE ISLANDS and the author's name, Iannis Antonaides. The book had been published some years ago in Kefalonia – self-published, to judge by the prose. Ray felt all the more touched that the woman had presented it to him, but when he made to thank her again he found that she was several tables away. "Could I have a look?" Doug said.

He leafed through the paperback, lingering over photographs and then at the start of a chapter. "You won't like this, Jules."

"The writing, you mean?" Ray said. "Most of us couldn't write a line in Greek, never mind an entire book."

"Not the writing." Doug glanced at William and held the open book towards Ray. "This part," he said.

Julian leaned across the table to frown at the book. All the bulbs on wires entwined like vines around the trellis overhead were lit now, and light glaring from the glossy page erased the title of the chapter. Ray had to take hold of the book to see that the page was headed *Vampire of Vasilema*. As he realised that he'd inadvertently turned the open pages towards the youngest member of the family, Jonquil said "Can you say a bug, William?"

"A bug," William said with a giggle of anticipation.

"Keep saying it."

"A bug a bug a bug," William said and giggled louder.

"Say it very fast."

"Please do nothing of the kind, William," Julian said. "Jonquil, everybody else can see exactly what you're trying to do. Kindly stop at once."

"I think she was trying to distract him for you," Sandra said.

"If that's genuinely the case I apologise." As Jonquil made to respond he said "All the same, I'd prefer you to find a more acceptable method."

"I wish sometimes you'd give her more of a chance," Sandra said. "Natalie, don't you?"

"I've told him so."

"Well, now I am. Will you do it for me, Julian?"

Ray was dismayed by the resemblance to a promise at a deathbed, and sensed that others heard it too. "Where it's appropriate," Julian said, and turned to Ray at once. "Perhaps you could keep your book to yourself while we're all together."

Ray felt as if he'd taken a rebuke on Jonquil's behalf, and

Doug's wink at him made him feel all the more conspiratorial. "I'll corrupt myself when you're done, dad," Doug said.

"No need for that," Natalie said more like her husband than herself.

"It's perfectly all right," Julian said. "I can take a joke. Now do you suppose we can close it?"

Doug pegged his lips together with a finger and thumb, rousing Julian's frown. "The book," he said.

As Doug shut the paperback Ray glimpsed a photograph of the monastery they'd visited. "Thank you," Julian said as he might have to an obedient child.

"Thank you very mutts," William said.

"Why are you speaking like that, William?" Natalie demanded.

The boy looked abashed by the failure of his joke. "That's how the waiter talks."

"It isn't nice to imitate people. You wouldn't like it done to you."

"The people in the church did."

"Which people?" Sandra said sharply enough to be expressing Ray's unease as well. "How were they imitating you?"

"The people that the man chased out. They weren't copying me, gran. I mean they all looked the same."

"I expect that means they're a family."

"Not just their faces." The boy shook his head for emphasis if not in frustration. "Like they were smiling," he insisted, "but it wasn't a smile."

"I saw nothing like that, William."

Ray felt anxious to support Julian. "Remember there were all the candles, William. I don't think any of us could see those people very well."

"I did. They were looking at grandma and Jonquil and Tim."

"Well," Sandra said, "someone must think I belong with the younger set."

"Of course you do. With all of us, and so does Ray," Pris said, only to appear to wonder if she'd said too much.

The teenagers had taken Sandra's hands, reaching across the remains of the meal, and Ray couldn't help being put in mind of a séance if not a secret sign. Julian cleared his throat to say "Shall we call for the bill?"

He beckoned to their waiter and mimed scribbling on his hand as if he'd had a thought he wanted to record. Once they had the reckoning and the contributions were gathered on the tray Julian added a gratuity. "Gosh, is that ten per cent?" Pris said. "They don't tip like that in Greece."

"Then perhaps we should set an example."

Natalie was urging William away, and Ray saw why when the waiter called "Thank you very mutts."

Tim and Jonquil weren't alone in visibly suppressing mirth, but William looked more than serious. "See, mummy, that is what he said."

"It's what he meant that counts, Will," Doug said. "Sometimes you have to look behind the words."

Just now this didn't sound like good advice – at least, Ray hoped the boy would leave quite a lot that he'd recently heard unexamined. Beyond the light from the taverna the way across the beach was unlit, and the sand felt as if the darkness were dragging at Ray's feet. As he trudged into the village, up an alley that eventually left the sand behind, he saw a bunch of elongated limbs reach down from a streetlamp at the end. It was only the magnified shadow of a spider flexing all its legs at the centre of its web, but he was glad when it stopped appearing to grope for Sandra and Jonquil and Tim.

★   ★   ★

"Do you mind if I read for a while?"

"Of course I don't, but you won't mind if I go to bed, will you? Then I shouldn't be so likely to nod off on the boat tomorrow."

"I'm only outside if you need me."

"And you know where I'll be."

"Just call if you need me for anything at all."

By now it was clear to them both that they were prolonging their moments together. As Ray kissed her eyes, the way he often used to before he and Sandra settled down to sleep, he felt how wrinkled the lids had grown. Weren't her wrinkles and his own a sketchy record of their lives together? "Rest well," he said and wished he weren't reminded of another version of the phrase.

Sandra switched on the balcony light for him and slid the window shut once he'd stepped out of the room. He would have liked her to leave the curtains open, but the light wouldn't help her to sleep. Did he really have to read the book right now? He wasn't even sure that he wanted to know why he felt he did. Perhaps he could glance through just the chapter that discussed the monastery. He sat by the outer wall, beyond which the waves were as slow and regular as sleeping breaths, and leafed through the book until he found the photograph.

It wasn't by any means recent. This was made plain by the car, presumably belonging to the photographer, that was parked at the end of the road between the trees. Ray guessed that the image was at least as old as himself. Why hadn't Iannis Antonaides taken a photograph of his own or chosen a more recent one? Perhaps the image was meant to illustrate a point, because it did. In the photograph the monastery was no less black than it was now, and the empty windows hinted at the deeper darkness underground, but the blackness grew paler as it spread down the ridge, and the lowest stretch of rock was no more than grey. All the nearest trees – indeed, all the trees in the photograph – were green.

So it hadn't been a fire that had destroyed them. Whatever had reduced them to their present state had come from the ridge, which was bare of vegetation in the photograph. Could it have become overgrown in the intervening years and then caught fire? Ray would have liked to show someone the picture, but Sandra had turned out the light in their room, and nobody was audible below. Straining to hear seemed to summon the night closer and transform the sound of the sea into rather too large and insistent a succession of breaths, perhaps because he'd realised that the photograph was meant to illustrate the chapter that began over the page, *Vampire of Vasilema.*

There came many years ago to the monastery of Agios Titus on the island of Vasilema a traveller from where nobody can tell...

It would be a legend, obviously. Certainly the prose was meant to sound like one. Ray thought Sandra might be amused and even touched by the author's bid to match style to content in a language not his own, and no doubt the legend would appeal to Doug and Pris – to the teenagers as well. The only one who absolutely mustn't see was William, who might mistake it for the truth.

There came many years ago to the monastery of Agios Titus on the island of Vasilema a traveller from where nobody can tell. He gave his name Proskynitis, means pilgrim. In all Greece a monastery must take in the pilgrim and those who seek shelter. The monks of Agios Titus offered hospitality for but a single night...

Perhaps the tale had a moral – that you shouldn't offer only token succour to those in need. It might almost be suitable for William, though Ray would rather the boy read books for fun and in general enjoyed himself without quite so much intervention by his parents – and then Ray saw how the sentence ended.

The monks of Agios Titus offered hospitality for but a single night, and the night Proskynitis brought them never saw the dawn.
He was said to tell the abbot he was wandering in search of solitude

where to contemplate eternal things. He vowed that on his death he would will riches to his benefactor who gave him what he sought. Some monks said that the monastery was not built to acquire fortune, but Proskynitis assured them that his riches would not be of the world but of eternity. They had put aside worldly matters, but their vanity was spiritual. So thus he won them to his cause. He became an inmate of the monastery, taking less sustenance than any monk while he fasted as a help to meditation. As well he counselled his brethren against distractions of the world and urged the dark upon them as the most true path to seeing the eternal...

Ray felt as if the dark was being wished on him as well. The waves on the beach might have been carrying it inland to gather below him, and he could have imagined that it was massing at his side, in the unlit room. He ought to go back to Sandra, but did the book explain why the monastery had gone underground? Perhaps once he knew that, he would be more able to sleep.

His example won him acceptance to the order, taking the name Brother Skiá, means shadow. He prevailed upon his brethren to help him build a cell deep in the rock, where no distraction of light could reach. Here he followed his ambition to embrace eternity, which is embrace the dark. Why could he not do this in real solitude, far from any man? He was said to have once, but eternity needs life to feed upon or it is only lifeless dark. He that learns secrets of the dark is caught in its embrace. If it brings unending life it fills its vessel with its hunger...

Ray wasn't sure how much of this he understood or cared to grasp. It didn't seem much like an aid to sleep. He wasn't far from blaming it for an impression that had begun to trouble him – a sense that more than waves were active on the beach. Of course only waves kept suggesting a lithe shape crouched almost on all fours and darting progressively closer to the Sunny View. When he peered at the beach he saw nothing restless apart from the water.

It was the abbot who invited the dark pilgrim within his door, and now the dark answered his invitation. Now the abbot fed the dark each night Skiá came to him. What promises the dark may whisper none can say who has not heard the dark, but by the day of Agios Titus some numbers of the brethren made their habitation in the depths. Yet Skiá must learn to moderate his thirst for the reason that the victim who dies rises thirsty from the dead to multiply the hunger. But those who feed on others for the vessel of the dark and choose to feed it while they live are rewarded with great age, and the pact may extend to their victims although they have not chosen. The blood is the exchange and the seal, and who may break the pact once it is sealed? ...

As Ray turned the page he felt he was being watched. When he glanced at the window he thought he'd just missed glimpsing someone who had looked out at him. Nobody was visible between the curtains now. He stood up so fast that the plastic chair almost toppled over, and went to the window. Through the meagre gap between the curtains he was able to distinguish that Sandra was asleep, one arm upturned on the thin quilt. No doubt because of his reading, her position reminded him of someone about to give blood. He blamed the book for making him imagine a face at the window as well. He was tempted to abandon the chapter until daylight, but he might as well finish it while Sandra was asleep. He would have that much more time to spend with her once she was awake.

Who will know what rites were celebrated each night in the chapel? Some who lived near in a village said the wind out of the trees brought a chanting in the language of the dark. Not every brethren made the dark his friend. Some few fled into the forest, but the dark brought them back to feed on, following all which they died and were burned before the hunger waked them. But Skiá's hunger had no bounds, whether being for victims or for knowledge of the dark. Did he seek the deepest blackness for his path to the eternal or for the reason he had become so monstrous none could bear to look upon him? The brethren who fed him dared to bring him no light, and in many years even their use to him was spent. Few travellers came to the monastery now, so the brethren still living must find others to feed...

Ray had had enough. The chapter was making him absurdly nervous, too aware of the unlit room beside him, too inclined to keep glancing towards it in search of the face he hadn't really glimpsed at all. He'd only seen Sandra alone in bed, and why wasn't he there with her? Suppose she felt lonely even if asleep? The thought made him close the book and drop it on the table like the irrelevance it was. It had nothing to do with either of them, and he didn't know why he'd given it so much of his time. He eased the window open and shut and crept into bed next to Sandra, who gave a sigh so heartfelt he could very well have taken it for a rebuke.

He'd hardly settled into bed when he heard a sound, though it didn't own up to being much of one. Was it in the room? It couldn't be Sandra, who hadn't moved in his loose embrace, unless her arm had shifted on the quilt. Surely he would have felt that movement too. No, the soft almost insubstantial activity was outside the window, and as he squinted across Sandra's silhouette Ray saw a dim shape at or on the section of the table that was visible between the curtains. In a moment it vanished, moving as fluidly as a wave. It had been a cat, of course, and to begin with he'd heard it leap onto the balcony. Now he wished he'd brought the book in with him.

Unless he did he mightn't sleep. Suppose the clouds turned to rain? He inched out of bed and padded across the room. He was sliding the window open with as little noise as the visitor had made when his hands jerked, and the window juddered in its frame. The book was nowhere to be seen.

Had the cat knocked it off the balcony? Ray glanced back at Sandra in case the rattle of the window had disturbed her, but she was lying as she had been, bare arm outstretched. He slid the window wide enough to let him out and hurried to the outer wall, clutching at the rough cold stone while he craned over. He couldn't see the book, either on the balconies below or in the undergrowth alongside them. He kept hold of the wall as he straightened up, fighting a surge of the dizziness that came with age. He was about to look under the table – his senses must be growing even more senile if he'd missed noticing the book was there – when he saw someone on the beach.

The figure was strolling towards Sunset Beach, practically gliding over the sand not too far from the edge of the glimmering waves. It was performing some action that seemed almost ritualistic, producing pale objects from an item in its hand before shying them into the water. Ray strained his eyes and narrowed them as well, and as the figure dodged with a sinuous motion out of reach of a wave he identified what it was holding – a book, from which it was tearing out pages to crumple them and fling them in the sea.

"What the devil?" Ray nearly yelled, but clapped a hand over his mouth instead. He knew which book it was, however the man had acquired it – presumably by picking it up once the cat had sent it off the balcony. He'd hushed himself so as not to waken Sandra, but he padded fast into the room and shut the window before grabbing his trunks. A hopping dance that felt as savage as absurd helped him find his way into them – he almost wished William could see him play the inadvertent clown – and he thanked whoever needed thanking that Sandra's sleep was so sound. He clutched his sandals in one hand while he retrieved the key from the slot by the door and let himself out of the apartment. Having eased the door shut, he sat on the steps to don the sandals while a host of flat unblinking eyes watched him from the play area. All the round faces met him with fixed toothy grins as he made a dash for the beach.

The road was deserted, not even a cat to be seen. The many-legged shadow that guarded the alley stirred as Ray sprinted panting under the lamp. Sand seemed to creep up the alley to meet him, and as it made him skid he bruised a hand against the spiky concrete wall. When he stumbled onto the beach the figure with the book was hundreds of yards away along the shoreline, and even harder to discern against the waves; its scrawny outline looked as unstable as the water. The man must be a reveller from Sunset Beach, quite possibly high on drugs and amused by the notion of destroying a book or else actively hostile to reading. He was still ripping pages out to throw into the sea, where numerous scraps of paper bobbed in his wake.

Or perhaps it wasn't quite his wake, for Ray had the wholly useless thought that the thief was staying well clear of the water. Ray floundered across the beach, where every step felt clogged with soft sand, to retrieve all the pages he could. Many, indeed most, were already well out to sea, too far away for him to risk paddling. He had a nightmarish vision of drowning out there in the dark, leaving Sandra alone because he'd cared more about a few bits of paper than he cared for her. Why, he'd already left her in the darkness by taking the key with him; while the fob wasn't in the slot the lights in the apartment wouldn't work. Just grab all the pages he could reach – the waves had even stranded a few on the sand – although were they worth salvaging? As he picked up the first sodden scrap he saw that the pages weren't even intact; they had all been torn raggedly in half. This was too much for him. "What do you think you're playing at," he shouted, "you damned vandal?"

He wasn't looking at the culprit, but when he straightened up from gathering a handful of crumpled scraps of paper he saw that the figure had turned to gaze at him. In a moment it shied the remains of the book into the sea and crouched towards him. He couldn't have said why he was grateful not to be able to make out its face. Its posture put him in mind of a runner at the start of a race, an idea that was all too appropriate. Before he could take a breath the figure came for him.

It moved as fast as any animal, practically flying across the soft sand. For a very short time Ray was determined to stand his ground and not be daunted, and then panic overtook him. He clutched the handful of paper so hard that moisture seeped between his fingers as he retreated towards the alley with all the speed he could achieve – not much at all. The sand felt as though his age had gathered underfoot, soft masses spilling into his sandals to grit between his toes, not merely retarding every step but weighing it down, sending heavy pains through the muscles of his legs. A backwards glance showed him that while he'd laboured halfway to the alley, where at least there was some light, the pursuer had almost halved the distance to him. Ray might have cried out if he'd had any breath to spare from struggling towards the feeble reassurance of the light. He couldn't even run, but had to take unsteady strides that came near to robbing him of balance. Another shaky stride that seemed more capable of kicking up sand than of bringing him any closer to the light, and another that let more aches dig deep into his legs, and one that nearly sent him stumbling headlong into the wall beside the alley – and then he was leaning against the prickly stone, and made himself twist around at once. As far as he could see, he was alone on the beach.

How reassuring could that be? Ray had a sudden awful notion that the pursuer might reach Sandra ahead of him. He dashed along the alley, barely managing not to collide with the walls. As he came to the end the spidery shadow reached for him, and he could have imagined the pursuer had leapt on him. He stumbled along the road to the Sunny View, where the unlit buildings and the glassy pool felt as if they were keeping quiet about an intruder, while the faces in the playground might have been sharing a secret grin. Ray hauled himself up the steps, every one of which demanded an effortful breath, and let himself into the lightless room.

He thought Sandra was asleep – she appeared not to have moved

– but she spoke as he looked for somewhere to put the bedraggled pages. "Ray, where were you? I thought you'd left me."

"Just with the book," he said in the hope that she hadn't fully wakened, "that's where I was," and felt as if he'd betrayed her by leaving her. Nothing would make him do that again, he vowed. He stowed the pages in his bedside table and slipped into bed to renew his embrace, but Sandra was asleep again well before him. He kept thinking that the soft fluid sound of waves had sneaked into the room, or another presence had – the pursuer from the dark beach.

THE NINTH DAY
28 AUGUST

"Sorry, everyone," Natalie said. "We needn't have got up quite so soon."

While Tim and Jonquil looked as if they might have answered this not just with dull-eyed blinks behind their sunglasses, it was Sandra who said "Not your fault. It's our transport that's late."

"Relax, you two," Doug said. "That's Greece."

"Perhaps we could have been warned about it," Julian said without quite identifying the culprit.

"The sooner I'm up seeing everyone," Sandra said, "the better I like it."

Her children and their partners produced a variety of smiles before they looked away, out of the courtyard. Beneath clouds growing pale with dawn, streetlamps cast shadows like emblems of the stillness of the road. Ray glimpsed movement at the near end of the alley leading to the beach, presumably the shadow of the spider that had the light for its lure – the retreating shape had been thin enough. He remembered last night, and was trying to make more sense of it than he had so far when William said "Please may I go on the swings while we're waiting?"

"If anyone would care to go with you I should think you may."

"I'll take you, William," Natalie said.

Ray thought Sandra would have offered if she hadn't joined the teenagers in a state close to dozing. All three were seated on the wall beside the entrance to the courtyard and already wearing hats as well as sunglasses. As Natalie and William disappeared through the gap in the apartment block the boy's absence let Ray blurt "Doug, you saw the photo in my book."

"The monastery, you mean? I got a glimpse," Doug said and visibly refrained from looking at Julian. "You should see it, Pris."

Ray felt robbed of whatever question he might have asked. "I don't know if you'll be able to. I'm afraid I've lost the book."

"Oh, Ray," Sandra said and made an effort to widen her eyes. "How?"

Her concern felt worse than an accusation. "I left it on the balcony," he said. "It must have fallen off."

"Haven't you looked for it?"

"I did last night. You won't believe this, well, you'll have to, but someone had run off with it."

By now Doug had acquired some of his mother's concern. "How do you know that, dad?"

"I saw them on the beach with it." Ray had a sense of abandoning reticence as he said "They were tearing it up."

"Well, that's awful," Pris declared. "What did you do?"

"I rescued some of it. That's where I was when you didn't know where, Sandra. I haven't had a chance to see what state the bits I saved are in."

"What kind of villain would destroy someone's book?" Julian demanded. "There was nothing objectionable in it, was there, Raymond?"

"Not unless someone objected to the legend of the monastery."

Ray saw Doug and Pris ready questions, but Julian was faster. "How long have we been waiting now? I'm somewhat tired of Greekness."

"It hasn't been half an hour yet," Pris said. "Maybe other people have kept the pickup waiting."

"I suppose we could call the rep," Doug said, though not as if he meant to.

"I have her number here."

"I'll see what she says, Jules," Doug said to forestall him. "Sam, it's Doug Thornton," he told his phone, having listened at length. "We're still waiting at the Sunny View. We're wondering if there's a problem."

"I'd like to hear what's said," Julian let him know.

" – really sorry," Sam said on the loudspeaker, "but the trip's been cancelled."

"How long have you been aware of that?"

Perhaps it was Julian's tone that made her pause. "I've just spoken to the tour operator, Mr Thornton," she said, presumably to Doug. "They say the sea's too rough. Of course you'll get a full refund."

"I think we should expect compensation for disappointment and inconvenience," Julian said.

"You'd need to take that up with our company when you're home. Now I have to let my other clients know about the cancellation if you'll excuse me, Mr Thornton."

"One moment," Julian said not far below a shout, then stared at Doug. "Have you let her go?"

"She went of her own accord, Jules. We'd better give Nat the sorry news."

Ray thought Sandra and the cousins might stay seated on the wall, but they stumbled in unison after him as if they hadn't quite woken up. He would have taken Sandra's arm if the teenagers hadn't been on either side of her. As everybody passed the office, Evadne called "Do you not go out today?"

"We've been let down," Julian informed her. "Kept in the dark as well."

Her gaze dodged from side to side as if nervous of settling. "Who is in the dark?"

"Jules is saying they didn't let us know."

"I don't need a translator, thank you, Douglas." In much

the same tone Julian told Evadne "Our day off the island has been cancelled."

"They do that often. That is their way."

"Well, it emphatically isn't ours," Julian said like a warning, "and it isn't what Samantha wanted us to think. She blamed the state of the sea."

"Maybe sea, maybe other troubles." Evadne seemed to make an effort to marshal her thoughts before saying "I expect the sea."

She'd left it too late to persuade Julian, and Ray felt oddly unconvinced as well. As everyone trooped past the pool Jonquil said "Maybe they don't want people getting off their island."

"That's a ridiculous idea, and I'll thank you not to tell William."

"I expect she means they want to keep us for themselves, don't you, Jonquil?" Ray said, only to find this less reassuring than he'd intended it to be.

In the play area William greeted everyone by flying into the air, while beside him the other three swings looked eager for occupants, which they might have been grinning wide-eyed to entice. "Natalie," Sandra said. "Don't be sad, but they've called off the trip."

"Oh, well." Ray glimpsed a hint of the wince that used to pinch their daughter's face whenever she was disappointed, and then he saw her recollect that they all had reason to be considerably sadder. "Never mind," she said.

"I'm sure you do, and you have every right to." As she gave him a reproachful look Julian said "Today is still your choice."

Natalie was letting William's swing subside to help her ponder when she said "Why don't we have your day today, William, since we're here in any case."

"Can we go to the beach with the big umbrellas instead?"

"As your mother said, you chose a day at, for the sake of peace let's call it a hotel."

Sandra and the teenagers had sat on the empty swings, and Ray thought she looked as if she was trying to recapture her youth while she could. As he turned away to dab at his blurred vision William said "I don't want the lady to have to play with me all by herself. It isn't fair."

"The other children went home yesterday, Julian," Natalie said. "I can't see any harm in Sunset Beach while it's so quiet."

"I'd like to," Sandra said enthusiastically enough to sway her perch.

"Then I suppose it's decided." As everyone headed for their apartments Julian detained Ray with a beckoning finger and then the same gesture of his hand. "If you see the fellow who stole your book, point him out," he murmured. "We should have a few words with him."

Ray increasingly suspected that the thief had been deranged, quite possibly by drugs. He wasn't eager to meet him again, and was glad to be able to say "I didn't really see what he was like. I doubt I'd recognise him."

Sandra was waiting by the steps to their apartment, and he was dismayed to think she needed help until she climbed them faster than he could. In the room she grabbed towels and swimming gear and sun cream. "I wouldn't mind a higher factor if we see any," she said.

"The forecast says another cloudy day."

"Then let's buy what we need before we need it," Sandra said so forcefully it disconcerted him.

He'd never known her to use a stronger sun cream as a holiday progressed than she'd begun by using. He shouldn't argue about it or over anything else, even if avoiding disagreements felt like invoking the unspoken. He had to devote himself to ensuring that all the time she had left was as untroubled as it could be. Years ago they'd decided that they didn't want to bequeath Natalie and Doug the burden of caring for them, even less the debt of doing so. If Ray weren't going to be left alone then Sandra would have been, and when he thought about that prospect he managed to feel it was even worse. "We're still a team," he said and saw his shadow fall across her face as he kissed her lined forehead.

Tim and Jonquil were on the swings, on another of which William was twisting back and forth. He jumped off when he saw his grandparents, and the teenagers followed at their own sleepy speed, increasing it somewhat when Julian urged them. Sandra felt lighter and swifter than Ray expected, so that he had to suppress the idea of holding a memory by the hand. On the bus the cousins found seats out of reach of the sun, though it was hidden by the clouds above the mountains. At least Julian didn't make an issue of it, which meant Ray didn't need to point out how Sandra had sought the unnecessary shade as well.

The neon signs of Sunset Beach were storing up the overcast. In some of the bars and tavernas staff were sweeping up litter, broken glass glinting amid dead leaves and crumpled plastic cups. The bus halted outside a taverna called Yummy's, which earned a giggle from William. "Excuse me," Julian said as he came abreast of the driver. "Where is the stop back?"

Presumably he meant to simplify his language, but the driver's eyebrows drew together to pinch a furrow above his porous swarthy nose. "Stop back."

"Yes, the stop back." When repetition didn't work Julian indicated the opposite side of the road and swept his hand leftwards. "The stop back," he said at half his previous speed.

"That's to say," Pris intervened, "where do we catch the bus back to Teleftaiafos?"

The driver's face cleared as if the hidden sun had found it. "Wait there," he said and pointed down the road to Sinatra's British Bar.

Pris was stepping off the bus when he resumed his frown. "No bus stop after eight."

"Where is it after that?" Julian said, displaying patience.

"No," the driver said and stared hard at him. "Bus don't stop."

"Where doesn't it?"

"Here," the driver said, throwing his arms wide to signify the whole length of the road. "Anywhere long here. Sunset Beach."

"That's not the case," Julian informed him. "We've seen the bus passing through our resort later than that."

The driver might have been staring at a backward pupil. "Bus comes, right. Won't stop."

"Are you telling us the people here get out of hand so early in the evening?"

"I say nothing about people." The driver looked as though he was trying to retreat behind his frown. "It is policy," he said. "And soon no stop after seven."

"Does it matter, Julian?" Natalie protested from the pavement. "We'll have gone back by then."

Julian descended the steps with a series of clanks like comments, eloquent though wordless, and seemed to feel he was regaining authority by finding a sign for the beach. It pointed down a concrete lane beside a supermarket called the Friendly Price. "Everyone go and get beds on the beach," Sandra said. "I won't be long."

Ray wasn't about to leave her. He watched her hurry to the racks of sunblock, where she found the largest plastic jar of the strongest preparation and hesitated over taking just one to the till. The large slow woman behind the desk gave the item an indifferent blink, and then her gaze strayed to the jar protruding from Sandra's bag. "You want more," she said.

"We're staying for a few days yet. I'll have run out by then."

"No, more." The woman jabbed a stubby finger at the jar in the bag and then jerked her curved fingertips upwards. "More better," she said.

"Stronger, yes, that's right. I expect I'm getting more sensitive to the sun in my old age."

The woman's eyelids drooped so nearly shut that Ray could have imagined she was dreaming or about to dream. "How you feel?"

"Oh, nothing much. Certainly nothing worth worrying about."

This was addressed mostly to Ray, who would have responded if the woman at the desk hadn't spoken. "Say how."

"Just a bit of a headache if I look at the sun too much." Since the woman seemed as dissatisfied with this as Ray was afraid he should feel, Sandra said "And I have to drink a lot of water. Don't fret, Ray, it isn't sunstroke. Remember it's given me back my appetite as well."

Ray had the odd impression that the woman found this less positive than he did. "You not stay here," she said.

Ray couldn't help reacting as Julian would have. "We aren't, but why shouldn't we?"

"I say you stay somewhere else. Sunny – "

Of course she hadn't cut herself off; the last word was the end of the sentence. "Somewhere sunny all right when it is," Ray said. "The Sunny View."

"Sunset Beach not for you. Not you or little boy." She must have seen the family outside, but Ray found her alertness disconcerting. "Not wanted," she said as if she was anxious to make her point clearer. "Too small."

Sandra might have been defending William by saying "He's growing every moment."

"Maybe he comes back."

"Not if his parents have anything to do with it." When the woman seemed uncertain how to take this Ray added "Aren't we wanted round here either? If he's too young we're too old."

"You must ask."

Ray might have retorted that he just had, but he was growing tired of the clumsy conversation; in fact, he'd begun to feel too much like Julian. "Shall we head for the beach, then?" he said to

Sandra. "We don't want them worrying what's happened to us."

He ought to have stopped at the question. Once she'd paid he followed her out of the supermarket, which faced a shop called Happy Snappy across the lane. As well as cameras and every other photographic need he could have thought of, the shop displayed prints of holiday photographs. No doubt the shot of a young woman in a minimal bikini had caught a few eyes besides Ray's, but he'd begun to feel a little disloyal to Sandra until the photograph made him falter. It showed the girl standing beside the bearded shaggy-haired proprietor outside the shop, and so did the photograph next to it on the wall. The trouble was that although the proprietor had aged quite a few years in the second photograph, acquiring wrinkles and a profusion of grey hairs, the girl didn't look a day older.

Of course that was easily faked. The shots of her had been taken at the same time, and one had been patched into a more recent image of the proprietor. No doubt the pair of photographs was designed to sell Sunset Beach, though Ray thought it odd that whoever had assembled the second one hadn't touched up an imperfection: wasn't that a bite on the girl's left forearm? The proprietor was behind the counter, and watching Ray as though he found his interest questionable. If Sandra had been close enough Ray would have pointed out the photographs, but she was well on her way to the beach, and he felt worse than unfaithful for lingering over his thoughts. He was wasting time that they ought to be spending together.

He caught up with her between two blocks of holiday apartments. Perhaps the clatter of his sandals in the alley disturbed a late sleeper, because a slatted blind shifted at a window to let a face peer out – a young man who looked uncommonly pale for Greece, even given the overcast day. He blinked at the clouds without bothering to don an expression, and then he sank back out of sight, no doubt slumping on a bed. Presumably Ray was put in mind of a prisoner because the slats of the blind bore some resemblance to the bars of a cell.

Following Sandra out of the alley felt oddly unlike emerging into the open – more like entering an artificial forest than stepping onto a seashore. The outsize umbrellas were so close together that for large stretches of the beach the shade was virtually complete. The beach was busier than Ray had expected, and the most adventurous folk had lowered their umbrellas to woo the sun or at any rate the clouds. When William's frantic waving let Ray locate the family – Sandra seemed hampered by her glasses – he saw that they'd settled on sunbeds under a cluster of open umbrellas. "Here we are," the boy called as if his grandparents might need extra help.

Julian was lowering an umbrella, a process that brought him to all fours while he clicked the lock on the shaft into place, and Ray couldn't help recalling someone else who had crouched on the beach. He glanced around, not entirely without nervousness, but none of the supine figures in the unnecessary shade seemed familiar or about to leap up. As Julian scrambled to his feet, dusting his knees like a servant impatient with a task, he said "You two will want yours down, will you?"

"I wouldn't mind some shade," Sandra said.

As if she'd awaited the cue Jonquil said "I wouldn't either."

Julian looked defeated even before Tim said "There's three of us."

"Don't worry, Jules," Doug said. "You aren't the only sunny person here."

"We'll have some sun if we can find it," Pris agreed. "And the shady trinity can share an umbrella, can't you? They're big enough."

When Jonquil dragged her sunbed under the umbrella her grandparents had selected Ray felt bound to vacate his lounger, even though this separated him from Sandra. "You have this one, Tim."

As Pris stood up from lowering her family's umbrella Jonquil said "What were you buying, gran?"

"Jonquil."

"It's perfectly all right, Julian," Sandra said. "Just some stronger sun cream for my poor old skin."

"I wish I had some," Jonquil said.

Ray didn't know why he held his breath until Tim spoke. "And me."

"Well then, you both shall. Just let me get protected and then you can. Could someone do my back for me?"

Ray always had. He found it a chore – both putting cream on Sandra and the dull process of smearing it on himself – but now he felt guilty for begrudging any help he could give her, and he was about to undertake it when Jonquil did. Her method differed from his, though he couldn't make out how. While she didn't take long over her grandmother's back, she used as much cream as he would have, and yet it seemed to be more readily absorbed, as if Sandra's skin was greedy for moisture. She dealt with the rest of herself and then with Jonquil's back as the girl did with her cousin's, and Ray had an odd sense of watching a ritual. He was distracted by Pris, who said "Shall I get your back, Ray?"

"I was going to," Natalie said.

"You haven't lost it, Ray," Sandra declared. "You've still got women fighting over you."

He tried not to hear a prediction – a wish for his lonely future. After an awkward silence Pris said "You keep it in the family then, Nat."

Ray managed not to flinch as Natalie's hand chill with cream found the back of his neck. Once she returned the jar to him he set about coating his torso and limbs, a lengthier task than Sandra had needed. He was silently cursing the grains of sand that somehow always managed to invade the ointment when Natalie said "Who's for a swim?"

"Grandad isn't."

"Never mind, William." Since it was plain the boy still did, Ray said "Someone has to watch out for the things and take the photographs."

"What things?"

Ray was beginning to wonder how few words were safe to utter around William, especially when Julian frowned. "All the belongings everyone's leaving here," Ray said and felt as if he'd needed a translator.

William seized his parents' hands to speed up the treat. "Isn't Jonquil coming in?"

As though she was somehow responding Sandra said "I'll have a swim while I can."

Presumably she meant while the sky was overcast, but Ray doubted he was alone in taking her remark another way, though that couldn't have been why Jonquil said "We'll come with you, gran."

As they followed the others into the sea, not quite holding hands, Ray was disconcerted to notice what the trio had in common: now Sandra had a bite on her arm. He remembered seeing that arm on the quilt last night, and wished he'd known there was an insect in the room. Why hadn't it bitten him as well, or preferably instead? He watched her wade into the shallows and eventually reach enough depth for a swim, and managed to relax to some extent when she didn't wince as the salt water found her arm. Now he was supposed to be playing the photographer.

The camera was small enough to fit in the palm of his hand. For years he'd found it entirely convenient, but now he wondered if the screen that was its only viewfinder was too small for his ageing vision. Even when he shaded his eyes he had to strain to focus on Sandra, and defining Tim and Jonquil on the screen was just as hard. Perhaps the ripples that surrounded all of them made their outlines difficult to capture, especially at the limit of the zoom. He was zooming out as gradually as his infirm fingers could manage when he saw a woman with a swollen midriff approaching him along the beach.

She was pregnant just with cash. The bulge was a bag that matched her black dress. As Ray dug money out of the tangled mesh that was the pocket of his trunks she said "How many?"

"Just the three, thanks."

Her long face grew thinner still as she sucked her cheeks in. "How many are you?"

"Nine," Ray said, which he thought should be evident from the items on the sunbeds. "Everybody else is in the drink."

She seemed not to like this answer much. "Maybe you need more."

"I shouldn't think so, not with your jumbo umbrellas. Is there a reason they're so big?"

"Some people want."

"I can imagine why when there's so much drinking."

"Drinking," she said like an undefined question.

"That's what people come here for, isn't it?" The money he was holding out had begun to feel absurdly like a bid to close the subject. "I don't mean we did," he said. "We're away from all this."

"You come for peace." Before he could determine whether she was saying he would have it she said "Nine beds, twenty euros."

"And we're here for the sun as well."

"Wanting will not bring." As Ray wondered if she meant some other wish was more likely to come true she took the cash and pointed at the nearest taverna. "Show your ticket at Aegean Taste," she said, "and you don't pay that much."

Ray had a sense of returning to the everyday from somewhere he was altogether less sure of. He stuffed the receipt into his pocket and peered at the sea to locate Sandra and the rest of them among the swimmers. He was about to switch on the camera when the pallid red-haired chubby man on the next occupied sunbed rolled onto his stomach to squint sideways at him. "Isn't what you're looking for, eh?"

"Sorry." While he wasn't, Ray felt obliged to add "What is?"

"You said you were after the sun. So you never saw what it's like here online."

"My wife and I had a look, yes. I believe most of the family did."

"That's what I'm saying. What it's really like, that's not there." With a grin Ray found less than appropriate the man added "You'd wonder why nobody's said."

"Perhaps they're too happy with the rest of it. Anyway, I think my son did find some reference eventually."

"Good for him." The grin rendered this equivocal. "We're not complaining, us," the man said. "We won't burn for once."

Ray saw he was including his wife and teenage son, both of whom were as red-haired and pale. "How long have you been here?"

"Got in yesterday like the rest of them."

"I think you may find the sun builds up despite the clouds. Some of my family have." Ray didn't know why he was anxious to learn "The rest of whom?"

"All this lot except for yours," the man said, encompassing the shore with a loose gesture. "If they weren't on our plane they were on the ferry."

Ray met the grin, though his own felt uncertain. "You don't mean everybody on the beach."

"I reckon, don't you, Madge? Shall we give them a yell?"

"I'll do it." His wife took a breath that stretched her capacious swimsuit top to shout "Who's here that just got in?"

Ray saw hands and in some cases entire bodies raised on both sides of him – dozens of them. The response spread as people further off asked what the question was and then joined in, until he could have thought the entire beach was being roused from slumber. "What's the survey for?" someone called.

"Just seeing we were right," Madge told her. "Everyone's new here."

"The day shift," her husband said.

Ray glanced out to sea – he'd begun to find the beach unsettling – and saw Sandra and the teenagers heading inshore. "Excuse me," he said and fumbled with the camera. "I'm meant to be the official photographer."

As Sandra and the cousins rose from the sleepy waves he tried to capture all three of them, but it didn't work. Perhaps they were too widely spaced for him to focus on, or just at different distances from the lens, but concentrating on Sandra didn't solve the problem. Whenever her image came close to growing sharp the manual focus shifted to another subject – one or more of the family, or someone unrelated, or even just the waves. Ray switched to automatic focus, but this failed to do the job, catching hold of any item in the frame except her. Perhaps his eyes rather than the camera were at fault, and he was so desperate for it to display more competence than him that he raised a hand in the impolite Greek gesture to detain Sandra and her companions. He took shots of them separately and together and with the rest of their party in the background as well, trusting the camera to do its automatic best even if he couldn't judge how efficiently it was performing. When the three began to look uncomfortable he beckoned them onto the beach. "Did you take some good ones?" Sandra said, grabbing her hat before she sank onto the bed beneath the umbrella.

"I hope so. Maybe it's the light, but I've been having trouble focusing." Ray thought of stopping there but said "You weren't in as long as usual."

"I started feeling a bit odd." As Ray wondered how much he could ask her while Tim and Jonquil would hear, she said "Nothing to worry about. I felt a bit watery again, that was all."

"How do you mean?"

"Like William's word." Disconcertingly, this didn't come from Sandra. "Like you're made of water," Jonquil said.

"We mostly are, aren't we? Everybody is." This was Tim, who threw Ray even more by saying "I felt like that as well."

Sandra uncapped a litre of water and took quite a swig before offering Ray the bottle, by which time the teenagers were drinking from their own. What was wrong with that? You were advised to avoid dehydration when you were anywhere like Greece. Ray was swallowing a mouthful cold enough to make him shiver – surely this was all that did – when his red-headed neighbour said "You've never gone and got yourself a lovebite, son."

"How can he have?" Madge protested. "He's been with us."

The teenager's pale face turned variously red. "An insect got me while I was asleep," he muttered.

"Was that what all the moaning was about?" his father said. "Sounded like you were having one hell of a dream."

"About that girl who looked at me when we was having dinner," the boy said lower and more red-faced still.

"Just you keep her in your dreams and nowhere else," his mother said. "You don't know what you could catch round here."

"Mam," the boy complained, fingering his neck, and Ray could have thought the reference to infection had darkened the overcast day as if the shade in which Sandra and the teenagers were lying had reached for him. The woman's remark had brought the state of the corpse in the cave to mind, but at least he was glad that Julian and Natalie appeared to have abandoned looking for signs of an epidemic. As for himself, he'd never even begun. With every day that passed he seemed to have less room in his mind to be concerned with anything but Sandra.

★   ★   ★

"Yes, come in, all my friends. Welcome to Aegean Taste."

Their host was expansive in every sense. His midriff strained at his white shirt as if eager to advertise the taverna. His rounded brown face was as glossy as his raked black hair, and his wide blue eyes glistened just as much. "Everywhere for you, my friends," he said. "Sit where is good."

They were the first customers for lunch. Like its neighbours, the taverna boasted umbrellas as large as the ones on the beach. When Sandra and the teenagers headed for the shadiest, everyone else followed them. "You will drink," the manager said, which stopped barely short of an assumption. "Wine for you?"

"At least two soft drinks, please," Julian said.

"Eat too, my friends. Catch of day is special."

"Pris is mine," Doug took the chance to say.

As Ray and Sandra awarded this a sigh each Natalie said "Then Julian must be my catch."

Ray saw Jonquil find somewhere else to look. Not least in a bid to leave any awkwardness behind he said "Sandra's always been mine."

None of the adults seemed to know how vigorously they should react, and the youngsters were growing more embarrassed. Perhaps Jonquil meant to change the subject by saying "They never have one of the night."

William giggled, if a little tentatively. "What can you catch at night?"

"Nothing at all, I hope," Natalie said.

"That's right, William," Julian said and stared at Jonquil. "Nights are for sleeping and that's all."

The manager's return with a stack of menus came as a relief. "Everything for you, my friends," he said.

Though Ray felt abashed for finding him a little too effusive, he could have thought the man was sweating with the performance. Wasn't he just being hospitably Greek? There was surely no reason to think the effort was conscious, and Ray didn't really glimpse a hint of guilt as their host glanced at the most shaded of the tables, unless the man felt Vasilema had let down its visitors by failing to provide more sun. Everyone ordered the catch of the day, including William. "We take bones away for you," the manager told him.

Having met this with a giggle, the boy seemed uncertain until Natalie said "The gentleman's going to bone your fish."

"You don't like head, my friend?" When William shook his the manager said "We take that too."

Ray couldn't help recalling the corpse in the cave, and saw Julian was reminded as well. He felt as if his thoughts were lying in wait for him without emerging into the open, and made a bid to quash them. "Here's something odd," he said. "Everybody on the beach has only just arrived."

"Now, Ray," Sandra said more mildly than he thought was called for. "How can you know that?"

"Someone asked and they all said they were."

"If you say so," Julian said, "but you'll forgive me, what's the significance?"

It seemed important to answer this, and Ray was struggling to think when Julian frowned at the beach. "Is that that fellow?"

"Who?" Jonquil said but didn't look.

"Not your follower. I've been keeping my eyes open for him, never fear. What's the fellow's name," Julian said more like a protest than a question. "The guide."

Natalie was on her feet. "Jamie," she said.

As Ray located him Jamie caught sight of them all. He was wearing shorts and an open shirt that revealed he hadn't bothered bleaching his chest hair. He glanced aside at once, fingering his lips to mime being overtaken by a thought, and turned away to retreat along the beach. "One moment, James," Julian called, and louder "James."

Perhaps Jamie didn't like this version of his name, since he kept on without looking back. At least he wasn't walking much faster than Ray, who followed Natalie and Julian to hear what might be said. "Jamie, hold on," Natalie shouted loud enough to raise the heads of a dozen sunbathers or whatever they'd be named at Sunset Beach.

This time Jamie had to turn, although Ray thought he briefly put on speed. By the time the guide faced the three of them he'd adopted a professional smile that seemed eager to suggest he hadn't previously noticed them. "Hi there again," he cried. "How's all the family? Having the time of your lives?"

"We're glad we came," Natalie said. "You remember us, then."

"I remember every last one of my clients." Perhaps Jamie decided this was too large a claim, because his smile wobbled for a moment. "Remind me where we met again," he said.

"We were on your cruise around the island."

"You were lucky with your day. We've had to cancel some trips since." With what Ray could have thought was haste Jamie added "Of course, your son was the clever little chap."

"He's the pride of the family," Julian said. "You'll remember you took us to your beach by the cave."

"I don't think we actually took you there. You can say we passed it if you want."

"We can say you were the reason we knew it was there. I assume you'll have heard we made our own way to it and what Mr Thornton and I found in the cave."

"Oh." Jamie seemed uncertain how the exclamation ought to sound. "That was you," he said.

"I should have thought you'd know that." When Jamie met this with a silence Ray would have called sulky if not adolescent, Julian said "What else have you heard?"

"I can't make out what you want to know."

"What happened to the man we found. Your client Mr Ditton."

"I knew who you meant." Ray was afraid Julian had antagonised Jamie beyond answering until he said "The poor guy drowned."

"There's more to it than that," Ray objected. "He wasn't even your age. I'm no swimmer, but I take it he was. How did he come to be drowned?"

"Some kind of attack." As though someone had misinterpreted him Jamie said "I'm not saying he was attacked. He had one in the water."

"At his age?" Natalie said. "Did he have a history of them?"

Ray could have thought he saw Jamie consider the notion before glancing around and lowering his voice. "I believe it may have been some kind of drug he took. I don't mean medication."

"What leads you to believe that?" Julian said.

"What else is it going to be?" When nobody supplied the answer Jamie said "Who else except the police?"

"I can't see how drugs explain the state he was in."

With a grimace that quivered his chubby cheeks Jamie muttered "It'd be the fish."

"Fish," Natalie said.

"Them and crabs and everything." Jamie waved his hands as if an unpleasant object had stuck to them. "If a body's in the sea it attracts them," he said, "and then, well, you two know what then."

Ray couldn't have said why he felt a trick had been played, and perhaps not the first one. He was trying to grasp the impression when Julian said "Will you give us your word that his condition wasn't infectious?"

Jamie's mouth appeared to be deliberating its shape. "My word."

"That still means something to some of us. Your word of honour."

"I'll swear on my grandmother's grave if you like. She brought me up a lot more than my mother did." Since this went some way towards impressing Julian, Jamie said "I'm swearing he couldn't infect anyone, because I know it's true."

"Well," Julian said to Natalie, "that improves the holiday, I think."

As she nodded Doug called "Here's lunch."

"Fish," Natalie remembered, and Ray saw a thought assail her. Then her eyes cleared, and she shook her head as though to evict the idea. "I need to stop being so ridiculous," she said. "How many fish are there in the sea? If I say anything else to spoil the holiday, dad, you tell me."

"You haven't spoiled a thing, and I'm sure your mother doesn't think so."

"Everything's hunky now, is it?" Jamie said without lingering for a response. "Have a splendiferous rest of your stay."

As Ray followed Julian and Natalie into the taverna Sandra said "What was all that about?"

Despite frowning at William, Julian seemed to feel bound to answer. "Ditton," he said. "No disease involved."

"I expect that's a relief."

Ray saw it ought to be and couldn't understand why he should demur. He was additionally troubled by feeling that Jamie's farewell had been as overstated as the welcome to Aegean Taste. He mustn't let his doubts show in case Natalie thought he was hesitating over the food. In fact the grilled fish was delicious, and he was heartened to see Sandra making a meal of hers along with digging into one of the communal bowls of Greek salad. He was poking his fork between the ribs of his fish to extract the last morsels before he consigned the skeleton to a plate heaped with bones and dead-eyed heads when he noticed someone striding along the beach.

Not just his robes made the man look out of place. The closer he approached, the darker his face seemed to grow. It was framed, not to say obscured, by hair as black as his cylindrical hat and his vestments — a fierce beard joined to a thick moustache and to sideboards that led to the pelt on his scalp. His boots kicked up sand that glittered on his trouser cuffs and the hem of his priestly costume. Ray thought the priest was clicking his teeth in case the glares he sent the occupants of sunbeds weren't sufficiently censorious, and then he saw that the sound came from a string of beads that dangled from the man's right hand. The priest continued thumbing them along the string while he stalked past the taverna, and the judgmental head swung towards the diners. As his glare found Sandra and the teenagers he raised his hand to click the beads at them. "Go back," he said.

His voice was unexpectedly thin and shrill. Before anybody could respond he strode onwards. Sandra and the cousins blinked at one another like sleepers not quite wakened, and seemed content to stay bemused by the incident until Ray stood up, almost flooring his chair. "Don't make a fuss," Sandra pleaded. "It doesn't matter."

"I'll see if it does," Ray said and tramped onto the beach.

He wasn't about to waste any breath in shouting after the man. The soft sand was enough of a hindrance, and his legs were aching by the time he managed to catch up with the priest and, thanks to an effort that left him breathless, overtake him. "Wait there," he gasped. "What did you, say to my, wife and our, grandchildren? What do you, mean by it?"

The priest had halted. Otherwise Ray would have been unable to keep up with him, let alone speak. He glared at Ray, and then his gaze softened, which Ray found no more appealing. It made him feel pitied, especially when the priest shook his head without speaking. "What exactly were you telling them to do?" Ray said, having recaptured his breath. "I know you understand me. You speak English."

How much like Julian did he sound? Just now he didn't care. The priest's gaze had grown softer still, but not in any reassuring sense. Compared to the expression he'd turned on the users of the sunbeds it looked enfeebled, and Ray was trying to define it more precisely when the priest said "Go back."

"You're saying that to them or you're saying it to me?" Ray's skull had begun to throb with frustration. "Go back where?" he begged.

The priest had already turned away, and now he recommenced his patrol of the beach. Ray might have followed him if he could have thought of more to ask, but he'd been thrown not just by the man's words but by his voice. This time it had been as deep as he would have expected a Greek priest's to sound. As he watched the man stride away he didn't know whether he was reminded of a thwarted child kicking up sand or somebody trying to uncover a burial. His thoughts in disarray, he trudged back to the taverna. "Did you get any sense from the fellow?" Julian said.

"I couldn't really make him out."

"I expect he thought we weren't as bad as everybody else," Doug said, "because we're only dining."

"That'll be it," Pris said. "We can still be saved."

Ray felt this was no more helpful than her laugh, but what else could he have said about the priest? Once Julian worked out the bill Doug left a bigger tip than Julian had at the previous meal, and Ray told himself the contest was harmless enough. Back on the beach he felt as though the priest had left him with a secret he couldn't define to himself, which might have involved the pallid overcast somehow if not the hundreds of people around him. However large that made it seem, he couldn't let it distract him from Sandra, however much it kept trying. It didn't even stay behind when at last they left the beach.

The sight of the Happy Snappy shop at the end of the lane was unexpectedly welcome. At least it gave Ray something to point out to the family, and he was about to speak when he saw that the first shot of the girl in a bikini had been replaced by a crimson sunset over the beach. "Where's the other photograph?" he blurted.

The proprietor was counting notes into a drawer of the till. Ray had to wait for him to look up, and then he seemed not to have heard the question. "The other photograph," Ray said and pointed at the wall.

The man rubbed his scalp as if he wanted to erase the grey that had invaded it. "No other."

"Yes, of you and that girl up there, only years ago."

"Too old. No use now," the man said as though he meant himself.

"You seemed to think it was before." When this gained no response Ray said "Could I just show it to my family?"

"No use," the man said and stared at Ray so hard his eyes grew blank. "Gone."

Ray felt exhausted and defeated. As he gestured everyone out of the shop Sandra murmured "What was all that about?"

"It was just a trick," Ray said, not knowing if he meant the photograph. Until he was thwarted he hadn't realised how much he wanted to show it to the family. It left him with a sense that he needed to confront at least the adults with something else, though he didn't know what or why. The impression felt like a shadow he couldn't shake off as he followed them to the bus stop.

THE TENTH DAY 29 AUGUST

A knock at the door of the apartment wakened Ray. "It's only me," Natalie called.

He was still sufficiently asleep to wonder who else it might have been and whether she felt bound to reassure him. Had something almost roused him earlier? He seemed to recall having heard a cry, unless that had been a dream. He was trying to grasp the impression when Natalie knocked louder. "Mum, dad? Are you awake?"

"I am," Ray said, and at once he violently was, having realised that Sandra had failed to respond. She was lying face up, and the quilt over her breasts didn't stir. Her right arm lay upturned on the quilt, and her limp hand appeared to be reaching out, away from him. Was the mark on her arm redder than it had been? He leaned across her to finger it, but there was no blood. Her face winced, tugging at the corner of her mouth, and she mumbled "Are you here again?"

"I'm always here," he protested, feeling not far from rebuffed. "It's Ray."

"Oh, Ray." Her eyes struggled open and found him. "I must have been very asleep," she said. "I thought you were someone else."

Ray had never been jealous in all their years of marriage, but now he felt he was for asking "Who?"

"I don't know." She clearly thought Ray was being as unreasonable as he felt. "I never see him," she said.

His mind was clamouring with questions, but they would have to wait. "Natalie's outside. I'd better see what she wants."

He limped quickly though not straight to the door and poked his head around it to find Natalie drumming on her pursed lips with a finger, the way she had before she'd even started school. "Sorry if I got you out of bed," she told him.

"We don't want to waste the day." As he saw her remember how little time might be left to her mother he hastened to ask "What's brought you up here?"

"We were wondering if you'd mind another trip on the road train. William would like one."

"Then I'm sure I would," Sandra called.

"It's a guided tour. Doug and Pris are in favour. The only thing is it leaves in an hour."

"I'm on my way," Sandra declared and shut herself in the bathroom. "Take the bread out of the fridge, Ray," she called.

He might have liked her not to be in quite such a hurry. He found a plate for yesterday's bread and then stood in front of the closed door. "What do you mean, you never see him?"

"I don't think I meant anything very much."

"Then can you tell me however much you did?"

"It was only a dream, Ray."

"You said never. You must have had it more than once."

"Just a couple of times, I think."

"Are you going to tell me what you dream?"

"Don't be upset, will you? We can't choose what we dream. It's only what the night sets free." She might have been awaiting some response from him before she said "Somebody came to me in the dark and gave me a kiss, that was all."

As Ray told himself that she wasn't responsible for the dream she opened the door and gazed into his eyes. Perhaps she was saddened by what she saw, because she took both of his hands. "I dreamed," she said, "he gave me some more life."

Ray wasn't sure what point there was to asking "How?"

"It was just my feeling in the dream. You know what it must be really, don't you? How our holiday with everyone has made me feel."

He couldn't argue with that, and yet when she withdrew into the bathroom he felt as though he'd left the issue uninvestigated. There was something else he'd neglected to examine, but he had time now. He pulled the drawer out of the bedside table and set it on the bed.

More than a day didn't seem to have done the remains of the book much good. He'd put them in the drawer for fear of waking Sandra, but in the morning he'd slipped a folded towel under them in case that helped. He couldn't tell whether it had. Most of the scraps of paper had stuck together in several wads, and as he set about peeling them apart he found that print had seeped through, blurring words. Many of the fragments had to be smoothed out as well, and the first of these was all that remained of the contents page, from which he saw that the only chapter concerned with Vasilema was the one he'd partly read.

As he separated the fragments he saw that they dealt with other islands: Crete, Zakynthos, Kefalonia, Kos... Hadn't he rescued anything about Vasilema? Yes, here was a jagged section of the first page of that chapter, which only made him anxious to find more. He'd coaxed almost all the damp wads apart, and his fingernail felt clogged with sodden pulp, by the time he identified another relevant fragment. It was torn from corner to corner, but an intact sentence caught his eye. They feed so Skiá feeds.

He was trying to imagine how the sentences above it might have been completed when Sandra came out of the bathroom. "You haven't time for that now, Ray," she said. "We don't want to disappoint William."

As Ray returned the scraps of paper to the drawer he saw

they'd left faint stains on the quilt, as if an ill-defined shape had been lying next to him. By the time he left the bathroom Sandra had arranged breakfast on the balcony – coffee, bread, salt, olive oil. He'd grown almost used to her wearing her hat and sunglasses in the shade. He was more concerned that she ate, and was heartened by her appetite. She was finishing the last crusty hunk of bread when Julian called "Five minutes, everyone."

They met in the play area, where Ray could have fancied that the faces on the equipment were grinning at a secret. The youngsters were being kept ignorant about their grandmother – that was where his sense of the unspoken came from. The silence seemed to grow more awkward as everybody crossed the courtyard of the Sunny View, until Julian said "What do you have to say, William?"

"I'm sorry if I woke anybody up."

"Your mummy did that," Sandra said. "Not that we're complaining."

"No, in the night. When I made a fuss."

"I wondered if I heard something," Ray said. "What was wrong, William?"

"I saw someone in our room."

"You didn't quite say that, did you? Tell grandma and grandad what you told us." When the boy looked embarrassed if not nervous Natalie prompted "Not in the room, in…"

"He was in the room." Just as stubbornly William said "Then he went in the window."

"Explain to everybody what you mean," Julian said.

"I expect you're saying he went out of it, are you?" Sandra said. "But we know it must have been a dream. I had one last night too."

Ray was hoping she wouldn't describe it when William said "It wasn't, gran."

"That's all it could have been." With dwindling patience

Julian said "You still have to say what you mean by going in the window."

"Like in the church. The pictures in the glass."

"Stained glass, do you mean?" Once the boy nodded Ray said "That's a dream if I ever heard one, William. Real people can't go inside glass."

"He did, and he was watching Jonquil. Then he sank."

"What do you mean," Julian objected, "sank?"

"Like the window was water, and then he wasn't there any more."

"And you don't think that was a dream?" When William was silent Julian said "Tell everybody who you thought he was."

"The man Jonquil was dancing with by the fire."

"Stop it, William," Jonquil said. "You know he couldn't have got in our room."

Julian turned from frowning at the Paradise Apartments to stare, but not at William. "Is he getting on your nerves? Then I hope you're satisfied."

Her voice took on more of an edge. "Why are you saying that?"

"Because I don't think there's any question who's responsible for William having these dreams."

"I don't think so either," Natalie said.

"Then we're in agreement, which is as it should be," Julian said and looked askance at her sigh. "Isn't that the case?"

"Julian, I wish occasionally you'd listen to someone besides yourself. I think you're giving William these dreams."

"Perhaps you'd care to explain how," Julian said and sucked his lips in to rid them of their pout.

"You've been harping on about Jonquil's boyfriend for days now. You even did it at the beach."

"He's not my boyfriend," Jonquil protested, though Ray thought he heard a hint of nervousness. "I've got one at home."

"All I'm saying," Natalie said, "is I'm surprised you aren't having dreams like William."

If Jonquil meant to speak, Julian didn't wait for her. "Any other complaints while I'm in the firing line?"

"You might like to remember we aren't just proud of William."

"I'm not aware of having said that was the case."

"You don't have to say, but you know you did. You told Jamie yesterday he was the pride of the family. As far as I'm concerned my daughter is as well."

"Don't you mean our daughter?"

Ray thought several people were suppressing their answers, but Sandra murmured "Do you want to say anything, Jonquil?"

"I try to be."

"Appreciated," Julian said. "I hope that's mutual."

Ray was on the edge of urging both of them to say more when William said "It isn't daddy's fault."

"I never said it was," Jonquil protested.

"Mummy did. It isn't fair."

"William, what I was actually saying – "

"You said daddy made me see the man in our room. Daddy didn't bring him there. I don't know who did."

Before Ray could judge how much the boy was striving to defend his father Julian said "William, would you prefer not to go on the train?"

"No, daddy," William said in dismay.

"Then kindly stop this nonsense. Everybody's had their fill of it. The train is to help you to forget all about it," Julian said and strode so fast towards the road train waiting in the square that he might have been determined to leave behind anybody's chance to speak. A few passengers were already seated in the open carriages, and their presence would inhibit any discussion of the kind the family had had or almost had. All the same,

Ray heard Julian mutter to Natalie "If it needs to be dealt with tonight I promise you I will."

★　　★　　★

As the train set off, the guide with the microphone introduced herself as Irene and the driver as Mikos in English and German and French. Her English was enthusiastic if somewhat ramshackle, which Ray suspected was the case with the other languages as well. By the time she finished speaking in them she hardly paused before starting the next section of her commentary in English. At least this helped to make it less apparent that Natalie and Julian had little to say to each other and were being ponderously polite. If their silences hadn't been infectious Ray might have pointed out that Irene was concentrating on the landscape the train was passing through – olive groves, depleted streams, hills decorated with goats – while neglecting the history of the island. He could have felt that the unspoken was an unacknowledged passenger on the train, and very close to him.

Might William lose interest in the ride when it was accompanied by so much language that he didn't understand? At least whenever it passed through a village he devoted himself to waving at everybody in the narrow convoluted streets. When the family joined in Ray thought William's parents were trying to outdo each other, which made them look as if they'd reverted to their son's age. William appeared to have communicated his zest to the villagers, who waved with such vigour that they might have been greeting royalty if not someone even more important to them.

The first stop on the outing was a vineyard. Once Irene had talked all three nationalities through the processes of making wine and raki, everyone had a chance to sample them. William seemed happy to be given a large bunch of grapes after Natalie had washed them at a sink. "Try some if you like," she told Jonquil, indicating the queue for drinks, and Julian said nothing at all. "Drink enough and you will sleep tonight," Irene told the girl, and Ray hoped William would do the latter.

Next on the tour was a ceramics factory. Russet jugs and varicoloured vases occupied a multitude of shelves, and Ray had never seen so many pottery depictions of the sun, ranging from red to a white that looked less radiant than drained of colour. Quite a few had faces, and of course their smiles couldn't seem anything other than fixed. A potter demonstrated shaping a vase and delighted William by letting him help with another, though the man was less successful at showing how to make a sun. He appeared to be distracted by more than one member of the audience — Ray couldn't tell who. The rays of the ceramic sun might have been the violent spikes of an explosion, while the smile the potter gouged wasn't too far from a grimace. "No good anyway," the man declared, crumpling the clay into a shapeless lump.

The excursion moved on to an embroidery workshop, where Ray was disconcerted to observe how many of the patterns resembled elaborate cobwebs. Had this been the case in Vasilema Town? When William said "Spiders" Ray thought he was being fanciful until he saw the boy didn't need to be. Any number of the intricate white cloths pinned to the walls were hiding spiders in their designs, as if the creatures were so inextricable from their webs that they could hardly be distinguished from them. "Why the spiders?" Doug asked the guide.

"They are emblem."

"An emblem of what?" Pris said.

"Our island."

"In that case," Julian said, "I'm surprised it isn't on a flag."

"It is to see when you are here."

"It might put people off coming, you mean?" Pris said.

Before Irene could answer, though she seemed uncertain how to, William said "Is it what the saint killed?"

The guide bowed her head as if to bring it closer to his meaning. "Saint, you say."

"St Titus," Doug said. "Will thinks we saw pictures of him fighting spiders."

"Or something like them," Pris said.

"Something." As Ray took this for a species of agreement Irene said "It has to be legend. He would not come back."

"No fight." This was contributed by a woman at a loom, whose black dress put Ray in mind of the priest on the beach. "Too much past now," she said.

"There you are, William," Julian said as Ray thought of asking Irene what either woman meant. "It was just a story, an old legend."

Ray supposed it was better for William to be concerned with this rather than his dream. Or could one have led to the other – the carvings on the trees by the path to the cave helping to inflame his imagination? Ray had lost the chance to question Irene, who was speaking to a solitary German couple in their language. He could have thought she was relieved to say "When we are all ready it is time for lunch."

They ate at a taverna next to a miniature waterfall and encircled by the stream it fed. The glade set with tables could have been the garden of the small house next to the taverna. The trees across the stream were as vitally green as the forest near the monastery of St Titus was black. A brawny woman welcomed everyone with sweeping gestures of her muscular bare arms, and brought brimming jugs of water to the tables. "Water your friend," she told William.

When he giggled at whatever he thought she meant she gave him a stern look and indicated how the stream surrounded them. "Water," she insisted. "Friend for life."

Ray thought Pris was saving the boy from any further misinterpretation as she said "Everyone's so friendly here."

"We need."

"That's your way, isn't it?" Doug was determined not to be puzzled by her response. "That's Greek," he said.

"Our way," the woman said and glanced at Sandra and the teenagers, who'd sat in the shade of several trees. "Yes."

She was moving away when Julian said "May we see the menu?"

"No menu. Freshest fish. You catch, we cook."

A wire mesh dammed an outlet from a large pool at the lowest section of the stream, trapping at least a dozen fish. Nets on poles lay on the stone rim of the pool. "Maybe boy don't like," she conceded. "I tell you other food."

"I like fish," William protested.

"Good boy. Grow up fine man," the woman said, ruffling his hair.

"We're a fine family," Julian said and nodded at Jonquil. "Both of them."

William was the first to pick up a net, and just as eager to wield it. "You can choose mine for me, Ray," Sandra said.

"Someone get mine too," Tim said, and Jonquil added "Please for me as well."

Ray caught their host sending all three a doubtful look. If they were comfortable where they were, he didn't see the problem, and why should he compound the anxiety that had become his constant companion? He watched William net a struggling fish, which the brawny woman took to the kitchen. Soon everybody's lunch was caught, and she brought out bowls of salad. "Do you live here, then?" Doug took the chance to ask.

"All the year."

"With your family?" When her gesture identified them as the waiter and the chef at the grill, Doug said "Doesn't it get lonely in the winter, all the same?"

"No visitors," the woman said, swinging her hand in a wide circle. "No problem."

Before long she and her son brought the grilled fish. Ray thought William might be dismayed by the blind head of his, but the boy seemed untroubled. "It's different now," he said calmly enough.

"That's because they've made it delicious for you," Sandra said, having sampled hers.

"It's dead," William declared as if this needed to be made plain. "It can't move any more."

"Of course it can't," Natalie said as she set about stripping the flesh from the bones for him. "Nothing can then, William."

Was the boy doing his best to look convinced? At least he seemed to enjoy his meal, even if he didn't match Sandra and the cousins for voraciousness. Ray kept growing aware of the perpetual monologue of the waterfall, which sounded like a meditation on endlessness. Despite its lack of words he could easily have fancied that it had some message for him, especially given their host's farewell to her English guests. "Water is good," she said with some force.

"Better than good," Pris said. "It's the best we've had."

Did Ray glimpse frustration in the woman's eyes? As Sandra and the teenagers stood up she gazed at them. "You remember."

"We do," Sandra assured her. "We make sure we don't get dehydrated."

This time Ray was sure she looked misunderstood. "Thank you," Sandra said as the woman turned to the German couple, but she didn't glance back. As the train left the taverna behind, the staff moved together to watch from just inside the watery boundary, and Ray wondered how often they crossed the stream. For an instant he felt close to grasping some point that the woman had tried to convey, and then it was gone.

Soon the train stopped at an olive oil factory. Irene showed everyone the massive old stone wheel that had been turned by four men or a quartet of donkeys, and then she led her party inside the factory for an extended look at the hydraulic equipment now in use. There were varieties of oil to sample, and Sandra might have been competing with Tim and Jonquil to prove who could dip the most bread. When Irene mentioned that olives were harvested in November, Doug said "What else happens in the winter? We've often thought we'd like to retire to an island like yours."

"I do not think so. You would find dead."

"It can't be as dead as all that, can it?" Pris objected. "Don't some places stay open for the locals?"

"Just enough to feed."

"That's enough then, isn't it? What else do you do till the spring?"

"Wait for sun."

"You'd have to do a lot of that round here." When this fell short of amusing her Doug said "There must be something to keep you on the island."

Irene looked away from him and indicated all the tourists. "We wait for you to come."

"That's hardly an activity, is it?" Julian said. "I believe Douglas was asking how you occupy yourselves."

"We are occupied," Irene said, turning back to Doug and Pris. "You would not want to be here. There is much dark."

"I should think Christmas is special," Pris insisted.

"The child is born to die and rise again."

"That's what it's all about," Doug said, if a little uncertainly. "My wife was asking how you celebrate."

"All we can for the dark."

Ray thought Doug was growing as frustrated as Julian visibly was. "It's related to that, isn't it?" Doug was determined to establish. "Christmas is, I mean. A way to remind us the light always comes back even when it's darkest."

"We have the darkest day."

To Ray this sounded like a grotesque boast, but perhaps Pris understood. "You mean you have another tradition."

"We light the fires. Fires to St Titus."

"Like the one we saw the other night, you mean."

"Not so much like. Fires, nothing else. They bring light but they don't bring sun." With a partial smile that looked not merely wry but half-hearted Irene said "Just more legends people can't let go. Fairy tales so children aren't afraid."

Ray assumed she meant superstitious folk. "St Titus again," he said. "His monastery, that must be the darkest place."

"What makes you say?"

"We've been there."

"But there is nothing to see." Irene might have been resolved if not anxious to persuade them. "Just dark," she said.

"There's plenty of that." As he saw her start to turn away he blurted "Don't people still live there, though?"

Julian scowled at him and jerked his head at William. By the time Natalie distracted the boy with chatter Irene had yet to respond. In case she was using William as an excuse for silence Ray murmured "I saw one."

"First we've heard," Doug objected.

"Are you sure, Ray?" Pris said too gently for his taste.

"Yes," Ray said and held Irene's gaze. "I am."

"Some of our oldest went there. It is a refuge always. Nowhere else for them." As Pris and Doug and Ray hindered one another with attempted questions she said "Now I must talk to my other guests." All the same, she lingered to add "We are happy when you come to our island."

Was this some form of apology for attempting to put Doug and Pris off? Ray gathered that was how they took it, and couldn't think what other interpretation there might be. "So what are you saying you saw, dad?" Doug said.

"Better not discuss it while William's around." Ray found he had too many incomplete thoughts to put in order if he could, but he was disconcerted to be using his grandson as a pretext. "We'll talk about it later," he said and felt as if he weren't admitting why he wanted to delay that, even to himself.

★   ★   ★

When they all heard a second splintering crash from a house opposite Chloe's Garden, Natalie gave William a worried look. "What's happening over there?"

"Nothing bad. It is his birthday," Chloe's daughter Daphne said.

"Happy birthday to him, then," Natalie said as if she were reassuring William. "How old is the birthday boy?"

"He is forty."

"I didn't think you did that any more," Doug said as they heard another item shatter.

"We break plates sometimes. We are Greek."

"No, I mean I thought you only celebrated children's birthdays. And your name day when you're his sort of age."

"We have the fun we can," Daphne said with an odd hint of defiance. "It is natural."

"I suppose nothing's more natural than growing old," Sandra said.

Natalie reached for her mother's hand as if she didn't trust herself to speak, and Ray saw Tim and Jonquil wonder why. Perhaps Pris intended to distract them by raising her glass towards the house across the road and calling "Hronia polla."

"Polyhronos," Doug shouted.

Daphne's eyes winced shut, and she shook her head. "We do not say that here."

"What aren't they meant to say?" Julian enquired.

"Live many years, apparently," Pris told him.

"Or live a thousand years," Doug said.

"Didn't somebody say something like that to us, Ray?" Sandra said.

As Natalie clasped her mother's hand with both of hers Daphne said "It is not the same. You are not from our island."

"I've no idea what difference that's supposed to make," Julian said.

"For you it is just a wish."

Jonquil was watching her mother and grandmother. Before anyone could answer Daphne the girl said "What's wrong?"

"Not a thing, Jonquil," Sandra said. "Really nothing at all, honestly."

Ray thought these were several words too many. "We've both been thinking something was," Tim said.

Natalie seemed unsure where to look, except not at William. "We weren't aware there had been any discussion," Julian objected, "and there's no need for any more."

"Gran ought to say," Tim said.

"Thank you both for caring. Nobody should tell you off for that. If anything was wrong," Sandra said, "it isn't worth bothering about any more, truly. Now I think Julian's right and we can put it to bed."

Ray saw that Jonquil wasn't entirely won over, and he thought Pris was trying to create another diversion. "If it's not a wish for you," she said to Daphne, "what is it, then?"

"More like a curse," Daphne said and glanced at the dim road, where nothing moved except the scrawny elongated limbs of the shadow of the spider in its web. "I will bring your drinks."

As she retreated, having scribbled down their food orders as well, Sandra said "I think I could live with that kind of curse."

Ray was hoping Tim and Jonquil couldn't sense how the

adults were suppressing their reactions when Doug said "Here comes somebody we know."

Neither of the cousins followed his gaze. Ray did, and saw the mute seller of trinkets approaching from the direction of the bridge. Might she have another copy of the book she'd given him? He pulled out a twenty-euro note and flourished it at her. Although she must have seen, she swung around as if she hadn't and tramped back the way she'd come. "Just a tick," Ray called. "Hang on."

"Ray," Sandra murmured. "She can't hear, can she?"

"She can see well enough," he said, pushing back his chair.

"Ray," Sandra protested more vehemently, but he hadn't time to make her understand. He ran out of the taverna and after the woman. If she couldn't hear his flapping sandaled footsteps he ought not to startle her, and so he was keeping to the opposite side of the road as he made to overtake her when his shadow did. She twisted around so fast that her bag thumped her hip. "It's all right," Ray said, though he felt absurd for speaking in a language she might not even know. "It's only me."

Presumably she saw that, even if it didn't seem to reassure her much. She held her cupped hands out to him, though only just, which he assumed was meant for a question. "The book you gave me," Ray said and saw from her eyes that she didn't understand, or could their blankness mean she was determined not to admit she did? He wasn't here to investigate how genuine her deafness was. He pointed at her bag and used both hands to mime pulling if not wrenching it wide.

How much like a bully did he look, if not a robber? She opened the capacious bag readily enough, but Ray had to crane over it to be certain in the dim light from the nearest streetlamp that none of the many items it contained was a book. He stuffed the note he was clutching back into his pocket and saw her face stay blank. No doubt she was used to that kind of rebuff, and Ray had to make her understand. "Book," he said. "Book."

He'd no business condemning Julian's impatience over language when he was behaving worse. He patted the air in front of the woman as if he were playing charades, and then indicated her with both hands before turning them upwards and cupping them towards himself vigorously enough to make his fingers twinge. He wished he'd learned signing, though would it be the same in Greece? He shook his head several times in the hope of conveying that he didn't want any items from her bag, and then held his folded hands in front of his face. He meant them to signify a book as he opened them while pressing their sides together, but might they look as though he had been praying or was now releasing some creature they'd trapped? He held out the left one and traced lines on the palm with his forefinger while he pored over the pretence of sentences. "Book," he said and stared at her in some desperation. "Book."

She nodded once, which surely meant she understood. Ray raised his fists and shook them, intending to communicate triumph, and then he showed her the backs of his hands as a kind of punctuation, a sign that he hadn't finished. How could he ask the question? He held out his hands with the fingers splayed and lifted his shoulders in an extravagant shrug and cocked his head on one side while widening his eyes and distorting the rest of his features into an interrogative grimace so fierce that his brows ached. "Why?" he didn't say but only mouthed, "why me?" and jerked all his fingers at himself.

He saw her grasp his meaning before her face reverted to illegibility. At first he thought she had no answer or refused to have one, and then she held up her right hand, bending the little finger against the palm to pin it with the thumb. Ray couldn't see what she was trying to communicate until she brandished the remaining fingers and then pointed them at the taverna, by which time he didn't know how much he cared to understand. "Three of what?" he demanded, feeling not just stupid but wilfully so. "Which three?"

He was dismayed to realise that he might have liked her not to comprehend, but she did. She nodded at the taverna, and was waiting for him to look when her gaze strayed past Chloe's Garden, along the road. Her hand sprang open and quivered while her mouth gaped as though straining to utter a cry. Ray turned so hastily to see what she was seeing that he almost fell.

Three figures stood beyond Chloe's Garden and the Sunny View, at the mouth of the alley under the streetlamp. Had she been pointing at them all the time? They were too distant for Ray to make out their faces or anything else of significance about them, and he might almost have been able to believe that nothing was wrong with the sight of them. Then a cat dashed out of the alley and fled together with its shadow across the road, and Ray saw what he ought to have noticed. The shadows of the figures were at least twice the length they should be, extending up the road as though in search of prey. As his pulse swelled in his ears his vision blurred, so that he couldn't be certain whether, even if the figures were staying utterly still, their shadows had begun to merge into a single mass of blackness.

He heard a clatter of footsteps behind him, and blinked his eyes clear barely in time to watch the mute woman disappear past the bend in the road. He swung around again to find that the road beyond the Sunny View was deserted apart from the dancing shadow of the spider. As he trudged back to Chloe's Garden he saw all the diners watching him, though quite a few turned away to pretend they hadn't been. Several of the family seemed to want to speak, and Doug was first. "Dad, what did you do to her?"

"I didn't do anything. I was just trying to make myself understood."

"Is that why she ran away?" Pris said with a tentative laugh.

"That wasn't my doing. Didn't you see?"

"See what?" Natalie said as if she mightn't want to know.

He mustn't unnerve William, especially since he was growing less sure what he'd seen. "That I didn't make her run," he said.

"If you say so," Doug said, "but what did you want from her?"

"Just to find out if she had another copy of that book."

"Maybe you can find it online. Shall I look?"

"I think I'm still capable, son," Ray said, not least because he felt slow for having failed to think of searching. He took out his phone and found nothing at all – no copies of *History of Greece Islands* for sale, and not a single reference to the book or its author. Though Ray had seen it was self-published, he wouldn't have expected it to be quite so unremarked. He could have fancied that every trace of it had been erased from the web.

"Let me try," Doug said, and Ray did his best not to feel patronised. As he watched Doug search he was aware of the darkness beyond the dim road, and felt as if the light of the phone were a feeble bid to hold it back. Before long Doug admitted defeat too. "Never mind," Ray said but did, which made him anxious to examine whatever was left of the book. Perhaps that was why he was on edge, though whenever he glanced along the road the scrawny restlessness turned out to belong to the shadow of the spider.

Once everyone had said goodnight while the faces watching from the playground grinned at them, he laboured upstairs after Sandra. She was inside the apartment by the time he reached it, and he might have thought she was eager for bed if not for making love. Just the same, he pulled out the drawer of the bedside table. "Do you mind if I finish sorting through all this?"

"Why is it so important to you, Ray?"

"I just want to see what I've managed to save. I'll do it outside if you like."

"I'll be in bed if you need me."

This sounded like an unmistakable hint, and he felt guilty for postponing his response. He gave her a smile that he hoped wasn't too abjectly apologetic as he carried the drawer onto the balcony. He switched on the outside light, which seemed to rouse a crouching shape on the beach – just a wave – before he slid the window shut behind him.

The fragments of the book were dry now, but this meant some of them were more thoroughly stuck together. However carefully he tried to part them, sections of one fragment clung to the other. He peeled them all apart as best he could and set about leafing through them. He was hoping to deduce why the woman had given him the book, and found that was as far as he could think.

There was nothing he could recognise as referring to Vasilema that he hadn't previously read, and nothing else that might explain the gift. The most substantial portion of the chapter was the first page, and even there the sentences were incomplete. As for the photograph of the monastery on the reverse, it had lost the section showing how unblackened the trees were. When he tried to recall the words missing from the sentences he felt as if he were drawing the darkness closer. Perhaps this was caused by the persistent sense he had of supine shapes creeping out of the night towards the Sunny View – still just waves on the beach.

Once he found he was rereading pages or rather their remains he decided he'd left Sandra by herself long enough. He eased the window open and saw she was asleep, though she'd stretched one arm towards the balcony as if to summon him in her dream. He replaced the drawer in the bedside table and used the bathroom as quietly as he could, then slipped into bed. As he slid an arm around Sandra's waist he was hoping to join her in sleep, but the fragmentary sentences were clamouring for completion, and the darkness only let them grow more insistent. The nearest he could come to quietening his mind was by concentrating on the single complete sentence that remained of the chapter on Vasilema — the last words of the chapter, on a page that had been largely blank. "They feed so Skiá feeds," he found himself repeating silently until it began to dull his awareness — until he lost the sense that it should waken him.

THE ELEVENTH DAY
30 AUGUST

Ray heard a cry and was awake at once, and lay trying to grasp what he'd heard. At least he was certain it hadn't been William. He was hoping it had nothing to do with the family until he managed to reconstruct the sound – Julian shouting in anger if not in disgust. What was the problem now? Should someone intervene? Ray blinked his eyes wide and was listening for any further commotion when Sandra sat up next to him in bed.

No, it wasn't Sandra. She was still lying beside him with his arm around her waist. Nobody had sat up, but a shape had risen from crouching over her. As Ray struggled to focus his eyes he saw a figure dart as swiftly as a spider to the window. It loomed like a scrawny shadow on the curtain, which stirred as though a wind no more substantial than a breath had touched it, and then the intruder was gone.

How could it be? Ray had grown uncertain what he'd seen by the time he floundered out of bed and stumbled to the window, which was shut and locked as well. As Sandra muttered an indistinct sleepy protest he dragged the window open and lurched onto the balcony. Light was streaming from below it, which meant he couldn't make out whether a thin shape had scuttled along the outer wall of the balconies before leaping from the furthest one into the dark. He craned over the wall and saw Julian outside the lower balcony, peering into the night. "What's going on down there?" Ray blurted, mostly in a whisper.

As Julian turned to stare up at him Doug called "Yes, Tim, what's happening? Was someone in your room?"

"Just me," Tim said as if he'd discarded a couple of consonants in his sleep.

Ray heard a confusion of voices in at least two rooms – Pris, Doug, Natalie, Jonquil, William – which didn't quite distract him from a glimpse of movement some way along the beach. By squinting he was just able to distinguish three receding figures. Perhaps because the dim shapes were silhouetted against the waves, their outlines looked not much more stable than the sea. "Who's that?" Ray demanded, stretching out a shaky arm. "Quick, Julian, look."

Julian shaded his eyes to gaze up at Ray before turning to face Sunset Beach. He'd made Ray glance at him, and when Ray returned his attention to the beach it was deserted. How was that possible when there was no concealment on the shore within hundreds of yards of where he'd just seen the figures? As Ray strained his eyes Julian said "What am I meant to be seeing?"

"There was somebody. I know I saw them, three of them. I don't know where they could have gone." Ray was still peering at the dark beach as he said "What are you doing out there, Julian?"

Julian moved close to the balconies and lowered his voice. "I wanted to prove once and for all that nobody could be getting into William's room."

Ray refrained from pointing out that it was Jonquil's too, and found he was nervous of asking "Did you?"

"Of course I did. What on earth do you think?" Having waited until Ray met his incredulous stare, Julian said "But I wanted to make certain he'd no reason to imagine it. I had my suspicions, and it's a damned good job I acted on them."

Ray felt compelled to drop his own voice further – he might

almost not have wanted Julian to hear. "Why was that?"

"The door and the windows were all locked, I saw to that, but I caught someone looking in."

"What happened?" Ray said more quietly still.

"I've been out here since William went to sleep. I came round from the front and caught the fellow on our balcony. I can even understand how William might have run away with the idea that he could come in through the glass. He had his face pressed against the window as if he meant to God knows what, squeeze through."

Ray was finding each question less easy to ask. "Do we know who he was?"

"I believe I already did. Perhaps I can be listened to in future." With a frown for anyone who'd earned the rebuke, Julian said "It was Jonquil's dancing partner."

Ray couldn't avoid realising that he'd already known as well. Before he could think of a response, Julian grimaced and wiped his hands on his shirt. "I had hold of him."

While Ray was by no means certain that he wanted to learn what Julian was recalling, he had to ask "Why are you looking like that?"

"I grabbed him when he hopped over the balcony. He showed me his teeth and gave me the slip." Julian's face writhed again as he said "Slippery isn't the word for him."

"What is, then?"

Julian pondered this, unless he was attempting not to. "Oily," he said. "Not just covered with it either."

Ray saw this too fell short of conveying Julian's experience. He felt as though his thoughts were creeping up on him while he said "Like William's word, do you think?"

"How could he know?" All the same, Julian's conviction appeared to falter. "I suppose," he conceded, "that's how a child might have described the fellow."

Ray's gaze strayed back to the beach, where the movements of the waves looked ominously surreptitious, too reminiscent of supine shapes biding their time. He was scarcely aware of muttering "Maybe that's how they are."

"Forgive me, what did you say?"

Ray was about to repeat the observation, though he was afraid to think where it might lead, until he heard Natalie. "Daddy and grandad are just chatting, William. Let's all try to get back to sleep."

"We'd better not discuss this any further," Julian murmured. "Perhaps we can continue at another time."

"I think we'll have to," Ray said but felt unhappily as though he'd lost a chance.

As Julian headed around the apartment block to his front door, Ray inched the window open. He was hoping Sandra hadn't wakened, but she mumbled "Who's out there?"

"Julian saw someone hanging about outside. I'll tell you about it later."

"I thought he'd got in," Sandra said quite clearly and at once was asleep. Ray knew he wouldn't be, but had to lie beside her and embrace her as well. When he tried to draw her arm into the safety of the quilt she moaned and moved it out of reach. He didn't know how much time passed before his eyes grew so tired that the lids slumped shut. Perhaps he needn't watch the window any longer – not tonight, at any rate. He still couldn't sleep, since far too many thoughts had caught up with him. Dismaying as they were, it was even worse to wonder how he could persuade everyone that he'd seen the truth.

★   ★   ★

Everyone had finished breakfast when Ray leaned over the balcony. "Shall we have our talk up here, Julian?"

"I think I've said all I have to say," Julian told him and patted William on the head.

"Some people won't have heard it. Sandra hasn't," Ray said, feeling bound for desperation before he'd thought he would.

"I should think you can tell her, Raymond."

"She's better hearing it from the man who knows most," Ray said more desperately still.

"I suppose there is that. Very well, we'll be up in a minute. Douglas and Priscilla may as well come too. Timothy, if you could help Jonquil with William we'll find you in the play area in due course."

"What aren't we allowed to hear now?"

"That's not the issue, Timothy. I hope you don't object to looking after your young cousin."

"I don't see why it needs both of us."

"Because he'll be safer with two of you, Tim," Natalie said. "Do you really mind?"

"Of course he doesn't, Nat," Doug said.

"He's just got a grump on because we had to wake him up," said Pris.

"You be good for Tim and Jonquil, William," Sandra called and tugged her hat down, shading her sunglasses further.

"You can help them both to finish waking up," Natalie said.

Ray glanced at Sandra, wondering how sleepy her eyes might be, but saw just his own shrunken reflection in the black lenses. As he and Sandra cleared the table on the balcony he heard the youngsters being sent on their way, and not many moments later there was a knock at the door, immediately followed by a lighter one. "That's two," Doug called, and Pris added "It's safe to let us in."

They thought they were joking or celebrating a local custom, but Ray was no longer amused. Sandra opened the door as he manhandled the two chairs out of the room to supplement the pair on the balcony, where he and Sandra and the other women sat down while Doug and Julian leaned against the outer wall. "So, Julian," Ray said, only to feel less prepared than he'd hoped to be. "What did you tell William and Jonquil?"

"Just that I was right and her follower had been loitering round here. And that I'd chased the fellow off and I doubt he'll be returning."

If Ray was closer to doubting the opposite, this wasn't the moment to argue. "Now can you say what you said to me?"

"I nearly had him but he was too fast for me."

"You said more than that, didn't you? You said you managed to grab him."

"I got my hands on him but he wriggled out of them."

"And you told me how he felt. You said…"

"Sweaty. You'll forgive me," Julian said with a glance at Doug and Pris, "but that's how quite a few of your locals smell."

"That isn't how you put it last night," Ray protested.

"I said he was oily, I believe. Pretty much the same thing. No, I'll grant you, a bit more. Oily in every sense."

"You said William's word applied as well."

"I don't think anyone would say I'd ever be so childish as to use it. Or if I thought about it that must show I have a little imagination after all."

As Ray struggled to think how to proceed Sandra said "Does any of this matter very much? How he felt, I mean. Have you been in touch with the police?"

"Natalie and I have decided against it, given my experience with them and Raymond's. I suspect they would feel we were wasting their time."

"But you wouldn't be, would you?" Doug said.

"All we could say was that the fellow was looking in the window." With a grimace not unlike the one Ray remembered from last night Julian said "I'm afraid we would have to admit that he may not have been entirely uninvited."

"Would you like to say what you mean by that?" Natalie demanded.

"I'm simply thinking of how Jonquil looked at him."

Ray thought Julian might have touched upon more of the truth than he knew. He was trying to think how to address this when Natalie said "She was just being teenage. It's about time you got used to it, Julian."

"I'm with Natalie," Pris said. "This doesn't seem much to bring us all up here for."

"It isn't everything." Ray felt as if he'd stepped over an edge or at any rate was about to be unable to step back. "I've got something you all need to see," he said and limped to the bedside table before he could find his actions impossibly foolish. He carried the drawer onto the balcony and, having dumped it on the table, found the remains of the first page about Vasilema. "Look at this," he urged.

As they examined the photograph everyone confirmed everybody else's silence. "It's the monastery," Natalie said at last in a tone like an audible shrug.

"Yes, but look properly, it's not as black. You can see how that's spreading from it, can't you? The rock underneath the monastery isn't nearly as black as we saw." Ray felt as if his words were insufficiently precise, just like the remnant of the photograph. "If we had the rest of it," he said, "you'd see the trees weren't even touched. Are you sure you didn't see that when I had the book, Doug?"

"I can't pretend I did."

As Natalie and Julian murmured similar denials Pris said "Why is it important to you, Ray?"

"Not just to me. It showed there was never a fire. The place was turning black, but not from that. It was coming out of the monastery, not from the woods at all."

Everyone seemed reluctant to speak, but Natalie did. "What was?"

Ray turned the page over and spread it on the table. "Read this and maybe you'll see what I think."

He very much hoped so, but their eyes looked unwilling to admit much into their thoughts. Once Doug and Julian straightened up from leaning over the table he couldn't tell who was waiting for the other to respond. It was Doug who said "I'm sorry, dad, I don't."

"Just look here," Ray said and saw how desperate he must seem.

There came many years ago to the monastery of Agios Tit
a traveller from where nobody can tell. He gave his name Proskynitis
Greece a monastery must take in the pilgrim and those who seek she
Titus offered hospitality for but a single night, and the night Prosky
saw the dawn.

He was said to tell the abbot he was wandering in search of sol
contemplate eternal things. He vowed that on his death he would will rich
who gave him what he sought. Some monks said that the monastery was not
fortune, but Proskynitis assured them that his riches would not be of the world
eternity. They had put aside worldly matters, but their vanity was spiritual. So
them to his cause. He became an inmate of the monastery, taking less sustenance
monk while he fasted as a help to meditation. As well he counselled his brethren
distractions of the world and urged the dark upon them as the most true path to
eternal.

His example won him acceptance to the order, taking the name Brother Skiá
shadow. He prevailed upon his brethren to help him build a cell deep in the rock, wh
distraction of light could reach. Here he followed his ambition to embrace eternity
embrace the dark. Why could he not do this in real solitude, far from any man? He
to have once, but eternity needs life to feed upon or it is only lifeless dark. He
secrets of the dark is caught in its embrace. If it brings unending life it fills its
hunger.

It was the abbot who invited the dark pilgrim within his door, and now
answered his invitation. Now the abbot fed the dar

"This said the abbot fed the dark. You can see it did," Ray insisted, poking the incomplete sentence with his fingertip so hard that the corner of the torn fragment humped up like a grub. "And it went on to say the man he'd invited in fed on the other monks as well. Shall I tell you what else it said?"

Nobody seemed eager to reply, but Sandra said "If you like, Ray."

"When the page was all there, it said how the man wanted to contemplate eternity but ended up being taken over by it somehow. I think you can see that was there if you look. I suppose it means he couldn't die, but he had to feed on other people to live. Only if they died of it they'd become like him, and so he tried to keep them alive. It's like one of the legends you're so fond of."

He was appealing to Doug and Pris. "That's right, dad, legends," Doug said, "but why are you – "

"There was more that I haven't got here any longer. As I read it he used people to feed on his behalf, and then he fed on them. You know what it means by feeding, don't you? Drinking their blood. And sharing like that extended their lives as well, because he needed them, or the dark did." As he realised that he might be saying too much too soon Ray said "Tell me one thing if you can. Why do you think anybody would want to destroy the book?"

He was asking everyone, which only earned a concerted silence. Eventually Doug said "I don't think we can know."

"Don't you remember what I suggested at the time, Doug? You seemed to think I could be right. I wondered if someone hadn't liked what it said about the monastery, but now I'm convinced it was more than that. They didn't want us to read what you say is just a legend. If that's all it is, why would anyone bother?"

He might have assumed nobody could think if Doug hadn't said "Is this why you went after that woman last night?"

"I wanted her to tell me why she'd singled me out for the book."

"Probably because you paid so much for William's cross."

"I don't mean why a present. Didn't you see how anxious she was for me to read it?" When this failed to find any agreement Ray pleaded "Then did really none of you see why she panicked last night?"

"Dad," Doug said, "we saw you harassing a disabled person when she wouldn't even have been able to tell you what you wanted to know. If we'd been at home you might easily have got yourself prosecuted."

"Do you imagine I'd have behaved like that unless I had good reason?" This revived the silence, which infuriated Ray. "Just take a look at this," he blurted.

He ought to have had the remnant of the other page to hand. As he searched through the ragged contents of the drawer his fingers made a sound like a rat scrabbling in litter. He found what survived of the last page of the chapter and brandished it. "See what this says?"

"There isn't much to see," Natalie reminded him.

"Just the last sentence. That's what I'm showing you."

Pris took hold of the scrap of paper to control its tremulousness. "I don't know what Skiá means."

"Do you, Doug?" Ray hoped.

"Not without looking it up," Doug said unlike any kind of promise.

"It means shadow. It said so on the other part of the first page. Check it on your phones if you like."

"I'm certain we can trust you, Raymond," Julian said.

"It's the name he took when he joined the monks, the traveller. Maybe they thought he was trying to be humble, but you can see it showed what he was actually like inside."

Nobody's eyes betrayed what they were seeing until Natalie

said "It's not a very likely name, is it? Not the kind you'd think monks would let someone use. What do you two think?"

"It shows it's just a legend," Doug said, and Pris visibly agreed.

"No, this shows a lot more." Ray jerked the scrap of paper, almost ripping it afresh until Pris let go. "You're leaving out the tense," he said. "It doesn't say he fed, it says he feeds. They still feed on his behalf, that's what it's saying."

In the midst of the latest silence Sandra said "Who are you talking about, Ray?"

"For pity's sake," Julian said before Ray could start to answer. "Please tell me someone else can see the reason."

"Which is…" Ray said without wanting to know.

"I don't think anyone would claim your writer is exactly fluent in our language. He can't even get his title right. *History of Greece Islands*, for heaven's sake. I'm quite willing to acknowledge that his English is streets ahead of my Greek, but all that tense means is he's got something else wrong."

Ray saw the others welcome the explanation, though he wasn't sure that Sandra did. Perhaps her uncertainty helped him to say "There's a lot more to the book."

Natalie let out a sigh that Doug might have been putting into words by asking "What else do you think there is, dad?"

"I think people here have been giving us hints ever since we arrived. Maybe even before that," Ray realised as a memory caught up with him. "Natalie was saying they told you on the mainland that people here aren't like them."

"And I told you that's what Greeks say about the Cretans," Doug said with a determined laugh. "You aren't trying to tell us everybody here is, I'm not even going to use the word."

"Not everybody, not even most, but I think we've seen a few of them."

"If you mean who I assume you mean," Julian said, "I think that's quite unnecessary."

"The one you grabbed last night sounds a lot like the one who stole my book. He was faster than you, wasn't he?" As Julian made his incredulity plain Ray grasped what he had to ask. "You told me he showed you his teeth," he said. "What were they like?"

"Good Lord above, why do you think I would take any notice of them? I was looking the fellow in the eye. That's how to deal with his sort."

Was Julian using too many words? Ray couldn't be sure they were meant to deny any nervousness. "You didn't notice them at all," he persisted.

"I saw he must have wanted me to. Exactly why I didn't look."

"All right, let's forget him for the moment," Ray said in a bid to leave his frustration behind. "Let's talk about what certainly did trouble you. The state Mr Ditton was in."

"You'll recall we were told fish were responsible for that."

"If you believe it." Ray saw that Julian and Natalie weren't alone in doing so, but surely he needn't despair. "I don't just mean how he was when we found him," he said. "I mean what they did to the corpse."

"I'm not sure what you have in mind."

"Oh, come along, Julian," Ray said, only to realise that offending anybody wouldn't help. "Sorry, but you know you were outraged because they'd removed the head. I believe you thought what I think now, it was the police who did."

"I'm certain I said nothing of the kind. I should think it goes to prove how bad a condition the body was in, which I'll remind you was exactly what you thought, Raymond. Now does anybody really need to hear any more about this?"

"Doug, you said you knew about it," Ray managed to remember. "You said it was how they made sure the victim didn't turn into — "

"That's just another legend, dad. I should never have brought it up. It wasn't in the best of taste, and I'm sorry I did."

Ray felt as if they were all turning off lights in his mind. As soon as he found a thought he blurted "You won't say nothing happened to you last night, will you?"

"I'm not sure what you're saying did."

"You thought they went in for a custom I believe they have all over Greece, wishing people on their birthdays a long life."

"Or a thousand years," Pris said. "Daphne asked us not to, but what are you thinking that shows?"

"Just that they know about people who live too long and why they do, and they don't want to be among them. We all heard her say it was like a curse."

He thought the silence meant he'd finally given his listeners a reason to ponder until Doug said "We shouldn't have said those things last night, but that isn't why."

"Why, then?"

"Because we should have thought of mum, and so should you. How can you waste your time with this stuff when she's dying?"

Ray's stomach constricted as if he'd been punched in the guts. He was trying to think of an answer when Julian twisted around to stare over the balcony wall. "Who's down there?"

For a moment Ray was able to imagine that some evidence had presented itself in support of his claims, and then Julian demanded "Is it you, Jonquil?"

The response came not quite from below him. "It's me."

"Tim," Pris said very little like a welcome. "What are you doing?"

"Getting my phone."

"Then why are you on the balcony?" Without waiting for a reply she said "How long have you been there? Have you been listening?"

"Wait a moment, Tim." Much lower Natalie said "Can you bring him up to talk? We don't want anyone else hearing, do we?"

"Tim, come up here," Doug called, "and make it quick."

Ray let him in. Even more than sometimes, Tim visibly wished he were smaller. He looked ready to let his height bow him down if this would make him less conspicuous, but even the hat couldn't obscure how much he was blushing. Behind the sunglasses his eyes were as wide as they could stretch, holding back a frown or fending off some other reaction. "I'm sorry," he muttered as Ray closed the door.

"I might have done the same in your place," Ray said for nobody but Tim to hear.

As he led the way onto the balcony Pris said "Well, Tim, what do you think you heard?"

Tim seemed to wish he could do without blinking. Barely audibly he admitted "What dad said about gran."

He sounded ten years younger – William's age – and Ray might have tried to comfort him if Sandra hadn't reached for their grandson's hand. "Oh, Tim, I wish you hadn't found out like this."

"Maybe things aren't as bad as I made out," Doug said. "That's what you've been saying, isn't it, mum?"

"That's right, Tim. We all have to go eventually, and I thought I was, but I feel as though someone's given me an extra lease of life."

"Forgive me," Julian said, "I don't believe we established whether Timothy was eavesdropping."

The teenager blinked – indeed, squeezed his eyes momentarily shut. "I'm sorry," he said as if he wished only his parents could hear. "I was."

"We can award you a mark for honesty at least."

"I won't blame you, Tim," Sandra said, "so I hope nobody else will."

As Doug and Pris confined their rebukes to their eyes Natalie said "Will you make me a promise, Tim?"

"What is it?"

"No harm in being careful," Natalie told Julian as he looked offended by Tim's response. "Tim, will you please not tell anyone what you heard?"

"All right," Tim said, but looked thwarted.

"We shouldn't be asking so much of you at your age." Sandra clasped his hand with both of hers while she said "It can be our secret, all right?"

Ray felt there were already too many of those – subjects the family wanted to ignore or refused to discuss. As Tim nodded, though without much vigour, Sandra said "Do you know what I've just thought, Tim? You haven't had your day yet."

"I shared mum's when we went off the road."

"Well, I think you're still owed one. Tell us what you'd like to do."

Ray saw she meant to reward their grandson for the demand that had been made on him. Perhaps he was passing on her generosity by saying "Auntie Nat, you never got your trip off the island."

"That's kind of you, Tim, but is it what you'd like yourself?"

"He's always liked that kind of jaunt," Doug said. "No reason he'd have changed."

As Tim's black lenses glinted in the shadow of his hat Julian said "That's settled, then. We'll go into the town and see where a boat will take us."

Ray felt events were moving faster than he liked – leaving too much behind or at any rate unacknowledged. "We'll come down with you now, Timothy," Julian said, only to linger as the rest of the family followed Tim out of the apartment. "I trust there'll be no further talk of legends and the rest of it," Julian said while Ray returned the drawer to the bedside table, and Ray felt robbed of the chance to voice a good deal more. He was dismayed by how close he was to resenting Tim as well as Julian for robbing him. He could almost have imagined Tim preferred him not to speak.

★　★　★

As the bus passed the Happy Snappy shop Ray said "I never explained properly about the photograph."

"You said it was a trick," Doug reminded him.

"I thought it was," Ray said, lowering his voice. "Now I'm not so sure."

"What's there to be sure of?" Sandra said.

"There were two of them, two photographs. You heard me saying so. The girl you saw was in both."

Pris leaned across the aisle and kept her voice low, which sounded to Ray like addressing an invalid. "We didn't see any girl."

"Yes, in the photo. The one the man in the shop left up."

"The cutie in the bikini," Doug murmured, earning Pris's elbow in his ribs. "Only trying to be certain who we mean."

"That's her. You saw how young she was, and you could see it was a recent photograph."

Doug looked not far from anxious. "How could we?"

"Because you saw the man behind the counter. You saw he was the same age in the photo."

"If you say so, dad. I expect he was close."

Ray became aware that Tim was chatting loudly if not chattering to William and Jonquil. He must be ensuring they didn't overhear in case the discussion was about their grandmother, a thought that made Ray more desperate to convince his listeners. "But he wasn't that age in the one he took down," he insisted. "He was years younger, I'd say at least ten, and yet she was exactly the same in both."

"As you said, Ray, it was a trick," Pris looked sad to have to tell him. "Anyone can do that kind of thing these days, not even just a photographer."

"I know that, but why did he hide the other photograph? He wouldn't give me an explanation."

"He didn't have to, did he?" More reasonably still Doug said "Maybe he'd decided it was sexist. Maybe somebody objected."

"In that case why didn't he take both the photographs down?" Ray saw Doug and Pris fail to find an answer, and the sight seemed to illuminate his mind. "Wait a moment," he said. "Did you notice the bite?"

"I didn't," Sandra said.

He didn't have time to examine her tone as Doug said reluctantly "Which bite?"

"On her arm in the photograph."

"I don't believe any of us did," Pris said.

"Well, it was there. I'll swear to it, in both of them. If he was playing tricks with the image, why wouldn't he have edited that out?"

Doug glanced at the youngsters two seats behind. "Dad, what are you trying to make out now?"

For the duration of a breath that he fought to take, Ray was on the brink of an admission he'd kept even from himself. Before he could speak Sandra took hold of his arm. "Maybe the photographer thought it made her look more real," she said.

He was trying to determine what the pressure of her grasp was intended to communicate when Pris said "I'm sure that's it, Ray."

He felt as if the energy to argue had deserted him. As the discussion petered out he heard Tim fall silent too. The bus sped out of Sunset Beach, where the virtually deserted streets felt like evidence he no longer had the will to cite. Before long he saw the shrine by the path to the beach, but couldn't judge if he was growing tense because he sensed how many people were willing him not to speak. The bus raced past the shrine, where the dim figure in the box had been overwhelmed by a restless mass of cobwebs. He didn't want to be alone with the glimpse, which was one excuse for muttering "Did everyone realise the monastery's linked to the cave?"

"Why should it be?" Pris said and clearly wished she'd asked a different question.

"I'm not saying they meant it to be. Maybe it said in my book if they did. All I'm saying is they must have dug so deep they broke into the cave."

"It looked as if they could have," Doug said. "Sounded that way too."

"So I'm wondering," Ray said in order to finish, "what might have ended up down there."

"We aren't," Doug told him.

"And you shouldn't," Pris said with just as concerned a look.

When Sandra squeezed his arm Ray didn't know if she was enjoining silence or trying to convey that she shared some of his thoughts. Nobody found anything more to say until the bus reached Vasilema Town, where several boats large enough to carry passengers were tied up beside the harbour. As William planted his hands with a thump against the window and greeted the boats with an enthusiastic cry, Julian said "May we get off here, please?"

Perhaps the driver didn't hear him. The bus carried on past the harbour while Julian searched for a bellpush anywhere around him. "I asked you to let us off," he said louder and tramped up the aisle, but the bus turned along the side street that led to the square. It didn't stop until it was opposite the ticket office, at which point the driver released the doors. "Do you not understand English?" Julian demanded.

The driver raised his eyes to the icon above the mirror. "Here you stop."

"Let it go, Julian," Natalie said. "We don't want to miss the boat."

"If that's the best you can do," Julian told the driver, "then I think the answer's no."

Natalie took William's hand as she made for the harbour, and Ray found Sandra's soft grasp. By the time everyone reached the wharf, Julian had strode ahead to examine the signboards in front of the boats. "This one goes in half an hour," he called.

While the boats were deserted, several men sat on folding chairs beside the furthest vessel. Ray saw one man stand up as Julian halted at the board, and then, having glanced at the rest of the party, the man resumed his seat before staring out to sea. "Does this appeal, Natalie?" Julian said. "Three hours on the mainland."

"I'd quite like the change if everybody else would."

When nobody dissented Julian called "Which of you gentlemen is responsible for this trip?"

Since they all seemed intent on the sea, Ray wasn't sure which of them spoke. "No trip today."

"Of course there is. It's advertised quite clearly here." When staring at them didn't earn him a response, Julian said "Very well, which boats belong to you fellows? What are you offering?"

Ray was just as unable to single out the next speaker. "He said no trip."

"None at all? That's utterly ridiculous. In that case why are your boards still up? Do you think it's amusing to waste people's time?"

"Julian," Natalie said. "It doesn't matter that much."

Ray thought it did, and not just the disappointment. He limped along the wharf to confront the man he'd seen stand up. "You were going to take us, weren't you?" he demanded. "What changed your mind?"

The man didn't quite meet his gaze, though Ray was standing in front of him. "See," he said.

Ray glanced at the family to make sure they could hear, only to find he was nervous of asking "See what? What did you see?"

Another boatman swept a hand in the direction of the water. "Sea."

"I don't believe that's what he was saying," Ray protested, but it was too late. Julian had joined him to enquire "What's wrong with the sea? It looks perfectly fine for a cruise."

"You can not say," the first man said. "We are fishermen."

"If that's the case where are your nets? Where's any tackle at all?"

Ray was afraid Julian was insulting the boatmen, not to mention commandeering the discussion. "I'd just like to ask you – "

"Let me handle this, Raymond. I'm doing it for my wife, you know." Before Ray could point out that she was his daughter too Julian said "Are you seriously all refusing to honour your commitments? Perhaps you ought to realise it doesn't help the image of your island."

"All we want to know," Ray said in desperation, "is why you've decided against taking us."

"Not you."

The voice was too muted for him to locate – almost too low to hear. "Then," Ray said and had to swallow, "who?"

"I'm sorry, Raymond, that's by no means all we're asking," Julian said and turned on the boatmen. "We can't see any excuse for you not to take us. Are you genuinely in the business of letting the public down? Is that even legal when you've attracted people with your advertising? Suppose we report you to the authorities, would that change your tune?"

"Hey," the oldest boatman threatened, brandishing his mobile phone. "I call."

"That really isn't necessary." Natalie had left William with Jonquil. "None of this is," she said. "I'm sure these gentlemen can judge what the sea's like better than we can. We haven't bought souvenirs yet. Let's do that instead."

She took Julian's arm to steer him away, and Ray felt

abandoned. What was the use of questioning the boatmen if nobody else could hear? As he trudged back to Sandra she said "What's the situation?"

"They're refusing to venture out to sea," Julian declared. "Every single one of them."

"Maybe they don't want us to go," William said.

"Don't you start that nonsense as well," Julian told him. "Did your sister give you her silly idea?"

"I never said anything about it," Jonquil cried. "And anyway, I'm not his sister. You sound like I don't even have a name."

Ray was a little less shocked by her outburst once he recalled that she didn't know about her grandmother. "Chill, Jonk," Tim said. "We know you wouldn't have."

"Tim's right, we do," Natalie said and gave her mother a sidelong blink. "We'll talk about the rest of it another time, shall we? While we're here we can shop for souvenirs instead."

Ray saw how Julian resented losing the opportunity to confront Jonquil. "Shall we look in at the bus station?" he was inspired to suggest. "You never did find out why the buses play that game at Sunset Beach."

"Do we even need to know about it? I can't imagine why any of us would be there that late."

"It isn't like you," Ray felt crafty for saying, "to leave anything unresolved."

At least this brought Julian with him while everyone else made for the toilets, but the queue for tickets was so long that he was afraid Julian might lose patience. He didn't want him to turn aggressive either, and so he blurted out his question as soon as they reached the booth. "Can you tell us what time the buses finish stopping at Sunset Beach?"

The uniformed young woman scrutinised him and Julian without displaying much of an expression. "What time do you go there?"

"We don't," Julian said, to Ray's dismay. "We want to be told why they won't stop."

"It is up to the driver."

"How can that be?" When she only stared at him Julian demanded "What sort of a way is that to run a public service?"

The woman shrugged, holding up her empty hands. "You are not at home."

"Believe me, you don't need to tell us that. Our two weeks are nearly up, at any rate."

Ray saw the woman take that as an insult to her island or her race. Almost too hastily to catch his breath he said "You haven't given us a time yet."

She glanced at a calendar that showed a swollen sun close to the horizon beyond an empty beach. "Tonight there may be no stop by eight."

"And soon it'll be earlier than that, won't it?"

"Your friend says you are not here then."

"For future reference," Ray said desperately. "In case we come back next year."

Some element of this persuaded her to say "Yes then, earlier."

"In other words, your drivers don't like to stop there after dark."

Her face grew even less expressive, as if she felt tricked. "I do not see you staying there."

"Because we're too old for it, you mean. Too old for what?" When she gave him silence for an answer Ray felt recklessly determined to provoke one that Julian would hear. "They want fresh blood, don't they? The kind that's easily replenished. Nothing too young, though. That might be too obvious to everyone else."

He'd said too much instead of forcing her to speak. She wasn't even looking at him, though Julian certainly was. Ray didn't realise why she was gazing past him until he heard a male voice at his back. "Problem here?"

"None that need concern you," Julian told the security officer.

"We've learned what we wanted to know."

Before Ray could speak Julian grasped him none too gently by the arm and ushered him out of the waiting-room. As they emerged into the square Julian murmured "I hope that's the end of that, Raymond. It's well past time you left it alone."

"I'll make certain I don't disturb William."

"It isn't only him, it's the entire family. In the circumstances, particularly Sandra."

"I'm doing it for her."

Julian released his arm and held Ray with his gaze instead. "How can that possibly be the case?"

Ray found he preferred not to answer, even in his mind. In any case they were too close to the others, and Natalie was asking "Did you sort it out?"

"We shouldn't expect any buses to stop there after sunset." Ray sensed how Julian was willing him not to say any more, but he'd already decided against it. "Let's look for things to take home, shall we?" he said and turned uphill.

Although the shade of the narrow streets closed over them at once, Sandra and the teenagers kept their sunglasses and hats on, even beneath the awnings overgrown with vines. Ray looked for the graffiti he remembered, but either he'd somehow missed the side street where he'd seen the remains of a word or the letters that were left had been erased. He hadn't previously noticed how much of the embroidery draped outside shops hid spiders, which made that street feel like walking through an enormous cobweb, while the street barnacled with leather goods put him uncomfortably in mind of ancient skin. Souvenir shops kept slowing the family down, and Ray did his best to feign interest until they reached the shop full of icons. "Doug, Pris," he murmured. "Stay here a minute."

While the proprietor had been eager to accost them last time, now she only glanced at them through the window before waddling at speed towards the back room. "Excuse me," Ray had to shout twice to make her turn, and gestured Doug and Pris to follow him into the shop. "You were telling us about your saint last week."

She might have been invoking the protection as she laid a hand on an image of St Titus. "Have you come to buy?"

"If you can tell us why again." As Doug and Pris looked at the very least bewildered he said "You were saying he might help some of us remember."

"Well, so."

While he hadn't quoted her precisely, he was gratified if he'd persuaded her that he had. "Who?" he said.

"I do not see them. Do you want to buy?"

"Possibly," Ray felt mean for saying. "Tell us this, then. What makes them forget?"

"Crossing water."

"Going home, you mean," Pris said.

"She doesn't just mean that, do you?" When the proprietor gazed at the icon as though seeking support Ray said "I'd have thought you two would be the first to see. You're fond of legends. You aren't like Julian."

"I wish you'd give him a break now and then, dad. He's doing his best in his way."

Ray mumbled in agreement, mostly to dismiss the subject, and Pris turned to the proprietor. "That's male solidarity for you. You've met the one they're trying to defend."

"Not defend, just understand. Don't you both do that at work?" Ray was distressed to think that the argument might divert them from the reason he was here. "Crossing water," he persisted. "How will it make them forget?"

"They leave memories here. Come back to find them."

"You're really saying they remember," Doug said in triumph that sounded like a good deal of relief. "Thanks for clearing that up. Come on, dad, if you're not buying anything. I can see the others waiting."

They hadn't quite left the shop when Pris murmured "You were right, Ray."

He was so heartened, even if nervously, that he didn't let her finish. "How?"

"As you say, we love legends and traditions and anything like that." She was the latest person to take hold of his arm. "Only you have to realise," she said, "that's all legends are."

Ray felt as if she'd laid a weight on him if not restored one. Perhaps that explained why climbing the streets was more laborious than ever, though he could blame his age as well. As he trudged from shop to shop he felt robbed of purpose, and then he saw the tattoo stall ahead. He couldn't tell how many of the family were willing him not to trouble the young woman. Would they even listen if he spoke to her? They seemed determined not to as they hastened past the stall, but he saw recognition flutter in her eyes as she noticed Tim. "You remember," Ray said.

If she recognised him, she was suppressing any sign. "You said your tattoos were no good," he reminded her. "Why?"

"He said."

Apparently she meant Julian, who was leading William uphill. "Dad," Doug said.

"Just bear with me," Ray said if not begged, and kept his eyes on the young woman. "You said more than he did. You told us it was too late."

Sandra had turned back now, and in a moment the teenagers did. Either the young woman had decided she wasn't being questioned or she was determined not to be, since her gaze had drifted to the stall. "Too late for what exactly?" Ray said, but when she didn't raise her eyes or speak he had to ask the question that he dreaded putting into words. "Too late for whom?"

Her gaze was flickering from Tim to Jonquil when Doug intervened. "Dad, you're harassing somebody again. We all know why you're feeling bad, but you mustn't let it make you act like this."

"That isn't why," Ray protested, but Doug had turned to the woman, having stepped between them. "Please excuse my father," he said. "He has a lot on his mind."

Ray thought Doug had no idea how much, but was there any use in saying? As he laboured uphill in the midst of the family he might have thought they were escorting him so that he wouldn't trouble anybody else. At least the route was leading them to the church, where he might have a last chance to gain some information – and then he remembered that the church was well beyond the highest shops, which meant they mightn't reach it. When the shops gave out he carried on. "I'm just going to the church."

"What do you want there?" Doug called after him.

"Maybe I'll pray," he said wildly and tramped panting up the hill.

As he crossed a junction he recognised a lane where a word had been sprayed on a wall, which was bare of letters now. From the square at the top of the hill he saw a distant island catch light from the sun behind the clouds above Vasilema. When he hurried into the church, having regained some breath, he had to blink his eyes clear of the dazzle that met them. Even once he succeeded in focusing, the wavering of air above the multitude of candle flames and the smell of hot wax felt like a threat of dizziness and nausea. At first he thought he was alone apart from the saints flattened on the walls and in the windows, grim figures too lacking in dimension to suggest any power, and then he glimpsed movement near the altar. It wasn't just the quivering of flames; the custodian had emerged from his room. "Hello?" Ray called – not too inappropriately loud, he hoped – and tramped along the aisle with an irrepressible clatter of sandals. "I was here last week when you chased those people out of your church."

The man greeted this with a scowl like a summation of the dimness that the flames failed to reach. At least he didn't retreat to his room, and Ray was about to question him when heard the door open behind him. He turned to see Sandra letting herself into the church. Surely she wouldn't try to silence him. "What did you say to those people?" he persisted.

The man glowered at his downturned hands and swept them apart. "Not welcome here."

"We saw they weren't, but why? What was it you called them?"

The man clasped his hands and rubbed them together with such force that the sound roused an echo, and Ray wondered if he could be sweating at the memory. When this was his only response Ray urged "What are they? Tell us that, then."

The man looked up to scowl at Sandra. "Not here. Shouldn't be in church."

"But why exactly?" As the custodian's disapproval stayed mute Ray abandoned caution. "Shall I tell you what they are?" he said, though his voice felt in danger of falling short of his words. "They feed so Skiá feeds."

Sandra was beside him now. Diminished flames trembled in the lenses of her sunglasses, and Ray wondered if this was the sight that seemed to fascinate the custodian. The man was licking his lips to separate them when Ray heard the door open again, and several people entering the church. "Dad," Doug called.

At the very least this was a warning. Ray swung around to see Doug and Pris and a pair of silhouettes behind them. Those didn't belong to Natalie and Julian, and even when they advanced into the candlelight he didn't immediately know why the men looked familiar. Then he made out their uniforms, and recognised the officers he'd seen behind the counter of the police station at Sunset Beach.

The door of the custodian's room shut with a decisive thud, disturbing so many flames that the golden figures seemed to start forward from the walls. When Sandra caught hold of his hand Ray thought she was going to lead him out of the church until he saw she wanted him to face her. She tilted her head towards him, emphasising the mark on her neck, while she whispered "I hope you're right, Ray."

THE TWELFTH DAY
31 AUGUST

As Ray leaned over the balcony in case he could determine how the night had treated everybody else, Sandra called "Come and see me."

He could have thought she had sex on her mind, but it seemed unlikely while she was in the bathroom. He straightened up too fast, which made the clouds above Vasilema appear to sink towards him and grow darker, putting out the hidden sun. He gripped the concrete wall until the bout of dizziness finished lingering, by which time he was afraid that Sandra might think he was ignoring her. "I'm on my way," he called as he opened his eyes and let go of the wall. He limped into the apartment and then faltered in the doorway of the bathroom.

Sandra was gazing at the mirror above the sink. For a moment that Ray couldn't help attempting to prolong, he was able to believe that nothing was amiss except a last trace of his dizziness. Couldn't this be why he found it hard to focus on the reflection in the glass? He took an uncertain step towards Sandra, which brought him too close to deny what she was seeing. It felt as if the wordless peace they'd shared last night – a calm that might have been the culmination of all their years together, of no longer needing to speak – had abruptly ended. His reflection was in focus, as it had already been, and so was the reflection of the bathroom. Only Sandra's image in the mirror was so indistinct that Ray felt as if he were straining to distinguish it in utter darkness.

Perhaps it wasn't quite that bad, he was desperate to think. As his eyes began to sting he managed to make out her face, even if the features were softened by the blur. Now it looked as if the section of the mirror within her outline had been transformed into mist or deep water, through which he was attempting to grasp the sight of her. He was struggling to recapture its clarity when Sandra reached for his hand. "You see it too," she said.

He thought she was reaching for solidity, and he hoped he could provide enough – hoped with a fervour that left words behind. As her hand closed on his he grew dizzy again, terrified that she might feel as her reflection looked. For a breath, or rather while he fought to draw one, he had the impression that she'd grown too fluid for him to take a firm hold – as indefinite as water. Then she gripped his hand tight, and her grasp seemed to regain substance. "That's all that's left of me," she whispered.

"What do you mean? You're still very much here." Dismay made his voice harsh until he brought it under control. "Never mind how it looks," he said and did his best to agree with his words. "How do you feel?"

"I've kept trying to tell you. More alive than I have for months."

"Isn't that what matters, then?" However absurdly grotesque it felt to say so while he gazed at her imprecise reflection, Ray added "Maybe we needn't care why too much."

"I wish it were that simple. What I said to you in the church, I wasn't thinking. I was being selfish."

This bewildered Ray as much as the sight in the mirror had. "Why should you think that?"

"It isn't only me, is it? It's Tim and Jonquil too."

Ray was dismayed to realise that he'd been so grateful to learn that she believed – indeed, welcomed – what he had deduced that he'd put the teenagers out of his mind. He was still more disconcerted to hear himself suggesting "If you don't think it's doing you any harm…"

"It's not the same or anything like it," Sandra said, turning from the mirror to give him a shocked look. "Maybe it's brought me more life, but they already have theirs, and they don't want that kind."

He felt pitifully glad of the excuse to look away from the mirror. "I shouldn't be so thoughtless."

"No wonder we both are with all this happening. I've got it to thank for taking away the pain and all the other bad things. It did that first night when I stayed on the balcony." Ray gathered this was meant to reassure him and perhaps herself as well before she said "But it's a bad thing too, isn't it? What are we going to do about Tim and Jonquil?"

"All we can do – " Ray said and winced as her hand clenched on his. Somebody was knocking at the door.

He was so confused by events that he was close to fancying the unacknowledged subject of their discussion had come to put a stop to it, and then Doug called "It's me and Nat. Is it convenient to have a word?"

"Don't you believe in knocking twice?" Ray said without managing to laugh.

"That's the sort of thing we want to talk about if you'll let us."

"Just give me time to get dressed," Sandra called as she left the bathroom and then released Ray's hand.

He waited while she donned not just a dress. He wondered if she'd put on her hat and sunglasses as a sign to Doug and Natalie, since she murmured "I'll help you convince them."

As soon as she opened the door she reverted to being maternal. "Doug, aren't you well?"

"Just a bit tired."

"Why, did something else happen in the night?" Ray said and rather hoped. "I'm afraid we were asleep."

"You shouldn't be afraid at all," Natalie protested. "If you're both sleeping, that's what we like to hear."

"You haven't told us what happened," Sandra said.

"Not a thing," Doug said in weary triumph. "Maybe Jules and I made sure it didn't. We've been up all night keeping watch."

"Why did it take both of you?" Sandra was eager to learn.

"Me at the front and him at the back. Maybe we nodded off in our chairs now and then, but we're certain nobody came anywhere near."

"You think that's why nobody did up here."

She might have been asking Natalie and Doug as well as Ray. The only response, if it could be called one, came from Doug. "Shall we talk inside?"

"Or outside if you like," Natalie said. "Everyone's by the pool."

As she brought an extra chair onto the balcony Ray asked Doug "So were you just helping to watch because of William?"

"Not just him."

"Jonquil?" Sandra prompted. "And Tim?"

"Not them at all. Especially not Tim. He's never been disturbed at night that we know of." As Sandra made to reply Doug said "We want to show dad he oughtn't to believe any of the stuff in that book."

"None of it?" Ray was taken aback by his own bitterness. "Not even all the chapters about the rest of Greece?"

"You know what we mean, dad. The kind of thing you've been bothering people with."

"The sort of question the police turned up to stop me asking at the church."

"I hope you don't think we had anything to do with that. And I don't believe you can say they meant to stop you either."

"They did, though, didn't they? You must have seen how fast the chap I was talking to fled when he saw them."

"Maybe he was running away from you," Natalie seemed sad to think, "like the disabled lady did."

"Sorry, Natalie, you weren't there," Sandra said. "Doug, why else do you think they came to the church?"

"We'll never know, will we? I should think they were looking for someone. They left speedily enough when they saw whoever it was wasn't there."

"That's because they scared off my informant." Having Sandra on his side emboldened Ray to add "I think they'd heard I was asking too many questions around the town. Perhaps someone called them. I wouldn't be surprised if the woman in the icon shop did."

"Actually," Natalie said, "maybe we did have something to do with them."

"How's that, Natalie?" Sandra said at once.

"That boatman was threatening to call them, wasn't he? It looks to me as if he did."

"And they just happened to be two of the police from Sunset Beach?" Ray saw this didn't prove much, and tried to think what did. "You should ask Julian about the way we were interrogated," he said. "Why we went to the beach with the cave, how we knew it was there, why I was in the cave – you'd have thought we were criminals. And I don't care what anybody says, you need to think why the man who questioned us lied about how long Ditton had been dead."

"Don't say that," Natalie pleaded. "You need to care what we're saying to you."

"We do," Sandra said, "but it has to go both ways."

"I'm not sure I understand you."

"Aren't you still afraid there might be some disease on the island?"

"Not since Jamie told us what must have happened to Mr Ditton, but I don't mind admitting that was a relief."

"Maybe you shouldn't feel so relieved." As Natalie's eyes widened to magnify her concern Sandra said "Maybe you should keep looking out for symptoms, just not the kind you thought."

"What kind, then?" Doug said before Natalie could.

"Sleepiness to start with," Sandra said, then touched her hat and glasses, a gesture that resembled a parody of an observance.

"Sensitivity to sunlight, but first of all this," she said, fingering the mark on her neck.

Now Doug seemed even less ready to speak than his sister, who was left to say "Symptoms of what?"

"I think you both have to know. What your father has been trying to tell you is the case."

Natalie closed her eyes as if this could shut off the situation. "Don't say dad has you thinking that as well," Doug protested.

"I'm quite able to think for myself at my age, thank you." Less sharply Sandra said "I gave it a lot of thought last night, and there are all sorts of things we should have noticed."

"Such as what?"

"You could try listening to yourself a bit more, and Pris too."

"I don't think we've said anything to give you the idea you seem to have."

"You did when you were translating. Don't you remember?" When Doug made his reluctance plain Sandra said "The man at the bonfire said those people were leeches, you told us. And the churchwarden if that's what we should call him, you said he was talking about transfusions. Don't you see that means they get blood on somebody else's behalf?"

"It doesn't have to mean that," Natalie said, "and I'm sure it doesn't. We've no reason to believe they were the same people either."

"That's because their faces wouldn't stay still in the church. I wonder if William saw them better than we did."

"Please don't bring him into it, mother, and certainly don't ask him."

"I wasn't about to." With enough frustration to be expressing Ray's as well Sandra said "But can you honestly think that man would have driven them out of his church just for giving blood?"

"I don't know what his beliefs may tell him to do. I don't suppose you do either, Doug."

As Doug gave his head a sad-faced shake Ray was provoked to

point out "There's something you both know that I haven't told your mother."

Only Sandra spoke. "What's that, Ray?"

"When we were under the monastery you both saw that cell with the marks on the wall."

Doug responded, though not immediately. "That's how some people keep track of the days."

"Not days down there, though. You saw what they were, Natalie, and you would have said except for William." When she closed her eyes once more Ray said "They were years, Sandra. Nearly four hundred of them."

"Just because they were in hundreds," Doug said, "it needn't mean that at all."

"But there was that motto in the chapel," Sandra reminded him. "Feed on the immortal and the immortal feeds on you."

"We weren't sure if it said that, and in any case all it has to mean is somebody who knew the legend wrote it on the wall."

"How much more are you going to dismiss like that? Do you really think we're so senile we're deluded?" Before Natalie or Doug could say what their faces already conveyed, Sandra said "And none of us knew about the monastery when Tim and Jonquil had their dreams. They dreamt about something that lived in the dark, if you remember."

"No need to bring them into it either," Doug said.

"What else are you going to refuse to look at?" As Ray grew tense in case she meant to talk about the teenagers Sandra said "People have been trying to let us know what's going on here ever since we came. We should have noticed how everyone is."

"You can't believe everyone is, I'm not going to say it," Natalie begged.

"Not even most of them. More likely just a few, but they all know. That's why they're ashamed of being glad we're here, can't you tell?"

"Likely," Doug repeated in despair as Ray said "And there are those names in the graveyard."

"Dad," Natalie said, "according to you they're supposed to be kept alive, not dead."

"They must have made some kind of mistake."

This seemed uselessly feeble, and he saw Sandra thought so. He shouldn't have mentioned the names at all. Perhaps they'd been victims of greed, he thought, and instantly knew that Ditton must have been one. He was wondering if he dared make the point when Sandra said "I'd like either of you to explain about the mirrors. How many have you seen since we came to the island?"

"Look, maybe some of the people believe the legend," Doug said. "That doesn't prove a thing except they do."

"Then here's some proof you won't be able to ignore," Sandra said and stood up. "Come and look at me in the mirror."

"Mother," Natalie pleaded, but Sandra was already on her way. "Yes, both of you," Ray managed to urge without faltering. "Go and see."

He sounded as if he didn't want to, which might well be the case. He limped hastily after them as Sandra opened the bathroom door wide and advanced to the mirror. He had scarcely joined them when Natalie turned away, immediately followed by her brother. "Mum, that's just a flaw in the glass," Doug said.

Sandra swung around, looking as triumphant as her sunglasses allowed. "What is?"

"The way you were a bit blurred," Natalie said. "That's what you meant, isn't it? Ask Evadne to replace the mirror."

"Can't you even bear to look?"

"We did," Doug said as he and Natalie moved away from the bathroom. "Please don't keep looking at it. It can't do you any good."

Sandra tramped out of the bathroom and slammed the door. "You really are determined not to see, both of you."

As Natalie dabbed at her eyes so fast and fiercely that she seemed bent on denying the action, Doug said "We just wanted to help if we could. We weren't expecting this."

"Not both of you," Natalie said almost to herself.

"We've been together too long to part now," Sandra said.

"We wouldn't want you to," Natalie cried. "But you don't have to agree about everything."

"We don't, but we do about this."

"Then I can't think what else we can do for you," Doug said as though exhaustion had overtaken him.

"Maybe you needn't do anything," Ray said. "You might remember we're still your parents. We can still know best now and then."

Though he felt embarrassingly banal, the rebuke appeared to work. Both their children looked defeated or at any rate resigned. "Come down when you're ready," Doug surrendered to saying, "and we can all decide what we're doing for the day."

Natalie followed him out of the apartment, only to turn to their parents. "If it helps you to believe all that," she said as best she could for the infirmness of her mouth, "I don't suppose we should take away your faith. But you shouldn't expect anyone else to believe, and I hope you won't try to make us any more."

Once the door closed Sandra said "Was there anything else we could have told them?"

"Nothing that was likely to convince them." Just the same, Ray felt encouraged to add "When I was at Sunset Beach and found out everybody was a newcomer I heard a young chap talking about a dream he'd had of being visited at night, and he had the mark on his arm."

"I don't think they would have given that much credence."

"But they ought to have seen what the priest on the beach meant. He was pointing at you and Tim and Jonquil, I'm certain. So was the woman I chased, if I'm not mistaken."

"They'd say you were."

"And then she saw three of those, those creatures waiting. Didn't you?"

"I'm sorry, Ray, I don't think anyone but you did."

The question had suggested one that made him more nervous. "Have you ever seen your, your visitor?"

"I think I dream when he comes instead."

Ray found the nonchalance of their discussion grotesque, which began to infuriate him. "But Julian saw one. He even touched it," he complained. "He simply won't admit what it was like."

"Maybe we shouldn't expect anyone to believe us. He was our best chance."

"We ought for Tim's and Jonquil's sakes." With mounting anger Ray said "Doesn't anybody realise what those women on the bus were doing? They were blessing just you three."

"Unless they were trying to fend us off."

"Don't say things like that, Sandra. Don't even think them." He took her hand and told himself it didn't feel even marginally less substantial than it should. "I wish somebody had seen what I saw under the monastery," he said. "That might have convinced them."

"What are you saying you saw?"

"Remember Irene on the train said the oldest folk took refuge there. When everybody else had gone back up I saw one run off into the dark." Ray took a firmer grip on Sandra's hand as he said "I can't tell you how old it was. Maybe as old as the marks on the wall of the cell."

Sandra matched his grasp for fierceness. "Do you think that's where I'll have to end up?"

"Of course I don't, and you won't be," Ray vowed. "You're coming home with me."

"If they'll let us go."

"Why wouldn't, wouldn't anyone? What's making you say that?"

"Evadne said they often cancel trips off the island, didn't she? Maybe William and Jonquil were right and they mean to keep anyone they want here."

His panic didn't quite rob Ray of thoughts, so that he was able to realise "We've seen people leaving. Certainly we'll be going home."

"Then Jonquil and Tim will, so we shouldn't have to worry about them after tomorrow night."

This only revived Ray's concern about the meantime. "We'd better go and find everyone," he said, "and let's try and think what we can do."

Did she brace herself in preparation for the sunlight as he opened the door? Surely she needn't when the sky was so overcast. As she followed him down the steps into the playground the eager faces showed their teeth at them. William was swimming up and down the pool in a flurry of ripples while his parents gave him their dutiful attention. They and the others were lying on sunbeds, and Tim and Jonquil each had the shade of an umbrella. Both wore hats and sunglasses, and Ray was tempted to declare why, but how could he while William would hear? "Sorry we kept you all waiting," he called instead.

"Blame me," Sandra said. "Another sleepy start. I expect I must be slowing down."

Ray sensed how relieved Doug and Natalie were that she seemed to have reverted to normal. William swam to the near edge of the pool and grabbed the top rung of a ladder. "How long are you going to live, gran?" he said.

For some moments there was silence while quivering ripples dissipated around him, and then Julian said low but harshly "Is that your doing, Jonquil?"

Jonquil turned her unreadable lenses towards him. "What am I supposed to have done now?"

"And Timothy's as well. I believe you undertook not to tell anyone."

"I didn't," Tim protested.

"Tell us what?" Jonquil pleaded. "Tim, what's wrong?"

"He heard someone say I was dying," Sandra said. "Don't worry, you haven't got rid of me yet."

"We don't want to," Jonquil cried, struggling to control the shape of her mouth.

"He heard me." With a visible effort Doug added "I hope I was wrong."

"You know you were now," Sandra said. "We just told you why upstairs."

As Ray saw Doug and Natalie avoid looking at each other William said "Why, gran?"

"Perhaps somebody comes in the night, William, and adds to my life."

Julian's face made his disbelief plain, and so did his outstretched hands. "Sandra, what on earth do you think you're doing?"

"Only answering William's question, aren't I, William?"

"Are we going to see you at Christmas, gran?"

"I'm sure you will if my extra life keeps up. Is that what you'd like?"

"How can you ask him that?" Jonquil said indistinctly, knuckling her eyes behind the sunglasses.

"I'm asking everyone." When this prompted a chorus of silence – Ray didn't trust himself to speak – Sandra said "I'll just have to invite it myself, then."

"What, gran?" William said.

Julian opened his mouth like a mime of incredulity and an exhortation of muteness, and Sandra glanced at him. "It's all right, William," she said. "I'm sure your dad and uncle will see you aren't bothered in the night."

For a moment Ray was as appalled by her behaviour as he

imagined everybody else must be, and then he grasped what she was trying to achieve on behalf of Tim and Jonquil. Last night Doug and Julian had kept any visitors away from them, and tonight they would as well. "They'll have to," he said.

As Doug sent him a mute reprimand Sandra said "So what are we doing today?"

"We may as well stay where we are now," Doug said.

If Ray had thought, he mightn't have remarked "That doesn't sound like you, Doug."

"I could use a lazy day, and I'm sure I'm not the only one who's tired," Doug told him, but Ray guessed this wasn't the whole of the truth. He had an inkling that his son meant to keep him and Sandra away from anywhere and anything they could interpret in terms of their secret belief. It wasn't so secret any longer, and yet he felt more oppressed by the unspoken than ever. The cloudy sky seemed to adumbrate the dark, but it was worse than that, and Doug couldn't distract him. It reminded him why his wife and Tim and Jonquil didn't welcome the sun.

THE THIRTEENTH DAY 1 SEPTEMBER

"Was that you, mum?" Doug called. "What did you say?"

Sandra leaned out of her chair and over the balcony. "Was what me?"

"I can't hear you properly. I'll come up."

Ray blinked at the view. While half a dozen people were swimming in the sea near the apartments, the shore was deserted all the way to Sunset Beach. "What did he think he heard?"

"Maybe…" Ray might have thought Sandra fancied someone unseen was at large beneath the pale overcast sky until she said "Maybe he's starting to imagine things if he's been up all night."

"You did what you thought you had to," Ray said, having seen that she blamed herself. "I don't know what else we could have done."

"At least there's only one more night and then they'll be safe at home."

"They will," Ray said, though it reminded him that he didn't know how leaving the island might affect her.

He opened the door to save Doug from knocking and was greeted by a gaping yawn. "How was your night?" he said.

"How do you think?" Doug said not far short of resentment. "The same kind Jules had."

"No encounters, though."

"None of those," Doug said as if the point needn't have been made. "I've got to speak to mum."

Ray hoped he didn't mean to try again to persuade her that she was mistaken. Outside the bathroom Doug said "Did Evadne change your mirror?"

"There's no need," Sandra said. "Have another look."

"I've already seen, thanks." Doug might have intended to rebuke them both by saying "Keep it how it is if that's what you want."

"You still haven't explained why we had to ask for them," Sandra said.

"Why don't you ask Evadne if you're so anxious to know?" At once Doug looked ashamed of his curtness. "On second thoughts leave it alone," he said. "We don't want her telling you more of that stuff."

"Maybe if you listened to her – "

"I won't be, and you shouldn't. Forget I said you ought." Doug had lowered his voice. "Let's not go on about it where people can hear," he said. "Nat and I have just been talking. Mum, you've lost some jewellery."

"Oh dear. I'll have to try and keep more of my wits about me," Sandra said, holding out a hand.

"No, I mean it's still lost. One of your earrings, it could be."

Sandra gazed at him as if she hoped to see a joke. "I know I've got all the ones I brought with me. I'll show you if you like."

"No," Doug said with patience not too distinguishable from weariness. "I'm saying you lost it at the monastery. We'll need to go and look for it."

Sandra laughed, though not as if she'd found much of a joke. "You mean you want us to look for something else."

"Yes, because you'll see there's nothing there."

Sandra didn't respond at once. "Who's supposed to be going?"

"Just me and Nat and you two. Everyone else will be down on the beach."

"I'm sorry, Doug, but I'll be joining them. That's how I'd like to spend our last day."

"Mum, you really ought to see."

"I'll trust you to tell me what you find," Sandra said, which seemed to make the situation clearer to her. "Just you take care, both of you. You've no idea what there may be. Ray, what are you going to do?"

He suspected she was urging him to protect their children. "I'll go with them."

"Then you be careful as well. At least you know to be." Ray thought she was looking for a hindrance as she said "How are you meant to be getting there, Doug?"

Doug fought to contain a yawn, an effort that tugged his jaw from side to side. "We've rung the place in Sunset Beach and booked a car."

"You won't be driving," Sandra pleaded, "when you're so tired."

"Nat's going to." Doug was plainly more anxious to say "Honestly, it would be a whole lot better if you came to see as well. That way there can't be any disagreement over what we've seen."

"I've already said I won't and that's the end of it. You hurry up and come back and then we can all be together."

"Yes, come along," Ray said to Doug, "or we'll miss the bus."

Natalie was perched on a swing in the play area and swaying very slightly back and forth. All around her the lifeless faces shared a grin, as if they were amused by somebody's behaviour. Ray remembered pushing her so high that she'd squealed with delight when she was William's age and some years older too. She was gazing at whoever was on the steps behind him, which he was sure was nobody only once she said "Are we waiting for mother?"

"They've decided she doesn't need to come," Doug said.

"Shouldn't that be her decision?"

"It very much was," Ray said, trying not to feel accused.

Natalie was silent until they'd left the Sunny View. "Is there much point in going without mother?"

"So long as we all agree what's there," Doug said.

To Ray this felt like being rebuked in advance. At least resentment helped him avoid imagining what they might find, and he hadn't too much room for dread while they were running or in his case limping at a fast trot to the bus stop. Doug reached it in time to halt a bus, where several black-clad women occupied the front seats. Once Ray was seated opposite Natalie and Doug he found the breath to whisper "Why do you think they didn't bless us?"

"Sounds like you're going to tell us," Doug said without enthusiasm.

Ray would have preferred them to see for themselves. "Because it was never us they meant."

"I don't think we want to know who," Natalie said.

He couldn't say it had been their mother, let alone Tim and Jonquil. They would only dismiss the idea and feel worse about him. He stayed quiet all the way to Sunset Beach, where the dead neon looked dusty with the overcast. Very few people were about, and he sensed that Natalie and Doug were watching how he reacted to any of them. While they looked ordinary enough, how reassuring could that be? He did his best to ignore them but saw this was obvious to his children as well.

Matthias Motors occupied a small block of the main street. Beyond a plate-glass window that contained an open door of the same material, a large tanned man sat behind an extensive white desk in a white-tiled room. His grey hair hung well over his ears, and Ray saw that the man had missed rubbing the tan into his pinkish hairline. As the proprietor looked up he brushed hair back from his right ear. "You have been once," he said.

Ray might have demanded how he knew they'd visited the monastery if Doug hadn't saved him from what must surely be a misunderstanding. "Yes, we hired from you last week."

"It is good you come back."

Ray wasn't far from wondering aloud whether this meant few of his customers from Sunset Beach did. As the man drew a pad of contracts towards himself he said "Where do you go today?"

"Your monastery," Ray said before anybody else could speak.

He was hoping to prompt a rejoinder, but the man only picked up a plump ballpoint pen. "Who has licence?"

Natalie passed him her driving licence, and he set about copying the details onto the form. The sight of the bent head veiled on both sides by hair frustrated Ray so much that he said "That's the monastery of St Titus."

The man didn't glance up, but as he crammed an elongated number into a thin box he said "Why you go there?"

"Will one of you answer that?"

As Natalie parted her lips Doug said "I think you ought to, dad."

He had to be hoping the man would refute whatever Ray told him. "It's a return visit," Ray said. "We didn't go all the way down."

"You will take care."

Ray was unnerved by the echo of Sandra's concern. "You're saying there's some danger there."

The man raised his head at last. "Take care with car off road."

Ray felt as if his children's skepticism had fed the man the answer. He was about to subside into silence when the proprietor brushed his hair back once more. "What's that on your neck?" Ray blurted.

"Old scar."

The man bent to the form again, and his hair covered the pink indentation on the side of his neck, surely not before Natalie and Doug had seen. "From what?" Ray persisted.

"Old bite."

"What bit you? Something big." When the man shrugged and kept his head down Ray said "When?"

"Years gone."

"Before tourists started coming to your island, would that be? Before there was someone else to bite?"

The man's lips stirred as he made the final entry on the contract form. They twisted into a faint wry smile, perhaps not too secret to be meant for Ray as well. It disappeared as the man lifted his head and held out the pen to Natalie. "You will sign," he said.

Ray was opening his mouth when Doug said "That's enough now, dad."

"Who's the parent here?" Ray muttered, but he'd already turned to leave the office. He would have felt ashamed, and not just for himself, to quarrel in front of the proprietor. The artificially swarthy man ushered Natalie and Doug outside and left them by an open jeep. As Ray climbed in the back he was unsurprised to see an icon of St Titus on the dashboard, and couldn't help thinking it symbolised powerlessness, the resignation that was the soul of Vasilema.

Natalie started the engine and eased the jeep out of the car park more warily than the deserted road seemed to call for. Ray could have thought she was afraid someone would appear without warning, but no doubt only he was. They encountered nobody until she turned the jeep along a road that led out of Sunset Beach, towards the forest on the horizon. As she drove across a junction Ray saw a couple in the side lane, which seemed not much brighter than twilit. "Slow down," he blurted. "Look what they're doing."

Natalie glanced along the lane and immediately put on speed. "For God's sake," Doug said. "What do you think they were?"

He didn't mean what Ray heard him ask. The young woman had been pressed against the wall of the alley with her eyes shut and her head thrown back while her thin companion mouthed her neck. "They were snogging, dad," Doug said. "It's that kind of place."

Ray might have been able to agree if he hadn't seen how the girl's arms had been outstretched in the manner of a crucifixion instead of embracing the man. There was no point in reminding Doug and Natalie of this, if they'd even noticed. Nobody spoke until they'd left the last apartments behind, and then Doug said "You mustn't think we don't know how you feel, dad."

"What are you telling me you know?"

"What all this is really about, all the things you've got mum believing now as well."

"You needn't think I did that. If you speak to her – "

"Didn't she accept how she was till she came here?" Natalie said, sending him an anguished look in the mirror.

"She'd managed to come to terms with it, we both had, but then – "

"Dad," Doug said, "you're the only one who hasn't. Maybe we know you better than you know yourself."

"I don't think I can be the only one."

"Yes, even William has. And Tim, and hasn't Jonquil too, Nat?"

"I believe it's helping her grow up. She's been doing everything she can to distract William."

"We know it must be harder for you than the rest of us, dad. But you mustn't get so desperate you start believing, well, you know."

"You've got it the wrong way round," Ray protested. "If I hadn't been so concerned for your mother I might have seen what was happening round here sooner."

"You always used to tell us not to be irrational, so don't be yourself."

"Doug's right," Natalie said.

"That isn't how you told me you felt yesterday."

"I've had more time to think about it, and I don't want the children to be led to believe that kind of thing. I'm sorry, that's the risk, and it can't do them any good at all."

Ray felt more alone than ever. His thoughts no longer seemed worth voicing, and he almost wished he could succumb to the drowsiness he saw overtaking his son, whose head kept sinking before it jerked vertical. He watched the forest appear to advance more gradually than the car was travelling, but at last the trees closed around the vehicle like silence rendered solid. The road had wound between the pines for miles before he wondered "When did we last see a bird? When did we even hear one?"

"Is he madder?" Doug mumbled too loosely to be quite awake, and Ray told himself that his son had asked "Does it matter?"

Perhaps Natalie was too intent on the twisted road to answer her father's question. As the scent of pines was invaded by another smell Ray could have taken the clouds that loured over the forest for an omen of the dark that lay in wait ahead. He wasn't smelling ash, he realised now, but desiccation. Beyond the next bend the silvery grey of the slim tree-trunks and the green of foliage gave way to blackness, and his mind seemed to darken in anticipation. Had the discolouration spread since his last visit? Now he saw how contorted the roots of the blackened trees were, as if they'd clutched at the soil in a convulsive bid to cling to life. Were those dead birds among the roots? Some of the dark lumps appeared to be covered with feathers, not leaves, and quite a few had collapsed, extruding twigs that might be bones. It wasn't worth drawing Natalie's attention to them, let alone Doug's drowsy awareness. Ray hoped he had something far more persuasive to show them, though the prospect threatened to rob him of breath.

When the car reached the end of the track he didn't feel as if it had emerged into the open. It might rather have been entering a place so innately dark that it rendered the daylight irrelevant, no more than an illusion. The monastery blocked off the dull sky like a shadow grown substantial, the essence of the blackness that steeped the ground beneath the car. The dozens of unglazed windows put Ray in mind of the multiple eyes of a spider, and their emptiness hinted at the deeper dark within. Natalie was parking the jeep at the foot of the steps that led up to the entrance when Doug uttered a slumbrous grumble. "A wither?"

"Yes, we're there," Ray told him. For a moment he thought his son sounded like a sleepy child, and then he recollected how much more Doug was – realised how he and Natalie were striving to protect their parents in every way they could believe might help. The handbrake rasped as Natalie hauled on the lever, and Doug mumbled "What chew dumb."

"It's the brake," Natalie said. "We're ready whenever you wake up."

It disconcerted Ray how much trouble Doug had with releasing his safety belt and clambering out of the jeep – more than he himself had. Doug blinked at the door when it failed to slam first time, and then he squeezed his eyes shut so fiercely that they seemed to tug his lips into a grimace while he slapped his cheeks with as much vigour as he shook his head. "All right, I'm back in the land of the living," he declared. "Somebody lead on."

He sounded too careless for Ray's liking, but then he and his sister thought the place was deserted. "Where do you want to look?" Ray said.

"We don't particularly want to look anywhere," Natalie retorted. "We thought you were convinced we hadn't gone down far enough."

"Even me and Pris," Doug said. "Even though we went nearly all the way and all we found were caves."

Ray had a foretaste of panic as he said "I thought you wanted me to see for myself."

"If that's what it takes."

"And while we can as well," Natalie said.

"That's the idea," Ray said and set about tramping to the entrance.

Doug and Natalie overtook him on the steps and helped him

to the top, and he tried not to let this make him feel enfeebled, less capable of facing whatever lay ahead. Had the door collapsed further? It was hardly even recognisable as the remains of one. As Ray ventured through the entrance, darkness seemed to close around his brain and parch his mouth, and he had an unpleasant sense that it was waiting for him and his children. Surely all this was apprehension, not evidence of a monstrous thirst that their presence had roused, but Ray had to swallow hard so as to ask "Shall I lead the way?"

"Let me," Natalie said and slipped past him.

Did she think she was the most competent of them, or was she simply eager to get the visit finished? At the end of the outer passage, where the walls looked even more oppressively black, she turned away from the chapel. The muffled daylight reached through the windows of the empty cells to impart some dimness to the corridor, but fell short of the steps leading downwards at the end. Natalie hesitated on the topmost step, though only to activate the flashlight on her phone. When Doug switched his on as well Ray said "I'll leave mine off for now. Better keep one in reserve."

He hadn't meant to sound nervous of the dark, but perhaps he was alone in thinking that he did. The flashlight beams found the close black walls and low sloping roof, and began to prance on them as Natalie led the way downwards. Doug's light was more wayward than hers, and he kept reaching for handholds. So did Ray, who was trying to ignore an impression that even when the beams converged the light stayed unhelpfully dim. To some extent he was glad when the steps came to an end, since the beams grew a little steadier, although this meant they showed how the corridor sloped as if the builders had been eager or at any rate compelled to reach a deeper darkness. "There's nothing to see along here, is there?" Doug said.

"There is," Ray said, "if you remember."

Neither of his children seemed to want to. As they preceded him down the corridor their lights blundered into the cells, awakening restless shadows. Were there any occupants to rouse, or had they fled into the depths? How many had last time, apart from the one he'd glimpsed? Doug's beam found the largest cell, where shadows swarmed away from scattered fragments of wood that might originally have belonged to furniture, and Natalie's light was hastening past the cells opposite when Ray said "That's what you should remember."

He had to point before both lights swerved into the cell where words had been scraped on the wall. "You thought that meant they fed him," he told Doug, "but Pris said it said they feed for him, and then you decided it could be both."

"But if you also recall," Natalie said, "we came to the conclusion it was religious."

"Did you, Doug?" When his son didn't answer at once Ray said "I think you were just trying to reassure William, weren't you, Natalie? Did you really think it would be God they'd be feeding down here?"

As he finished speaking he wondered whether by persuading Doug and Natalie he might make the dark more vital — lend it life. Did he actually need to show them whatever might be hiding in the farthest dark? Couldn't he pretend they'd convinced him there was nothing to see? He suspected that wouldn't satisfy them, but he mustn't let them go ahead without him. He no longer knew what he hoped to achieve by indicating the next cell. "That bothered you, Doug, if you recall."

The lights groped through the uneven entrance to settle on the back wall — on the bunches of more or less vertical lines strung together by slashes that weren't quite horizontal. To Ray they looked very much like marks of desperation even before they started to twitch like insects, borrowing movement from the unsteady lights. "Bothered me how?" Doug said.

"You thought it looked as if whoever lived in there felt they were serving a sentence."

"We can't know that, can we? It was just something I said."

"But it does look like that, doesn't it, Natalie? Only then we have to wonder why a monk would feel that way."

"As Doug says, we'll never know. We've already talked about it once. It isn't what we've come to see."

Was Ray making them nervous? Perhaps they were simply unhappy with his insistence; he doubted they were feeling as he'd begun to feel – that his behaviour was an invitation to the dark or whatever it concealed. He could easily have fancied that his words and theirs were being overheard. Natalie was right to imply that he was delaying the exploration, because his unacknowledged dread was growing as they advanced into the dark. He had to swallow more than once to make his parched voice work. "Then let's see why we've come," he said.

He was unnerved to think this could be taken as an invitation too. As he trailed his children down the sloping corridor he peered uneasily into each cell and had to restrain himself from asking for the lights to linger. All too soon everybody was by the lowest cell, from which he'd previously seen an occupant dart forth. The dark shape that lurched up from the crude stone bench inside the cell was just the shadow of the entrance – no more than a final distraction. They'd reached the steps that led down into the deepest dark. "I'll go first," Natalie said. "You two watch your step."

"I ought to lead," Ray told her as protectiveness overcame his dread.

"I'm the fittest one just now." Before he could protest again, Natalie stepped down. "And I want to get this over with," she said.

Doug followed her at once, and Ray felt pathetically inadequate for calling after her "You watch where you're going as well."

He stayed two steps behind Doug so as not to crowd him, which left Ray surrounded by darkness. Natalie and Doug kept their flashlight beams on the increasingly uneven steps, an action that appeared to jerk the roof lower still. Could the batteries be failing? Surely that wouldn't enfeeble the lights, but even before the beams reached the bend in the narrow passage they didn't seem to extend as far as they should. As he clambered around the bend Ray clung to rough handholds on the wall. Ahead of his children the steps led down into a blackness that the beams seemed unable to relieve. The passage shut their footfalls in and amplified them while dulling them, and Ray felt as if the clutter of sound was obscuring some other noise. "Did you hear that?" he blurted.

Natalie halted, and as Doug stumbled to a standstill the flashlight beams came more or less to rest. "It's just water, dad," Doug said. "Pris and I told you last time there are caves down here."

"I don't mean that. Wasn't there something else?" It seemed too little to put into any more words – the noise that he was almost sure he'd heard somewhere ahead, sounding more solid than water. "Keep listening," he said and at once was nervous for his children. "Take care where you're walking, though."

He'd begun to hope this might be all the danger they were in, though a careless step down here would be perilous enough. As the flashlight beams wobbled downwards they appeared to be miming precariousness, while the dark that they left untouched might have been playing a secretive game, pretending coyly to retreat ahead of them and then welling up to await the intruders. Was that the only movement down below? Ray was growing surer by the moment that the crowd of footfalls and their echoes were hindering everyone from hearing another sound, more substantial than water and yet not quite sufficiently solid, an impression he was by no means eager to understand. Did he and his children really have to see what was stirring in the dark? Why couldn't just hearing convince them? He was close to praying, however desperately, that it would. "Stop and listen," he pleaded. "You must be able to hear. That's never only water."

Doug twisted impatiently round. "Look, dad, if – "

Ray threw out his hands to steady him as Doug made a grab at the wall, but they were both too late. Doug had lost his footing and missed the handhold as well. He collided with Natalie, who cried out and stumbled down the steps so fast she looked utterly helpless. As Doug managed to regain his balance she clutched at both walls to halt herself, and her phone flew out of her hand. It skittered down the steps as if it might never come to rest, and by the time it did the illuminated screen was no bigger than a fingernail. The phone had lodged on the edge of a step, from which the microscopic flashlight beam reached down into the dark. Ray took a breath to replace his dismayed gasp. "Are you all right?" he called.

"I'm not sure." Natalie let go of the walls, only to seize hold at once. "No, I'm not," she said.

"What have you done to yourself?"

"I think it's what someone else did." As Ray told himself that at least she'd retained her spirit she said "It's my ankle."

"How bad?"

"I don't think it's broken." She shifted her weight on the step and sucked in such a hiss of air that it made Ray's teeth ache. "I'm afraid it's sprained," she said.

"For heaven's sake don't go any further."

"I wasn't about to. I'm going to have to come back up."

Ray watched her turn with painful carefulness. She was being wary of her ankle, not of the darkness at her back. All at once he was afraid of seeing a shape dart or lurch or flounder into the distant flashlight beam, to pursue her up the steps faster than she could scramble. The sight of her efforts was distressing enough, even when Doug extended a hand, which she grabbed before supporting herself on his arm while she inched past him. "Thanks," she said not entirely unlike a rebuke.

"You stay with dad while I get your phone."

As Natalie grimaced at having put too much weight on her ankle Ray saw Doug start downwards and immediately stumble, almost slithering down a step. "Doug, you've already fallen once," he protested. "Let me."

Doug's flashlight beam swung around as he did, and the darkness rose up behind him. "I don't think that's such a good idea, dad."

"We can leave it if we have to," Natalie said. "It's only a phone."

Ray wondered if they were concerned just about his safety on the steps. Might they sense more about the depths than they cared to admit to themselves? At least he was no longer hearing any sounds down there, and was able to think that the light from Natalie's phone might have driven away any lurkers. "You don't want to lose your photographs, do you?" he said.

"I'd rather lose them than you."

"No need for either," Ray said, gripping her shoulders as he eased himself past her. "Let's take everything home that we can."

As he sidled past Doug his son took him by the arm. Ray couldn't help hoping he meant to accompany him after all until he realised Doug was only steadying him. Doug sent his flashlight beam downwards while Ray switched on his own. "Take your time," Natalie urged him.

"That's right, there's no hurry," Doug said. "We'll be here."

They were doing their best to look after him but only aggravating his nervousness. He didn't need to be reminded how wary he should be. He would have liked to use both hands for steadying himself, but he couldn't risk losing hold of his phone. Its light wobbled around him as he kept groping at the wall, setting one foot and then the other on every step he had to descend. All he could hear were his effortful breaths and the thudding of his pulse, which felt as if it were expanding in his guts. Was there anything else he should hear? The dark beyond the supine beam of Natalie's flashlight looked lifeless enough, but he could easily have thought it was collaborating with the light to entice him into the depths. He took the last few steps down to it more slowly than ever, and not just to make certain of his balance. As he stooped to retrieve the phone he sent his own beam as far into the dark as it would reach.

The beam lit up the foot of the steps, though dimly. They ended at a passage that bent left into the dark. Ray was straightening up with a mobile in each hand, bruising his shoulder against the wall as his balance almost deserted him, when he heard a sound along the passage – a surreptitious shifting. "Are you okay, dad?" Doug shouted.

"I'm all right. I'll be fine." He would have said so just to quieten Doug, who had prevented him from identifying the sound. As he turned off Natalie's flashlight and stowed the phone in a pocket of his shorts he heard the noise again. It was the lapping of water, which he guessed was at the near end of the cave by the secluded beach, but wasn't there more to the sound? Ray might have fancied something large and sluggish was wallowing in the water. He grasped a protruding chunk of wall in order to look up at Natalie and Doug. They and Doug's light were so tiny that he was reminded of using a telescope the wrong way round, but he mustn't let that daunt him. "I won't be long," he called. "I'm just going down to see."

"Dad," Doug protested. "What's the point if we don't as well?"

"If there's anything to show you I'll take a photograph," Ray said and immediately thought that some things mightn't show up on camera. If it hadn't managed to focus on Sandra and the teenagers, how much more trouble might it have down here? He mustn't use that as an excuse not to look. He ought to see, and he made himself descend the steps as fast as planting both feet on each of them would let him.

As he reached the entrance to the passage the black walls gleamed at him, so that he could have imagined that the dark was celebrating his arrival. He gripped his wrist with his other hand to stabilise the flashlight beam, which didn't prevent the walls from appearing to quiver. One hand was as shaky as the other, and together they were twice as bad. Now he felt as if the passage was magnifying his nervousness and shutting him in with it, and he let go of his wrist as he ventured to the bend.

Beyond it the passage straightened, and water glinted at the far end. Ray glimpsed ripples and heard them lapping at rock, and the other noise again – activity that wasn't quite so fluid. Were the acoustics of the place transforming the sound of the sea? As he urged himself towards it he passed several alcoves too shallow to be called caves, a large one opposite several not much broader than he was. The flashlight beam strayed into them, producing the impression that the wall of the largest had grown pallid and unstable, a notion Ray wasn't anxious to linger over. He hurried to the end of the passage and shone the beam across the water.

He had indeed reached the cave he'd visited last week. He could see the narrower stretch that he'd followed back to the sea, and was even able to identify the rocks that had snagged Ditton's corpse. He didn't rest the light on them any longer than it took him to be sure, but swept the beam around the cave. It was deserted, and the ripples that were subsiding on the water had obviously come in from the sea, the furthest traces of waves. He felt relieved by the lack of any presence and yet unsettlingly disappointed, as if he'd been robbed of a belief on which he'd depended more than he knew. He was giving the cave a final sweep of the beam when Doug called "Dad, are you all right?"

His voice was disconcertingly remote. "I'm fine," Ray shouted so loud that his lungs ached. The shout roused echoes in the caves, and as the echoes faded he saw the ripples grow still. He was watching the last of them disappear when he remembered what he'd heard and seen last week in the cave – the shrill giggling that he'd ascribed to the ripples, and the whitish movement that had receded into the dark. As he realised he was standing just where that activity had been, he heard the restless sluggish sound again. It was behind him.

He could hear it more clearly now – more than he liked. It put him in mind of an enormous bag full of some soft material, slithering across rock. As he twisted to face it the light flailed at the walls, so that he wasn't immediately sure what he was seeing in the passage. Even if there was no movement other than the trembling of the light, this didn't reassure him much, since the sound had unquestionably originated somewhere along the passage. Just as dismaying in another way, Doug was calling out to him. "What did you say, dad?"

"I'm coming now," Ray cried, so afraid for his children that it almost overcame his more immediate dread. Suppose Doug stumbled down to find him, what might happen then? He limped at all his speed towards the bend, struggling to prepare himself for whatever might be there, but he wasn't even close to it when he began to grasp how much he'd overlooked or misperceived. The largest of the chambers off the passage wasn't just an alcove after all. He'd perceived it as shallow only because it was full of a swollen bulk, which wasn't pale just from the flashlight beam. The mass was at least as wide as the entrance to the cave it filled – a dozen limping strides wide. Ray had no time to examine it more closely or even to wonder what species of underground growth it might be. Telling himself that it was restless only with the movement of the flashlight beam occupied his mind just now – indeed, strove to be his solitary thought. He very much wished that he hadn't explored quite so far. He wasn't even at the midpoint of the cave that he was growing more than anxious to pass when the pale bulk thrust its face and arms towards him.

The face was a man's, or had been. Now it resembled a bloated mask, almost engulfed in a mass of flesh so pallid it might never have been touched by the sun. The nose resembled a colourless tuber, and the thick broad lips were just as white. It was impossible to judge what expression the face bore, not just since the lips appeared to have swelled together in an immobile straight line but because the eyes had atrophied, puckering so deep that they'd sucked the lids inwards. All the same, as Ray shrank back from the sight, having staggered to a paralysed halt in the corridor, he had a sense that the face was aged by more than centuries – by some awful knowledge around which it had closed to keep it from the world. Then the eyes opened in the depths of the whitish sockets, and the arms stretched out to cut off his escape.

All he could see in the tiny glinting eyes was hunger so voracious it was mindless. At once Ray knew what had befallen Ditton, who must have strayed into the lair, from which his drained remains had been flung into the water. For a moment Ray imagined he would be able to dodge Skiá's clutches, since even though the arms were at least twice the breadth of his own, they were dwarfed by the mass from which they protruded several yards apart. But they were on either side of him, and before he could move, the gigantic pallid body squeezed forward to extend the arms across the passage, trapping him.

As the face surged towards him, a tongue like a great white slug poked the lips apart, revealing a solitary fang. The moist white eyes were so enlivened by thirst that they were creeping forwards in the sockets. Loathing indistinguishable from panic overwhelmed Ray's thoughts, so that he was scarcely aware of backing away until he found himself in an alcove nowhere near as deep as a cell. The vast body was still emerging from the cave, not so much like flesh as a vast sack of fluid. The face crept into the alcove, together with a distended portion of the bulk in which it was embedded, and Ray shrank against the rock, which felt implacably chill. The greedy eyes bulged forth from their sockets while the fanged mouth gaped as wide as a fist, and Ray heard Doug and Natalie calling out to him.

Their voices were muffled by the fleshy obstacle that filled the entrance to the alcove. Ray was appalled by not knowing how close they were – not knowing whether Doug was on his way to find him. His terror clarified his thoughts, and he realised he might have a weapon. He thrust his phone at the advancing face, shining the flashlight beam into the eyes. He didn't know he meant to speak until words spilled out of his mouth. "Let us live and we'll let you live."

The eyes shrivelled into the head, and the towering body dragged itself back into the passage. Ray thought it had given him the chance to flee until he saw it was only making space for an arm to reach into the alcove. The writhing fingers groped for him and closed around his wrist. They felt as they looked: like cold dead grubs. As Ray jerked free with a convulsion that involved his entire body he almost dropped the phone that the enormous hand was searching for. The eyes were venturing forth again like snails emerging from their shells, and this time they didn't wither so much when he aimed the beam at them. As Ray bruised his shoulders against the unyielding wall he remembered he had Natalie's phone too, but how much difference could that make? He had a last despairing idea, and fumbled for her mobile as the mass that had crammed itself into the alcove slithered forward to let the hand at him. The fingers hadn't quite found him when he heard Doug calling him again. His son sounded closer – distressingly close.

"Stay there," Ray yelled, struggling to wield the second phone with his left hand. He couldn't simply use his own mobile when he would need to switch off the light first, leaving him with Skiá in the dark. As he managed to retreat a very few more inches, if even that far, the arm emerged further from the wad of flesh, and the fingers squirmed in search of him. He was so desperate to avoid them that he nearly touched the wrong icon on the mobile – the one that would activate the phone – which, in the midst of his breathless panic, made him yearn to be speaking to Sandra. Then he succeeded in activating the camera, and held it towards the face that was bulging at him. In such haste that he nearly lost hold of the phone, he set off the flash.

The eyes wizened and the face recoiled, sinking into the mass of flesh. The colossal body flinched into the passage, not by any means as far as Ray would have liked. All the same, this looked as if it was his only chance. As he lurched out of the alcove he saw the eyes beginning to stir in their sockets. The hands had jerked up to cover them, but the width of the body meant they weren't even nearly within reach. Ray thrust the camera at them again and used the flash. As the eyes dwindled, the arm closer to the steps swung towards him, and the soft cold almost fluid fingers brushed his cheek. But the body had withdrawn further, and there was space for Ray to sidle past, scraping his shoulders on the wall. He dashed around the bend and saw Doug almost at the bottom of the steps. "I said I was coming," Ray gasped. "I'm here. Go up."

"What was all the noise? What did you photograph?"

"I'll show you both when we're out of here. Don't leave your sister like that. I told you, go up."

He switched off the camera and shoved it in his pocket as Doug started upwards. Ray was mutely urging his son to climb faster in the hope of keeping pace with him when Doug swung around with one hand on the wall. "What did I just hear?"

"Nothing," Ray protested, but perhaps the truth was in his eyes. "Just water, like you said."

Doug hesitated before resuming his climb, and Ray felt as if this let the darkness or its contents grow more solid behind them. In one sense he was glad if their footfalls were blotting out any further sounds that might tempt Doug to investigate, but he kept having to glance back to reassure himself that they weren't being followed. Nothing was visible except the dark, and the only noise he could hear was the lapping of ripples in the cave, even if it put him in mind of a huge puffy tongue licking bloated lips.

As the flashlight beams found Natalie she began gingerly to climb. Despite the relative silence behind him, Ray had to resist exhorting her to put on speed, though it wasn't her fault that he was slowing down. Each step upwards seemed to rob him of more energy, until he felt as if he were being dragged back by the darkness — by its insubstantial weight that was gathering on him. He could have thought he was being drained of strength by the hunger of the dark, which would never let him reach the light again.

At last Natalie and Doug emerged into the subterranean corridor full of cells, and Ray toiled after them. Making their variously hampered way along it took rather more time than he cared for, despite the silence at his back. There was still the upper flight of steps to conquer, and before he reached the top Ray's entire body was shaking with his pulse, which seemed to be stealing his breath. He had to lean against the wall in the top corridor for some minutes while he regained a modicum of strength, and he felt barely capable of helping Doug support Natalie down the steps from the monastery. Just the same, as the blackened trees rose up in front of them like a reminder of the buried darkness, Ray grew more than eager to be away from the place and what it harboured. "I'll drive," he said.

"May I have my phone now?" Natalie said, having sunk with a wince onto the back seat of the jeep.

"You were going to show us what you found," Doug reminded his father, taking the seat beside him.

"It's on there," Ray said and handed Natalie her mobile. "Look for yourselves."

She opened the album and examined the most recent image while Ray started the car. Having looked at the previous photograph, she passed Doug the phone. "There's nothing," she said.

She was gazing at Ray in the mirror, searching for his reaction. As Doug peered at the mobile Ray glanced at the screen. The most recent photographs showed a blurred image of the cave off the lowest passage – no more than a dark vague emptiness. "You were right," he said as he sent the jeep along the track towards the unblackened trees. "There was nothing at all."

THE LAST DAY
2 SEPTEMBER

"You may go first, William," Julian said.

The boy stepped forward with enough drama for a school play and handed Evadne the bouquet tied up with a ribbon. "Thank you for having us."

"He picked those for you himself."

"He wanted to give you his own present," Natalie said. "And Jonquil donated the ribbon."

"I haven't worn any for years," Jonquil wanted everyone to know. "It was hiding in my case from a long time ago."

"Well, you are kind," Evadne told her and William. "I shall put them somewhere."

Ray had a passing notion that she meant or ought to mean the graveyard. Might she place them on the graves of visitors who had never left the island? Just now all that mattered was that Sandra and the teenagers were about to leave it. When Evadne laid the flowers on the counter in her office Julian cleared his throat as a preamble to planting a fifty-euro note beside them. "For your hospitality. From the family," he said.

Ray wondered if this sounded like ensuring she didn't think he personally valued her that much. "From all of us," Doug said.

"You are kind again." It wasn't clear exactly who she was addressing, nor when she said "You will come back."

"You've got to be asking that," Pris said. "We've had an eventful stay."

"I've liked my time here," Sandra said.

"If we made you welcome, tell your friends."

This seemed to silence most of her listeners, leaving Tim to promise "I'll tell mine."

As Jonquil nodded, darkening her sunglasses with the shadow of her hat brim, Evadne said "And come back for your memories." "You've all given me a few I wouldn't mind revisiting," Sandra said.

Ray was troubled by a sense that she'd misunderstood Evadne somehow. As he thought of asking what Evadne meant, Julian said "I believe our transport is here."

A man and woman at least as old as Ray were the only passengers so far. While the driver piled luggage in the belly of the bus Sam ushered the newcomers on board. Did she seem oddly relieved by the sight of them or to be sending them home? Ray took Sandra's hand to help her up the steps onto the coach, only to feel as though she was lending him some of her vigour. When she squeezed his hand he wished she would put whatever thoughts she was having into words, but he suspected that mightn't be advisable while the family could hear.

William waved goodbye if not a mime of hoping to return. As the coach left the Sunny View behind, Ray glanced at the streetlamp where he'd so often noticed the spider. He couldn't see it or its web, and he wondered if they were among the aspects of Vasilema that were seldom visible by day. Would they have shown up in a photograph? Surely they ought to, since they'd cast a shadow – and then he remembered that the figures under the lamp had cast one, which didn't reassure him at all.

Soon the bus arrived at Sunset Beach. As it collected passengers Ray recognised accommodations where people had failed to show up for a tour they'd booked. Like Sandra and the teenagers, and despite the overcast sky, most of the young folk wore sunglasses and outsize hats. Quite a few were visibly reluctant to leave the shade of trees or awnings, and some left it as late as possible to sprint to the coach as though fleeing a storm. While Ray didn't look too hard for bites, he noticed several. "That's the last," Sam eventually told the driver and picked up her microphone. "Have we all had a good stay? Looking forward to next year?"

The chorus of agreement was mostly a mumble. "I'll tell you when we're coming to the ferry," she announced. "Looks as if some of us would like a snooze."

Ray saw she didn't mean just Doug and Julian, though both of them were dozing in their seatbelts. As Sam laid down the microphone Sandra leaned across the aisle to murmur to Natalie and Pris. "I'm sorry I was a pain last night. I've changed my mind."

Natalie glanced around to see that Tim and Jonquil had set about distracting William from the conversation. "So long as you're happy in yourself."

"I should have believed the photographs you brought back." Sandra looked ashamed and then more so. "How's your ankle now?" she said.

"I told you, better than it was. Honestly, don't worry, and certainly don't blame yourself."

"I do for making Doug and Julian have to go on patrol again, though."

"They were just being men," Pris said. "Nat and I offered to keep watch but they were having none of it."

"You could have, couldn't you," Sandra said and gazed at Ray. "Especially since there wasn't anyone to keep a lookout for."

"We've agreed to that now," Ray said.

They had, but only so as to reassure the family. Last night Sandra had pretended she believed the uninhabited photographs had been taken just to disprove his fancies and her own. He'd already told her how he'd ventured into the depths beneath the monastery, but had stopped short of describing what he'd found. He'd heard the movements of something that still lived down there, far from any light: that was enough for her to know. He didn't want to associate it with her, however remotely. Whenever he'd wakened in the night, and too often while he was asleep, he'd seen the dwarfed although swollen arms poking out of the immense bloated body, reaching to drag him towards the pallid practically eyeless face, the fanged voracious mouth.

As the coach passed the shrine that marked the start of the path to the beach and the cave, he saw the image of St Titus brandishing his rotten splintered lance, the cocoon bulging out of the spear. It seemed to sum up the secret of Vasilema – the ineffectual dead saint nurturing the occupant of the cell under the monastery that bore the saint's name, the saviour only managing to prolong Skiá's unnatural life by figuring in rituals that epitomised resignation. Before the coach left the path behind, Ray had the horrid thought that the pallid body concealed somewhere in the darkness beneath the landscape was all too reminiscent of a cocoon. Suppose it was ripe to burst open, releasing a multitude of thirsty progeny? He managed to shudder the notion away, hoping Sandra wouldn't ask why he'd grimaced at the window. The truth about Skiá was dreadful enough, though perhaps not so awful that he couldn't bear it for her sake.

He did his best to concentrate on her needs until he was distracted by a throaty rattle from the microphone Sam had picked up. "We're nearly at the ferry," she said. "Make sure you all have your tickets to show."

As the coach drove down to the harbour Ray saw masts rise and fall as if they were making a bid to tug the clouds lower. Among them the ferry was less agitated, almost still. The coach driver released the doors, but even when he opened the luggage compartment some of the passengers seemed by no means eager to leave the bus. Once they'd retrieved their luggage they made a dash for the ferry, where they took refuge in the enclosed saloon, having barely waited for the crew to check their tickets. As he and

Natalie competed at limping to the gangplank, Ray observed that Sandra and the teenagers weren't in quite such of a hurry to reach the saloon as the contingent from Sunset Beach had been. It was enough to let him murmur words under his breath.

The family had hardly found seats in the saloon when William said "Are we coming back next year?"

"Don't you want to see more of the world?" Ray hoped aloud.

"I wouldn't mind coming here again," Tim said.

"Nor me," said Jonquil.

As Julian looked ready to object Sandra said "You can't say what you'll want a year from now, can you? You shouldn't, either."

Having seen what she intended, Ray joined in. "There's so much more to your lives."

"What are you going to be doing before then?" Sandra asked them.

"Some friends and me, we've started a band," Tim said. "And I've got my art project for school."

"Mine's all the history of our town, my project," Jonquil said. "And I'm being Ariel in the play."

Ray thought they were starting to recollect their lives off the island. He was certain there was more to them – surely enough to divert them from yearning to return to Vasilema. He and Sandra would be striving to ensure they didn't, though without admitting why. As the ferry edged away from the wharf he gazed out at the town, and then he leaned close to the window. Dozens of watchers had gathered beyond the harbour, peering out of the streets that were shaded by overgrown awnings. While the faces were too distant for Ray to be able to make out their features, he was sure that if they were closer he would recognise several of the watchers. Even at that distance he fancied that he sensed their thirst, which all of them were suffering on behalf of the denizen of the dark. When he glanced at Sandra he glimpsed longing in her eyes, but the instant she noticed that he was looking at her she smiled and clasped his hand.

The ferry swung away from the harbour, and the faces withdrew into the streets on the hill as though retreating into a lair. For a while he listened to the chugging of the engines, until he began to feel as soporific as Doug and Julian continued to be. The ferry had been at sea for most of half an hour when Sandra said "What did we do with all those days?"

She sounded wistful but also not far from confused. "Oh, mum," Doug said.

"So long as they gave you some benefit," Julian said.

"You said they did you good," Natalie reminded her, and Pris contributed "We could see they did."

They all must think her age was catching up with her, but Ray knew how wrong they were. He'd seen Tim and Jonquil agree with her question, and they might have supported it if Doug and the others hadn't responded first. So this was how Vasilema enticed back its visitors: not to relive their memories but in search of them, if they even realised. Crossing water erased the memories — that was one of the hints the family had been given on the island. At once he hoped it could do more, and took out his phone to activate the camera while he trotted down the aisle to face his family. "Is there enough light for that?" Pris said.

"We'll soon find out." However hard he squinted at the miniature screen, Ray wasn't sure. He took one photograph and used the flash to take another, which made several of the other passengers grimace despite their sunglasses. "You're right," he said, having examined the images. "I'll try for a better one later."

He was able to believe it would indeed be better. While Sandra and the teenagers weren't in focus, he was certain that their outlines were significantly sharper than the last time he'd tried to photograph them. "Some people aren't helping," Julian said. "Do you seriously still need to keep those on, Jonquil?"

Jonquil snatched her hat off, further tousling her hair, and dropped her sunglasses into it. "Maybe not just now."

"Well then," Sandra said, "I don't think I do either."

She removed her hat and glasses as Tim did. "Welcome back to the light," Natalie said to them all.

Ray heard more than she'd meant, but wondered if this was a little premature. "I'm just going up for a last look," he said.

Nobody followed him up the stairs to the open deck, and so he couldn't judge whether Sandra and the teenagers were still wary of sunlight. As he emerged onto the deck, where a very few people were seated at the rail, the clouds unveiled the sun. It felt like sailing free of the shadow of Vasilema, but he knew that its influence lingered within Sandra and Jonquil and Tim. The clouds seemed to shrink back towards Vasilema, and he realised that he was seeing the entire length of the island for the first time in his life. He thought the elongated mound looked like a colossal grave, but it was more than that too. He watched it sink beneath the horizon as if it were retreating into hiding. As it vanished, drawing the clouds with it, he repeated the words he'd breathed before stepping off the island, and wondered how much he was inviting for himself as well. "Let us come back," he murmured like a prayer.

ACKNOWLEDGEMENTS

This book has seen the world. It was worked on at the splendid Shangri-La's Rasa Sentosa Resort and Spa across the bridge from Singapore. It went to the always delightful Deep Blue Sea Apartments in Georgioupolis on Crete, where you are advised to stay well clear of the Fereniki complex (TripAdvisor tells you more). Fantasycon in York played host too, as did the Festival of Fantastic Films in Manchester.

Jenny was my inspiration as ever, but I owe the seed of the entire book to the gentleman who runs off-road trips on Zakynthos, where we were staying in 2014 at the wonderful Roula Apartments in Alykes. As he drove through a young folk's resort he made a passing comment, and in less than a minute I had the idea that grew into this novel. I spent much of our day trip scribbling notes. His name, I believe, was Iannis Tepmoneras. Thank you once again, Iannis!

FLAME TREE PRESS
FICTION WITHOUT FRONTIERS
Award-Winning Authors & Original Voices

Flame Tree Press is the trade fiction imprint of Flame Tree Publishing, focusing on excellent writing in horror and the supernatural, crime and mystery, science fiction and fantasy. Our aim is to explore beyond the boundaries of the everyday, with tales from both award-winners and original voices.

•

Other titles available include:

Think Yourself Lucky by Ramsey Campbell
The House by the Cemetery by John Everson
The Toy Thief by D.W. Gillespie
The Siren and the Specter by Jonathan Janz
The Sorrows by Jonathan Janz
Kosmos by Adrian Laing
The Sky Woman by J.D. Moyer
Creature by Hunter Shea
The Bad Neighbor by David Tallerman
Ten Thousand Thunders by Brian Trent
Night Shift by Robin Triggs
The Mouth of the Dark by Tim Waggoner

•

Join our mailing list for free short stories, new release details, news about our authors and special promotions:

flametreepress.com